Pelvic Organ Dysfunction in Neurological Disease

Clinical Management and Rehabilitation

Pelvic Organ Dysfunction in Neurological Disease

Clinical Management and Rehabilitation

Edited by

Clare J. Fowler FRCP
Professor of Uro-Neurology, Institute of Neurology, University College London, UK; Consultant, National Hospital for Neurology & Neurosurgery, London, UK

Jalesh N. Panicker MD DNB DM MRCP(UK)
Consultant Neurologist, Department of Uro-Neurology, National Hospital for Neurology & Neurosurgery, London, UK; Honorary Research Associate, Institute of Neurology, University College London, UK

Anton Emmanuel BSc MD FRCP
Senior Lecturer in Neurogastroenterology, Department of Gastroenterology, University College Hospital, London, UK

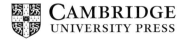

CAMBRIDGE UNIVERSITY PRESS
Cambridge, New York, Melbourne, Madrid, Cape Town, Singapore,
São Paulo, Delhi, Dubai, Tokyo, Mexico City

Cambridge University Press
The Edinburgh Building, Cambridge CB2 8RU, UK

Published in the the United States of America by
Cambridge University Press, New York

www.cambridge.org
Information on this title: www.cambridge.org/9780521198318

First published 2010

Printed in the United Kingdom at the University Press, Cambridge

A catalogue record for this publication is available from the British Library

Library of Congress Cataloging-in-Publication Data

Pelvic organ dysfunction in neurological disease : clinical management
and rehabilitation / editors, Clare J. Fowler, Jalesh N. Panicker, Anton
Emmanuel.
    p. ; cm.
    Includes bibliographical references and index.
    ISBN 978-0-521-19831-8 (Hardback)
1. Urinary organs—Diseases.   2. Urinary organs–Innervation.
3. Nervous system–Degeneration–Complications.   I. Fowler, Clare J.
II. Panicker, Jalesh N.   III. Emmanuel, Anton.   IV. Title.
    [DNLM: 1. Nervous System Diseases–complications.   2. Fecal
Incontinence–etiology.   3. Fecal Incontinence–therapy.   4. Sexual
Dysfunction, Physiological–etiology.   5. Sexual Dysfunction,
Physiological–therapy.   6. Urinary Incontinence–etiology.   7. Urinary
Incontinence–therapy. WL 140 P393 2010]
    RC919.P45 2010
    616.6–dc22
                                                               2010016806

ISBN 978-0-521-19831-8 Hardback

Contents

*The colour plates will be found between
pages 178 and 179.*

Contributors

Apostolos Apostolidis PhD FEBU
Lecturer in Urology-Neurourology,
2nd Department of Urology,
Papageorgiou General Hospital,
Aristotle University,
Thessaloniki, Greece

Charlotte Chaliha MA MD MRCOG
Consultant Obstetrician & Gynaecologist,
Subspecialist Urogynaecologist,
Department of Obstetrics & Gynaecology,
The Royal London & St Bartholomew's Hospitals,
London, UK

Maureen Coggrave PhD MSc RN
Clinical Nurse Specialist,
The National Spinal Injuries Centre,
Stoke Mandeville Hospital,
Aylesbury, UK;
Lecturer,
The Burdett Institute of Gastrointestinal Nursing,
King's College,
London, UK

Catherine M. Dalton MD MRCPI
Clinical Research Associate,
Department of Uro-Neurology,
National Hospital for Neurology & Neurosurgery,
London, UK

Ranan DasGupta MBBCh MA MD FRCS[Urol]
Consultant in Urology,
Imperial College Healthcare NHS Trust,
London, UK

Soumendra Nath Datta MBBS(Hons) BSc(Hons) MRCS(Eng) MSc(Urol)
Specialist Registrar in Urology,
Imperial College Healthcare NHS Trust,
London, UK

Marianne de Sèze MD PhD
Consultant,
Physical Medicine & Rehabilitation Unit,
Urology Department of Saint Augustin Clinic,
Bordeaux, France

Sohier Elneil PhD FRCOG
Consultant in Uro-Gynaecology,
Department of Uro-Neurology,
National Hospital for Neurology & Neurosurgery,
London, UK

Anton Emmanuel BSc MD FRCP
Senior Lecturer in Neurogastroenterology,
Department of Gastroenterology,
University College Hospital,
London, UK

Clare J. Fowler FRCP
Professor of Uro-Neurology,
Institute of Neurology,
University College London, UK;
Consultant,
Department of Uro-Neurology,
National Hospital for Neurology & Neurosurgery,
London, UK

Xavier Gamé MD MSc
Consultant in Urology,
Department of Urology,
Kidney Transplantation and Andrology,
University Hospital Rangueil,
Toulouse, France;
Honorary Clinical Assistant,
Department of Uro-Neurology,
National Hospital for Neurology & Neurosurgery,
London, UK;
Honorary Research Assistant,
Institute of Neurology,
University College London, UK

Gwen Gonzales RGN
Clinical Nurse Specialist in Neurostimulation,
Department of Uro-Neurology,
National Hospital for Neurology & Neurosurgery,
London, UK

Derek J. Griffiths PhD
Geriatric Continence Research Unit,
University of Pittsburgh, USA;
Honorary Senior Research Fellow,
Institute of Neurology,
University College London, UK

Rizwan Hamid FRCSEd FRCS (Urol)
Consultant Neuro-Urologist,
Department of Neuro-Urology,
Royal National Orthopaedic Hospital,
London, UK;
Department of Uro-Neurology,
National Hospital for Neurology & Neurosurgery,
London, UK

Collette Haslam BSc RGN
Clinical Nurse Specialist in Uro-Neurology,
Department of Uro-Neurology,
National Hospital for Neurology & Neurosurgery,
London, UK

Jeanette Haslam MPhil MCSP
Clinical Specialist Physiotherapist in Continence &
Women's Health

Takamichi Hattori MD PhD
Professor Emeritus,
Department of Neurology,
Chiba University Graduate School of Medicine,
Chiba City, Japan

Vinay Kalsi MRCS
Specialist Registrar in Urology,
Department of Urology,
Frimley Park Hospital,
Frimley, UK

Rajesh B. C. Kavia BSc(Hons) MBBS MRCSEd
Specialist Registrar in Urology,
Wexham Park Hospital,
Slough, UK

Thomas M. Kessler MD FEBU
Consultant in Urology,
Department of Urology,

University of Bern,
Bern, Switzerland

Shahid Khan MS DNB MRCS
Registrar & Honorary Research Assistant,
Department of Uro-Neurology,
National Hospital for Neurology & Neurosurgery,
London, UK

Gustav Kiss MD
Head, Neuro-Urology Unit,
Department of Neurology,
University Hospital Innsbruck,
Austria

Klaus Krogh MD PhD DMSc
Associate Professor,
Neurogastroenterology Unit,
Department of Hepatology & Gastroenterology,
Aarhus University Hospital,
Aarhus, Denmark

Hadi Manji MA MD FRCP
Consultant Neurologist,
National Hospital for Neurology & Neurosurgery,
London, UK

Jalesh N. Panicker MD DNB DM MRCP(UK)
Consultant Neurologist,
Department of Uro-Neurology,
National Hospital for Neurology & Neurosurgery,
London, UK;
Honorary Research Associate,
Institute of Neurology,
University College London, UK

Simon Podnar MD DSc
Neurologist & Clinical Neurophysiologist,
Institute of Clinical Neurophysiology,
Division of Neurology,
University Medical Centre,
Ljubljana, Slovenia

Giuseppi Preziosi MBBS MRCS
Research Fellow,
Division of Surgery & Interventional Sciences,
University College Hospital,
London, UK

Ryuji Sakakibara MD PhD
Associate Professor,
Neurology Division,

Department of Internal Medicine,
Sakura Medical Center,
Toho University,
Toho, Japan

Prateesh M. Trivedi BSc MD MRCS
Research Fellow,
Division of Surgery & Interventional Sciences,
University College London, UK

Foreword

Excretory and sexual functions are mediated by the coordinated activity of multiple pelvic organs and by complex neural circuitry in the brain and spinal cord. Accordingly, injuries or diseases at various sites in the nervous system can produce prominent changes in micturition, defecation, and sexual activity. Thus basic knowledge of the neurobiology of the lower urinary tract, distal bowel, and sexual organs, which is provided in this book, is essential for urologists, gastroenterologists, neurologists, and urogynecologists who are caring for people with neurological disorders affecting the pelvic viscera.

The book is divided into three sections that contain: (1) comprehensive reviews of the neural control of the pelvic organs; (2) methods for evaluation and management of neurogenic disorders of individual organs; and (3) descriptions of the impact of specific conditions such as Parkinson's disease, multiple sclerosis, and spinal cord injury on pelvic organ functions. The book brings together diverse information from many basic science and medical disciplines, including neurophysiology, neuropharmacology, neurology, urology, and gastroenterology, allowing the reader to compare the pathophysiological mechanisms underlying neurogenic dysfunctions of the different organs. These comparisons can be useful clinically in evaluating neurogenic disorders, because the pelvic organs exhibit similar afferent and efferent innervations carried by autonomic and somatic nerves arising at the lumbosacral level of the spinal cord. The organs also exhibit common unique properties not shared by other visceral organs including: (1) complete dependence on central neural control; (2) functions such as, micturition, defecation, emission-ejaculation, that are initiated in an all-or-none, switch-like manner;

(3) functions requiring neurally mediated coordination between multiple smooth and striated muscles; and (4) voluntary control of micturition and defecation in contrast to the involuntarily control of other visceral functions.

The high quality of this book is attributable to the broad clinical and research expertise of the contributing authors, who are based in neurology, urology, gastroenterology, urogynecology, neurosurgery, and uro-neurology departments. This group of clinical scientists, which was organized by Professor Fowler at the National Hospital for Neurology and Neurosurgery, Queen's Square, London, is recognized internationally for its studies of the neural mechanisms underlying pelvic organ dysfunctions. Professor Fowler's laboratory has played a key role in identifying the pathophysiological mechanisms underlying overactive bladder symptoms and the mechanisms involved in idiopathic urinary retention in young women (Fowler's Syndrome). Professor Fowler's pioneering studies of intravesical vanilloid therapy established bladder afferent nerves as an important targets for drugs, and her studies of the effects of botulinum toxin and sacral neuromodulation identified mechanisms by which these therapies influence bladder function.

The experience of Professor Fowler's Uro-Neurology Department at Queen's Square in integrating basic and clinical research has clearly served as a model for the preparation of this excellent book, which efficiently links basic neuroscience information with the diagnosis and management of neurogenic pelvic organ dysfunctions.

William de Groat
University of Pittsburgh

Preface

This book has been edited and written by, and for, clinicians with a special interest in the management of bladder, bowel and sexual problems in neurological disease. Based soundly on knowledge of basic science, the first section outlines the separate neurological control of bladder, bowel and sexual function. The next section describes the investigation and generic management of each type of organ dysfunction, dealing predominantly with medical treatments, although a chapter on surgical interventions is included as well. Not attempted in any other single volume, a unique feature of the approach taken in this book is the description of the impact of neurological dysfunction on each pelvic organ.

The Department of Uro-Neurology was established at the National Hospital for Neurology and Neurosurgery, Queen Square, London 20 years ago and all the authors of this book have had a close association there, either contributing to its research or developing the clinical service. Over this period much has been learnt from basic science as well as clinical studies about the neurological control of the pelvic organs and possible treatment of their disorders. *Pelvic Organ Dysfunction in Neurological Disease* brings together that knowledge in an easy-to-read text. Each chapter makes sense on its own but if the reader wants to know more, for example about the treatment of symptoms in a specific condition, they will find good internal referencing to the relevant chapter. The book is directed towards any healthcare professional managing patients in whom pelvic organ functions have been compromised by neurological disease. These patients present with complex pelvic organ symptoms, and it is our intention that the clinician who sees such a patient can now source helpful information from a single book, not separate textbooks on urology, gynecology, andrology and gastroenterology.

Neurological control of the bladder in health and disease

Derek J. Griffiths and Apostolos Apostolidis

Peripheral control of micturition

A dense network of nerves lies immediately below the bladder urothelium (in the "suburothelium"; Fig. 1.1), with occasional fibers penetrating the basal lamina. Afferent nerve endings in the bladder wall are important in conveying the sensations associated with various degrees of bladder fullness and also bladder pain to the spinal cord. Two main types of afferent axons are involved in this process: the myelinated Aδ-fibers and the unmyelinated C-fibers. Most Aδ-fibers are sensitive to mechanical stimuli, e.g. distension and stretch, whereas most C-fibers are not, due to a higher mechanical threshold. Thus, in conditions of health it is the Aδ-fibers which convey information about bladder filling, while C-fibers remain largely quiescent, responding only to noxious, chemical and cooling stimuli (Fig. 1.2).

Excitatory input to the bladder is conveyed by efferent parasympathetic nerves, whose axons originate in the S_2–S_4 intermediolateral column of the spinal cord. The S_2–S_4 roots contain the preganglionic parasympathetic fibers destined for ganglia in the pelvis, from which short postganglionic fibers originate to innervate the detrusor smooth muscle (Fig. 1.2).

The latter release acetylcholine (ACh), which acts on muscarinic receptors in the detrusor muscle and results in its contraction (see Fig. 1.3 and "Spinal control" below) [1]. A smaller contribution to detrusor contraction comes from the purinergic pathway, via release of adenosine triphosphate (ATP) by parasympathetic postganglionic terminals, which in health only achieves a fast, short-lived bladder contraction.

Important for continence is the contraction of the striated element of the urethral sphincter

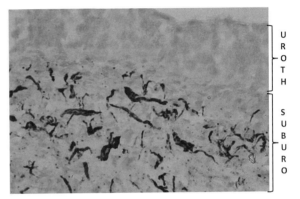

Fig. 1.1. Immunohistochemical staining of a human bladder specimen obtained via flexible cystoscopy with the pan-neuronal marker PGP9.5 depicts the dense network of suburothelial nerve fibers laying immediately below the basal lamina of the urothelium. Abbreviations: UROTH = urothelium, SUBURO = suburothelium. See plate section for color version.

and the pelvic floor muscles, due to activation of nicotinic receptors by ACh released by somatic efferents originating at Onuf's nucleus in the anterior horn of the S_2–S_4 spinal cord. Afferent activity which increases as the bladder fills enhances efferent output to the sphincter, the basis of the "guarding reflex" (see Fig. 1.4 and "Spinal control" below).

A further contribution to storage and voiding comes from the sympathetic innervation. The bladder base and the urethral smooth muscle are innervated by sympathetic neurons originating at the intermediolateral cell column of the T_{11}–L_2 spinal cord (Fig. 1.5). The main sympathetic neurotransmitter is norepinephrine, which acts on α-adrenoreceptors resulting in contraction of the bladder base and urethral smooth muscle to

Pelvic Organ Dysfunction in Neurological Disease: Clinical Management and Rehabilitation, ed. Clare J. Fowler, Jalesh N. Panicker & Anton Emmanuel. Published by Cambridge University Press. © Cambridge University Press 2010.

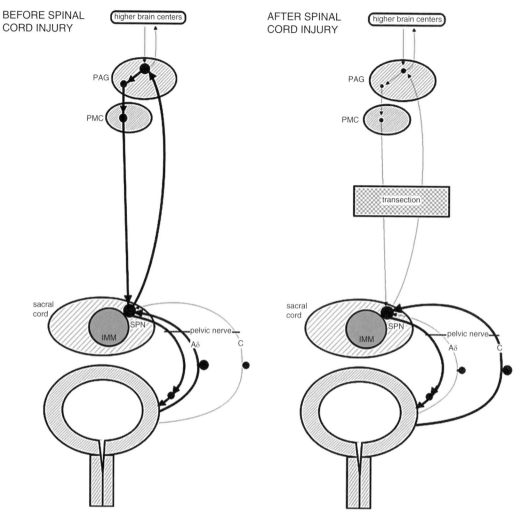

Fig. 1.2. These cartoon representations of simplified micturition pathways in health (left) and spinal cord lesions (right) aim to demonstrate the role of the types of bladder afferents in micturition reflexes. In conditions of health, Aδ-fibers convey information about bladder filling, whereas C-fibers remain largely quiescent. Both types of afferents run via the pelvic nerve. Sensory input to the spinal cord ascends to the PAG, where stimuli are filtered under the influence of higher brain centers to provide input to the PMC. Excitatory input descends via the spinal cord and the peripheral parasympathetic efferent nerve fibers running through the pelvic nerve to the detrusor. Thus a bladder contraction begins. Following a suprasacral spinal lesion, the formerly quiescent C-fiber afferents change their properties and hypertrophy and become highly excitable by mechanical stimuli. Consequently, they respond with increased afferent firing to the spinal cord at low urine volumes during bladder distension. This, in turn, produces increased parasympathetic input to the bladder and results in detrusor overactivity. Abbreviations: PAG = periaqueductal gray; PMC = pontine micturition center; SPN = sacral parasympathetic nucleus; IMM = sacral intermediomedial cell group.

contribute to continence during urine storage, and on β-adrenoreceptors resulting in relaxation of the detrusor muscle. The urethral smooth muscle also receives sacral parasympathetic efferents releasing nitric oxide (NO), which exerts an inhibitory effect on the muscle; this achieves urethral relaxation during contraction of the bladder (see Fig. 1.3 and "Spinal control" below) [1].

Cellular signaling pathways in normal bladder function

The detrusor muscle

The abundance of intercellular mechanical adhesions, known as "adherens" junctions, in detrusor muscle cells [2, 3] probably underlies the mechanical cell coupling between those cells and contributes to the generation of both spontaneous and normal detrusor contractions. The actions of ACh, the main neurotransmitter of detrusor contractions in health, are mediated by five subtypes of muscarinic ACh receptors in the detrusor muscle (M_1–M_5). Although the M_2 subtype is predominant in density, it is the M_3 subtype which mediates detrusor contraction in health in all species [4]. However, the M_2 receptor may also have a supportive role in detrusor contraction and efficient voiding via inhibition of the cyclic adenosine monophosphate (cAMP)-mediated smooth muscle relaxation as well as via opposition of the sympathetic activation of β-adrenoreceptors [4]. In addition, M_1 receptors expressed in prejunctional cholinergic nerves appear to have a facilitatory role in the release of ACh, thus enhancing detrusor contraction and assisting efficient voiding function [4]. ATP, a co-transmitter with ACh in parasympathetic nerve terminals, is responsible for the atropine-resistant component of detrusor contraction in conditions of health [5]. Urine storage, on the other hand, is facilitated by the detrusor muscle relaxation via activation of a subpopulation of β-adrenoreceptors ($β_3$) [6].

The urothelium and suburothelium

Both ACh and ATP are released by the bladder urothelium during urine storage, in increasing concentrations as the bladder wall distends [7, 8]. Muscarinic, nicotinic and purinergic receptors have been identified in the bladder urothelium and/or suburothelium in human or animal studies [9–13] (Fig. 1.6). It has been proposed that ACh released from the urothelium during bladder storage acts on muscarinic receptors in the suburothelium and the detrusor to stimulate a constant muscle tone [14] and an additional autocrine role for urothelially released ACh cannot be excluded. Stimulation of urothelial muscarinic receptors has been shown to be associated with the release of an as yet unidentified urothelium-derived inhibitory factor with a relaxing effect on the detrusor [15]. Moreover, ACh released by the urothelium appears to activate two opposing nicotinic signaling pathways mediated by type $α_7$ (inhibitory) and type $α_3$ (excitatory) nicotinic receptors, which facilitate urine storage and bladder emptying respectively (Fig. 1.6) [13].

A role in bladder mechanosensation has been identified for the ATP-gated purinergic receptor $P2X_3$ [16]. It is thought that ATP released from the urothelium during bladder stretch activates $P2X_3$ receptors on suburothelial afferent nerve fibers to stimulate afferent firing to the spinal cord (Fig. 1.6) [17]. Recent studies have also confirmed the presence of the sensory receptor Transient Receptor Potential Vanilloid 1 (TRPV1, formerly known as the capsaicin or vanilloid receptor VR1) in urothelial cells [18] and suburothelial nerves (presumably C-fiber afferents) (Figs. 1.6 and 1.7) [19]. TRPV1 is necessary for the release of ATP and NO from the urothelium, and its gene depletion in a knockout mouse resulted in a number of changes in normal bladder function, supporting its role in normal bladder mechanosensation [20].

C-fiber afferents are also thought to be responsible for thermal perceptions; TRPV1 is activated by temperatures higher than 43°C. From the same family of transient receptor potential channels, the "menthol" TRPM8 receptor is sensitive to low temperatures and menthol [21], is expressed in suburothelial fiber-like structures in the human [22], and appears to mediate the bladder cooling reflex which emerges following a spinal injury [23].

Sensory neuropeptides, namely substance P (SP) and calcitonin gene-related peptide (CGRP), are also abundantly found in suburothelial afferents (Fig. 1.7) [24, 25]. Although primarily associated with neurogenic inflammation and pain, both SP and CGRP appear to also be involved in lower urinary tract neuromodulation via complex interactions (Fig. 1.6). In brief, SP and CGRP may induce the expression of the neurotrophic growth factor (NGF) [26], regulate the expression of TRPV1 and $P2X_3$ [27], activate non-selective cation channels in afferent neurons [28], and sensitize P2X receptors to the action of ATP [29]. In turn, activation of TRPV1 promotes the release of SP and CGRP from afferent nerves via an ATP-mediated pathway [30]. In the rat bladder, SP levels were found to inversely correlate to the micturition threshold [31].

Recently, functional cannabinoid CB1 and CB2 receptors were identified in the human bladder [32, 33]. CB2 receptors were identified in sensory suburothelial nerves, and also in cholinergic neurons in the detrusor. Their activation decreased the nerve-evoked contractions of the bladder and increased the micturition intervals and bladder pressure, suggesting a modulatory role of CB2 in both afferent signaling and cholinergic nerve activity [33].

As the bladder urothelium expresses a large range of receptors and neurotrophic factors, and releases tachykinins, prostaglandins, NO, ACh and ATP, the

VOIDING REFLEX

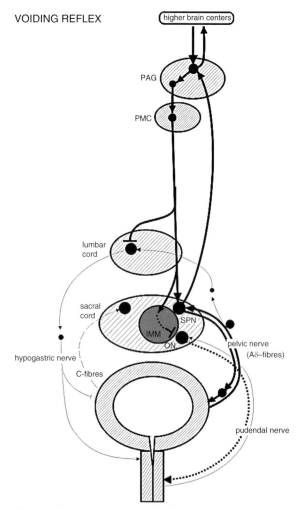

Fig. 1.3. Voiding depends on a bladder-to-bladder excitatory reflex, whereby increasing wall tension or detrusor pressure stimulates bladder afferents which synapse at the SPN. From there, afferent stimuli travel via the spinal cord to brain centers – the PAG and the PMC. From the latter, excitatory stimuli descend via the spinal cord. One branch inhibits the sympathetically mediated storage reflex (shown in Fig. 1.5) and another descends to the SPN and then via the pelvic nerve to the bladder wall, inducing detrusor contraction. At the same time, it excites an inhibitory interneuronal connection at sacral level and thus relaxes the striated urethral sphincter, so that voiding can occur. During the storage phase, excitation of this voiding reflex is blocked by inhibition of the PAG by higher centers (Fig. 1.10). When voiding is appropriate the inhibition is lifted so that the voiding reflex is excited, emptying the bladder.

older notion that it serves as a plain protective barrier has now been superseded by the view that it is a sensory organ [34]. Its functional properties robustly support a complex interaction with the suburothelial space (Fig. 1.6). A recently identified cell entity, the suburothelial "myofibroblast" or interstitial cell, has become the focus of attention as an integral part of

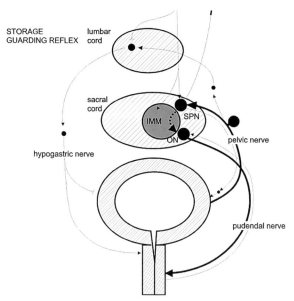

Fig. 1.4. During the storage phase somatic efferents originating from Onuf's nucleus (ON) in the anterior horn of S_2–S_4 spinal cord and running in the pudendal nerve are being stimulated by afferent firing from the bladder via a synapse with sacral interneurons.

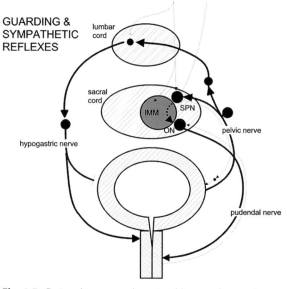

Fig. 1.5. During the storage phase, in addition to the guarding reflex (Fig. 1.4), sympathetic neurons originating at the intermediolateral cell column of the T_{11}–L_2 spinal cord and running through the hypogastric nerve convey efferent stimuli to the bladder and the smooth muscle of the urethra. These stimulate α-adrenoreceptors in the bladder base and urethral smooth muscle resulting in contraction and thus contributing to continence during urine storage, whilst other efferent stimuli act on β-adrenoreceptors in the body of the bladder resulting in relaxation of the detrusor muscle.

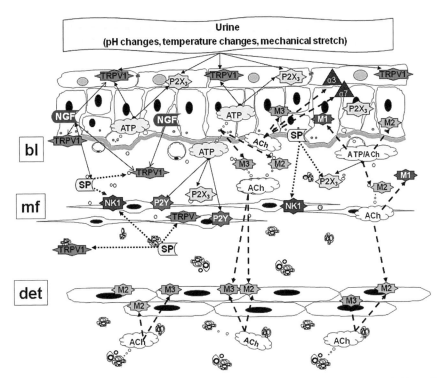

Fig. 1.6. In this cartoon representation of the ultrastructural components of the human bladder wall, the known or proposed location of receptors and sites of release of neuropeptides, neurotransmitters and growth factors thought to be involved in bladder mechanosensation are shown (updated from figure in [117]). A complex system of interactions has been proposed between the neurotransmitters and neuropeptides released and their respective receptors, which are thought to be up-regulated in DO. Fine-line arrows refer to the proposed activation of urothelial and suburothelial purinergic receptors and potentiation of the response of TRPV1 to irritative stimuli by urothelially released ATP. Dotted arrows refer to the proposed activation of suburothelial and detrusor muscarinic receptors by ACh released from the urothelium and suburothelial nerves. Dashed arrows refer to proposed activation of NK1 receptors on myofibroblasts and potentiation of suburothelial TRPV1 and P2X$_3$ receptors by SP. A reciprocal relationship appears to exist between SP and NGF, also identified by such arrows. Finally, thick-line arrows refer to the known effect of NGF on the expression of TRPV1. Abbreviations: bl = basal lamina of urothelium; mf = myofibroblast layer; det = detrusor muscle; TRPV1 = transient receptor potential vanilloid 1; P2X$_3$ = ionotropic purinergic receptor type 3; P2Y = metabotropic purinergic receptors types 2, 4 and 6; M2/M3 = muscarinic acetylcholine receptors types 2 and 3; α_3/α_7 = nicotinic acetylcholine receptors types 3 and 7; NK1 = neurokinin receptor type 1 (SP receptor); SP = substance P; NGF = nerve growth factor; ACh = acetylcholine; ATP = adenosine triphosphate. See plate section for color version.

the urothelio-suburothelial functional syncitium. In the human bladder, myofibroblasts were found to attach to each other and lay in close apposition to vesicle-packed unmyelinated nerve fibers [35] (Fig. 1.6). It has been shown that suburothelial myofibroblast-like cells are extensively linked by connexin-43-containing gap junctions [36], have high membrane capacitance, show spontaneous spikes of electrical activity and respond to ATP by an increase in intracellular Ca^{2+} sufficient to activate contractile proteins and generation of an inward current [37]. Further studies suggest the presence of muscarinic [11], purinergic [38] and TRP channel receptors [39] in myofibroblasts as well as expression of neuronal nitric oxide synthase (nNOS) [39]. It was thus hypothesized that the myofibroblasts and the closely associated nerve axons

could collectively function as a bladder stretch receptor, where intracellular electrical signaling could pass from cell to cell, while contraction of that cell layer could exert stretch-dependent activation of the sensory nerves [37].

Changes in peripheral control of micturition in bladder disease states

Detrusor overactivity

Afferent pathway changes: the vanilloid and purinergic pathways

In animal models of suprasacral spinal lesions, a series of changes, including body hypertrophy and increased excitability, render the C-fiber

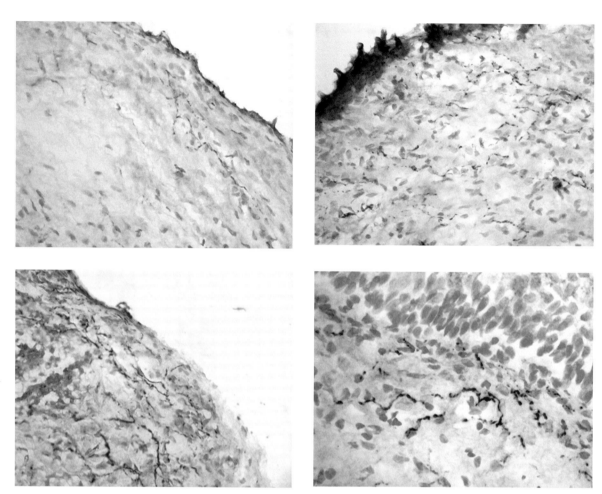

Fig. 1.7. Immunohistochemical staining of human bladder specimens obtained via flexible cystoscopy with specific antibodies to the vanilloid receptor TRPV1 (top left – suburothelial fiber-like staining, magnification x20), substance P (top right – urothelial cell and suburothelial fiber-like staining, magnification x20), vesicular acetylcholine transporter VAChT (bottom left – suburothelial fiber-like staining, magnification x20) and CGRP (bottom right – suburothelial fiber-like staining, magnification x40). See plate section for color version.

afferents in the bladder wall sensitive to mechanical stimuli (mechanosensitive) [1]. Consequently, the C-fibers become excited at low urine volumes in the bladder and respond with increased afferent firing to the spinal cord during bladder distension. This, in turn, induces increased parasympathetic input to the bladder, which results in detrusor overactivity (DO) [40] (Fig. 1.2).

Evidence exists for a similarly augmented afferent limb of the micturition reflex in humans with DO due to spinal lesions [1, 40] and is thought to be associated with the symptoms of urgency (defined as "a sudden, compelling desire to void, which is difficult to defer" [41]), urgency incontinence and also in part increased daytime micturition frequency and nocturia (the symptom of waking up at least once to pass urine).

Increased density of suburothelial innervation and, in particular, sensory nerve fibers expressing TRPV1 and P2X$_3$ was found in patients with MS or suprasacral injury and was greatly reduced following intravesical instillations of C-fiber toxins, such as capsaicin and resiniferatoxin (RTX), in patients who benefited from treatment, but not in those who failed to respond [42–44].

Although increased daytime frequency and incontinence can be largely explained as consequences of the reflex detrusor contractions, the pathophysiology of urgency and nocturia remains to be elucidated. The sensation of urgency, which is distinct from the normal sensation of even strong desire to void, is thought to occur when a barrage of afferent activity, deriving from pathologically sensitive bladder stretch-sensing receptors which increase in number, ascends via a sufficiently preserved spinal cord to consciousness. This should imminently precede the reflex detrusor contraction. To support this notion, peripheral afferent neuromodulation could suppress the sensation of urgency and associated incontinence [45]. Levels of suburothelial nerve $P2X_3$ receptors were decreased in parallel with the number of urgency episodes following successful treatment of DO [19]. Urgency and associated incontinence showed an earlier response to treatment than frequency (Fig. 1.8), [46] suggesting different pathophysiological mechanisms for the symptoms of the overactive bladder (OAB) syndrome [41]. Treatment of DO also improves nocturia but the pattern of post-treatment changes in nocturia is more unpredictable compared to other OAB symptoms. This implies that neural changes leading to DO may only partly contribute to the pathophysiology of nocturia.

The role of the urothelium in the dysfunction of the proposed urothelio-suburothelial functional syncitium appears crucial in bladder pathophysiology. Urothelial cell TRVP1 levels followed similar changes to suburothelial TRPV1 in patients with neurogenic DO (NDO) [47]. Similarly, an increase in urothelial cell $P2X_3$ was found in patients with DO in comparison with controls [19]. The function of urothelial $P2X_3$ is not known, but implies there may be an autocrine role for ATP released from the urothelium. The latter was found to be significantly increased in conditions of spinal NDO [48], but also via interactions with ACh [49].

Cholinergic pathway changes

Recent findings support the hypothesis that DO could be partly due to an increased urothelial release of ACh during bladder filling, which may excite afferent nerves in the suburothelium and within the detrusor and increase detrusor smooth muscle tone [14]. The evidence includes:

- an increase of distension-evoked urothelial ACh release with age [7] and the increased prevalence of DO in the elderly
- an effect of anticholinergic drugs on the bladder afferents [50, 51], which may explain why they reduce urgency and increase bladder capacity
- suppression of the muscarinically mediated inhibitory influence of the urothelium on the detrusor in patients with DO [15].

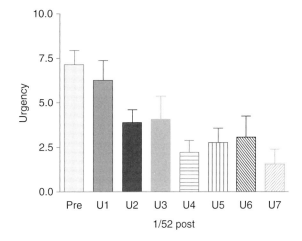

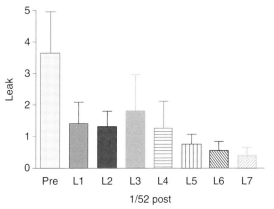

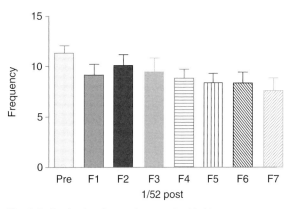

Fig. 1.8. Day-by-day changes in overactive bladder symptoms during the first week after treatment with intravesical BoNT/A injections. A more rapid onset of the therapeutic effect noted for urgency and incontinence episodes compared to micturition frequency implies differences in the pathogenesis of those symptoms.

Reports, however, on the changes of urothelial and suburothelial muscarinic receptors in bladder disease states have been conflicting [4, 11, 52], but suggest a possible role of the M_2 receptor.

A number of changes have been identified in the detrusor of ageing or obstructed human bladders, including:

- an age-related decrease in M_3 receptor mRNA
- a decrease in detrusor contractility with ageing [10]
- a decrease in the cholinergic component of bladder contraction as opposed to an increase in the atropine-resistant (purinergic) component in the ageing human detrusor [7] and the obstructed human bladder [56]
- denervation accompanied by hypersensitivity of the detrusor to ACh in obstructed bladders [56].

Such findings became the basis of the myogenic theory of overactive bladder pathophysiology, where local denervation of bladder smooth muscle leads to increased excitability of ACh receptors and facilitates signal transmission between smooth muscle cells, thus stimulating the propagation of coordinated contractions [57] or micromotions. This hypothesis is contradicted by studies showing no difference in response to ACh between detrusors with and without overactivity [58].

The role of cell junctions

It has been shown that suburothelial myofibroblasts and detrusor smooth muscle cells are electrically coupled via gap junctions [37, 59]. Increased expression of the gap junction protein connexin-43 was found in suburothelial myofibroblasts [60] and in the detrusor [61] of patients with DO. In addition, there is evidence that cadherin, one of the proteins constituting the adherens junction complex, mediates cell-to-cell interactions between suburothelial myofibroblasts as between detrusor smooth muscle cells [62]. Cadherin-11 expression was found to be up-regulated in the suburothelium, but was unchanged . in the detrusor of patients with DO [63]. Co-localization of cadherin-11 and connexin-43 implied that gap and adherens junctions may form a functional unit. Animal studies have linked both normal detrusor function and DO with the modulation of spontaneous activity by myofibroblasts [64]; inappropriate activation was proposed to result in pathological localized contractions and "sensory urgency" [65]. However, human detrusor cells are also known to possess properties that allow the development of spontaneous activity which may affect adjacent cells and thus produce a stronger myogenic response [59].

Bladder pain

Recent findings support a neurogenic basis for the "bladder pain syndrome" (BPS), especially its most studied form, interstitial cystitis (IC). In feline IC, bladder afferents exhibit increased firing in response to intravesical pressure, suggesting increased mechanoreceptor sensitivity [66]. Stretch-evoked urothelial ATP release and urothelial $P2X_3$ expression are increased in patients with IC [67, 68]. In support of neuroplastic changes, NGF levels and suburothelial SP-expressing fibers were found to be increased in IC bladders [69, 70]. Significant attenuation of pain and urgency in IC patients treated with intravesical instillation of lidocaine, which in addition to its known local anesthetic effect is also known to have an inhibitory effect on neurite regeneration and synapse formation, further supports a role of bladder afferents in the pathophysiology [71].

Detrusor underactivity

The least studied of bladder dysfunctions may have a variety of neural etiological associations, including sacral and infrasacral spinal lesions. However, the neurological concept of "upper and lower motor neuron" lesions, which is fundamental for understanding neurogenic skeletal muscle weakness, is not directly applicable to neurogenic bladder disorders because, although damage to an anterior horn cell in the cord or its motor axon in ventral root or peripheral nerve will result in denervated striated muscle and flaccid paralysis, a sacral root lesion does not produce detrusor denervation. This is because the S_2–S_4 roots contain the preganglionic parasympathetic fibers destined for ganglia in the pelvis, from which short postganglionic fibers originate to innervate the detrusor smooth muscle (Fig. 1.2). The bladder is innervated by both extramural and intramural ganglion cells [72] although the relative proportions of each type of ganglia are not known. Following loss of the parasympathetic innervation, it was shown in cats that preganglionic sympathetic nerves reinnervated the parasympathetic ganglion cells [73]. Subsequent bladder contractile activity was then demonstrated following hypogastric nerve stimulation so that it was proposed that the "autonomous hyperactive bladder" [74] seen following sacral root injury was due to plasticity in adrenergic innervation of the ganglia changes [73]. It seems likely that intrinsic activity of the smooth muscle driven by urothelial-detrusor mediated reflexes may also contribute.

So it is that infrasacral cord or cauda equina lesions (Chapter 17) may produce an insensate "decentralized" bladder, with poor compliance or detrusor overactivity, presumably due to the mechanisms outlined above, as well as an underactive detrusor and urinary retention [75]. Retention can result from damage to the ganglia as may occur in the condition of pure autonomic failure with ganglionic autoantibodies, or surgical damage to the ganglia and postganglionic fibers during radical pelvic surgery (Chapter 18). Detrusor under activity expressed with incomplete bladder emptying or complete retention, reduced bladder sensation, increased bladder capacity, reduced micturition frequency and voiding difficulty can also result from the small fiber involvement of diabetic or amyloid neuropathy, which affect both the pre- and postganglionic innervations (Chapter 18).

Detrusor underactivity may also be associated with chronic bladder outlet obstruction; in men it is usually represented by the "decompensated" detrusor caused by benign prostatic enlargement. In women it has been described as part of Fowler's syndrome, characterized by a primary disorder of external urethral sphincter relaxation, possibly due to a hormonal channelopathy (Chapter 19) [76].

"Idiopathic" detrusor overactivity/overactive bladder

Although the term "idiopathic" is used in cases where detrusor overactivity cannot be associated with obvious neurology or bladder outlet obstruction, changes in the neural control of micturition have been identified, both in the afferent bladder pathways and the detrusor in IDO. IDO is the commonest cause of the OAB syndrome, in which urgency is considered the driving symptom for frequency, incontinence and (in part) nocturia. Up-regulation of sensory receptors [19] and neuropeptides [25] as well as increased release of excitatory neurotransmitters occurs in both neurogenic and idiopathic DO/OAB. Neural plasticity in idiopathic DO can be presumed from the successful regulation of bladder symptoms via both electrical neurostimulation of the afferents and chemical neuromodulation with the use of botulinum toxins and resiniferatoxin [45, 19, 46, 77]. The

properties of suburothelial cell junctions are also affected, with changes in the expression of muscarinic receptors [11] and gap [60] and adherens junction proteins [63]. Further to evidence for the augmentation of the peripheral part of the afferent limb in idiopathic DO, assumptions about concurrent alteration of spinal reflexes can be drawn from the improvements made in urgency and urgency incontinence by peripheral and sacral nerve stimulation [45, 78]. Thus there is abundant evidence of various types of demonstrable peripheral pathologies in different types of IDO. Reconciliation of the view that IDO has peripheral causes with the view that the condition has its cause in the brain (see pp. 14–15) is difficult and the matter is as yet unresolved, with the "centralist" arguing that detrusor overactivity represents a loss of voluntary control of the bladder and control is exercised from the brain. The solution may lie with the more precise definition of different types of IDO.

Spinal control of bladder function

A series of spinal reflex mechanisms are involved in the control of the urethro-vesical unit. These promote urine storage and micturition via sympathetic, parasympathetic and somatic nerves mediating efferent and inhibitory input to the urethral sphincter and the bladder accordingly [1].

A bladder-to-urethral sphincter reflex, named the "guarding reflex," has a central role during bladder filling; pudendal urethral efferents are stimulated by afferent firing from the bladder via a synapse with sacral interneurons during the storage phase (Fig. 1.4). An increase in urethral electromyographic activity as the bladder progressively fills during urodynamic investigations provides evidence for the presence of this reflex in humans [79]. The low detrusor pressure achieved until micturition threshold is reached is maintained via an additional, *sympathetically mediated reflex* which inhibits detrusor contraction while promoting urethral smooth muscle contraction during bladder filling (Fig. 1.5) [78, 80].

When the bladder is full, activation of a *bladder-to-urethral sphincter inhibitory reflex* interrupts urethral sphincter activity, an event timely followed by a rise in detrusor pressure (detrusor contraction), which is promoted by a *bladder-to-bladder excitatory reflex* [78, 80]. Thus, voiding begins. In healthy adults these reflexes form part of the spinobulbospinal voiding reflex, with connections to the brainstem and midbrain as shown in Fig. 1.3. This enables higher brain centers to exert control of the voiding phase, as discussed in the section on central control which follows.

The emerging role of interneurons

Interneurons at various levels of the spinal cord may represent a crucial element in the regulation of reflex activity, serving as integrating areas of afferent projections from both the bladder and the urethra [78, 80]. Urine storage is facilitated by the activation of a *bladder-sphincter-bladder reflex* pathway in which the *bladder-to-external urethral sphincter excitatory reflex* (Fig. 1.5) activates the *urethral sphincter-to-bladder inhibitory reflex* (Fig. 1.9) via interneuronal synapses. Suppression of bladder activity and urine storage are additionally facilitated by inhibition of excitatory interneurons and preganglionic parasympathetic neurons [80].

During the voiding phase, activation of excitatory interneurons and preganglionic parasympathetic neurons promotes detrusor contraction until the bladder empties (Fig. 1.9). Pudendal afferent activity from urogenital sites can inhibit the excitatory parasympathetic outflow to the bladder via interneuronal pathways (Fig. 1.9). At the same time, activation of interneurons by bladder afferents stimulates parasympathetic efferent inhibitory activity to the urethral smooth muscle.

Spinal reflexes and bladder pathophysiology

It is now proposed that augmented "excitatory" or "inhibitory" function of spinal interneurons could be etiologically involved in conditions of either bladder overactivity or urinary retention. Supporting evidence comes from the successful use of peripheral and central neurostimulation in the treatment of human bladder dysfunction: sacral nerve stimulation (SNS) can be effective in the treatment of both intractable DO [78] and urinary retention [81]. In the former, it is believed that SNS suppresses detrusor contraction via activation of the bladder-sphincter-bladder reflex pathway mentioned above (Fig. 1.3) [78, 80]. In the latter, SNS has been proposed to suppress inhibitory interneurons and release the bladder from an augmented sphincter-bladder reflex (Fig. 1.9). Finally, stimulation of pudendal afferents can suppress urgency and alter bladder function in patients with idiopathic DO (Fig. 1.9) [45].

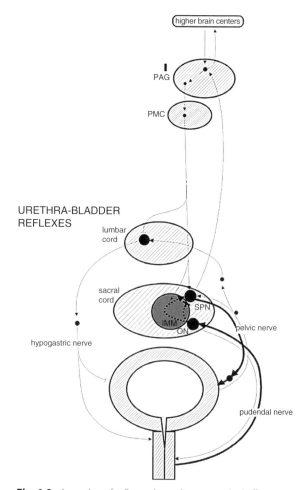

Fig. 1.9. A number of reflexes depending on urethral afferent signals utilize sacral interneurons to help regulate the coordination between the bladder and the urethra. Further to the "guarding reflex," urine storage is facilitated by the activation of a *urethral sphincter-to-bladder inhibitory reflex*, where pudendal afferents terminating at the ON synapse via inhibitory interneurons with parasympathetic efferents at the SPN. The latter activate β-adrenoreceptors in the bladder wall, resulting in detrusor relaxation. In contrast, during voiding, stimulation of urethral afferents by the urine passing through the urethra stimulates excitatory interneurons and preganglionic parasympathetic neurones, which in turn act on muscarinic acetylcholine receptors in the bladder wall to further promote detrusor contraction until the bladder empties completely.

The peripheral elements of the segmental bladder-sacral spinal cord-bladder reflex, which emerges following suprasacral spinal lesions, have been discussed in detail in a previous section. Further to DO, which develops as a result of this augmented reflex after the initial phase of spinal shock and results in reflex voiding (Fig. 1.2), the striated urethral sphincter becomes dyssynergic, i.e. it contracts

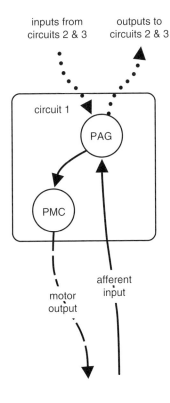

inputs from circuits 2 & 3

outputs to circuits 2 & 3

Fig. 1.10. Midbrain and brainstem control of the voiding reflex (circuit 1).

circuit 1

PAG

PMC

afferent input

motor output

simultaneously with a detrusor contraction, allowing only partial emptying of the bladder.

Fig. 1.2 represents simplified micturition pathways in health (left) and spinal cord lesions (right). In conditions of health, Aδ-fibers convey information about bladder filling, whereas C-fibers remain largely quiescent. Sensory input to the spinal cord ascends to the periaqueductal gray (PAG), where stimuli are filtered under the influence of higher brain centers (see Fig. 1.10) to provide input to the pontine micturition centre. Excitatory input descends via the spinal cord and the peripheral parasympathetic efferent nerve fibers to the detrusor and a bladder contraction begins. In suprasacral spinal lesions, C-fiber afferents change their properties, hypertrophy and become highly excitable to mechanical stimuli. Consequently, they respond with increased afferent firing to the spinal cord at low urine volumes during bladder distension. This, in turn, produces increased parasympathetic input to the bladder and results in detrusor overactivity. Interneuronal connection to Onuf's nucleus may facilitate dyssynergic excitation of the urethral sphincter.

Lower lesions, on the other hand, may result in reduced contractility of the striated urethral sphincter

in conjunction with either a decentralized or denervated detrusor.

Current concepts of brain control of the bladder

As described in the first part of this chapter and in a recent review [82], the behavior of the lower urinary tract is governed by a number of spinal reflexes and also by a long-loop spinobulbospinal reflex concerned specifically with voiding (Fig. 1.3). This voiding reflex is driven by mechanical receptors in the bladder wall. If it operated in isolation, it would lead to involuntary bladder emptying (incontinence) whenever the bladder volume reached a critical level. Although such behavior is tolerated in infants and may recur in the latest stages of life, in continent adults the firing of the reflex is under strict voluntary control, exerted by a supraspinal network.

The ultimate function of the network is to prevent the voiding reflex from firing automatically and to allow urination only if and when desired, while ensuring that voiding occurs sufficiently often to maintain homeostasis. To this end, the brain network maintains constant inhibition of the voiding reflex during urine storage. Meanwhile it generates a sensation (desire to void) that increases in intensity with bladder filling, and it allows excitation of the voiding reflex only if excitation would be (1) mechanically appropriate (i.e. bladder volume is adequate), (2) emotionally safe, and (3) in the judgment of the individual, socially appropriate.

The midbrain PAG plays a pivotal role between the voiding reflex and supraspinal control because (1) it is the rostral terminus of the reflex, receiving and generating ascending bladder afferents and descending efferents (Fig. 1.10), and (2) it transmits and receives signals to and from the higher parts of the brain, the realms of emotion and consciousness. The PAG receives projections from many brain and spinal regions, enabling it to organize and coordinate the behavior of all basic bodily systems, not just the urinary tract. In the case of the bladder, the PAG exercises control via a brainstem nucleus, the pontine micturition center (PMC, also referred to as the "M-region" or "Barrington's nucleus"), which seems to be specialized for lower urinary tract control and coordination [82]. (It may also coordinate fecal and urinary elimination; see Chapter 3.) Stimulation of neurons in the PMC activates a spinal efferent pathway to the sacral cord which, via spinal circuitry, both inhibits (relaxes) the urethral sphincter mechanism and excites detrusor contraction, causing voiding. The strongest projecting pathway to the PMC is from the PAG. The only other monosynaptic input comes from the hypothalamus. In cats and probably in humans, ascending spinal afferents from the bladder bypass the PMC [83] and synapse first in the PAG (Fig. 1.10). Thus the PMC is critical for organizing synergic bladder contraction and urethral relaxation, but actual control of voiding appears to be the province of the PAG, perhaps with some input from the hypothalamus.

Prior to the application of functional brain imaging to urinary problems, clinical observations and animal experiments had shown that numerous brain regions were concerned with bladder control (Chapter 11) and had excitatory or inhibitory effects on voiding (Fig. 1.11) [84].

Use of functional brain imaging (SPECT) to examine the neural control exerted by these regions on the human bladder and urethra was first reported by Fukuyama et al. in 1996 [85]. In the following year Holstege's group published a PET study of brain activation during filling and voiding in men [86], which established a framework of thinking that has informed studies in this area ever since. Activation was demonstrated in the dorsal pons, the presumptive location of the PMC, in subjects who were able to void in the scanner. In those who tried to void but could not do so, there was activation in a more ventrolateral pontine "L-region," previously postulated to be important for continence [87]. A review of human functional brain imaging experiments conducted since these early studies [88] summarizes the midbrain and pontine locations of activation that have been found (Fig. 1.12A). Activations are clustered near the PMC (mostly during voiding), more rostrally near the PAG, and also near the putative L-region. In the early PET imaging experiments the PAG was activated on both bladder filling and voiding. Subsequent studies confirmed prominent activation on bladder filling [89]. One potential problem that should be borne in mind when interpreting these functional imaging studies is that observed activations represent neuronal activity which may be either excitatory or inhibitory: without further information it is not possible to distinguish these two possibilities. Moreover, in some brain

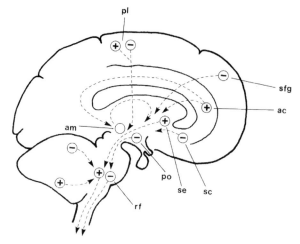

Fig. 1.11. Simplified representation of cerebral areas involved in micturition. Abbreviations: + = facilitation; − = inhibition; ac = anterior cingulate gyrus; am = amygdala; pl = paracentral lobule; po = preoptic nucleus; rf = pontine reticular formation; sc = subcallosal cingulate gyrus; se = septal area; sfg = superior frontal gyrus. From reference [84] with permission.

regions, deactivations are observed; their interpretation is discussed below. Nevertheless the observations provide general support for the arrangement of reflex bladder control shown in Fig. 1.10, which is referred to in this chapter as circuit 1 of the control system. Note that urethral afferents and efferents and also the L-region have been omitted from this figure.

Bladder sensation and the concept of "interoception"

Fig. 1.10 suggests that in normal adults information about the bladder is passed from the PAG to higher regions of the brain. A critical element of that information is an appreciation of the degree of bladder filling, ultimately resulting in the desire to void. This type of interoception is mediated by afferent input through small-diameter fibers in lamina 1 of the spinal cord. These neurons carry homeostatic information ("the sense of the physiological condition of the entire body") about many different tissues [90]. They project via the spinothalamic tracts to subcortical homeostatic centres including the hypothalamus and PAG. In humans and higher order primates they relay in the thalamus and converge on the nondominant anterior insula. Indeed the insula has come to be regarded as the homeostatic afferent cortex that registers visceral sensations [91, 92].

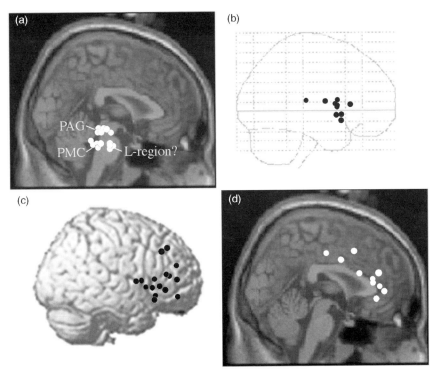

Fig. 1.12. Reported locations of peak activation (deactivation in a few cases). A. Brainstem areas activated during withholding of urine or full bladder, or during voiding, projected on a medial section of the brain. B. Insular areas activated during withholding of urine or full bladder, in a lateral view through a glass brain (activations are 20–30 mm deep below the lateral surface of the cortex; see Fig. 1.13). C. Lateral frontal areas activated during withholding of urine or full bladder, or during voiding, projected on a lateral view of the brain. D. Anterior cingulate gyrus activated during withholding of urine or full bladder, or during voiding. Based on PET, fMRI and SPECT studies in healthy controls. Adapted from reference [88] with permission.

Consistent with this concept, insula activation has been observed in most studies of urine storage (Fig. 1.12B), and in healthy controls activation increases with bladder filling and therefore with desire to void [89, 92]. It is also relatively weaker in older subjects, who correspondingly have less pronounced bladder sensation [93]. The pathways are presumably bilateral, possibly with a right-sided preference [86, 89]. The role of the thalamus in processing and relaying bladder signals to the cortex (including the insula) is supported by several imaging studies that have shown thalamic excitation in response to bladder filling [94].

A key feature of interoceptive sensations is their association with an affective, motivational aspect and hence their value in homeostasis. For example, as discussed above, increasing desire to void as the bladder fills ensures that the bladder is regularly emptied, even though the exact time and place are under voluntary control. The anterior cingulate cortex (ACC) can be considered as the limbic motor cortex [95],

responsible for motivation and context-driven modulation of bodily arousal states [96]. ACC activation has been demonstrated in many functional imaging bladder experiments [88] although, as shown in Fig. 1.12D, the precise location depends on the paradigm used to evoke brain responses. The part of the ACC most clearly associated with motivation to void is the dorsal part (dACC, also described as the posterior midcingulate [97]) shown in Fig. 1.12D. In patients with urge incontinence this area is strongly activated when a nearly full bladder is further distended (without detrusor contraction) (Fig. 1.13), giving rise to an extremely strong sensation that is probably equivalent to the "urgency" complained of by such subjects and formerly defined by the International Continence Society as "a strong desire to void accompanied by fear of leakage" [98]. The dACC is activated by bladder filling in normal subjects also, but much less strongly. Since it is responsible for autonomic motor arousal [96] it probably recruits mechanisms that enable voiding or allow it to be postponed [82].

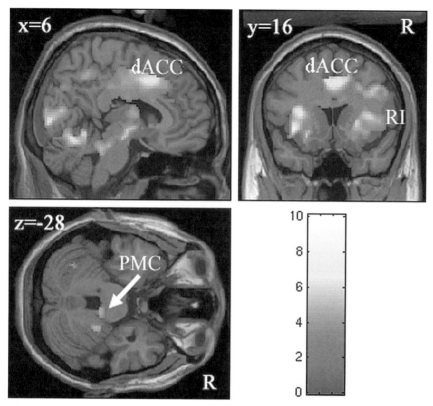

Fig. 1.13. Activation in response to bladder filling in subjects with urge incontinence (P < 0.01 uncorrected). Abbreviations: dACC = dorsal anterior cingulate cortex; RI = right insula; x, y and z are Montreal Neurological Institute (MNI) coordinates for the three sections shown. Adapted from reference [118] with permission. See plate section for color version.

It thus appears that, whereas insula activation principally represents bladder afferent signals, activation of the dorsal ACC provides the neural substrate for the motivational aspect of bladder sensation and the corresponding motor output that is essential to a homeostatic emotion such as desire to void or urgency [99].

Prefrontal cortex and bladder control

The prefrontal cortex lies anterior to the motor strip and supplementary motor areas. Ventromedial regions are involved in decision-making in an emotional and social context. They have extensive interconnections with the limbic system – the hypothalamus and amygdala – as well as the insula and ACC. The more lateral parts of the prefrontal cortex are involved in aspects of cognition, especially working memory [100]. Connections with the ventromedial PFC give them access to the limbic system and other parts of the brain [101].

The importance of the prefrontal cortex in bladder control was established by clinical studies by Ueki [102]. Subsequently Andrew and Nathan [103] highlighted that the location of lesions which were clinically demonstrated to have long-term effects on bladder function was in white matter tracts in the medial prefrontal regions. Medial prefrontal gray-matter lesions led to relatively short-term incontinence (Fig. 1.14; see also Chapter 11).

Whether the primary abnormality in IDO is in the prefrontal cortex and its connecting pathways (representing a change in how the brain handles afferent signals from the bladder) rather than in the afferents themselves is not resolved. Cerebral white-matter changes are associated with diminished bladder control in older people and also, paradoxically, with increased activation of the dorsal anterior cingulate gyrus referred to above (unpublished observation). The white-matter changes are presumably a cause of impaired control, while the increased cingulate

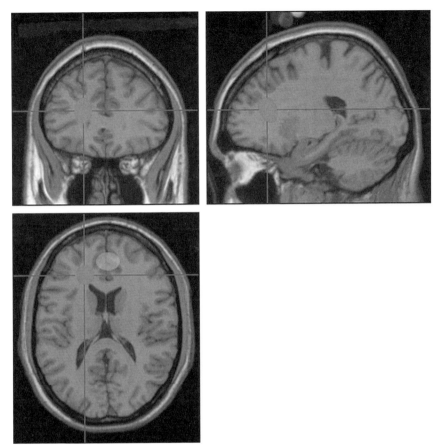

Fig. 1.14. Location of lesions causing incontinence (or occasionally retention) in the group of patients studied by Andrew and Nathan [103]. The red ellipse shows where white-matter lesions caused lasting urinary tract dysfunction. The cyan ellipse shows the location of gray-matter lesions that caused transient dysfunction. (Nathan, personal communication.) See plate section for color version.

activation appears to be an attempt to cope with imminent loss of control. Therefore it seems likely that in some cases IDO is mainly of peripheral origin and in others central. Presumably, in reality, both central and peripheral changes contribute to IDO and incontinence, implying that different types of IDO should be distinguished [104] and further that the condition may not really be "idiopathic" DO.

The medial prefrontal area is activated during voiding as shown by a PET study [86]. Unfortunately this observation is unlikely to be confirmed by fMRI in the near future because of the difficulty of designing a protocol to study voiding in the repetitive manner desirable for fMRI. During withholding of urine or with full bladder, however, few if any observations have shown medial prefrontal activation, although many have shown lateral activation (Fig. 1.12C). Indeed, recent observations indicate that the medial parts of the prefrontal cortex show a

trend to deactivation in response to bladder filling (Fig. 1.15) [88]. The interpretation of deactivation is controversial [105] and requires explanation. It means that, in response to an event such as bladder filling, activity in the given location falls to below its resting value. Deactivation is commonly observed in a specific "default mode network" that is active during resting conditions and includes the medial frontal cortex [106]. Deactivation of this network is a sign that default mode activity is suspended while the brain uses other resources to process an event that requires attention, such as bladder filling.

In the medial prefrontal cortex the almost unique deactivation response, together with the lesion data of Andrew and Nathan, confirms the critical importance of this region for control of voiding. Indeed it has been hypothesized that the region "plays a role in making the decision about whether [voiding] should take place" [107].

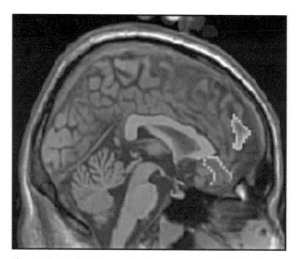

Fig. 1.15. Medial PFC deactivation in response to bladder filling in patients with urge incontinence (P < 0.05 uncorrected). Two regions appear to be involved: the medial prefrontal cortex (BA 9) and the orbitofrontal cortex (BA 11/32 plus pregenual ACC). The medial prefrontal cortex is near the cyan ellipse shown in Fig. 1.14. See plate section for color version.

Brain-bladder control network

The observations outlined above suggest that the most important brain structures in bladder control are the PMC and PAG, the insula and dACC, and the dorsolateral and ventromedial prefrontal cortices. They also provide some indication of function. However, these six regions are very much fewer in number than the regions recognized clinically (Fig. 1.11) and indeed brain imaging itself shows that numerous other regions respond to bladder events. To understand this complexity it helps to place the various brain regions in a systematic framework – a tentative model of the cerebral control system, its centers and interconnections, which is based on clinical and experimental observations with some imaginative extensions.

As outlined above, the brain network maintains constant inhibition of the voiding reflex during urine storage. Meanwhile it generates a sensation (desire to void [41]) that increases in intensity and unpleasantness with bladder filling but allows excitation of the voiding reflex if it is mechanically appropriate, emotionally safe and socially appropriate. Corresponding to these three conditions, three modules or control circuits can tentatively be identified. Working essentially in parallel (although with some mutual interaction), it is postulated that their net result determines whether voiding occurs or not.

Circuit 1: mechanical (midbrain/brainstem)

Circuit 1 comprises the midbrain and pontine structures supporting the voiding reflex (Fig. 1.10). The afferent arm of the reflex ascends from the bladder via the spinal cord to terminate in the central PAG [108]. The efferent arm originates in the lateral PAG and descends via the PMC to the sacral cord. Interneuronal connections between the central and lateral PAG presumably enable the signal processing needed for the PAG to exert basic control of voiding and integrate it with other bodily functions. During bladder filling the efferent pathway to the PMC is turned off, preventing voiding, but at a certain level of bladder distension afferent activity from the bladder exceeds a critical threshold in the PAG and switches the pathway to maximal activity [82] so exciting the PMC and causing voiding, as described in the first part of the chapter. Thus the PAG, acting via the PMC, is able to control and coordinate voiding in a mechanical, automatic way, so forming control circuit 1 (Fig. 1.10). Circuit 1 does not provide for voluntary control of the lower urinary tract, nor for conscious bladder sensation.

Circuit 2: safety (limbic)

During voiding the organism is vulnerable and so, from an evolutionary perspective, safety is an important issue. Circuit 2 (Fig. 1.16) assesses safety against a background of innate responses and learned experience, preventing voiding if it would not be safe. Safety is concerned with fear (and the derived concept, anxiety), and this primary emotion is available for modification by circuit 3 to form more complex secondary emotions such as urgency, which has a fear component (see Bladder sensation and the concept of "interoception" above).

Primary emotions involve the limbic (emotional) nervous system, whose fundamental regions are the amygdala/parahippocampal complex and hypothalamus [109]. The septal region (Fig. 1.11), in particular the nucleus accumbens, is usually considered to be limbic also; it is close to the head of the caudate nucleus, part of the basal ganglia. These and possibly other regions would be expected to form the basis of any control circuit concerned with safety (Fig. 1.16).

Functional brain imaging shows that, during urine storage in healthy subjects, bladder filling causes increased fMRI activity [88] or changes in the PET signal [110] in a location that probably represents the

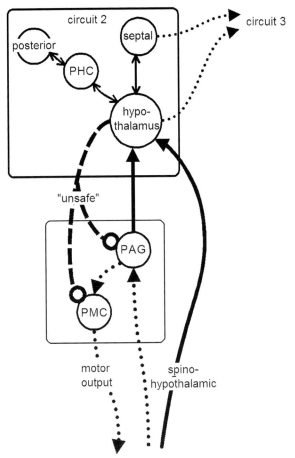

Fig. 1.16. Cerebral control: circuit 2 and circuit 1. Solid lines = principal connections of circuit 2. Dashed lines = descending output from circuit 2. **O**= inhibitory synapse. PHC = parahippocampal complex; posterior = posterior cingulate and (pre)cuneus.

preoptic hypothalamus. Since this region has direct access to the PAG and the PMC [108], it is plausible that, in the unnatural surroundings of the scanner, bladder filling gives rise to an "unsafe" signal from the hypothalamus that inhibits the PMC and PAG (Fig. 1.16), with consequences that are discussed below.

Other imaging evidence for the structure and function of circuit 2 is mainly indirect and dependent on pathological behavior. In women with urge incontinence, for example, responses to bladder filling include a trend to deactivation of the parahippocampal complex and inferior temporal cortex; both are limbic regions expected to belong to circuit 2 (Fig. 1.16). Bladder filling also causes deactivation in the ventromedial prefrontal cortex and nearby pregenual ACC, regions that are strongly connected with

the limbic system [101]. The head of the caudate nucleus (close to the septal region) is also deactivated.

A study of young women with urinary retention and impaired bladder sensation (Fowler's syndrome) has shown highly abnormal responses to bladder filling characterized by widespread deactivations instead of the normal activations (Chapter 19) [111]. Restoration of sensation and voiding ability by treatment with sacral neuromodulation is accompanied by replacement of these deactivations by more normal positive responses, especially in a circuit that includes the parahippocampal gyrus and inferior temporal cortex (extending medially towards the PAG), as well as the caudate nucleus and the posterior cortex (cuneus and precuneus). The inference is that these limbic and related regions form parts of circuit 2.

Circuit 2 apparently receives bladder information from the PAG after preprocessing in circuit 1 and also directly via spinohypothalamic tracts (Fig. 1.16) [82, 108]. The information is provided with emotional content [112] by comparison with innate and learned responses in the parahippocampal region and the (pre)cuneus. If the situation is judged not to be safe, an "unsafe" signal is sent to circuit 1 (Fig. 1.16). Other output, with its emotional content, is sent to circuit 3 to form the basis of the bladder-specific homeostatic and social emotions that underlie the sensations associated with bladder filling: desire to void and urgency [99]. Circuit 2 still makes no provision for voluntary control of voiding. Indeed it can readily override voluntary control. For example, about half of trained subjects are unable to void on command in the scanner [86]. Similarly, many people have difficulty in voiding in public at all, even with adequate bladder filling and desire to void, and in a socially appropriate location, because they unconsciously judge it to be unsafe. Among urge-incontinent subjects, even involuntary detrusor contraction (detrusor overactivity) is difficult to provoke in the scanner [89], presumably because the voiding reflex is suppressed by circuit 2.

Circuit 3: social (cortical/cingulate)

Embarrassment about inappropriate voiding and feelings of shame about incontinence are deeply embedded in human behavior. The neural basis for these social emotions is dependent on cortical and cingulate brain functions (circuit 3 in Fig. 1.17). The function of circuit 3 is to provide bladder filling sensation and its motivational aspect, to assess them in the social

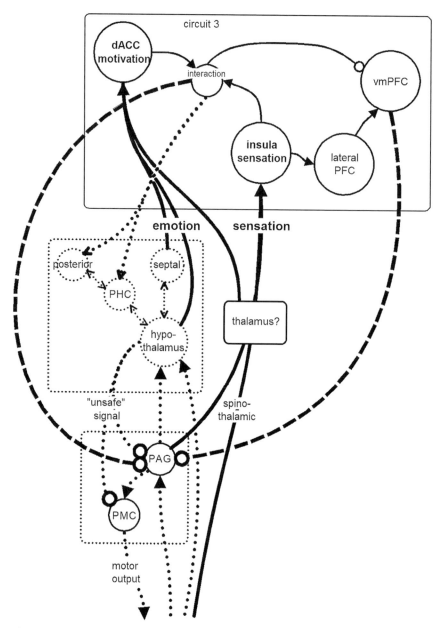

Fig. 1.17. Cerebral control: circuit 3 and circuits 1 and 2. Solid lines = principal connections of circuit 3. Dashed lines = descending output from circuit 3. **O**= inhibitory synapse. PFC = prefrontal cortex; vmPFC = ventromedial prefrontal cortex. The "interaction" region in circuit 3 may be the thalamus, although it is shown separately.

context and to decide whether voluntary voiding is appropriate or not. The final determination of whether voiding actually occurs of course depends also on the results of processing in circuits 1 and 2.

These complicated functions involve the cortical and cingulate brain regions already identified, including insula, dACC and parts of the prefrontal cortex.

The insula and dACC receive bladder information via various pathways, which in the case of the dACC is accompanied by an appropriate emotional response from circuit 2, the basis of the sensation of urgency. Parietal and temporal cortical regions have been identified in some experiments but are omitted from Fig. 1.17.

The afferent pathways shown in Fig. 1.17 follow two main tracks. One track labeled "emotion" and concerned mainly with emotional aspects travels via circuit 2 and culminates in the dACC, which deals with motivation and ultimately motor output. This track is similar to the feed-forward pathway postulated by Phillips et al. [101], which leads from the parahippocampal/amygdala complex to the ventromedial prefrontal cortex and supports automatic regulation of emotion. The other track, labeled "sensation," bypasses circuit 2 and terminates in the insula, concerned principally with strength of sensation. Many different efferent pathways might be taken by the signals from insula and dACC, to many different target regions inside and outside the prefrontal cortex. However, a connectivity analysis [113, 114] has identified a few regions which are effectively connected (via an interaction region) with both the insula and dACC. These target regions include putamen (not shown in Fig. 1.17 but, like the caudate nucleus, part of the basal ganglia), cuneus and hippocampal gyrus (in circuit 2), and PAG and PMC (in circuit 1; presumably PMC is inhibited when sensation and motivation to void increase, so as to maintain continence).

Fig. 1.17 also includes pathways from the cortex and dorsal ACC to the parahippocampal complex, as well as to PAG and PMC (dotted and dashed lines). These may be part of a feedback pathway originating in the lateral prefrontal cortex, which is believed to support voluntary regulation of emotion [101].

The ventromedial PFC and pregenual ACC are deactivated by bladder filling (Fig. 1.15) and are also effectively connected with the insula and dACC (Fig. 1.17).

The effective connection referred to in the previous paragraph implies that if RI and dACC are both strongly activated (e.g. during urgency provoked by bladder filling) then deactivation is reinforced. Correspondingly, deactivation increases with the clinical severity of urge incontinence [115]. A plausible interpretation is that the deactivation of the medial frontal cortex observed in urge-incontinent women represents a reaction aimed at maintaining continence by inhibiting the voiding reflex. Thus this region apparently delivers to the PAG and PMC the output from circuit 3 which, with circuits 1 and 2, determines whether voiding is to occur. When the decision to void is made, inhibition of the voiding reflex by the mPFC is lifted and, if the other circuits concur, voiding takes place.

Conclusion: central control

The model of central control of lower urinary tract function shown in Fig. 1.17 reflects reasonably faithfully the results of functional brain imaging relevant to bladder function. Moreover it has a plausible structure reminiscent of that of many other natural networks: modules (circuits) with dense internal connections are joined to each other by relatively few connector hubs [116]. Nevertheless it has obvious limitations. It is greatly oversimplified: in circuit 1 all spinal reflexes such as those shown in Figs. 1.2–1.5 have been ignored despite their importance in infant development [82] and possibly again in old age; in circuit 3 there are in reality dense bi-directional interconnections between many different regions of the prefrontal cortex which have been omitted from Fig. 1.17. Furthermore, the model is mainly concerned with storage, not voiding. Urethral afferents and efferents are not included; nor are urethral sphincter control regions such as the paracentral lobule or pontine L-region. The basal ganglia and parietal and cerebellar regions are for the most part omitted, although functional imaging and the older observations shown in Fig. 1.11 and described in Chapter 11 show that they are involved in bladder control. Thus details will change as new knowledge accumulates, but this model may provide a starting point for further work, improved understanding and ultimately better treatment of functional bladder disorders.

Acknowledgements

Derek J. Griffiths is greatly indebted to Dr Stasa Tadic and Professor Clare Fowler for stimulating discussions that led to many of the ideas expressed here. Without their help and the help of many colleagues and co-workers in Pittsburgh and London, none of these ideas would have been developed. He gratefully acknowledges support from the University of Pittsburgh Competitive Medical Research Fund and from the US Public Health Service, grants R03AG25166 and R01AG020629.

References

1. Yoshimura N. Bladder afferent pathway and spinal cord injury: possible mechanisms inducing hyperreflexia of the urinary bladder. *Prog Neurobiol* 1999;**57**:583–606.

2. Elbadawi A. Functional pathology of urinary bladder muscularis: the new frontier in diagnostic uropathology. *Semin Diagn Pathol* 1993;**10**:314–54.

3. Carey MP, De Jong S, Friedhuber A, Moran PA, Dwyer PL, Scurry J. A prospective evaluation of the pathogenesis of detrusor instability in women, using electron microscopy and immunohistochemistry. *BJU Int* 2000;**86**:970–6.

4. Abrams P, Andersson KE, Buccafusco JJ, et al. Muscarinic receptors, their distribution and function in body systems, and the implications for treating overactive bladder. *Br J Pharmacol* 2006;**148**:565–78.

5. Harvey RA, Skennerton DE, Newgreen D, Fry C. The contractile potency of adenosine triphosphate and ecto-adenosine triphosphatase activity in guinea pig detrusor and detrusor from patients with a stable, unstable or obstructed bladder. *J Urol* 2002;**168**:1235–9.

6. Tyagi P, Thomas CA, Yoshimura N, Chancellor MB. Investigations into the presence of functional Beta1, Beta2 and Beta3-adrenoceptors in urothelium and detrusor of human bladder. *Int Braz J Urol* 2009;**35**:76–83.

7. Yoshida M, Miyamae K, Iwashita H, Otani M, Inadome A. Management of detrusor dysfunction in the elderly: changes in acetylcholine and adenosine triphosphate release during aging. *Urology* 2004;**63**:17–23.

8. Ferguson DR, Kennedy I, Burton T. ATP is released from rabbit urinary bladder epithelial cells by hydrostatic pressure changes – a possible sensory mechanism? *J Physiol* 1997;**505**:503–11.

9. Mansfield KJ, Chandran JJ, Vaux KJ, et al. Comparison of receptor binding characteristics of commonly used muscarinic antagonists in human bladder detrusor and mucosa. *J Pharmacol Exp Ther* 2009;**328**:893–9.

10. Mansfield KJ, Liu L, Mitchelson FJ, Moore KH, Millard RJ, Burcher E. Muscarinic receptor subtypes in human bladder detrusor and mucosa, studied by radioligand binding and quantitative competitive RT-PCR: changes in ageing. *Br J Pharmacol* 2005;**144**:1089–99.

11. Mukerji G, Yiangou Y, Grogono J, et al. Localization of M2 and M3 muscarinic receptors in human bladder disorders and their clinical correlations. *J Urol* 2006;**176**:367–73.

12. Elneil S, Skepper JN, Kidd EJ, Williamson JG, Ferguson D. Distribution of P2X(1) and P2X(3) receptors in the rat and human urinary bladder. *Pharmacology* 2001;**63**:120–8.

13. Beckel JM, Kanai A, Lee SJ, de Groat WC, Birder LA. Expression of functional nicotinic acetylcholine receptors in rat urinary bladder epithelial cells. *Am J Physiol Renal Physiol* 2006;**290**:F103–10.

14. Andersson KE, Yoshida M. Antimuscarinics and the overactive detrusor–which is the main mechanism of action? *Eur Urol* 2003;**43**:1–5.

15. Chess-Williams R. Muscarinic receptors of the urinary bladder: detrusor, urothelial and prejunctional. *Auton Autacoid Pharmacol* 2002;**22**:133–45.

16. Cockayne DA, Hamilton SG, Zhu Q-M, et al. Urinary bladder hyporeflexia and reduced pain-related behaviour in P2X3-deficient mice. *Nature* 2000;**407**:1011–15.

17. Burnstock G. Purine-mediated signalling in pain and visceral perception. *Trends Pharmacol Sci* 2001;**22**:182–8.

18. Lazzeri M, Vannucchi G, Zardo C, et al. Immunohistochemical evidence of vanilloid receptor 1 in normal human urinary bladder urothelium. *Eur Urol* 2004;**46**:792–9.

19. Apostolidis A, Popat R, Yiangou Y, et al. Decreased sensory receptors P2x3 and Trpv1 in suburothelial nerve fibers following intradetrusor injections of botulinum toxin for human detrusor overactivity. *J Urol* 2005;**174**:977–83.

20. Birder LA, Nakamura Y, Kiss S, et al. Altered urinary bladder function in mice lacking the vanilloid receptor TRPV1. *Nat Neurosci* 2002;**5**:856–60.

21. Peier AM, Moqrich A, Hergarden AC, et al. A TRP channel that senses cold stimuli and menthol. *Cell* 2002;**108**:705–15.

22. Mukerji G, Yiangou Y, Corcoran SL, et al. Cool and menthol receptor TRPM8 in human urinary bladder disorders and clinical correlations. *BMC Urol* 2006;**6**:6.

23. Geirsson G. Evidence of cold receptors in the human bladder: effect of menthol on the bladder cooling reflex. *J Urol* 1993;**150**:427–30.

24. Wakabayashi Y, Tomoyoshi T, Fujimiua M, Arai R, Maeda T. Substance P-containing axon terminals in the mucosa of the human urinary bladder: pre-embedding immunohistochemistry using cryostat sections for electron microscopy. *Histochemistry* 1993;**100**:401–7.

25. Smet PJ, Moore KH, Jonavicius J. Distribution and colocalization of calcitonin gene-related peptide, tachykinins, and vasoactive intestinal peptide in normal and idiopathic unstable human urinary bladder. *Lab Invest* 1997;**77**:37–49.

26. Burbach GJ, Kim KH, Zivony AS, et al. The neurosensory tachykinins substance P and neurokinin A directly induce keratinocyte nerve growth factor. *J Invest Dermatol* 2001;**117**:1075–82.

27. Priestley JV, Michael GJ, Averill S, Liu M, Willmott N. Regulation of nociceptive neurons by nerve growth factor and glial cell line derived neurotrophic factor. *Can J Physiol Pharmacol* 2002;**80**:495–505.

28. Oh EJ, Gover TD, Cordoba-Rodriguez R, Weinreich D. Substance P evokes cation currents through TRP

channels in HEK293 cells. *J Neurophysiol* 2003;**90**:2069–73.

29. Paukert M, Osteroth R, Geisler HS, et al. Inflammatory mediators potentiate ATP-gated channels through the P2X(3) subunit. *J Biol Chem* 2001;**276**:21077–82.

30. Huang H, Wu X, Nicol GD, Meller S, Vasko MR. ATP augments peptide release from rat sensory neurons in culture through activation of P2Y receptors. *J Pharmacol Exp Ther* 2003;**306**:1137–44.

31. Maggi CA, Gepetti P, Santicioli P, Spillantini M, Frilli S, Meli A. The correlation between sensory-efferent functions mediated by the capsaicin-sensitive neurons and substance P content of the urinary bladder of the rat. *Neurosci Lett* 1987;**76**:351–6.

32. Tyagi V, Philips BJ, Su R, et al. Differential expression of functional cannabinoid receptors in human bladder detrusor and urothelium. *J Urol* 2009;**181**:1932–8.

33. Gratzke C, Streng T, Park A, et al. Distribution and function of cannabinoid receptors 1 and 2 in the rat, monkey and human bladder. *J Urol* 2009;**181**:1939–48.

34. Birder LA, de Groat WC. Mechanisms of disease: involvement of the urothelium in bladder dysfunction. *Nat Clin Pract Urol* 2007;**4**:46–54.

35. Wiseman OJ, Fowler CJ, Landon DN. The role of the human bladder lamina propria myofibroblast. *BJU Int* 2003;**91**:89–93.

36. Sui GP, Rothery S, Dupont E, Fry CH, Severs NJ. Gap junctions and connexin expression in human suburothelial interstitial cells. *BJU Int* 2002;**90**:118–29.

37. Sui GP, Wu C, Fry CH. Electrical characteristics of suburothelial cells isolated from the human bladder. *J Urol* 2004;**171**:938–43.

38. Wu C, Sui GP, Fry CH. Purinergic regulation of guinea pig suburothelial myofibroblasts. *J Physiol* 2004;**559**:231–43.

39. Ost D, Roskams T, Van Der Aa F, deRidder D. Topography of the vanilloid receptor in the human bladder: more than just the nerve fibers. *J Urol* 2002;**168**:293–7.

40. de Groat WC, Kawatani M, Hisamitsu T, et al. Mechanisms underlying the recovery of urinary bladder function following spinal cord injury. *J Auton Nerv Syst* 1990;**30**:S71–7.

41. Abrams P, Cardozo L, Fall M, et al. The standardisation of terminology of lower urinary tract function: report from the Standardisation Sub-committee of the International Continence Society. *Neurourol Urodyn* 2002;**21**:167–78.

42. Brady CM, Apostolidis A, Harper M, et al. Parallel changes in bladder suburothelial vanilloid receptor TRPV1 (VR1) and pan-neuronal marker PGP9.5 immunoreactivity in patients with neurogenic detrusor

overactivity (NDO) following intravesical resiniferatoxin treatment. *BJU Int* 2004;**93**:770–6.

43. Brady C, Apostolidis A, Yiangou Y, et al. P2X3-immunoreactive nerve fibres in neurogenic detrusor overactivity and the effect of intravesical resiniferatoxin (RTX). *Eur Urol* 2004;**46**:247–53.

44. Dasgupta P, Chandiramani VA, Beckett A, Scaravilli F, Fowler CJ. The effect of intravesical capsaicin on the suburothelial innervation in patients with detrusor hyper-reflexia. *BJU Int* 2000;**85**:238–45.

45. Oliver S, Fowler CJ, Mundy A, Craggs M. Measuring the sensations of urge and bladder filling during cystometry in urge incontinence and the effects of neuromodulation. *Neurourol Urodyn* 2003;**22**:7–16.

46. Kalsi V, Apostolidis A, Gonzales G, Elneil S, Dasgupta P, Fowler CJ. Early effect on the overactive bladder symptoms following botulinum neurotoxin type A injections for detrusor overactivity. *Eur Urol* 2008;**54**:181–7.

47. Apostolidis A, Brady CM, Yiangou Y, Davis J, Fowler CJ, Anand P. Capsaicin receptor TRPV1 in the urothelium of neurogenic human bladders and the effect of intravesical resiniferatoxin. *Urology* 2005;**65**:400–5.

48. Khera M, Somogyi GT, Kiss S, Boone TB, Smith CP. Botulinum toxin A inhibits ATP release from bladder urothelium after chronic spinal cord injury. *Neurochem Int* 2004;**45**:987–93.

49. Birder LA, Barrick SR, Roppolo JR, et al. Feline interstitial cystitis results in mechanical hypersensitivity and altered ATP release from bladder urothelium. *Am J Physiol Renal Physiol* 2003;**285**: F423–9.

50. Yokoyama O, Yusup A, Miwa Y, Oyama N, Aoki Y, Akino H. Effects of tolterodine on an overactive bladder depend on suppression of C-fiber bladder afferent activity in rats. *J Urol* 2005; **174**:2032–6.

51. De Laet K, De Wachter S, Wyndaele JJ. Systemic oxybutynin decreases afferent activity of the pelvic nerve of the rat: new insights into the working mechanism of antimuscarinics. *Neurourol Urodyn* 2006;**25**:156–61.

52. Tong YC, Chin WT, Cheng JT. Alterations in urinary bladder M2-muscarinic receptor protein and mRNA in 2-week streptozotocin-induced diabetic rats. *Neurosci Lett* 1999;**277**:173–6.

53. Tong YC, Cheng JT. Alteration of M(3) subtype muscarinic receptors in the diabetic rat urinary bladder. *Pharmacology* 2002;**64**:148–51.

54. Mansfield KJ, Liu L, Moore KH, Vaux KJ, Millard RJ, Burcher E. Molecular characterization of M2 and M3 muscarinic receptor expression in bladder from

women with refractory idiopathic detrusor overactivity. *BJU Int* 2007;**99**:1433–8.

55. Datta SN, Roosen A, Popat R, et al. Cholinergic signalling pathways in the superficial layers of the human bladder; comparing health, disease and the effect of botulinum toxin type A. *J Urol* 2009;**181**:676–7.

56. Harrison SC, Hunnam GR, Farman P, Ferguson DR, Doyle PT. Bladder instability and denervation in patients with bladder outflow obstruction. *Br J Urol* 1987;**60**:519–22.

57. Turner WH, Brading AF. Smooth muscle of the bladder in the normal and the diseased state: pathophysiology, diagnosis and treatment. *Pharmacol Ther* 1997;**75**:77–110.

58. Yokoyama O, Nagano K, Kawaguchi K, Hisazumi H. The response of the detrusor muscle to acetylcholine in patients with infravesical obstruction. *Urol Res* 1991;**19**:117–21.

59. Fry CH, Sui GP, Severs NJ, Wu C. Spontaneous activity and electrical coupling in human detrusor smooth muscle: implications for detrusor overactivity? *Urology* 2004;**63**:3–10.

60. Roosen A, Datta SN, Chowdhury RA, et al. Suburothelial myofibroblasts in the human overactive bladder and the effect of botulinum neurotoxin type A treatment. *Eur Urol* 2009;**55**:1440–8.

61. Haferkamp A, Mundhenk J, Bastian PJ, et al. Increased expression of connexin 43 in the overactive neurogenic detrusor. *Eur Urol* 2004;**46**:799–805.

62. Kuijpers KA, Heesakkers JP, Jansen CF, Schalken JA. Cadherin-11 is expressed in detrusor smooth muscle cells and myofibroblasts of normal human bladder. *Eur Urol* 2007;**52**:1213–21.

63. Roosen A, Apostolidis A, Elneil S, et al. Cadherin-11 up-regulation in overactive bladder suburothelial myofibroblasts. *J Urol* 2009;**182**:190–5.

64. Roosen A, Wu C, Sui G, Chowdhury RA, Patel PM, Fry CH. Characteristics of spontaneous activity in the bladder trigone. *Eur Urol* 2009;**56**:346–53.

65. Gillespie JI. The autonomous bladder: a view of the origin of bladder overactivity and sensory urge. *BJU Int* 2004;**93**:478–83.

66. Roppolo JR, Tai C, Booth AM, Buffington CA, de Groat WC, Birder LA. Bladder Adelta afferent nerve activity in normal cats and cats with feline interstitial cystitis. *J Urol* 2005;**173**:1011–5.

67. Sun Y, Keay S, De Deyne PG, Chai TC. Augmented stretch activated adenosine triphosphate release from bladder uroepithelial cells in patients with interstitial cystitis. *J Urol* 2001;**166**:1951–6.

68. Tempest HV, Dixon AK, Turner WH, Elneil S, Sellers LA, Ferguson DR. P2X2 and P2X3 receptor expression in human bladder urothelium and changes in interstitial cystitis. *BJU Int* 2004;**93**:1344–8.

69. Lowe EM, Anand P, Terenghi G, Williams-Chestnut RE, Sinicropi DV, Osborne JL. Increased nerve growth factor levels in the urinary bladder of women with idiopathic sensory urgency and interstitial cystitis. *Br J Urol* 1997;**79**:572–7.

70. Pang X, Marchand J, Sant GR, Kream RM, Theoharides TC. Increased number of substance P positive nerve fibres in interstitial cystitis. *Br J Urol* 1995;**75**:744–50.

71. Parsons CL. Successful downregulation of bladder sensory nerves with combination of heparin and alkalinized lidocaine in patients with interstitial cystitis. *Urology* 2005;**65**:45–8.

72. Dixon JS, Jen PY, Gosling J. The distribution of vesicular acetylcholine transporter in the human male genitourinary organs and its co-localization with neuropeptide Y and nitric oxide synthase. *Neurourol Urodyn* 2000;**19**:185–94.

73. de Groat WC, Kawatani M. Reorganization of sympathetic preganglionic connections in cat bladder ganglia following parasympathetic denervation. *J Physiol* 1989;**409**:431–49.

74. Bors E. Neurogenic bladder. *Urol Surv* 1957;**7**:177–250.

75. Podnar S, Trsinar B, Vodusek DB. Bladder dysfunction in patients with cauda equina lesions. *Neurourol Urodyn* 2006;**25**:23–31.

76. Fowler CJ, Christmas TJ, Chapple CR, Parkhouse HF, Kirby RS, Jacobs HS. Abnormal electromyographic activity of the urethral sphincter, voiding dysfunction, and polycystic ovaries: a new syndrome? *BMJ* 1988;**297**:1436–8.

77. Silva C, Ribeiro MJ, Cruz F. The effect of intravesical resiniferatoxin in patients with idiopathic detrusor instability suggests that involuntary detrusor contractions are triggered by C-fiber input. *J Urol* 2002;**168**:575–9.

78. Leng WW, Chancellor MB. How sacral nerve stimulation neuromodulation works. *Urol Clin North Am* 2005;**32**:11–18.

79. Morrison J, Birder L, Craggs M, et al. Neural control. In: P Abrams, L Cardozo, S Khoury, A Wein, eds. *Incontinence*. Jersey: Health Publications, Ltd; 2005:363–422.

80. de Groat WC. Integrative control of the lower urinary tract: preclinical perspective. *Br J Pharmacol* 2006;**147** (Suppl 2):S25–40.

81. Dasgupta R, Wiseman OJ, Kitchen N, Fowler CJ. Long-term results of sacral neuromodulation for women with urinary retention. *BJU Int* 2004;**94**:335–7.

82. Fowler CJ, Griffiths D, De Groat WC. The neural control of micturition. *Nature Reviews Neuroscience* 2008;**9**:453–66.

83. Blok BF, Holstege G. The neuronal control of micturition and its relation to the emotional motor system. *Prog Brain Res* 1996;**107**:113–26.

84. Torrens M, Feneley RC L. Rehabilitation and management of the neuropathic bladder. In: LS Illis, EM Sedgwick, HJ Glanville, eds. *Rehabilitation of the neurological patient.* Oxford: Blackwell Scientific Publications; 1982.

85. Fukuyama H, Matsuzaki S. Neural control in man examined with single photon emission computer tomography using 99m Tc-HMPAO. *Neuroreport* 1996;**7**:3009–12.

86. Blok BF, Willemsen AT, Holstege G. A PET study on brain control of micturition in humans. *Brain* 1997;**120**:111–21.

87. Griffiths D, Holstege G, Dalm E, de Wall H. Control and coordination of bladder and urethral function in the brainstem of the cat. *Neurourol Urodyn* 1990;**9**:63–82.

88. Griffiths D, Tadic SD. Bladder control, urgency, and urge incontinence: evidence from functional brain imaging. *Neurourol Urodyn* 2008;**27**:466–74.

89. Griffiths D, Derbyshire S, Stenger A, Resnick N. Brain control of normal and overactive bladder. *J Urol* 2005;**174**:1862–7.

90. Craig AD. How do you feel? Interoception: the sense of the physiological condition of the body. *Nat Rev Neurosci* 2002;**3**:655–66.

91. Craig AD. A new view of pain as a homeostatic emotion. *Trends Neurosci* 2003;**26**:303–7.

92. Kuhtz-Buschbeck JP, van der Horst C, Pott C, et al. Cortical representation of the urge to void: a functional magnetic resonance imaging study. *J Urol* 2005;**174**:1477–81.

93. Pfisterer M, Griffiths D, Schaefer W, Resnick N. The effect of age on lower urinary tract function: a study in women. *J Am Geriatr Soc* 2006;**54**:405–12.

94. Kavia RB, Dasgupta R, Fowler CJ. Functional imaging and the central control of the bladder. *J Comp Neurol* 2005;**493**:27–32.

95. Devinsky O, Morrell MJ, Vogt BA. Contributions of anterior cingulate cortex to behavior. *Brain* 1995;**118**:279–306.

96. Critchley HD, Mathias CJ, Josephs O, et al. Human cingulate cortex and autonomic control: converging neuroimaging and clinical evidence. *Brain* 2003;**126**:2139–52.

97. Kuhtz-Buschbeck JP, Gilster R, Van der Horst C, Hamann M, Wolff S, Jansen O. Control of bladder sensations: an fMRI study of brain activity and effective connectivity. *Neuroimage* 2009;**47**:18–27.

98. Abrams P, Blaivas JG, Stanton S, Andersen JT. The standardisation of terminology of lower urinary tract function. *Neurourol Urodyn* 1988;**7**:403–26.

99. Damasio AR. *Looking for Spinoza: joy, sorrow, and the feeling brain.* Orlando, FL: Harcourt, Inc; 2003.

100. Bechara A, Damasio H, Damasio AR. Emotion, decision making and the orbitofrontal cortex. *Cereb Cortex* 2000;**10**:295–307.

101. Phillips ML, Ladouceur CD, Drevets WC. A neural model of voluntary and automatic emotion regulation: implications for understanding the pathophysiology and neurodevelopment of bipolar disorder. *Molecular Psychiatry* 2008;**13**:833–57.

102. Ueki K. Disturbances of micturition observed in some patients with brain tumour. *Neurol Med Chir* 1960;**2**:25–33.

103. Andrew J, Nathan PW. Lesions of the anterior frontal lobes and disturbances of micturition and defaecation. *Brain* 1964;**87**:233–62.

104. Fall M, Geirsson G, Lindstrom S. Toward a new classification of overactive bladders. *Neurourol Urodyn* 1995;**14**:635–46.

105. Shih YI, Chen CV, Shyu B, et al. A new scenario for negative functional magnetic resonance signals: endogenous neurotransmission. *J Neurosci* 2009;**29**:3036–44.

106. Raichle ME, Snyder AZ. A default mode of brain function: a brief history of an evolving idea. *Neuroimage* 2007;**37**:1083–90.

107. Blok BF. Central pathways controlling micturition and urinary continence. *Urology* 2002;**59**:13–7.

108. Holstege G. Micturition and the soul. *J Comp Neurol* 2005;**493**:15–20.

109. LeDoux JE. Emotion circuits in the brain. *Annu Rev Neurosci* 2000;**23**:155–84.

110. Athwal BS, Berkley KJ, Hussain I, et al. Brain responses to changes in bladder volume and urge to void in healthy men. *Brain* 2001;**124**:369–77.

111. Kavia RB, DasGupta R, Critchley HD, Fowler CJ, Griffiths D. An fMRI study of the effect of sacral neuromodulation on brain responses in women with Fowler's Syndrome. *BJU Int* 2010;**105**:366–72.

112. Damasio AR. The somatic marker hypothesis and the possible functions of the prefrontal cortex. *Philos Trans R Soc Lond B Biol Sci* 1996;**351**:1413–20.

113. Tadic SD, Griffiths D, Schaefer W, Resnick NM. Abnormal connections in the supraspinal bladder control network in women with urge urinary incontinence. *Neuroimage* 2008;**39**:1647–53.

114. Griffiths D, Tadic S, Schaefer W, Resnick N. Cerebral control of the lower urinary tract: how age-related changes might predispose to urge incontinence. *Neuroimage* 2009;47:981–6.

115. Tadic SD, Griffiths D, Schaefer W, Cheng CI, Resnick NM. Brain activity measured by functional magnetic resonance imaging is related to patient reported urgency urinary incontinence severity. *J Urol* 2010;183:221–8.

116. Bullmore E, Sporns O. Complex brain networks: graph theoretical analysis of structural and functional systems. *Nat Rev Neurosci* 2009;**10**:186–98.

117. Apostolidis A, Dasgupta P, Fowler CJ. Proposed mechanism for the efficacy of injected botulinum toxin in the treatment of human detrusor overactivity. *Eur Urol* 2006;**49**:644–50.

118. Griffiths D, Tadic SD, Schaefer W, Resnick NM. Cerebral control of the bladder in normal and urge-incontinent women. *Neuroimage* 2007;**37**:1–7.

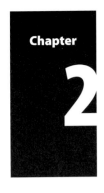

2

Neurological control of the bowel in health and disease

Prateesh M. Trivedi and Derek J. Griffiths

Introduction

There are a number of neurological diseases which have an effect on bowel function. These include spinal cord injury (SCI; worldwide prevalence 2.5 million), spina bifida (1 in 1000 livebirths), multiple sclerosis (MS, greater than 1.3 million), Parkinson's disease (PD, 4 million) and stroke (worldwide incidence 15 million per year). The most common symptoms are constipation, difficulty with evacuation and fecal incontinence. Whilst urological problems have been extensively documented and researched in these groups, very little in comparison is known about the epidemiology and pathophysiology of bowel dysfunction. The underlying mechanisms are unclear due to incomplete knowledge of gastrointestinal (GI) physiology, the role of enteric neural networks and their interplay with the central nervous system.

Improvements in acute medical care and rehabilitation have led to increased survival of these individuals. This has led to an even greater need to investigate the causes of bowel dysfunction secondary to neurological disease.

This chapter will provide an overview of GI physiology, with particular reference to the hindgut and pelvic floor, and in addition will address the problems caused by common neurological diseases.

Neurological control of the bowel in health

Anatomy of the bowel

The intra-abdominal GI tract is structurally varied, and divided into the organs of the stomach, small intestine and large intestine. These organs subserve a functionally distinct role in the digestive process: food

material exits the stomach, enters the small bowel, where it is broken up into smaller compounds, some of which are then absorbed. Material then passes into the large bowel. The first part of the large bowel is the cecum. This is followed, downstream, by the ascending, transverse, descending and sigmoid colons. The GI tract culminates in the rectum and anal canal. The cecum, ascending colon and first half of the transverse colon are referred to as the right, or proximal, colon. The distal half of the transverse colon, the descending colon and the sigmoid colon are referred to as the left, or distal, colon. The main functions of the colon and rectum are to absorb water and salts, degrade short-chain fatty acids and store feces until a socially appropriate opportunity for defecation. Transit from the ileocecal valve to the rectum takes between 12 and 30 hours.

The outer layer of the bowel wall is formed by the longitudinal muscle. Immediately inside and perpendicular to this is the circular muscle layer (Fig. 2.1). The thickness of the two layers varies between different parts of the GI tract and between species. The longitudinal layer is formed into three discrete symmetrical bands called the tenia coli from the cecum to the sigmoid colon. The tenia coli merge at the rectum to form a continuous layer.

The smooth muscle cells are embedded within connective tissue, which also contains glial cells, fibroblasts and the interstitial cells of Cajal (ICCs). They are connected by gap junctions, allowing them to function as a syncitium.

The pelvic floor and anal sphincter complex

The pelvic floor is made of the three parts of levator ani, namely puborectalis, pubococcygeus and ileococcygeus, in addition to the coccygeus. These form the pouch within which the pelvic organs sit (Fig. 2.2).

Pelvic Organ Dysfunction in Neurological Disease: Clinical Management and Rehabilitation, ed. Clare J. Fowler, Jalesh N. Panicker & Anton Emmanuel. Published by Cambridge University Press. © Cambridge University Press 2010.

The internal anal sphincter (IAS) is made up of predominantly slow-twitch, fatigue-resistant smooth muscle which is a continuation of the circular muscle layer of the bowel wall and not under voluntary control (Fig. 2.3). The IAS maintains a constant tone to prevent the leakage of feces [1]. Tonic contraction of the IAS produces 80% of the resting anal pressure [2]. However, when the rectum is constantly distended, the IAS only contributes approximately 60% to resting pressure [1]. IAS closure is maintained by a tonic sympathetic discharge as suggested by sphincter tone reduction in high spinal anesthesia or by infusing the α-adrenergic antagonist phentolamine [3]. The remainder of resting anal pressure is made up with contributions from the external anal sphincter (EAS), the anal mucosal folds and the puborectalis muscle. The IAS is surrounded by a thin muscle called the conjoint longitudinal coat. The functional significance of this coat is unknown.

The EAS is made up of striated muscle derived from the pelvic floor and is partly under voluntary control. Like the striated urethral sphincter (Chapter 1), it is innervated from Onuf's nucleus in the ventral horn of the sacral spinal cord via the pudendal nerves supplied by sacral roots S_2 and S_3 [4]. The predominant excitatory neurotransmitter is acetylcholine working via nicotinic receptors [5]. The EAS provides continence until a convenient time and place for defecation is available. There is additionally a reflex component which maintains continence when intra-abdominal pressure is raised, for example during the Valsalva maneuver. The EAS is one of the few striated muscles which are tonically active; the other in the pelvic floor is puborectalis [6]. The EAS can contribute up to 50% of resting pressure when the rectum is distended [1].

The puborectalis forms a sling around the rectum and is attached anteriorly to the pubic symphysis. It is responsible for maintaining the anorectal angle, and in this way contributes to maintaining continence [7]. It was originally thought that the puborectalis was also innervated by the pudendal nerve, but electrophysiological studies suggest its nerve supply is from the sacral plexus [8].

The intrinsic (enteric) nervous system

The nerve supply to the bowel is complex because the bowel wall contains all the elements necessary for peristalsis via the intrinsic, or enteric, nervous system.

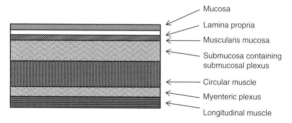

Fig. 2.1. Innervation of the bowel wall. The myenteric (Auerbach's) plexus is a ganglionated plexus between the longitudinal and circular muscle layers. Interior to the circular layer is the submucosa, followed by the very thin muscularis mucosa, then the mucosa. The submucosal (Meissner's) plexus is the second ganglionated plexus, which is situated in the submucosal layer.

Labels for Fig. 2.1:
- Mucosa
- Lamina propria
- Muscularis mucosa
- Submucosa containing submucosal plexus
- Circular muscle
- Myenteric plexus
- Longitudinal muscle

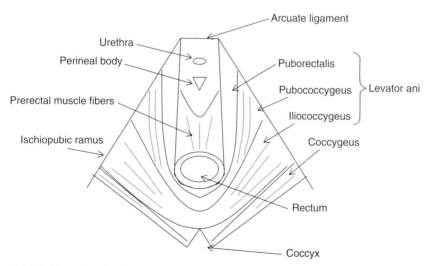

Labels for Fig. 2.2:
- Arcuate ligament
- Urethra
- Perineal body
- Puborectalis
- Pubococcygeus
- Levator ani
- Iliococcygeus
- Prerectal muscle fibers
- Coccygeus
- Ischiopubic ramus
- Rectum
- Coccyx

Fig. 2.2. The male pelvic floor.

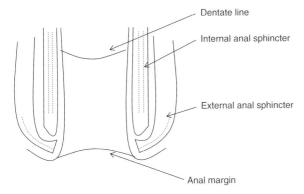

— Dentate line

— Internal anal sphincter

— External anal sphincter

— Anal margin

Fig. 2.3. The anal sphincters.

It is estimated that the intrinsic system contains 80–100 million neurons, a number not dissimilar to estimates of neurons within the entire spinal cord itself [9].

The myenteric and submucosal plexuses

The enteric system is divided into two ganglionated plexuses, namely myenteric and submucosal, with numerous other connections called interneurons. The sites of these two plexuses within the bowel wall are described above.

Myenteric and submucosal neurons have different targets; the myenteric motor neurons innervate the circular and longitudinal layers with additional secretomotor innervation to the mucosal layer. The submucosal neurons tend to be secretomotor especially in the small intestine, but they also innervate the muscularis mucosa and submucosal vessels, in addition to having a sensory component.

Neuropeptides

In addition to the conventional neurotransmitters acetylcholine (ACh) and noradrenaline (NAdr), the neurons of the intrinsic system contain substance P (SP), vasoactive intestinal peptide (VIP), γ-amino butyric acid (GABA), serotonin (5-HT), somatostatin and nitric oxide (NO) [10, 11]. Many are still labeled as putative neurotransmitters or neuropeptides as they have not fulfilled the criteria to be accepted as neurotransmitters.

Peptides are synthesized within the neuronal cell body and are transported via the axon to be stored in synaptic vesicles in the nerve endings. SP, the first gut neuropeptide to be discovered in 1931 [12], is an excitatory neurotransmitter present within the myenteric plexus acting upon cholinergic neurons and directly upon smooth muscle to cause contraction of both circular and longitudinal muscle layers. It increases gut motility, increases blood flow within the gut, binds to pancreatic acinar cells associated with enzyme secretion and inhibits acid secretion and intestinal absorption [13]. VIP stimulates intestinal secretion and relaxes the GI tract. Myenteric VIP neurons project in a caudal manner and may have a role in descending inhibition [13].

Classification of enteric neurons

The enteric neurons can be classified according to their relative roles [10]:

Intrinsic afferents are the sensory pathways of the intrinsic motor and secretomotor reflexes and project to interneurons in both plexuses. They tend to be cholinergic and may contain neuropeptides such as SP.

Interneurons project between the afferent and efferent (motor and secrotomotor) nerves. They are subgrouped according to which neurotransmitters are expressed but their roles remain largely unknown.

Motor neurons may be excitatory or inhibitory. The excitatory neurons project locally or to the circular muscle in a cephalad direction and contain ACh or SP. The inhibitory neurones innervate the circular muscle caudally; they contain VIP and NO.

The extrinsic nervous system

The intrinsic nervous system is modulated by the autonomic nervous system (ANS) and central nervous system (CNS), which comprise the extrinsic system. Sensory fibers travel from the bowel to communicate with the ANS in the spinal cord and higher centers in the brain. The nature of these pathways is still unclear. The ANS is classically divided into the parasympathetic and sympathetic systems (Fig. 2.4).

Parasympathetic innervation

The parasympathetic innervation of the proximal colon is via the vagus nerve (cranial nerve X) which originates in the brainstem and supplies the esophagus through to the splenic flexure of the colon. The remainder of the colon is supplied by parasympathetics arising from the sacral nerve roots $S_2–S_4$, forming the pelvic plexus. The precise point in the colon at which the parasympathetic innervation changes from vagus to pelvic nerves is unclear as some suggest vagal innervation down to the rectum, while others claim pelvic nerves innervate the entire

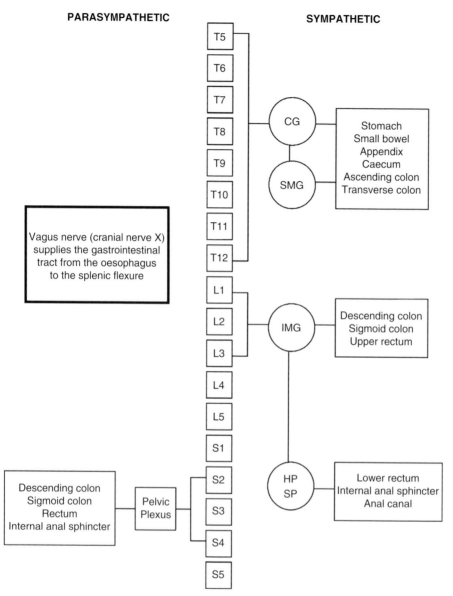

Fig. 2.4. Autonomic innervation of the bowel. Abbreviations: CG = celiac ganglion; SMG = superior mesenteric ganglion; IMG = inferior mesenteric ganglion; HP = hypogastric plexus; SP = sacral plexus.

colon [14, 15]. The IAS is innervated by parasympathetics from the sacral roots.

There are two types of preganglionic axons; one to intramural cholinergic excitatory neurones, and the other to intramural non-adrenergic non-cholinergic inhibitory neurones. The sacral input is mediated by nicotinic cholinergic receptors and is thought to reinforce mass contractions by contraction in both circular and longitudinal layers, but if the cholinergic fibers are blocked using atropine then there is an inability to contract due to muscle cell hyperpolarization. Sphincter relaxation is caused by activation of non-cholinergic non-adrenergic neurons.

In summary, the parasympathetic system is thought to increase contractility and motility of the large bowel and cause relaxation of the IAS.

Sympathetic innervation

The sympathetic supply to the small bowel, ascending colon and transverse colon arises from T_5–T_{12} roots synapsing at the celiac and superior mesenteric ganglia. The left colon and upper rectum are supplied by L_1–L_3 roots synapsing at the inferior mesenteric ganglion. The lower rectum and anal canal are supplied by aortic and lumbar splanchnics via the hypogastric and sacral plexuses. The IAS is innervated by postganglionic fibers from the inferior mesenteric ganglion via the hypogastric nerves. The postganglionic sympathetic nerve endings contain a variety of neuropeptides such as VIP, SP, encephalin and cholecystokinin (CCK).

The sympathetic system is inhibitory to the colon and rectum; by preventing excitatory transmitter release from presynaptics, it reduces blood flow to the colon and slows motility by relaxing the colonic wall to increase compliance [16]. The spinal cord is responsible for tonic inhibition mediated via the sympathetic system. Removal of the spinal cord and lumbar ventral roots in cats leads to a decreased efferent lumbar colonic nerve firing with a parallel increase in colonic motility, suggesting efferent inhibition from T_{12} to L_5 [17]. In contrast to the colon and rectum, the sympathetic effect on the IAS is excitatory; a tonic discharge maintains its closure.

In summary, the sympathetic system slows colonic motility, increases colonic compliance and causes constriction of the IAS.

Gut hormones

In addition to the intrinsic and extrinsic nervous systems, the GI hormones also play a role in colonic motility. For example, CCK is produced by the duodenum in response to fat and protein-rich chyme. Its function is to stimulate the release of digestive enzymes and bile. It delays gastric emptying and inhibits small intestinal motility. Conversely, gastrin, produced in the gastric antrum and duodenum, promotes gastric and intestinal motility, whilst relaxing the pyloric sphincter. SP and VIP have been discussed above.

Colonic activity

The control of colonic activity is autonomous. The rhythmic changes in electrical activity which are observed in smooth muscle cells are called slow waves. These are due to ionic movements regulated by ion channels. If these slow waves reach a certain threshold then an action potential is generated which leads to contraction via activation of L-type calcium channels [18].

The pacemaker cells have been identified as not being smooth muscle cells, but the ICCs [19]. These cells with prominent nuclei were first described by Cajal over 100 years ago [20]. He initially thought they were neurons, but it has subsequently emerged that the fibroblast-like cells are a separate entity. Very little was known about the ICCs until it was discovered that they expressed a c-kit tyrosine kinase receptor. This made it possible to visualize the cells using immunocytochemistry [21]. Gap junctions join ICCs both to each other and to smooth muscle cells. The spontaneous slow waves that are developed are conducted to the smooth muscle cells. The frequency of the slow wave determines the rate of contractions, and both the amplitude of the slow wave and resting membrane potential of the smooth muscle determine the magnitude of contraction. The ionic channel responsible for the pacemaking ability in the ICCs has not been determined. The ICCs are present very early in embryonic development: from 14 weeks' gestation in the proximal small bowel, 23 weeks' in the colon and 34 weeks' in the colon [22].

Colonic motility comprises many factors including myoelectric activity, contractile activity, tone and transit. Colonic contractile activity can be divided into three groups: segmental phasic contractions, low-amplitude phasic contractions (LAPCs) and high-amplitude propagated contractions (HAPCs). Segmental contractions usually occur with a frequency of three cycles per minute and serve to mix stool. LAPCs occur about 100 times daily, typically with pressures less than 50 mmHg (70 cmH$_2$O) and result in organized propulsion of small regions of colon, sending waste material towards the anus. HAPCs occur approximately five times a day with pressures exceeding 100 mmHg, cause propulsion of large volumes of feces and may stimulate defecation [23].

Peristalsis is brought about by contraction of a proximal segment of bowel (contraction of circular muscle and relaxation of longitudinal muscle) with simultaneous relaxation of a more distal segment of bowel (relaxation of circular muscle and contraction of longitudinal muscle) and its function is to move ingested material towards the anus. It can occur in an isolated segment of bowel in vitro. It is predominantly a function of circular muscle. It has been estimated that circular muscle shortening of 17% reduces the luminal cross sectional area by 59% in the presence of tenia coli [24]. Peristalsis occurs in response to circumferential stretch as it is inhibited by longitudinal muscle stretch via nitric oxide release in guinea pigs [25]. It is thought that the longitudinal muscle distally contracts due to ACh release from the myenteric plexus and relaxation of the circular muscle is due to increased discharge from inhibitory interneurons [26]. The evidence for this is found in Hirschsprung's disease (absence of myenteric ganglion cells in the rectum or distal colon), as there is no spasm in an aganglionic section of bowel. There is no reflex relaxation due to a lack of inhibitory interneurons containing VIP and NO; the aganglionic segment thereby causes mechanical bowel obstruction [27].

Specialized aspects of gut motility include various gut reflexes. The gastrocolic response, first described by Hertz and Newton in 1913, occurs when food ingestion stimulates colonic motor activity [28]. This response is most marked in the descending and sigmoid colon and is not triggered by the stomach as it occurs if food bypasses the stomach. It is thought to be mediated by the vagus nerve, enteric reflexes and gut hormones. The enteric system also mediates a colonic-induced peristalsis, which is triggered in response to stretch or distension of the colonic wall. The rectocolic reflex occurs in response to rectal distension and causes colonic peristalsis.

Disturbances of colonic activity can lead to disrupted function. There are tests which can measure varying aspects of colonic activity. For example, myoelectric activity can be measured using electromyography (EMG), tonic and phasic contractile activity using an electromechanical barostat, and transit by utilizing radio-opaque markers or nuclear medicine techniques.

Defecation

The process of defecation depends on a number of steps occurring consecutively and as yet not all of these are well understood. Afferent sensory fibers from mechanoreceptors in the pelvic floor running in the dorsal and anteromedial columns of the spinal cord relay the extent of rectal distension. The central processing remains unclear and some have suggested the existence of a brainstem defecation center [29] analogous to the pontine micturition center (PMC; Chapter 1). There is coordination between the extrinsic and intrinsic nervous systems in order to relax the anal sphincter complex whilst simultaneously

contracting abdominal musculature and initiating peristalsis to evacuate the rectum. This is accompanied by concomitant relaxation of the pelvic floor. The relative contributions of raising abdominal pressure and rectal contraction in order to generate the propulsive force required to defecate are unknown. Defecation is the ultimate effect of the colonic propagating HAPCs. A median of 2.2 HAPCs in the 15 minutes prior to defecation has been reported [30]. There is a cycle of antegrade propulsion which is then followed by retrograde propulsion.

A small amount of straining to initiate defecation is normal. However, excessive straining and use of the Valsalva maneuver impedes evacuation as although rectal contraction is stimulated, the pelvic floor musculature contracts, thereby increasing the resistance to evacuation [31]. Defecation can be postponed if it is inconvenient, by contraction of the EAS, as well as accommodation of the rectum [6].

Cerebral control of bowel function

Despite their elaborate and extensive character, the intrinsic and extrinsic neural control systems described above do not provide for voluntary control, i.e. for conscious decision about when and where to defecate. The decision to defecate depends not only on sensation, the volume of stool in the rectum and perhaps the presence of HAPCs, but on whether the social and environmental circumstances are judged appropriate. Such assessments and decisions are presumably made in the cerebral cortex, the seat of conscious control.

Following earlier animal and clinical studies, in the past decade neuroimaging of the brain-gut axis has shown us how and where the sensations emanating from the gut are modulated and registered in the brain [32, 33]. As in the bladder control system (Figs. 1.2 and 1.10, pp. 2 and 11), afferent signals from the gut travel in the spinal cord to synapse in the midbrain periaqueductal gray (PAG) and the thalamus, passing thence to the insula and the limbic and cortical mechanisms shown in Fig. 2.5; however, there are differences between the neural control of gut and bladder. The enteric nervous system, which is able independently of any central input to propel colonic contents and relax the internal anal sphincter, is unique to the GI tract. Moreover the PAG and Barrington's nucleus (PMC) seem to play a more limited role in defecation than in micturition.

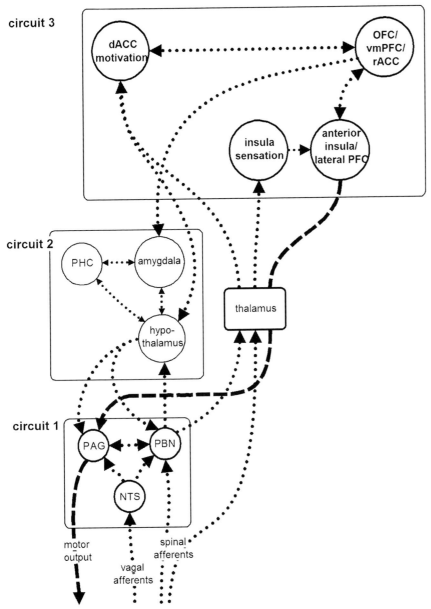

Fig. 2.5. Sketch of some of the brain pathways involved in control of the gut and defecation, based on [32]. Circuit 1: pontine and midbrain; circuit 2: limbic; circuit 3: cortical. Abbreviations: NTS = nucleus tractus solitarius; PAG = periaqueductal gray; PBN = parabrachial nucleus; PHC = parahippocampal cortex; PFC = prefrontal cortex; vmPFC = ventromedial prefrontal cortex; dACC = dorsal anterior cingulated cortex; rACC = rostral anterior cingulate cortex; OFC = orbitofrontal cortex.

Together these observations suggest that the CNS may exert control over the gut less tightly (or at least in a more distributed fashion) than over the bladder. Correspondingly, the gut brain-imaging literature is concerned with sensation rather than control: many experiments have been directed at the modulation of visceral sensations such as pain and urgency by emotional and cognitive stimuli (e.g. attention) [32], but control over defecation has been less well studied.

These visceral sensations depend on afferent signals from the distal gut that travel in lamina 1 of the spinal cord and also on afferents from the proximal gut that travel in the vagal nerve to the medullary nucleus tractus solitarius. The two types of afferents are integrated in the midbrain parabrachial nucleus and pass via the thalamus to the insula. Insula activation has been a consistent feature of nearly all studies that provoked afferent activity by distension of the gut. Conscious perception of the state of the gut is the end result of this visceral input to the insula, together with other inputs from cognitive and emotional circuits. As in the bladder, signals are processed in the prefrontal cortex, and there is some evidence that the lateral prefrontal and orbitofrontal cortices, especially on the right, are concerned with top-down modulation of responses to gut sensations although prefrontal activations are less consistent than for the insula [32]. The nearby rostral (perigenual) anterior cingulate cortex (rACC) also plays an important role. Perhaps these prefrontal regions of the brain may be ultimately responsible for voluntary initiation of defecation. The dorsal anterior cingulate cortex (dACC, responsible for the affective aspects of sensation, including motivation and motor organization) is consistently activated in different studies [32]. Presumably it reflects the urge to defecate, as it does for micturition. Indeed, all these regions are implicated, in rather similar ways, in urinary tract sensation and control (compare Fig. 2.5 with Fig. 1.17, p. 18). It is not clear whether the interconnections between the regions are excitatory or inhibitory and these are therefore not detailed in Fig. 2.5.

The efferent signals descending from the cortex and hypothalamus are responsible for the motor aspects of control of defecation. However, that control seems not to be concentrated in just one or two nuclei (like the PMC in the case of the bladder) but to be exerted through a hierarchical series of reflexes at midbrain, medullary, spinal and peripheral levels. Thus the "center of gravity" of neural control may be more caudal for the gut than for the bladder. Consequently the diagram shown in Fig. 2.5, with its division of CNS control into midbrain/brainstem, limbic and cortical circuits, may offer a helpful classification but is incomplete in principle because it omits the spinal and enteric parts of this complex control system.

The effects of neurological disease on bowel function

Constipation, evacuation difficulties and fecal incontinence

Bowel dysfunction affects approximately 80% of those with SCI and causes more of a problem than urinary

and sexual dysfunction in approximately a third of individuals with SCI [34]. In those with MS, bowel and bladder dysfunction are rated third after spasticity and incoordination [35]. In addition to constipation, difficulty with evacuation and fecal incontinence, other complaints include abdominal pain, hemorrhoids, gastro-esophageal reflux and, in SCI, autonomic dysreflexia [36]. The proportion of SCI persons who suffer constipation varies from 43% to 58% [37]. The modified Rome criteria have been used as a definition of constipation; two or fewer bowel movements a week, or the use of laxatives or an enema at least once a week, or digital evacuation of feces on all occasions [38]. The prevalence of constipation increases with a higher level of SCI. In order for the true prevalence of constipation to be determined it is important to have universally agreed definitions. Evacuation disorders ought to be categorized separately from constipation, as the latter implies a motility problem, whereas the former could be anatomical, physiological or psychological.

Fecal incontinence (FI) is the inability to control when and where to defecate, resulting in individuals soiling themselves. FI tends to be less common than constipation in those with neurological disease, although it is not without considerable psychological morbidity. Being afraid of having FI episodes in public is a common reason for not leaving the home or engaging in daily activities. FI is experienced at least once per year by 75% of those with SCI and daily by 5% [39, 40].

There are limited symptomatology data for bowel dysfunction in other neurological diseases. A study of those with cauda equina lesions reported that 86% had fecal incontinence to varying degrees and 76% had constipation [41]. Approximately a third of MS patients complain of constipation and one quarter suffer from FI once a week [42]. Up to 78% of those with spina bifida have bowel dysfunction, and 53% have frequent episodes of FI. Constipation is the predominant symptom affecting those with PD, with up to 37% complaining of evacuation difficulties [43]. Of those who survive a stroke, 12% complain of fecal incontinence [44].

Abdominal pain

A postal study reported that 34% of SCI individuals had chronic abdominal pain [45]. Furthermore they reported that in 53%, the abdominal pain began five years after the initial injury. This was associated, although not linked causally, with a reduction in defecation frequency. The mechanism of visceral pain in SCI is poorly understood, although there are several theories which include continuous C-fiber discharge caused by altered visceral function, changes in the sympathetic chain and the activation of high-threshold afferent impulses [46, 47].

Bowel dysfunction over time

Studies have suggested that bowel dysfunction deteriorates over time elapsed since SCI [36, 40, 48]. A prospective study reported a significant deterioration over a 10-year period from 1996 to 2006, with those reporting bowel dysfunction increasing from 25% to 38%. This finding is echoed in those with MS [49]. As life expectancy increases, bowel dysfunction is more likely to become a problem.

Bowel dysfunction and autonomic dysreflexia

Autonomic dysreflexia (AD) occurs in persons with SCI when there is uncontrolled sympathetic activation in response to a stimulus. It is thought to be due to a lack of descending neuromodulation (Chapter 15). The most common manifestation of this is high blood pressure causing headache, flushing of skin and sweating. If left untreated the high blood pressure can lead to potentially life-threatening seizures or intracranial bleeds.

The main stimuli for AD are urological and GI. The commonest urological causes are bladder distension (up to 85% of cases), urinary tract infection and instrumentation [50]. GI problems are the second most common stimuli for AD. These include fecal impaction, rectal distension, hemorrhoids and fissure-in-ano [51, 52].

Gut pathophysiology in neurological disease

Gut motility and the gastrocolic reflex

The mean mouth-to-cecum transit time is approximately 55 minutes and the mean colonic transit time has been estimated at 36 hours.

Gastric emptying is not delayed in those with SCI. However, mouth-to-cecum transit time is prolonged in subjects with quadriplegia, but not in those with

tetraplegia [53]. Cisapride is a synthetic benzamide which enhances the release of ACh in the myenteric plexus. It has a prokinetic action which has been shown to increase gastric emptying in patients with dyspepsia [54]. Early enthusiasm for cisapride waned after double-blind trials reported minimal efficacy in SCI [55]. In those with PD, its effects did not last more than six months [56]. Prior to the introduction of cisapride, another prokinetic, metoclopramide, was shown to enhance gastric emptying in those with SCI, but its extrapyramidal side-effects have limited its use.

Colonic transit time can be measured either using radiological techniques or physiological tools. Radiological techniques include ingesting radio-opaque markers followed by serial plain abdominal x-rays, ingesting three distinct markers on successive days followed by a single plain abdominal x-ray and finally ingesting a radio-isotopic compound contained within a capsule to prevent disintegration until it reaches the ileocecal region [57–59]. Physiological methods include deriving a motility index from measuring phasic pressure peaks using manometrical devices [60].

There have been several studies using radiological techniques to measure colonic transit.

Those with supraconal SCI have increased transit times. However there is some debate as to the part of the colon responsible for delayed transit. Some studies have reported a global colonic delay [61, 62], whereas others have found that the majority of the delay is due to abnormal motility in the left colon and rectum [63, 64].

Delayed colonic transit is a feature of many other neurological diseases. A key feature is that the delay is predominantly in the left colon and rectosigmoid. This is the case in lower motor neurone spinal cord injury, such as cauda equina injury, MS, spina bifida and PD [65–69].

Baseline colonic activity in SCI is reduced by way of these subjects having a reduced motility index as well as a reduced wave amplitude, a finding echoed in those with PD [68, 70]. The delay in transit is thought to be mediated via the autonomic nervous system [71]. The explanation in PD is thought to be the presence of Lewy bodies in the myenteric plexus, in addition to the reduction in dopamine-producing cells in the colonic wall [72, 73].

The gastrocolic reflex describes increased colonic motor activity after food ingestion. In SCI, this normal increase in postprandial colonic activity is attenuated, and this attenuation is reversed with

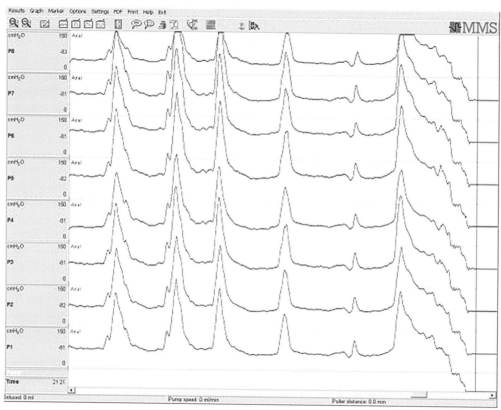

Fig. 2.6. Eight-channel anorectal physiology recording.

neostigmine [34, 71]. Neostigmine is a reversible anticholinesterase inhibitor and indirectly stimulates muscarinic parasympathetic receptors, which serve to augment colonic motor activity and enhance colonic transit. Individuals with MS and spina bifida fail to demonstrate a postprandial increase in colonic myoelectrical activity [69, 74].

Anorectal manometry and dysfunction

Anorectal manometry is typically performed in a GI physiology unit using a water-perfused catheter or solid-state catheter with the subject lying in the left lateral position (Fig. 2.6). The step pull-through technique is usually employed. The measurements recorded are as follows: resting anal pressure (RP), anal squeeze pressure (SQP), cough pressure, whether or not the subject can sustain a squeeze and the recto-anal inhibitory reflex (RAIR).

Tonic contraction of the IAS produces 80% of the RP, and therefore measurement of RP is a marker for the assessment of IAS tone [2]. Some have reported

a reduced RP in supraconal SCI [75–77], whilst others have reported an unchanged RP [1, 65, 78]. RP is also unchanged in both cauda equina syndrome, MS and PD [79, 80], but is reduced in spina bifida [81].

SQP is recorded when the subject is asked to voluntarily squeeze and is a marker of EAS activity and function. Those with complete supraconal SCI do not have a recordable squeeze. SQP is reduced in incomplete supraconal SCI, cauda equina lesions, MS and spina bifida [1, 75, 79, 82–84]. Sustained SQP is reduced in those with PD [80].

Sensation testing is traditionally carried out by inflating a balloon in the rectum. The recorded volumes are first sensation, urge sensation and finally the maximal tolerable volume. Sensation to rectal distension is reduced in those with SCI, cauda equina injury and MS, but is preserved in PD.

Neurological disease may lead to difficulties with evacuation. This problem may be attributed to difficulty in increasing intra-abdominal pressure and anorectal dyssynergia. In healthy individuals, a rise in intra-abdominal pressure leads to a coordinated

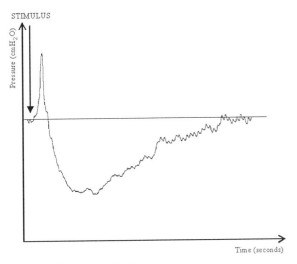

Fig. 2.7. The recto-anal inhibitory reflex.

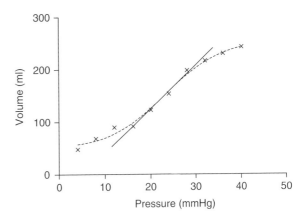

Fig. 2.8. A compliance curve.

contraction of the rectum with simultaneous relaxation of the EAS resulting in defecation. The dyssynergia results from contraction of both muscle groups simultaneously, thereby preventing expulsion of feces.

The recto-anal inhibitory reflex

The RAIR is a transient relaxation of the IAS in response to rectal distension and was first described by Gowers in 1877 (Fig. 2.7) [85]. The reduction in anal pressure is thought to be due to the IAS because studies have shown the RAIR is associated with reduced electrical activity in the IAS but not the EAS [86]. The amplitude of the RAIR depends on the initial anal resting pressure and characteristics of the stimulus [87]. Its function is thought to be to allow sampling of rectal contents in the upper anal canal in order to differentiate between flatus and feces and has been reported to occur up to seven times daily.

The mechanism of the RAIR remains unclear. There are thought to be rectal mucosal receptors which induce it since local anaesthetic applied topically abolishes the reflex [88]. There is indirect evidence to suggest the RAIR pathway is intramural [87] and it has been proposed that nitric oxide may mediate it [4]. This is supported by studies which have shown the RAIR is present in those with SCI [89] and in children with spina bifida [90].

The correlation between an abnormal RAIR and fecal incontinence in otherwise healthy subjects has led some investigators to study its constituent parameters [91]. The amplitude of the RAIR is defined

as the maximal reduction in the resting pressure from baseline ARP. Its amplitude is increased in those with SCI, which suggests that the extrinsic nervous system plays a role in modulating it [92]. There are no differences in the RAIR amplitude in PD [80].

Compliance

Compliance is a measure of how distensible a hollow viscus is and is defined as the change in volume per change in unit pressure ($\Delta V/\Delta P$). It is determined by measuring the pressure–volume (P–V) relationship over a series of pressures using an electromechanical barostat (Fig. 2.8). The P–V relationship is sigmoidal, and compliance is determined by measuring the gradient of the steepest part of the curve. The P–V relationship reflects a combination of passive properties (connective tissue), muscle tone ("static properties") and phasic responses to distension ("dynamic properties"). It is for this reason that it is preferable to calculate compliance from a curve, as opposed to using values at a particular distension threshold. It is unclear whether or not structures extrinsic to the rectum (e.g. bladder, uterus) affect the P–V relationship.

The first proponents of measuring filling pressure of the large bowel were Joltrain et al. in 1919 [93]. The method was rediscovered independently by White et al. in 1940. They reported the first study of the P–V relationship to investigate neurological abnormalities [94]. They called the resulting P–V curve a colonmetrogram. They derived this by filling the rectum with water, and then measuring the pressure.

This study suggested that supraconal SCI was associated with a rapid rise in the volume pressure curve (reduced compliance), whereas lower motor neuron SCI was associated with a flat volume pressure curve (increased compliance).

The traditional view is that those with a supraconal spinal injury have a stiff, hyper-reflexive bowel (reduced compliance), which mirrors the findings on clinical examination of the limbs, with a floppy hyporeflexive bowel in lower motor neuron SCI. Earlier studies of rectal and colonic compliance have reflected this theory. More recent evidence using the electromechanical barostat has shown that both rectal and sigmoid compliance are increased in supraconal SCI [92], with rectal compliance being reduced in lower motor neuron injury [95]. Rectal compliance is also reduced in MS [79] but remains unchanged in PD [68].

The sympathetic nervous system increases bowel compliance and the mechanism in supraconal SCI may be due to uncontrolled sympathetic activity in the absence of supraspinal modulation. A reduction in rectal compliance in lower motor neuron injury and in MS also suggests a loss of extrinsic modulation.

These abnormalities in colorectal compliance may partly explain the symptoms of constipation in supraconal SCI, and fecal incontinence in MS and lower motor neuron SCI.

Dysfunction of CNS control

Neurological diseases such as SCI or MS frequently impair CNS control of the gut. The difference between the neural control systems for bowel and bladder is underlined clinically by the differing effects of such diseases on the two systems.

Supraconal SCI tends to cause difficulty with evacuation of feces in addition to fecal incontinence, but predominantly difficulty with urinary continence. Therefore defecation may require some central stimulus to initiate it, while the voiding reflex in contrast requires tonic suppression in order to maintain urinary continence (see Chapter 1).

Functional bowel disorders, classified as being "non-neurological," are common. Irritable bowel syndrome, for example, is a functional bowel disorder characterized by sensory abnormalities (chronic abdominal pain, discomfort, bloating) and motor abnormalities (alteration of bowel habits) in the

absence of detectable organic cause. Diarrhea or constipation may predominate, or they may alternate. Thus there may be problems with containment as well as evacuation. One influential view is that such disorders may be related to changes in central modulatory circuits shown in Fig. 2.5 rather than to peripheral processes such as inflammation that are traditionally considered important [33]. Thus such problems may be the result of rather subtle neurological changes that have not yet been recognized.

Conclusion

Individuals with neurological disease suffer from bowel dysfunction. The physiological basis of the symptoms has not been clearly established. The literature is incomplete with regards to both the epidemiology and the pathophysiology. The causes are multifactorial, and bowel regimens need to be tailored on an individual basis depending on symptoms and the results of radiology studies and physiology investigations. There is still much work to be done to identify which tests are most useful in predicting the severity of bowel dysfunction and deciding further treatment plans. Further research needs to be done to address these issues in order to ameliorate these significant quality-of-life-impairing symptoms.

References

1. Frenckner B. Function of the anal sphincters in spinal man. *Gut* 1975;**16**:638–44.

2. Schweiger M. Method for determining individual contributions of voluntary and involuntary anal sphincters to resting tone. *Dis Colon Rectum* 1979;**22**:415–16.

3. Frenckner B, Ihre T. Influence of autonomic nerves on the internal and sphincter in man. *Gut* 1976;**17**:306–12.

4. Craggs MD, Balasubramaniam AV, Chung EA, Emmanuel AV. Aberrant reflexes and function of the pelvic organs following spinal cord injury in man. *Auton Neurosci* 2006;**126–127**:355–70.

5. Schroder HD. Onuf's nucleus X: a morphological study of a human spinal nucleus. *Anat Embryol (Berl)* 1981;**162**:443–53.

6. Bharucha AE. Pelvic floor: anatomy and function. *Neurogastroenterol Motil* 2006;**18**:507–19.

7. Parks AG, Porter NH, Hardcastle J. The syndrome of the descending perineum. *Proc R Soc Med* 1966;**59**:477–82.

8. Percy JP, Parks AG. The nerve supply of the pelvic floor. *Schweiz Rundsch Med Prax* 1981;**70**:640–2.

9. Furness JB, Costa M. *The enteric nervous system.* Edinburgh: Churchill Livingstone; 1987.

10. Goyal RK, Hirano I. The enteric nervous system. *N Engl J Med* 1996;**334**:1106–15.

11. Olsson C, Holmgren S. The control of gut motility. *Comp Biochem Physiol A Mol Integr Physiol* 2001;**128**:481–503.

12. Von Euler US, Gaddum JH. An unidentified depressor substance in certain tissue extracts. *J Physiol* 1931;**72**:74–87.

13. Dockray GJ. Physiology of enteric neuropeptides. In: Johnson LR, ed. *Physiology of the gastrointestinal tract.* Second edn. New York: Raven Press; 1987:41–66.

14. Stiens SA, Bergman SB, Goetz LL. Neurogenic bowel dysfunction after spinal cord injury: clinical evaluation and rehabilitative management. *Arch Phys Med Rehabil* 1997;**78**(Suppl 3):S86–102.

15. De Groat WC, Krier J. The sacral parasympathetic reflex pathway regulating colonic motility and defaecation in the cat. *J Physiol* 1978;**276**:481–500.

16. Brading AF, Ramalingam T. Mechanisms controlling normal defecation and the potential effects of spinal cord injury. *Prog Brain Res* 2006;**152**:345–58.

17. De Groat WC, Krier J. The central control of the lumbar sympathetic pathway to the large intestine of the cat. *J Physiol* 1979;**289**:449–68.

18. Tomita T. Electrical activity (spikes and slow waves) in gastrointestinal smooth muscle. In: Bulbring E, Brading AF, Jones AW, Tomita T, eds. *Smooth muscle: an assessment of current knowledge.* London: E. Arnold; 1981.

19. Sanders KM. A case for interstitial cells of Cajal as pacemakers and mediators of neurotransmission in the gastrointestinal tract. *Gastroenterology* 1996;**111**:492–515.

20. Cajal SR. Sur les ganglions et les plexeux nerveux de l'intestin. *CR Soc Biol* 1893;**45**:217–23.

21. Ward SM, Sanders KM. Physiology and pathophysiology of the interstitial cell of Cajal: from bench to bedside. I. Functional development and plasticity of interstitial cells of Cajal networks. *Am J Physiol Gastrointest Liver Physiol* 2001;**281**:G602–11.

22. Hansen MB. Neurohumoral control of gastrointestinal motility. *Physiol Res* 2003;**52**:1–30.

23. Sarna SK. Physiology and pathophysiology of colonic motor activity (1). *Dig Dis Sci* 1991;**36**:827–62.

24. Bharucha AE. Lower gastrointestinal functions. *Neurogastroenterol Motil* 2008;**20**(Suppl 1):103–13.

25. Dickson EJ, Spencer NJ, Hennig GW, et al. An enteric occult reflex underlies accommodation and slow transit in the distal large bowel. *Gastroenterology* 2007;**132**:1912–24.

26. Wood JD. Physiology of the enteric nervous system. In: Johnson LR, ed. *Physiology of the gastrointestinal tract.* Second edn. New York: Raven Press; 1987.

27. Lynch AC, Antony A, Dobbs BR, Frizelle FA. Bowel dysfunction following spinal cord injury. *Spinal Cord* 2001;**39**:193–203.

28. Hertz AF, Newton A. The normal movements of the colon in man. *J Physiol* 1913;**47**:57–65.

29. Weber J, Denis P, Mihout B, et al. Effect of brain-stem lesion on colonic and anorectal motility. Study of three patients. *Dig Dis Sci* 1985;**30**:419–25.

30. Herbst F, Kamm MA, Morris GP, Britton K, Woloszko J, Nicholls RJ. Gastrointestinal transit and prolonged ambulatory colonic motility in health and faecal incontinence. *Gut* 1997;**41**:381–9.

31. Sapsford RR, Hodges PW, Richardson CA, Cooper DH, Markwell SJ, Jull GA. Co-activation of the abdominal and pelvic floor muscles during voluntary exercises. *Neurourol Urodyn* 2001;**20**:31–42.

32. Mayer EA, Naliboff BD, Craig AD. Neuroimaging of the brain-gut axis: from basic understanding to treatment of functional GI disorders. *Gastroenterology* 2006;**131**:1925–42.

33. Birder L, Drake M, De Groat WC, et al. Neural control, committee 3 of incontinence. In: Abrams P, Cardozo L, Khoury S, Wein A, eds. *4th international consultation in incontinence.* Paris: Health Publications Ltd.; 2009:225–53.

34. Glick ME, Meshkinpour H, Haldeman S, Hoehler F, Downey N, Bradley WE. Colonic dysfunction in patients with thoracic spinal cord injury. *Gastroenterology* 1984;**86**:287–94.

35. Bauer HJ, Firnhaber W, Winkler W. Prognostic criteria in multiple sclerosis. *Ann N Y Acad Sci* 1965;**122**:542–51.

36. Stone JM, Nino-Murcia M, Wolfe VA, Perkash I. Chronic gastrointestinal problems in spinal cord injury patients: a prospective analysis. *Am J Gastroenterol* 1990;**85**:1114–19.

37. Ng C, Prott G, Rutkowski S, et al. Gastrointestinal symptoms in spinal cord injury: relationships with level of injury and psychologic factors. *Dis Colon Rectum* 2005;**48**:1562–8.

38. De Looze D, Van Laere M, De Muynck M, Beke R, Elewaut A. Constipation and other chronic gastrointestinal problems in spinal cord injury patients. *Spinal Cord* 1998;**36**:63–6.

39. Glickman S, Kamm MA. Bowel dysfunction in spinal-cord-injury patients. *Lancet* 1996;**347**:1651–3.

40. Krogh K, Nielsen J, Djurhuus JC, Mosdal C, Sabroe S, Laurberg S. Colorectal function in patients with spinal cord lesions. *Dis Colon Rectum* 1997;**40**:1233–9.

41. Podnar S. Bowel dysfunction in patients with cauda equina lesions. *Eur J Neurol* 2006;**13**:1112–17.

42. Hinds JP, Eidelman BH, Wald A. Prevalence of bowel dysfunction in multiple sclerosis. A population survey. *Gastroenterology* 1990;**98**:1538–42.

43. Krogh K, Ostergaard K, Sabroe S, Laurberg S. Clinical aspects of bowel symptoms in Parkinson's disease. *Acta Neurol Scand* 2008;**117**:60–4.

44. Kuptniratsaikul V, Kovindha A, Suethanapornkul S, Manimmanakorn N, Archongka Y. Complications during the rehabilitation period in Thai patients with stroke: a multicenter prospective study. *Am J Phys Med Rehabil* 2009;**88**:92–9.

45. Finnerup NB, Faaborg P, Krogh K, Jensen TS. Abdominal pain in long-term spinal cord injury. *Spinal Cord* 2008;**46**:198–203.

46. Donovan WH, Dimitrijevic MR, Dahm L, Dimitrijevic M. Neurophysiological approaches to chronic pain following spinal cord injury. *Paraplegia* 1982;**20**:135–46.

47. Cervero F, Laird JM. *Visceral pain. Lancet* 1999;**353**:2145–8.

48. Kogos SC, Jr., Richards JS, Banos JH, et al. Visceral pain and life quality in persons with spinal cord injury: a brief report. *J Spinal Cord Med* 2005;**28**:333–7.

49. Munteis E, Andreu M, Tellez MJ, Mon D, Ois A, Roquer J. Anorectal dysfunction in multiple sclerosis. *Mult Scler* 2006;**12**:215–18.

50. Shergill IS, Arya M, Hamid R, Khastgir J, Patel HR, Shah PJ. The importance of autonomic dysreflexia to the urologist. *BJU Int* 2004;**93**:923–6.

51. Widerstrom-Noga E, Cruz-Almeida Y, Krassioukov A. Is there a relationship between chronic pain and autonomic dysreflexia in persons with cervical spinal cord injury? *J Neurotrauma* 2004;**21**:195–204.

52. Lindan R, Joiner E, Freehafer AA, Hazel C. Incidence and clinical features of autonomic dysreflexia in patients with spinal cord injury. *Paraplegia* 1980;**18**:285–92.

53. Rajendran SK, Reiser JR, Bauman W, Zhang RL, Gordon SK, Korsten MA. Gastrointestinal transit after spinal cord injury: effect of cisapride. *Am J Gastroenterol* 1992;**87**:1614–17.

54. Edwards CA, Holden S, Brown C, Read NW. Effect of cisapride on the gastrointestinal transit of a solid meal in normal human subjects. *Gut* 1987;**28**:13–16.

55. Geders JM, Gaing A, Bauman WA, Korsten MA. The effect of cisapride on segmental colonic transit time in patients with spinal cord injury. *Am J Gastroenterol* 1995;**90**:285–9.

56. Jost WH, Schimrigk K. Long-term results with cisapride in Parkinson's disease. *Mov Disord* 1997;**12**:423–5.

57. Metcalf AM, Phillips SF, Zinsmeister AR, MacCarty RL, Beart RW, Wolff BG. Simplified assessment of segmental colonic transit. *Gastroenterology* 1987;**92**:40–7.

58. Arhan P, Devroede G, Jehannin B, et al. Segmental colonic transit time. *Dis Colon Rectum* 1981;**24**:625–9.

59. Proano M, Camilleri M, Phillips SF, Brown ML, Thomforde GM. Transit of solids through the human colon: regional quantification in the unprepared bowel. *Am J Physiol* 1990;**258**(6 Pt 1):G856–62.

60. Bruninga K, Camilleri M. Colonic motility and tone after spinal cord and cauda equina injury. *Am J Gastroenterol* 1997;**92**:891–4.

61. Devroede G, Arhan P, Duguay C, Tetreault L, Akoury H, Perey B. Traumatic constipation. *Gastroenterology* 1979;**77**:1258–67.

62. Keshavarzian A, Barnes WE, Bruninga K, Nemchausky B, Mermall H, Bushnell D. Delayed colonic transit in spinal cord-injured patients measured by indium-111 Amberlite scintigraphy. *Am J Gastroenterol* 1995;**90**:1295–300.

63. Menardo G, Bausano G, Corazziari E, et al. Large-bowel transit in paraplegic patients. *Dis Colon Rectum* 1987;**30**:924–8.

64. Nino-Murcia M, Stone JM, Chang PJ, Perkash I. Colonic transit in spinal cord-injured patients. *Invest Radiol* 1990;**25**:109–12.

65. Beuret-Blanquart F, Weber J, Gouverneur JP, Demangeon S, Denis P. Colonic transit time and anorectal manometric anomalies in 19 patients with complete transection of the spinal cord. *J Auton Nerv Syst* 1990;**30**:199–207.

66. Krogh K, Mosdal C, Laurberg S. Gastrointestinal and segmental colonic transit times in patients with acute and chronic spinal cord lesions. *Spinal Cord* 2000;**38**:615–21.

67. Weber J, Grise P, Roquebert M, et al. Radiopaque markers transit and anorectal manometry in 16 patients with multiple sclerosis and urinary bladder dysfunction. *Dis Colon Rectum* 1987;**30**:95–100.

68. Sakakibara R, Odaka T, Uchiyama T, et al. Colonic transit time and rectoanal videomanometry in Parkinson's disease. *J Neurol Neurosurg Psychiatry* 2003;**74**:268–72.

69. Di Lorenzo C, Benninga MA. Pathophysiology of pediatric fecal incontinence. *Gastroenterology* 2004 Jan;**126**(1 Suppl 1):S33–40.

70. Fajardo NR, Pasiliao RV, Modeste-Duncan R, Creasey G, Bauman WA, Korsten MA. Decreased colonic motility in persons with chronic spinal cord injury. *Am J Gastroenterol* 2003;**98**:128–34.

71. Aaronson MJ, Freed MM, Burakoff R. Colonic myoelectric activity in persons with spinal cord injury. *Dig Dis Sci* 1985;**30**:295–300.

72. Singaram C, Ashraf W, Gaumnitz EA, et al. Dopaminergic defect of enteric nervous system in Parkinson's disease patients with chronic constipation. *Lancet* 1995;**346**:861–4.

73. Kupsky WJ, Grimes MM, Sweeting J, Bertsch R, Cote LJ. Parkinson's disease and megacolon: concentric hyaline inclusions (Lewy bodies) in enteric ganglion cells. *Neurology* 1987;**37**:1253–5.

74. Glick ME, Meshkinpour H, Haldeman S, Bhatia NN, Bradley WE. Colonic dysfunction in multiple sclerosis. *Gastroenterology* 1982;**83**:1002–7.

75. Greving I, Tegenthoff M, Nedjat S, et al. Anorectal functions in patients with spinal cord injury. *Neurogastroenterol Motil* 1998;**10**:509–15.

76. Tjandra JJ, Ooi BS, Han WR. Anorectal physiologic testing for bowel dysfunction in patients with spinal cord lesions. *Dis Colon Rectum* 2000;**43**:927–31.

77. Krogh K, Mosdal C, Gregersen H, Laurberg S. Rectal wall properties in patients with acute and chronic spinal cord lesions. *Dis Colon Rectum* 2002;**45**:641–9.

78. Lynch AC, Anthony A, Dobbs BR, Frizelle FA. Anorectal physiology following spinal cord injury. *Spinal Cord* 2000;**38**:573–80.

79. Nordenbo AM, Andersen JR, Andersen JT. Disturbances of ano-rectal function in multiple sclerosis. *J Neurol* 1996;**243**:445–51.

80. Ashraf W, Pfeiffer RF, Quigley EM. Anorectal manometry in the assessment of anorectal function in Parkinson's disease: a comparison with chronic idiopathic constipation. *Mov Disord* 1994;**9**:655–63.

81. Arhan P, Faverdin C, Devroede G, Pierre-Kahn A, Scott H, Pellerin D. Anorectal motility after surgery for spina bifida. *Dis Colon Rectum* 1984;**27**:159–63.

82. Correa GI, Rotter KP. Clinical evaluation and management of neurogenic bowel after spinal cord injury. *Spinal Cord* 2000;**38**:301–8.

83. Jameson JS, Rogers J, Chia YW, Misiewicz JJ, Henry MM, Swash M. Pelvic floor function in multiple sclerosis. *Gut* 1994;**35**:388–90.

84. Agnarsson U, Warde C, McCarthy G, Clayden GS, Evans N. Anorectal function of children with neurological problems. I: Spina bifida. *Dev Med Child Neurol* 1993;**35**:893–902.

85. Gowers WR. The automatic action of the sphincter ani. *Proc R Soc Lond* 1877;**26**:77–84.

86. Kerremans R. Electrical activity and motility of the internal anal sphincter: an "in vivo" electrophysiological study in man. *Acta Gastroenterol Belg* 1968;**31**:465–82.

87. Penninckx F, Lestar B, Kerremans R. The internal anal sphincter: mechanisms of control and its role in maintaining anal continence. *Baillieres Clin Gastroenterol* 1992;**6**:193–214.

88. Gaston EA. The physiology of fecal continence. *Surg Gynecol Obstet* 1948;**87**:280–90.

89. Denny Brown P, Roberston, E. An investigation of the nervous control of defecation. *Brain* 1935; **58**:256–310.

90. Varma KK, Stephens D. Neuromuscular reflexes of rectal continence. *Aust N Z J Surg* 1972; **41**:263–72.

91. Kaur G, Gardiner A, Duthie GS. Rectoanal reflex parameters in incontinence and constipation. *Dis Colon Rectum* 2002;**45**:928–33.

92. Trivedi PM, Bajwa A, Boulos PB, Craggs MD, Emmanuel AV. Increased sigmoid compliance may explain gut symptoms and response to treatment in supraconal spinal cord injury [abstract]. *Gut* 2009;**58** (Suppl 1):A34.

93. Joltrain E, Baufle P, Coope R. Essai de measure de la pression du gros intestin. *Bull et Mem Soc Med Hop de Paris* 1919;**43**:211–19.

94. White JC, Verlot MG, Ehrentheil O. Neurogenic disturbances of the colon and their investigation by the colonmetrogram: a preliminary report. *Ann Surg* 1940;**112**:1042–57.

95. Trivedi PM, Thoua N, Boulos PB, Craggs MD, Emmanuel AV. Lower motor neurone spinal cord injury reduces rectal compliance whilst preserving sigmoid compliance [abstract]. *Gut* 2009; **58**(Suppl 1):A35.

Neurological control of sexual function in health and disease

Clare J. Fowler, Jalesh N. Panicker and Rajesh B. C. Kavia

Introduction

The neurology of human sexual responses is poorly understood, not only because it is a highly complex process involving much of the nervous system, but also because in comparison to the extent to which research has been carried out in experimental animals, humans have been relatively little studied. Whereas in animals the central and peripheral nervous system control of penile erection and copulatory behavior have been intensively examined, our knowledge about human function and the brain is based mainly on a synthesis of observations of reported abnormalities resulting from disease [1]. Now, however, functional brain imaging data have begun to complement those data.

Homology between primates and rodents has been shown for many aspects of sexual responses but there remains much that is unknown about the more complex human processes, especially the neurological determinants of sexual desire.

After defining the various phases of the human sexual cycle, this chapter outlines the roles of the subcortical and cortical regions, spinal connections and peripheral innervation involved in those phases, with reference to the experimental animal literature and mention of the dysfunctions that can result from neurological disease at each level. Findings from recent functional imaging experiments are discussed in the context of the role of the cortical regions in human neurological control of sexual function.

Phases of the human sexual cycle

Scientific rigor was brought to the study of human sexual function when 40 years ago the different phases of the response cycle were defined by Masters and Johnson. Based on observations under laboratory conditions of over 300 couples, they identified four discrete phases of the human sexual response as arousal (excitement), plateau, orgasm and satisfaction [2]. This sequence was subsequently modified to include the phase of sexual drive: Kaplan proposed a triphasic response model, each phase with a distinct underlying neurophysiological basis (Fig. 3.1) [3]. This has since proved a valuable framework for the scientific study of human sexual behavior although the premise that sexual responses progress only in sequence has since been revised.

It is now acknowledged that phases overlap and that the sequence can vary, particularly in women. The frequency with which surveyed women reported "low sexual desire" led Basson to rethink the relationship between desire and sexual activity in women [4]. Basson observed that many women frequently begin a sexual experience for intimacy-based reasons in a sexually neutral state, finding or receiving sexual stimuli then move her to a state of arousal, and she then develops the desire to continue the experience. This means than many women do not experience desire ahead of sexual experience although some do, particularly those in new relationships who may be driven by sexual hunger as in the traditional male model. This has had important implications for the pharmaceutical industry when considering treatment for female "hypoactive sexual desire disorder" [5].

Physiology of sexual functions

Libido is defined as the biological need for sexual activity (sex drive) and depends upon hypothalamic and temporal lobe functioning. Although little is known about the physiological basis of libido, previous sexual activity, psychosocial background, brain

Pelvic Organ Dysfunction in Neurological Disease: Clinical Management and Rehabilitation, ed. Clare J. Fowler, Jalesh N. Panicker & Anton Emmanuel. Published by Cambridge University Press. © Cambridge University Press 2010.

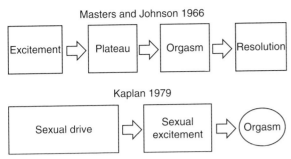

Fig. 3.1. Phases of human sexual response according to Masters and Johnson and subsequently revised by Kaplan.

and brainstem dopaminergic receptor activation, and gonadal hormones are believed to be involved in its regulation.

Male sexual responses

Penile erection depends on a complex interaction of psychological, neural, vascular and endocrine factors. The penis is innervated by somatic and autonomic nerves which travel in the pudendal and cavernosal nerves respectively. The pudendal nerve conveys penile sensations and is responsible for contraction and relaxation of the striated ischiocavernosus and bulbospongiosus muscles. The cavernosal nerves are derived from both the sympathetic and parasympathetic system and innervate the corpora cavernosa, corpus spongiosum and glans penis, regulating blood flow during erection and detumescence. The two main vasodilator neurotransmitters involved in erection are nitric oxide (NO) and cyclic guanosine monophosphate (cGMP). During erection, relaxation of the trabecular smooth muscle of the corpora cavernosa results in vasodilatation of the arterioles with a several-fold increase in blood flow and expansion of the sinusoidal spaces. The outflow of blood is minimized by compression of the subtunical venular plexus against the tunica albuginea and compression of emissary veins by the stretched tunica. This combination of factors increasing penile blood supply results in its lengthening and enlargement.

It is now well established that there are two separate pathways for erection, a reflexive and a psychogenic erection mechanism [6, 7]. Reflex erections resulting from genital stimulation are mediated by sacral segmental pathways and are short-lived and inadequate for penetration. These are preserved in men with suprasacral spinal lesions. Psychogenic erections occur in response to perceived erotic stimuli

and are mediated by the thoracolumbar sympathetic outflow. Psychogenic erections may be preserved in men with lumbar cord lesions below the level of the sympathetic outflow, although only if there has not been additional damage to the sacral segments of the cord or the sacral roots. In men with intact spinal cords these two types of erectile responses fuse to produce an adequate erection for penetration and one that can be maintained throughout intercourse. Neural pathways involved in night-time erections have not yet been fully elucidated, but to achieve nocturnal erections of normal quality, the preservation of thoracolumbar and sacral neural control is required, as well as partially intact spinal connections to higher brain centers responsible for arousal [8].

Ejaculation has two phases: emission and true ejaculation. The emission phase (i.e. deposition of seminal fluid into the posterior urethra) is under control of the sympathetic nervous system, while the ejaculatory phase (expulsion of the seminal fluid from the posterior urethra through the penile meatus) is under control of a spinal reflex at the level of the spinal nerves S_2–S_4 mediated via the pudendal nerve.

Orgasm is controlled by the autonomic nervous system and involves smooth muscle contraction of the accessory sexual organs, contraction of the urethral bulb and perineum, rhythmic contractions of the pelvic floor muscles, semen emission and ejaculation. This is accompanied by a sudden release of endorphins generating a feeling of euphoria. It is possible for men to have orgasm without erection and/or ejaculation, and to ejaculate without reaching orgasm.

Detumesence is the result of sympathetic discharge during ejaculation, cessation of neurotransmitter release or breakdown of second messengers by phosphodiesterases. Contraction of the trabecular smooth muscle reopens the venous channels and expels the trapped blood, resulting in the penis becoming flaccid.

Female sexual response

The female sexual response cycle follows a similar pattern as in men. The homologous response to erection in women is increased vaginal blood flow [9] and vaginal lubrication [10]. These receptive responses are initiated by neurotransmitter-mediated smooth muscle relaxation involving substances such as vasoactive intestinal polypeptide (VIP) and NO, resulting in increased pelvic blood flow, transudative vaginal lubrication, and clitoral and labial engorgement.

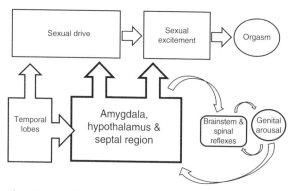

Fig. 3.2. Neural input to the human sexual response cycle.

Subcortical and cortical inputs

Fig. 3.2 summarizes the role of various neural inputs in the human sexual response cycle based on the Kaplan model.

Evidence from animal experiments

Animal experimental data and limited clinical observations together point to a complex of forebrain structures comprised of the amygdala and nuclei within the hypothalamus as having a central role in determining sexual drive. Using stimulation and ablation techniques, regions of the hypothalamus, specifically the medial preoptic area (MPOA) and the paraventricular nucleus (PVN) were shown to effect penile erection and copulatory behavior in several species of monkey [11–13] and rats [14]. Indeed, the male rat model of penile physiology has contributed in a major way to knowledge of the peripheral and central mechanisms controlling erectile function [15].

In the rat, the paraventricular nucleus was found to be one of the most sensitive brain areas for the pro-erectile effect of oxytocin [15] and neurons from there project to the hippocampus, medulla oblongata and the lumbosacral region of the spinal cord (Fig. 3.2). Synaptic connections have been demonstrated between the PVN and the hypogastric, pelvic and corporeal nerves [16]. It is thought that when cells in the PVN are excited, primarily by oxytocin (although a number of other neurotransmitters are also active at this site [15]), they also release oxytocin and induce penile erection.

A hypothalamic lesion involving in the MPOA severely attenuates or abolishes male copulatory behavior in all species assessed [17]. In the rat the

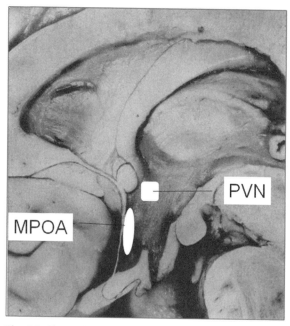

Fig. 3.3. The medial preoptic area (MPOA) and paraventricular nucleus (PVN) drawn on a diagram of the human hypothalamic region originally created by Andrew and Nathan [24], used with permission.

MPOA contains a high density of neurons which concentrate gonadal androgens and is widely connected with the PVN, limbic system and brainstem [18]. The MPOA is thought to coordinate autonomic events associated with sexual responses [19] and it has been proposed that in both genders in the rat, the MPOA is involved in mate selection [20]. Animal lesions of the medial amygdala in rats had no effect on erections during copulation but facilitated reflexive erections and depressed "non-contact" erections [21].

A nucleus in the rat rostra medulla, the nucleus paragigantocellularis (nPGi), has been found to be inhibitory for erection [22]. Serotonergic projections from this region reach the lumbosacral cord and serotonin applied to the spinal cord has been shown to inhibit sexual reflexes.

Human data

In man the PVN contains large neurosecretory cells which secrete vasopressin and oxytocin. It is situated in the medial region of the hypothalamus in the wall of the third ventricle and projects both to the posterior pituitary (the neurohypophysis), extrahypothalamic brain areas and the spinal cord (Fig. 3.3) [23].

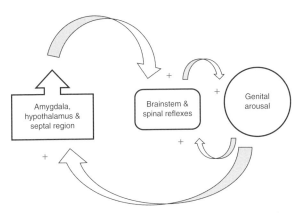

Fig. 3.4. Forebrain activation of spinal reflexes results in genital arousal. Genital afferents enhance the spinal reflex responses and also modulate forebrain activity, creating a positive feedback loop. The inhibitory connections from the nucleus paragigantocellularis (nPGi) to the spinal cord are not shown.

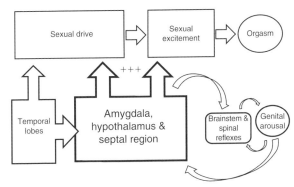

Fig. 3.5. The effect of "irritant" hypothalamic or septal lesions on sexual drive.

Current evidence suggests there is not a single "erection center" in the hypothalamus [19] but rather a series of densely interrelated pathways between the MPOA and PVN in the hypothalamus, the medial amygdala, the periaqueductal gray (PAG) of the midbrain and nPGi in the rostral medulla [25], the concerted action of which modifies spinal sexual reflexes resulting in genital arousal. All these regions have been shown to contain neurons whose activity is modulated by pelvic sensory input [25], so that it has been proposed that these nuclei which modify the spinal sexual reflexes are in turn modulated by genital sensory input in a positive feedback fashion (Fig. 3.4). However, these regions are also known to be implicated in the control of a variety of other homeostatic functions and motivated behaviors [26].

Evidence in man from the "lesion literature," reviewed in Chapter 11, supports the view that there is some homology between the rat and human neural organization of sexual function. Pathology which has an "irritant" effect in the hypothalamic or "septal region" (see Table 11.3, p. 169) has been described as resulting in a marked increase in sexual drive (Fig. 3.5). Conversely, damage in this area has resulted in instances of loss of libido. When psychosurgical procedures were used to treat patients with addictions including "sexual deviations," stereotactic hypothalamotomy seemed to help them regain their self-control and reduce sexual drive [27].

Following the observation of the facilitatory effect of dopamine on sexual behavior in man, the effect of dopamine agonists was studied in rodents. Apomorphine injected into the PVN in rats induced penile erection [28] and further studies showed this effect was mediated by D2 receptors on the cell bodies of oxytocinergic neurons. The MPOA and PVN are known to receive projections from the nigral dopaminergic neurons. The role of these receptors in the hypersexuality which may be a feature of the dopamine dysregulation syndrome in patients with Parkinson's disease who have been treated with long-term dopamine agonists or l-dopa (Chapter 12) has yet to be elucidated, although an excessive stimulation of D3 receptors at these sites has been implicated [29].

Although the nature and exact site of pathology in Kleine-Levin syndrome is not known, several of the episodic features, which include hypersomnia, megaphagia and hypersexuality principally in men, suggest hypothalamic involvement [30].

Neuroendocrine effects

An experimental neuroscientist Beach, some 40 years ago, wrote a highly influential paper on the central nervous system control of male copulatory behavior in animals and put forward a series of postulates [31]. These have since been intensely scrutinized but largely upheld [32], [25]. Amongst his postulates, Beach proposed that gonadal hormones have relatively little or no direct effect on spinal cord or lower brainstem centers but exert an effect by modifying cerebral control of lower reflexive mechanisms. Exceptions to this postulate have been identified since and sex hormone receptors have been found in the brainstem and spinal cord [32], although activation at these sites appears to affect sexual performance rather than sex drive in animals [33].

43

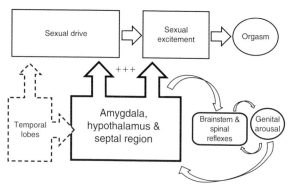

Fig. 3.6. Loss of the regulating effect of the temporal lobes results in the clinically observed "altered sexuality" together with other behavioral changes seen in humans with the Kluver-Bucy syndrome.

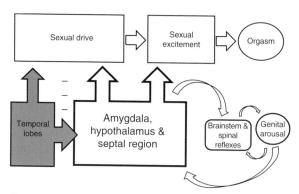

Fig. 3.7. A proposed mechanism for hyposexuality in TLE. In some cases sexuality can be normalized or increased following temporal lobectomy.

Neurons within the midbrain, hypothalamus, and amygdala have been shown in rats to contain receptors for gonadal hormones and it is thought that it is by activation of receptors at these levels that hormones regulate sexual behavior and motivation [25]. Similar findings have been shown in man, and the amygdala in particular is linked to regions of the hypothalamus that are involved in the regulation, production and secretion of gonadal steroids [34].

Temporal lobes and amygdala

The importance of the temporal lobes in regulating sexual function in primates was recognized by Kluver and Bucy who demonstrated that bilateral temporal lobectomy including the uncus, amygdala and hippocampus in rhesus monkeys produced a constellation of symptoms including hypersexuality [35], a condition which became known as the Kluver-Bucy syndrome (KBS) (Fig. 3.6). Less than full-blown cases have been described in clinical medicine in patients with bilateral temporal lobe disease following neurosurgery [36], trauma, encephalitis, or neurodegenerative diseases [37, 38] (Chapter 11). Not all the features of KBS seen in the monkey have been described in these cases although all the patients showed very profound behavioral changes. However, the occurrence of their "altered sexuality" supports the notion of the integral role of the temporal lobes in the regulation of human sexual behavior.

The precise structure within the temporal lobe which is responsible for the syndrome has not been delineated but based on animal studies it was suggested that the amygdala is critical, although as Baird points out, bilateral amygdala lesions in humans do not consistently produce hypersexuality [1].

The role of the amygdala in human sexuality appears significant although much about this remains to be discovered. It is relevant to acknowledge here Swanson's observation that the amygdala "is neither a structural nor a functional unit; instead, it is a collection of adjacent cell groups in the medial temporal lobe that was defined on gross anatomic terms" [39]. The work of Baird and her colleagues showed that amygdala volume on the contralateral side of a temporal lobectomy was a key determinant for increased postoperative sexual drive. It was proposed that the mechanism for this was either amygdalo-hypothalamic connections' control over the endocrine substrates of sexual behavior or that the amygdala has a crucial role in processing potentially significant sexual stimuli [40]. Either way, patients in whom sexual drive increased following temporal lobectomy did not show the inappropriate or indiscriminate sexual behaviors which have characterized patients with KBS but rather simply an increase in "normal" sexual drive [40].

Interictal hyposexuality in patients with temporal lobe epilepsy was a phenomenon first observed by Gastaut and Collomb in 1954 [41]. They noticed hyposexuality in several hundred institutionalized patients with psychomotor seizures and characterized the disorder in 26 out of 36 patients studied in detail. These patients had a "profound disinterest in all the usual libidinous aspects of life" with the onset of their global hyposexuality developing 2–4 years after the onset of seizures. Gastaut hypothesized that "due to the effect of an irritative lesion, the rhinencephalon of the epileptic was in a state of excitation" having a sustained tonic inhibitory effect on the diencephalon (Fig. 3.7). The pioneering neurosurgeon Earl Walker, in a tribute lecture, described the enhancing effect on

Table 3.1. Changes in human sexual behavior which have been described in association with TLE

Interictal	Ictal	Postictal
Hyposexuality/asexuality	Orgasmic aura	Postictal sexual arousal
Less commonly hypersexuality	Genital automatisms	
Paraphilias	Sexual automatisms	
paedophilia	simulated intercourse	
fetishisms	exhibitionism	
	masturbation	

sexual behavior of the successful removal of temporal lobe foci in some patients and posed the rhetorical question "where is the seat of lust?" continuing "obviously not in the tissue removed, but in the parts released from control of the second and inferior temporal gyri and the medial temporal structures – uncus, amygdale and rostral hippocampus" [42]. The explanation he proposed was that the structures he had removed had had an inhibitory effect on the septum and hypothalmus and removal of these regions may have caused a hypersensitivity of the deafferented nuclei (Fig. 3.7).

The complex role of the temporal lobes in mediating human sexual response is evident from the various effects that can characterize disease of this region, and are commonly associated with epilepsy. The changes that have been observed are summarized in Table 3.1 and some details of clinical cases with features of these various disorders are given in Chapter 11.

Some authors have pointed to the fact that there appears to be an asymmetry in the contribution made by the left and right hemispheres to sexual drive. In a review of the literature it was found that a significantly higher number of patients with hyposexuality were found to have a left hemisphere lesion whereas those with hypersexuality had a right hemisphere lesion, leading to the conclusion that the normal right hemisphere probably inhibits libido and the normal left hemisphere probably enhances it [43]. Orgasmic epileptic auras have been shown to result almost exclusively from ictal foci in the right hemisphere, most commonly from within the right mesiotemporal region [44].

A study of the relationship between sexual dysfunction, epilepsy laterality and reproductive hormone levels in women found that sexual dysfunction was significantly more common in women with right-sided epileptiform discharges than in controls and was inversely correlated with bioactive testosterone levels [45]. Further investigation of the neuroendocrine disorders that occur in TLE has suggested distinct abnormalities of biochemical and reproductive profiles are associated with left and right foci respectively [46].

Frontal lobes

Baird et al. [1] make the distinction between true hypersexuality and disinhibition. It is the latter that characterizes frontal lobe damage with a loss of social inhibition of sexual activity, particularly lesions affecting the orbitofrontal region of the limbic system [1]. Observations on the effect of frontal lobotomy are given in Chapter 11.

Sexual motor behaviors with pelvic and truncal movements are a form of "genital automatism" and appear to be peculiar to frontal lobe epilepsy [47]. In many species, but particularly well studied in the cat, copulatory behaviors can be induced by stimulation of the PAG [48]. A speculative hypothesis is that in health, the frontal regions exert a tonic inhibitory function over motor patterns which exist in structures such as the PAG, and paroxysmal loss of this allows expression of primitive behaviors.

Parietal

For the last 60 years the cortical representation of the penis has been illustrated by the sensory homunculus drawn by Penfield and Rasmussen [49], which shows the organization of the primary sensory cortex along the postcentral gyrus. This map was based on observations made during surgery when the cortex was

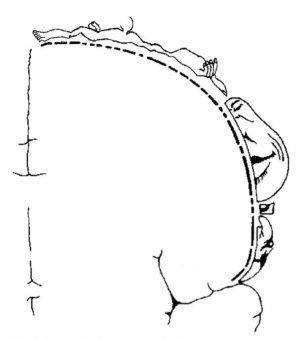

Fig. 3.8. A modified version of Penfield and Rasmussen's sensory homunculus. From [52], with permission.

know that Penfield was in the audience because it was recorded that he contributed to the discussion. It must be for this reason that the male genitalia have appeared on the mesial surface of the parietal lobe beneath the toes for so many years.

Although the canonical sensory homunculus has been reproduced in textbooks ever since, the position of genital representation was questioned [51]. Recently the situation has been clarified by a functional neuroimaging experiment [52]. In healthy male volunteers, activation to light touch on the left side of parts of the penis without any sexual content to the stimulus was seen to result in activation of in the medial edge of the convexity of the contralateral post-central gyrus. The region of activation lay lateral to that of the toe representation and the lower abdominal wall. No indication of a penile representation was found in the mesial wall (Fig. 3.8). Bilateral activation clusters were also found in the opercular secondary somatosensory cortices.

The few clinical cases that have been reported with parietal lesions causing genital symptoms, either ictal or non-ictal, are described in Chapter 11.

Representation of the penis on the primary sensory cortex would be the expected neurological substrate for exteroceptive stimuli, and that somatosensory evoked potentials can be readily recorded with surface electrodes from this region in response to electrical stimulation of the dorsal nerve of the penis [53] or clitoris [54] is consistent with that observation. However, genital sensations associated with sexual arousal presumably have a different neurological basis. Since in animal studies pelvic sensory input has been shown to modulate activity in many of the forebrain structures which have a critical role in controlling sexual function, genital afferent stimulation is thought to have a positive feedback effect on the structures which in turn further excite spinal reflexes [25] (Fig. 3.4). Sensations perceived as erotic are presumably the result or part of that process and are interpreted by the interoceptive sensory system, a hypothesis which emerging evidence from functional brain imaging experiments supports.

directly stimulated and the awake patient asked to report what they sensed. The authors comment that reported genital sensations were "rare" and in fact found only one man out of 400 subjects, who reported sensation on the contralateral side of his penis in response to stimulation of a region adjacent to areas which had produced sensation in the upper leg and buttock. Although the homunculus when drawn showed the male genitalia on the mesial surface of the parietal lobe beneath the toes, the authors do express some uncertainty; "while data do not permit exact location of the representation of the genitalia in the cortex," they go on to say "the clinical evidence already available suggests the area in question is the general region of the paracentral lobule" [49], citing Erickson [50]. Erickson had presented, at a meeting in Chicago in 1944, the case of a woman with a hemangioma at the upper end of the Rolandic sulcus between the medial surface of the hemisphere and the falx, who had been troubled by episodic intense vaginal sensations and also "passionate feelings" and stated that "the sensory representation of the genitalia has been demonstrated in monkeys to lie in the paracentral lobule at the upper lip of the callosomarginal sulcus" and so explained his patient's symptoms. We

Functional brain imaging of sexual activity

Functional brain imaging is already providing a better understanding of the neural basis of human sexual function and it is a technique which has enormous potential in this area. Although animal experiments have provided a wealth of data on the forebrain and spinal neural pathways involved in sexual function (and the limited evidence from observations in human disease appears to confirm a legitimate homology), such studies cannot provide subjective insight. Functional brain imaging offers the opportunity for the subjective and emotional aspects of human sexual activity to be explored, and work to date promises an interesting future for such research.

Compared to the state of knowledge about functional brain imaging and bladder control and the relatively simple processes determining bladder sensation on filling and the decision and process of voiding as outlined in Chapter 1, the same framework of thinking has yet to be formulated in relation to the much more complex behaviors of sexual function. So far, publications have related mostly to sexual excitation with lesser attention to the neurology of sexual desire and orgasm.

Imaging of sexual desire

The experimental difficulties of defining sexual desire and correlating brain imaging mean that this has proved to be a difficult area to study. Mouras et al. used subjective ratings of sexual desire in normal men and showed that regions in the parietal lobe, the right parieto-occipital sulcus, the left superior occipital gyrus and the precentral gyri were activated when the response to viewing sexual video clips was compared to that of watching sports clips [55] but no correlation between sexual desire and change in activity in a specific region was made.

Middle-aged men showed no activation of the hypothalamus and thalamus in response to erotic visual stimuli, possibly accounting for the lower levels of arousal in the older subjects [56]. In two hypogonadal patients, brain activation in response to erotic film clips was decreased compared to that of healthy controls, but was improved by testosterone supplementation [57].

Women have been investigated by looking at the brain response evoked by erotic films at different stages of their menstrual cycle [58, 59]. Both studies showed that activation is different between the ovulatory and menstrual phases, providing neurological evidence for the ovulatory cycle's modulation of the processing of sexual arousal in the female human brain.

A comparison between women with hyposexual desire and controls suggested differences between the groups in encoding arousing stimuli, retrieval of past erotic experiences, or both [60]. The women with hyposexual desire disorder appeared to allocate significantly more attention to monitoring and/or evaluating their responses than controls, and it was suggested that this might interfere with their sexual response.

Activation in limbic, temporal association areas and the parietal lobe was approximately 8% greater on average in premenopausal women than in menopausal women and postmenopausal women. Signal enhancement was maximized in the genu of the corpus callosum and superior frontal gyrus [61].

Imaging of sexual excitement

Table 3.2 lists the functional studies that have been performed evaluating sexual excitement. The table includes the imaging modality that was used, the nature of the subjects and the modality of stimulation. Stimulation took the form of either erotic still photographs or video clips, sometimes with additional sound, and a few studies used genital stimulation. One study used only women's perfume. The degree of resulting sexual arousal has mostly been assessed by subject rating, although in some experiments more objective measures of penile erection were employed.

Fig. 3.9 summarizes the regions of activation that were reported during sexual excitation from the publications listed in Table 3.2. The image was created using MRIcro [62] which allows placement of a 1 cm diameter circle where published coordinates with the highest "z" scores were given. The figure therefore illustrates the distribution of regions of activation rather than the intensity.

Fig. 3.9 shows that regions of activity included prefrontal, orbitofrontal cortex, insula, anterior cingulate gyrus, occipitotemporal area, parietal lobes, amygdala, hypothalamus, thalamus, claustrum, putamen and caudate. The observed activation of the amygdala and hypothalamus is in keeping with the established role of these structures in the male erectile response and furthermore, the magnitude of hypothalamic activation was positively correlated with reported levels of sexual arousal [65], [72] in men.

Table 3.2. Functional imaging studies evaluating sexual excitement

Author	Date of publication	Imaging modality	Subjects	Modality of stimulation used
Redoute et al. [63]	2000	PET	9 heterosexual males	Visual stimulation Sexual video clips of graded intensity Control clips – neutral and humorous
Arnow et al. [64]	2002	fMRI	14 heterosexual males	Visual stimulation Sexual video clip Control video clips – relaxing and sports
Karama et al. [65]	2002	fMRI	20 heterosexual males 20 heterosexual females	Visual stimulation Erotic video clips Control – emotionally neutral
Mouras et al. [55]	2003	fMRI	8 heterosexual males	Visual stimulation Sexual photographs Control – emotionally neutral
Holstege et al. [66]	2003	PET	11 heterosexual males	Tactile penile stimulation by sexual partner Control – rest
Hamann [67]	2005	fMRI	14 heterosexual males 14 heterosexual females	Visual stimuli Sexual photographs Controls – non-sexual couple photographs
Georgiadis et al. [68]	2005	PET	11 heterosexual males	Tactile penile stimulation by sexual partner Control – rest Re-analysis of [66] data
Moulier et al. [69]	2006	fMRI	10 heterosexual males	Visual stimuli Sexual – nude photographs Controls – non-sexual dressed women
Kim et al. [56]	2006	fMRI	10 heterosexual males	Visual stimuli Erotic film clip Control – sports/relaxing video clip
Georgiadis et al. [70]	2006	PET	12 heterosexual females	Tactile stimulation Clitoral stimulation by sexual partner Control – rest
Huh et al. [71]	2008	fMRI	8 heterosexual males	Olfactory stimulation Sexual stimulation – women's perfume Control – rest
Georgiadis [72]	2009	PET	11 heterosexual males 12 heterosexual females	Reanalysis of 2003, 2005 and 2006 data

In general, hypothalamic activation was found to be significantly greater in male than female subjects. Connections between the thalamus, insula, anterior cingulate gyrus and orbitofrontal cortex form a network important for processing interoceptive stimuli [73] (Chapter 1) so that activations of these regions would be expected with genital arousal, generating a combination of interoceptive and exteroceptive sensations. Greater activation in the parietal lobe was seen in women compared with men, possibly reflecting stimulation of the vestibulo-vaginal region rather than only the glans of the clitoris but the greater

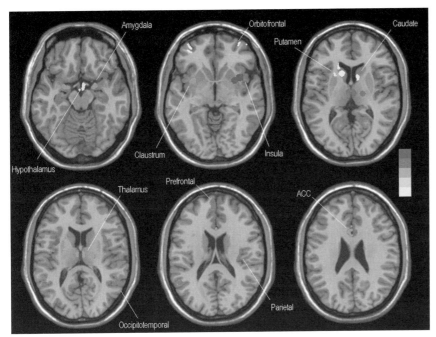

Fig. 3.9. Summary of patterns of brain activity with sexual stimulation (visual, olfactory, auditory or tactile). Dark red seen in 8, light red in 7, orange in 5, dark yellow in 4 and light yellow in 3 out of 13 published reports (listed in Table 3.2). See text for further explanation. See plate section for color version.

activation of the claustrum and occipitotemporal regions in men is thought to be due to the male methods of processing visual imagery rather than perception of penile sensation [72].

Imaging of orgasm

PET studies of orgasm in both sexes were carried out at Groningen and the data sets from 11 men and 12 women comprehensively analysed and compared [66, 70, 74, 72]. Whereas notable differences between men and women were found during tactile genital stimulation (see above), the differences between men and women during orgasm were relatively minor and completely different from the pattern of activation of genital stimulation (Fig. 3.10). In both gender groups, orgasm was characterized by marked deactivation in the prefrontal cortex and left temporal lobe and activation of the anterior lobe of the cerebellum and pontine regions. Stronger activation of the PAG was found in men than women, and in women there was stronger activation of the right posterior insula compared with men, although this latter finding was the result of deactivation in the male group.

The interpretation of deactivation is controversial but arithmetically it means there is less activity during the event, in this case orgasm, than during the contrast phase, in this case genital stimulation (deactivation should not be confused with inhibition). The prominent deactivation of the prefrontal cortex seen in both women and men at orgasm has been attributed to release from behavioral inhibition and a carefree state of mind [72]. The pontine and anterior cerebellar activation seen may relate to cardiovascular arousal.

In the original presentation of the data in men, much was made of the activation seen in the ventral tegmental area (VTA) of the mesencephalon [66]. This region contains dopaminergic cells, and is an area known to play a crucial role in rewarding behaviors including the orgasm-like rush heroin addicts experience when injecting. It was proposed that the VTA might represent the anatomical substrate for the strongly reinforcing nature of sexual activity in humans – "it would be critical for reproduction of the species to favour ejaculation as a most rewarding behavior" [66]. Although reanalysis of the data showed that much of the originally observed activation was

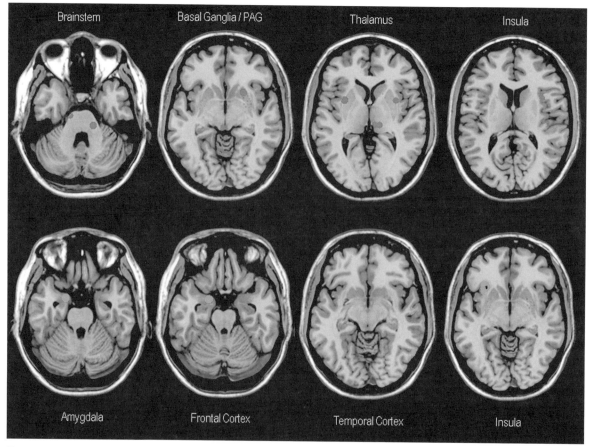

Fig. 3.10. Brain activations (red) and deactivations (blue) seen with orgasm in 16 males and females. Summary figures created using MNI coordinates from three datasets [68, 70, 75]. Figure created using MRIcro. See plate section for color version.

artefactual, some activation was still apparent in the left transition zone of the midbrain and thalamus related to ejaculation [74], perhaps permitting Holstege's eloquent explanation of the powerful hedonic properties of orgasm to survive.

Imaging of the resolution stage

A single study so far has investigated the resolution stage following ejaculation in men [76]. Using fMRI for 30 minutes beginning three minutes after ejaculation, the amygdala, temporal lobes and septal areas were maximally active just after ejaculation. The amygdala and temporal lobe remained active for 20 minutes, whilst the septal regions were activated for 15 minutes post-ejaculation. It was suggested that the amygdala and temporal lobe activity account for the post-ejaculatory refractory period in men.

Brainstem and spinal cord

The first of Beach's four proposals was that reflexive mechanisms for sexual function involve highly complex patterns of activation and the coordination of activity is largely organized in the spinal cord [31]. Because sexual function is so severely affected by spinal cord damage in humans, this may surprise those principally acquainted with clinical medicine, but the evidence from experimental animals clearly demonstrates that erection and ejaculation are preserved following spinal cord transection [77].

Central pattern generators in the spinal cord coordinate the output of the parasympathetic, sympathetic and somatic innervation of the genital region for erection and ejaculation in males and arousal responses in the female, and reduce blood flow to extragenital regions as well as inhibit activity of the bladder and bowel in response to genital stimulation.

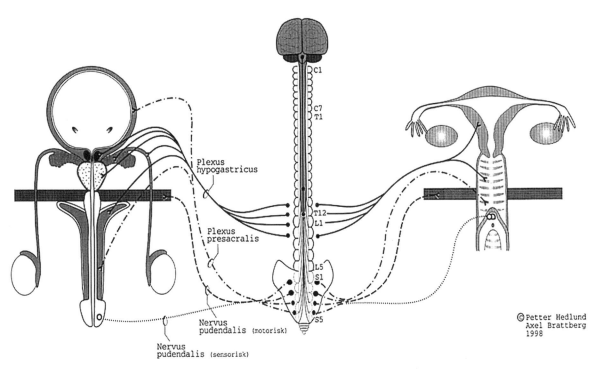

Fig. 3.11. Innervation of the genitalia in men and women illustrates the spinal levels of origin of the parasympathetic (S_2–S_4) and sympathetic (T_{11}–L_2).

In the spinally intact animal, the stimuli to activate or enhance these complex patterns of response come not only from genital afferents but also from higher centers including the hypothalamic nuclei, mesial amygdala and PAG of the midbrain. It appears that there is a positive feedback loop with genital stimulation increasing the spinal responses and the central drive which in turn increases the conditions of the genitals to be more responsive (Fig. 3.4). It is presumably because of a greater dependence on the interaction between central activity and spinal reflexes in humans compared to other species that spinal deficits have such a deleterious effect on their sexual function. That an erectile response may occur in only a few neurologically intact men in response to tactile penile stimulation whilst solving arithmetical problems, but is much enhanced during erotic fantasizing, illustrates the role of human forebrain structures in providing the central drive for erection [78].

The lumbosacral segments of the spinal cord are the site of coordination of many genital afferent-mediated pelvic and sexual responses. Afferent activity enters the cord through the sacral roots in the pudendal and pelvic nerves and the thoracolumbar region via the hypogastric nerves (Fig. 3.11). The simplest demonstrable reflex is the bulbocavernosus reflex whereby a transient stimulation of the glans of the penis results in a contraction of the perineal striated muscles, the bulbocavernosus muscle and also the anal and urethral sphincters – all responses which can be clinically detected or recorded electrophysiologically (Chapter 10). The bulbocavernosus reflex is an oligosynaptic response with a pudendal nerve-mediated input and output and few spinal interneurons [79].

Sustained stimulation of the penis, the glans in particular, results in penile erection, and a homologous process occurs in women following stimulation of the clitoris. The reflex for this process is preserved in men with complete spinal cord transection at levels above T9 [80], although the erection is usually not adequate for penetration, and likewise vasocongestion responses in spinal cord injured women [81] (Chapter 15). The afferent limb for this response is from genital afferents conveyed in all three innervating systems, with penile erection being mediated by the parasympathetic outflow, principally S_2 in man [82]. Little is known about the spinal interneurons which are involved in these reflexes but animal studies to date have suggested these are in the central region of the lumbosacral cord [25]. The pharmacology of spinal cord control of sexual responses is highly complex [33] but it seems likely there is considerable functional redundancy [15].

In men who have sustained injury to the lower lumbar spine without extensive damage to the sacral roots (an uncommon scenario), psychogenic erections may be more readily induced than erection following genital stimulation [83]. This is evidence for a sympathetically mediated pathway, although Brindley points to evidence that the parasympathetic innervation can also mediate psychogenic erections [78]. In women following spinal cord injury, vasoactively mediated genital congestion and vaginal lubrication (a nitric oxide mediated response) are preserved or lost in a pattern comparable to that seen in men [81]. Following damage above the lower thoracic region, reflex responses to genital stimulation are preserved and women with incomplete spinal cord injury who are able to perceive pinprick in the T_{12}–L_2 segment may retain the ability for psychogenic genital vasocongestion [81].

In spinal health, reflex and psychogenic responses in men fuse to produce an erection adequate for penetration and leading on to ejaculation and in women receptive responses, culminating in orgasm. The duplication in these systems seems likely to be the result of evolutionary forces creating safety factors for preserving the means of reproduction.

In the non-sexually aroused state in health, higher centers are largely inhibitory and an important pathway has been demonstrated from the nPGi in the brainstem. This has serotonergic neurons which project to the spinal cord and spinal centers, mediating tonic descending inhibition of sexual reflexes, probably by a direct serotoninergic pathway [22]. The demonstrated inhibitory effect of serotonin may explain the observed negative effects of antidepressant serotonin reuptake inhibitors on sexual activity.

Ejaculation can be elicited in many species of spinalized animals [31] and an "ejaculator generator" has been demonstrated in the rat lumbar spinal segments, L_3 and L_4. The neurons are activated by ejaculation but not other components of male sexual behavior and have projections which extend to the posterior thalamus [84]. The spinal ejaculation generator coordinates sympathetic, parasympathetic and motor outflow to induce the two phases of ejaculation, emission and expulsion in the rat. The generator is

under the influence of supraspinal sites in the brainstem, hypothalamus and preoptic area and sensory information related to ejaculation is processed in the spinal cord and brain [85].

In humans these processes require coordinated sympathetic and parasympathetic activity to close the bladder neck and induce contractions in the ductus deferens and expulsion of semen into the urethra. Rhythmic contractions of the striated perineal muscles, innervated by the pudendal nerves, results in expulsion of semen. The striated muscle contractions have been shown to occur at the same time as the pleasurable sensation of orgasm [86]. Few men with a spinal cord lesion can ejaculate but a strong vibratory stimulus can be applied to the glans penis to obtain semen (see Chapter 15). The vibration acts by stimulating spinal reflexes whereas Brindley deduced that transrectal "electroejaculation" worked by direct stimulation of the preganglionic sympathetic innervation in front of the bifurcation of the aorta and between the rectum and the obturator nerve [87].

In a study which used physiological measurements and written accounts of sensations to record orgasm, 44% of women with spinal cord injuries were able to achieve orgasm in the laboratory setting although the time to do so was much longer than in control, able-bodied women [81]. It has been suggested that the preserved vaginal–cervical "awareness" is provided by vagal innervation which provides a "spinal cord bypass" [75].

In the rat, ejaculation-related signals from pelvic organs are relayed in spinothalamic pathways [85]. The evidence from men who have undergone bilateral anterolateral cordotomies for relief of pain is that "erotically coloured" sensations are conveyed in the spinothalamic tracts since they lose the orgasmic sensations which formerly accompanied ejaculation [88] and patients with selective damage to these tracts may complain of anorgasmia and ejaculatory failure [89]. Loss of orgasmic capacity in women with MS commonly occurs as a consequence of spinal cord involvement (Chapter 14) and is the sexual dysfunction for which they most commonly seek medical treatment [90].

Although there has been research focusing on the rewarding properties of ejaculation in the rat, many questions remain [85]. In the PET study of ejaculation in man, activation was seen in the VTA of the mesencephalon, a finding that survived a reanalysis of the data [74]. The VTA contains dopaminergic

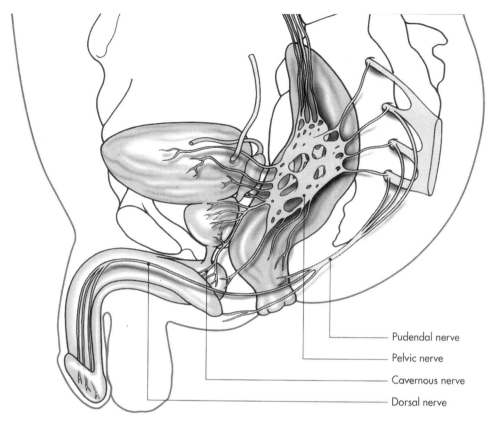

Fig. 3.12. Penile innervation by pelvic (cavernosal) and pudendal (dorsal) nerves. Reproduced from Carson et al. (1999) [103].

cells, and is an area known to play a crucial role in rewarding behaviors. It was proposed that the VTA might represent the anatomical substrate for the strongly reinforcing nature of sexual activity in humans [66].

Peripheral innervation

In both genders the innervation of pelvic organs is derived from the superior hypogastric plexus. This is situated anterior to the aortic bifurcation at the level of the fifth lumbar vertebral body and sacral promontory between the common iliac arteries. Caudally it divides into the right and left hypogastric nerves which are major conduits of sympathetic innervation into the pelvis. These pass down into the inferior hypogastric plexus, also known as the pelvic plexus, where they are joined by the pelvic nerves, the major source of parasympathetic innervation. The pelvic plexus lies lateral to the rectum, seminal vesicle, prostate and posterior part of the urinary bladder in men (Fig. 3.12) and in the pararectal space in close

approximation to the cervix and posterior bladder in women (Fig. 3.14).

Male genital innervation

The main penile parasympathetic innervation originates from the S_2–S_4 spinal segments and passes through the pelvic plexus to form the cavernosal nerves which enter the base of the penis in the midline and innervate erectile tissue (Fig. 3.12). These nerves also contain sympathetic fibers.

It is at the apex of the prostate that the cavernosal nerves are at risk of damage when the prostatic capsule is removed as part of a radical prostatectomy (see Chapter 18). Because these nerves mainly subserve erectile function rather than somatic penile sensation, this explains why neurogenic erectile failure can occur following surgery which damages the cavernosal nerves while penile sensation remains intact. Furthermore this explains why neurophysiological tests which were mostly based on eliciting responses in the large diameter myelinated somatosensory fibers

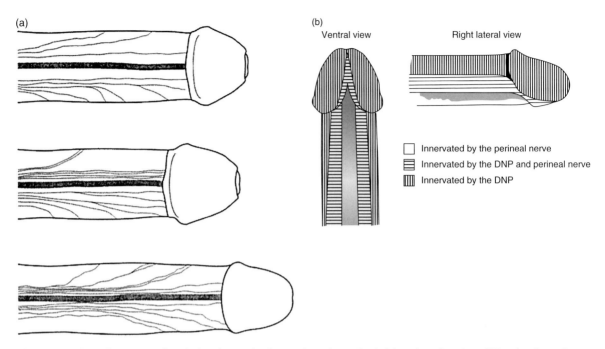

Fig. 3.13. **A** shows the patterns of penile dorsal nerve distribution along the penile shaft based on dissection of 22 cadaveric specimens. The deep dorsal vein is shaded [92]. **B** shows the sensory distribution of the dorsal nerve of the penis. The hatched area on the ventrolateral aspect of the penis represents the transition zone where pinprick sensation was appreciated but dulled compared to the ventral aspect. This area is innervated by the dorsal nerve of the penis and the perineal nerve. The area not anesthetized is innervated solely by the perineal nerve. From [92] and [93] with permission.

of the pudendal nerve correlated poorly with erectile dysfunction (Chapter 10) [91].

The somatic innervation of the genitalia, which is predominately sensory, is conveyed in the pudendal nerves. These bilaterally originating nerves arise from the S_3–S_4 sacral segments and form as branches off the sacral plexus. In the male the pudendal nerve gives off a number of branches in the pelvis (Fig. 3.12). It divides into two terminal branches – the perineal nerve, and the dorsal nerve of the penis (males) or the dorsal nerve of the clitoris (females). The dorsal nerve of the penis enters the base of the penis in the midline, on either side of the dorsal vein. The axons of the dorsal penile nerve have been shown to segregate into two populations: one with a constant course along the dorsal midline (after branching in the glans) and the other with a variable arcade of branches along the shaft of penis (Fig. 3.13A). The right and left dorsal nerves were in close proximity to each other in the dorsal midline but no symmetry was observed between sides and no nerves crossed the midline. The fibers had an undulating configuration which allows for the distensibility

necessary to accommodate the 40 per cent elongation that occurs with erection [92].

By injecting local anesthetic in the pudendal nerves of healthy volunteers, Yang and Bradley established that the dorsal nerve is the sole innervator of the glans and dorsal shaft of the penis. The ventral surface is innervated by perineal nerve (Fig. 3.13B). [93].

The glans has a high receptor density; up to 80–90% of the nerve endings are free, in the most superficial layer of mucosa. There are also corpuscular-type endings beneath the mucosal layer. The receptors are of two types: slowly adapting distally and rapidly adapting proximally, with afferents C and Aδ-fibers [94]. Surrounding the cavernous bodies are large nerve endings which resemble onions, with thick lamellae and a central nerve fiber connected to thick, myelinated nerve fibers. These nerve endings respond to deep pressure and vigorous movement. Receptors close to the cavernous bodies are influenced by the amount of engorgement of cavernous tissues so that touch may thus be experienced as just touch or as sexual stimuli depending upon the degree of engorgement.

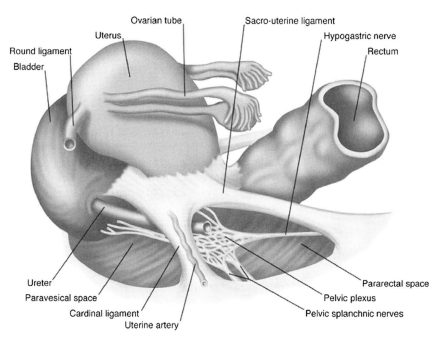

Fig. 3.14. The female pelvic organs showing the nerves that are vulnerable to damage during radical hysterectomy. From [95], with permission.

Female genital innervation

The pelvic plexus in women lies in the pararectal space where it receives sympathetic fibers via the hypogastric nerve and gives rise to the cavernosal nerves which pass anteriorly to innervate the clitoris (Fig. 3.14). These structures can be damaged by radical pelvic surgery for cervical, bladder or rectal tumors resulting in female sexual dysfunction [95] (Chapter 18).

Comparatively, the innervation of the clitoris has been much less researched than that of the male counterpart. Indeed the constituent parts of the clitoris have only recently been defined, the anatomy of the clitoris being deemed a topic of lesser noteworthiness according to many standard textbooks – but much twentieth century controversy [96]! O'Connell et al. suggested that the term "clitoris" be used to describe the cluster of erectile tissue responsible for female orgasm. This has five definite components, the paired bulbs, paired corpora (which are continuous with the cura) which form the body, and the glans, although the distal vagina and distal urethra may also have a contributory role [96]. The glans is the only external manifestation of the clitoris, the other components being deep to the labial

fat. The components exist in a three-dimensional configuration, a factor which has contributed to the poor documentation of the clitoris, its anatomy being difficult to display and illustrate [97]. Although illuminating three-dimensional reconstructions of the fetal clitoris have been published [98], at this point in time the best illustrations of healthy, premenopausal female genitalia are probably those that were obtained by unenhanced MRI and shown in Figs. 3.15 and 3.16. The axial section (Fig. 3.15) shows the structures parallel to the ischiopubic rami but a sagittal view (Fig. 3.16) is required to show the clitoral body, crura and glans, which project into the fat of the mons.

The ultrastructure of the female corporeal bodies is similar to that of the penis. The glans clitoris forms a cap on top of the distal end of the narrowed corporeal bodies [98].

The cavernous nerves originate from the vaginal plexus of the pelvic plexus and travel along the anterior vaginal wall. Although their distribution in the human fetus [100] and the mouse [101] have been explored, this has been difficult to define in adult cadaveric specimens [96].

The pudendal nerves bifurcate into perineal and clitoral divisions, the former to innervate the sphincter

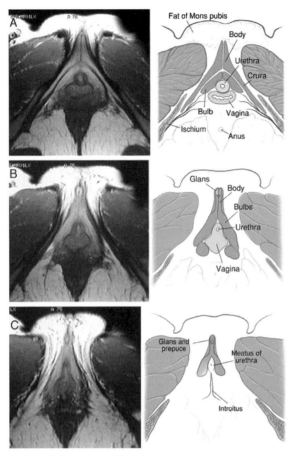

Fig. 3.15. The clitoris and its components including bulbs, crura, and corpora demonstrated in axial plane MRI [99]. **A:** Cluster formed by bulbs, crura, and corpora and forming a complex with the urethra and vagina. **B:** Clitoral glans ventral to the remainder of the clitoris. **C:** Most caudal section. Reproduced with permission.

in the perineal triangle. The somatic nerve supply to the glans clitoris is from the dorsal clitoral nerves which ascend along the ischiopubic rami to meet each other and travel along the superior surface of the clitoral body passing largely undivided into the glans. These nerves are at least 2 mm in diameter and are "impressive" even in infancy [98]. Although there has been speculation as to the density of innervation of the glans – "such a small structure which such abundant innervation" [96] – there does not appear to have been a recent formal study of this. The threshold for perception of vibration on the glans clitoris is extremely low, of the order of 2–3 microns [102].

Conclusion

Significant progress has been made over the last 10 years in understanding the neurology of human sexual function. This has been due to a number of factors, including the recognition that sexual function is an important determinant of quality of life and the advent of effective therapies to treat erectile dysfunction (Chapter 10). The application of functional imaging experiments is allowing visualization of brain activation during human sexual responses and is a technique with immense future research potential. It seems very likely that using this and future methods of imaging brain activity humans will appropriately supplant the rat as being the prime source of knowledge about the neurology of their sexual function in health and disease.

Acknowledgement: the authors would like to thank Dr Amee Baird for her comments on the manuscript when it was in the early stages of preparation.

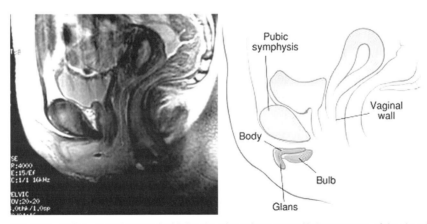

Fig. 3.16. Midline, sagittal section highlights the "almost boomerang-like" appearance of the clitoral body, crura and glans [99]. Reproduced with permission.

References

1. Baird AD, Wilson SJ, Bladin PF, Saling MM, Reutens DC. Neurological control of human sexual behaviour: insights from lesion studies. *J Neurol Neurosurg Psychiatry* 2007;**78**:1042–9.

2. Masters WH, Johnson VE. *Human sexual inadequacy*. Boston: Little Brown; 1970.

3. Kaplan HS. Sexual medicine. A progress report. *Arch Intern Med* 1980;**140**:1575–6.

4. Basson R. Female sexual response: the role of drugs in the management of sexual dysfunction. *Obstet Gynaecol* 2001;**98**:350–3.

5. Basson R, Berman J, Burnett A, et al. Report of the international consensus development conference on female sexual dysfunction: definitions and classifications. *J Urol* 2000;**163**:888–93.

6. Sachs BD. Placing erection in context: the reflexogenic-psychogenic dichotomy reconsidered. *Neurosci Biobehav Rev* 1995;**19**:211–24.

7. Bernabe J, Rampin O, Sachs BD, Giuliano F. Intracavernous pressure during erection in rats: an integrative approach based on telemetric recording. *Am J Physiol* 1999;**276**(2 Pt 2):R441–9.

8. Schmid DM, Hauri D, Schurch B. Nocturnal penile tumescence and rigidity (NPTR) findings in spinal cord injured men with erectile dysfunction. *Int J Impot Res* 2004;**16**:433–40.

9. Levin RJ. VIP, vagina, clitoral and periurethral glans – an update on human female genital arousal. *Exp Clin Endocrinol* 1991;**9**:61–9.

10. Mattson D, Petrie M, Srivastava DK, McDermott M. Multiple sclerosis. Sexual dysfunction and its response to medications. *Arch Neurol* 1995;**52**:862–8.

11. MacLean PD, Ploog DW. Cerebral representation of penile erection. *J Neurophysiol* 1962;**25**:29–55.

12. Dua S, Maclean PD. Localization for penile erection in medial frontal lobe. *Am J Physiol* 1964;**207**:1425–34.

13. Robinson BW, Mishkin M. Penile erection evoked from forebrain structures in Macaca mulatta. *Arch Neurol* 1968;**19**:184–98.

14. Marson L, List MS, McKenna KE. Lesions of the nucleus paragigantocellularis alter ex copula penile reflexes. *Brain Res* 1992;**592**:187–92.

15. Argiolas A, Melis MR. Central control of penile erection: role of the paraventricular nucleus of the hypothalamus. *Prog Neurobiol* 2005;**76**:1–21.

16. Wagner CK, Clemens LG. Projections of the paraventricular nucleus of the hypothalamus to the sexually dimorphic lumbosacral region of the spinal cord. *Brain Res* 1991;**539**:254–62.

17. McKenna KE. The neural control of female sexual function. *NeuroRehabilitation* 2000;**15**:133–43.

18. Simerly RB, Swanson LW. The organization of neural inputs to the medial preoptic nucleus of the rat. *J Comp Neurol* 1986;**246**:312–42.

19. Steers WD. Neural pathways and central sites involved in penile erection: neuroanatomy and clinical implications. *Neurosci Biobehav Rev* 2000;**24**:507–16.

20. McKenna K. The brain is the master organ in sexual function: central nervous system control of male and female sexual function. *Int J Impot Res* 1999;**11** (Suppl 1):S48–55.

21. Kondo Y, Sachs BD, Sakuma Y. Importance of the medial amygdala in rat penile erection evoked by remote stimuli from estrous females. *Behav Brain Res* 1998;**91**:215–22.

22. Marson L, McKenna KE. The identification of a brainstem site controlling spinal sexual reflexes in male rats. *Brain Res* 1990;**515**:303–8.

23. Nolte J. *The human brain: an introduction to its functional anatomy*. Sixth edn. Philadelphia: Mosby Elsevier; 2008.

24. Andrew J, Nathan PW. The cerebral control of micturition. *Proc RSM* 1965;**58**:553–5.

25. McKenna KE. Some proposals regarding the organization of the central nervous system control of penile erection. *Neurosci Biobehav Rev* 2000;**24**:535–40.

26. Swanson LW, Sawchenko PE. Hypothalamic integration: organization of the paraventricular and supraoptic nuclei. *Annu Rev Neurosci* 1983;**6**:269–324.

27. Dieckmann G, Schneider H. Influence of stereotactic hypothalamotomy on alcohol and drug addiction. *Appl Neurophysiol* 1978;**41**:93–8.

28. Melis MR, Argiolas A, Gessa GL. Apomorphine-induced penile erection and yawning: site of action in brain. *Brain Res* 1987;**415**:98–104.

29. Fenu S, Wardas J, Morelli M. Impulse control disorders and dopamine dysregulation syndrome associated with dopamine agonist therapy in Parkinson's disease. *Behav Pharmacol* 2009;**20**:363–79.

30. Arnulf I, Lin L, Gadoth N, et al. Kleine-Levin syndrome: a systematic study of 108 patients. *Ann Neurol* 2008;**63**:482–93.

31. Beach FA. Cerebral and hormonal control of reflexive mechanisms involved in copulatory behavior. *Physiol Rev* 1967;**47**:289–316.

32. Rose JD. Forebrain influences on brainstem and spinal mechanisms of copulatory behavior: a current perspective on Frank Beach's contribution. *Neurosci Biobehav Rev* 1990;**14**:207–15.

33. Giuliano F, Rampin O. Neural control of erection. *Physiol Behav* 2004;**83**:189–201.

34. Herzog AG, Fowler KM. Sexual hormones and epilepsy: threat and opportunities. *Curr Opin Neurol* 2005;**18**:167–72.

35. Kluver H, Bucy PC. Preliminary analysis of functions of the temporal lobes in monkeys. *J Neuropsychiatry Clin Neurosci* 1997;**9**:606–20.

36. Terzian H, Ore GD. Syndrome of Kluver and Bucy; reproduced in man by bilateral removal of the temporal lobes. *Neurology* 1955;**5**:373–80.

37. Lilly R, Cummings JL, Benson DF, Frankel M. The human Kluver-Bucy syndrome. *Neurology* 1983;**33**:1141–5.

38. Miller BL, Cummings JL, McIntyre H, Ebers G, Grode M. Hypersexuality or altered sexual preference following brain injury. *J Neurol Neurosurg Psychiatry* 1986;**49**:867–73.

39. Swanson LW. The amygdala and its place in the cerebral hemisphere. *Ann N Y Acad Sci* 2003;**985**:174–84.

40. Baird AD, Wilson SJ, Bladin PF, Saling MM, Reutens DC. The amygdala and sexual drive: insights from temporal lobe epilepsy surgery. *Ann Neurol* 2004;**55**:87–96.

41. Gastaut H, Collomb H. Sexual behavior in psychomotor epileptics. *Ann Med Psychol (Paris)* 1954;**112**:657–96.

42. Walker AE. The libidinous temporal lobe. *Schweiz Arch Neurol Neurochir Psychiatr* 1972;**111**:473–84.

43. Braun CM, Dumont M, Duval J, Hamel I, Godbout L. Opposed left and right brain hemisphere contributions to sexual drive: a multiple lesion case analysis. *Behav Neurol* 2003;**14**:55–61.

44. Janszky J, Szucs A, Halasz P, et al. Orgasmic aura originates from the right hemisphere. *Neurology* 2002;**58**:302–4.

45. Herzog AG, Coleman AE, Jacobs AR, et al. Relationship of sexual dysfunction to epilepsy laterality and reproductive hormone levels in women. *Epilepsy Behav* 2003;**4**:407–13.

46. Herzog AG. Disorders of reproduction in patients with epilepsy: primary neurological mechanisms. *Seizure* 2008;**17**:101–10.

47. Williamson PD, Spencer DD, Spencer SS, Novelly RA, Mattson RH. Complex partial seizures of frontal lobe origin. *Ann Neurol* 1985;**18**:497–504.

48. Holstege G. The emotional motor system in relation to the supraspinal control of micturition and mating behavior. *Behav Brain Res* 1998;**92**:103–9.

49. Penfield W, Rasmussen T. *The cerebral cortex in man.* New York: Macmillan; 1950.

50. Erickson TC. Erotomania (nymphomania) as an expression of cortical epileptiform discharge. *Arch Neurol Psych* 1945;**53**:226–31.

51. Feinsod M. Kershman's sad reflections on the homunculus: a historical vignette. *Neurology* 2005;**64**:524–5.

52. Kell CA, von Kriegstein K, Rosler A, Kleinschmidt A, Laufs H. The sensory cortical representation of the human penis: revisiting somatotopy in the male homunculus. *J Neurosci* 2005;**25**:5984–7.

53. Haldeman S, Bradley WE, Bhatia N, Johnson BK. Pudendal evoked responses. *Arch Neurol* 1982;**39**:280–3.

54. Vodusek DB. Pudendal SEP and bulbocavernosus reflex in women. *Electroencephalogr Clin Neurophysiol* 1990;**77**:134–6.

55. Mouras H, Stoleru S, Bittoun J, et al. Brain processing of visual sexual stimuli in healthy men: a functional magnetic resonance imaging study. *Neuroimage* 2003;**20**:855–69.

56. Kim SW, Sohn DW, Cho YH, et al. Brain activation by visual erotic stimuli in healthy middle aged males. *Int J Impot Res* 2006;**18**:452–7.

57. Park K, Seo JJ, Kang HK, et al. A new potential of blood oxygenation level dependent (BOLD) functional MRI for evaluating cerebral centers of penile erection. *Int J Impot Res* 2001;**13**:73–81.

58. Gizewski ER, Krause E, Karama S, et al. There are differences in cerebral activation between females in distinct menstrual phases during viewing of erotic stimuli: a fMRI study. *Exp Brain Res* 2006;**174**:101–8.

59. Zhu X, Wang X, Parkinson C, et al. Brain activation evoked by erotic films varies with different menstrual phases: an fMRI study. *Behav Brain Res* 2010;**206**:279–85.

60. Arnow BA, Millheiser L, Garrett A, et al. Women with hypoactive sexual desire disorder compared to normal females: a functional magnetic resonance imaging study. *Neuroscience* 2009;**158**:484–502.

61. Jeong GW, Park K, Youn G, et al. Assessment of cerebrocortical regions associated with sexual arousal in premenopausal and menopausal women by using BOLD-based functional MRI. *J Sex Med* 2005;**2**:645–51.

62. Rorden C, Brett M. Stereotaxic display of brain lesions. *Behav Neurol* 2000;**12**:191–200.

63. Redoute J, Stoleru S, Gregoire MC, et al. Brain processing of visual sexual stimuli in human males. *Hum Brain Mapp* 2000;**11**:162–77.

64. Arnow BA, Desmond JE, Banner LL, et al. Brain activation and sexual arousal in healthy, heterosexual males. *Brain* 2002;**125**(Pt 5):1014–23.

65. Karama S, Lecours AR, Leroux JM, et al. Areas of brain activation in males and females during viewing of erotic film excerpts. *Hum Brain Mapp* 2002;**16**:1–13.

66. Holstege G, Georgiadis JR, Paans AM, et al. Brain activation during human male ejaculation. *J Neurosci* 2003;**23**:9185–93.

67. Hamann S. Sex differences in the responses of the human amygdala. *Neuroscientist* 2005;**11**:288–93.

68. Georgiadis JR, Holstege G. Human brain activation during sexual stimulation of the penis. *J Comp Neurol* 2005;**493**:33–8.

69. Moulier V, Mouras H, Pelegrini-Issac M, et al. Neuroanatomical correlates of penile erection evoked by photographic stimuli in human males. *Neuroimage* 2006;**33**:689–99.

70. Georgiadis JR, Kortekaas R, Kuipers R, et al. Regional cerebral blood flow changes associated with clitorally induced orgasm in healthy women. *Eur J Neurosci* 2006;**24**:3305–16.

71. Huh J, Park K, Hwang IS, et al. Brain activation areas of sexual arousal with olfactory stimulation in men: a preliminary study using functional MRI. *J Sex Med* 2008;**5**:619–25.

72. Georgiadis JR, Reinders AA, Paans AM, Renken R, Kortekaas R. Men versus women on sexual brain function: prominent differences during tactile genital stimulation, but not during orgasm. *Hum Brain Mapp* 2009;**30**:3089–101.

73. Craig AD. Interoception: the sense of the physiological condition of the body. *Curr Opin Neurobiol* 2003;**13**:500–5.

74. Georgiadis JR, Reinders AA, Van der Graaf FH, Paans AM, Kortekaas R. Brain activation during human male ejaculation revisited. *Neuroreport* 2007;**18**:553–7.

75. Komisaruk BR, Whipple B. Functional MRI of the brain during orgasm in women. *Annu Rev Sex Res* 2005;**16**:62–86.

76. Mallick HN, Tandon S, Jagannathan NR, Gulia KK, Kumar VM. Brain areas activated after ejaculation in healthy young human subjects. *Indian J Physiol Pharmacol* 2007;**51**:81–5.

77. McKenna KE. Neural circuitry involved in sexual function. *J Spinal Cord Med* 2001;**24**:148–54.

78. Brindley G. Neurophysiology. In: Kirby R, Carson C, Webster G, eds. *Impotence: Diagnosis and management of male erectile dysfunction.* Oxford: Butterworth-Heinemann; 1991:27–31.

79. Vodusek DB, Janko M. The bulbocavernosus reflex. A single motor neuron study. *Brain* 1990;**113** (Pt 3):813–20.

80. Bors E, Comarr A. Neurological disturbances of sexual function with special references to 529 patients with spinal cord injury. *Urol Survey* 1960;**10**:191–222.

81. Sipski ML, Alexander CJ, Rosen R. Sexual arousal and orgasm in women: effects of spinal cord injury. *Ann Neurol* 2001;**49**:35–44.

82. Brindley GS. The Ferrier lecture, 1986. The actions of parasympathetic and sympathetic nerves in human micturition, erection and seminal emission, and their restoration in paraplegic patients by implanted electrical stimulators. *Proc R Soc Lond B Biol Sci* 1988;**235**:111–20.

83. Comarr AE. Sexual function among patients with spinal cord injury. *Urol Int* 1970;**25**:134–68.

84. Truitt WA, Coolen LM. Identification of a potential ejaculation generator in the spinal cord. *Science* 2002;**297**:1566–9.

85. Coolen LM, Allard J, Truitt WA, McKenna KE. Central regulation of ejaculation. *Physiol Behav* 2004;**83**:203–15.

86. Gerstenberg TC, Levin RJ, Wagner G. Erection and ejaculation in man. Assessment of the electromyographic activity of the bulbocavernosus and ischiocavernosus muscles. *Br J Urol* 1990;**65**:395–402.

87. Brindley GS. Electroejaculation: its technique, neurological implications and uses. *J Neurol Neurosurg Psychiatry* 1981;**44**:9.

88. White JC, Sweet WH, Hawkins R, Nilges RG. Anterolateral cordotomy: results, complications and causes of failure. *Brain*;**73**:346–67.

89. Beric A, Light J. Anorgasmia in anterior spinal cord syndrome. *J Neurol Neurosurg Psychiatry* 1993;**56**:548–51.

90. Dasgupta R, Wiseman OJ, Kanabar G, Fowler CJ, Mikol DD. Efficacy of sildenafil in the treatment of female sexual dysfunction due to multiple sclerosis. *J Urol* 2004;**171**:1189–93.

91. Fowler CJ. The neurology of male sexual dysfunction and its investigation by neurophysiological methods. *Br J Urol* 1998;**81**:785–95.

92. Yang CC, Bradley WE. Peripheral distribution of the human dorsal nerve of the penis. *J Urol* 1998;**159**:1912–16.

93. Yang CC, Bradley WE. Innervation of the human glans penis. *J Urol* 1999;**161**:97–102.

94. Halata Z, Munger BL. The neuroanatomical basis for the protopathic sensibility of the human glans penis. *Brain Res* 1986;**371**:205–30.

95. Rees PM, Fowler CJ, Maas CP. Sexual function in men and women with neurological disorders. *Lancet* 2007;**369**:512–25.

96. O'Connell HE, Sanjeevan KV, Hutson JM. Anatomy of the clitoris. *J Urol* 2005;**174**(4 Pt 1):1189–95.

97. O'Connell HE, Hutson JM, Anderson CR, Plenter RJ. Anatomical relationship between urethra and clitoris. *J Urol* 1998;**159**:1892–1897.

98. Baskin LS, Erol A, Li YW, et al. Anatomical studies of the human clitoris. *J Urol* 1999;**162**(3 Pt 2):1015–20.

99. O'Connell HE, DeLancey JO. Clitoral anatomy in nulliparous, healthy, premenopausal volunteers using unenhanced magnetic resonance imaging. *J Urol* 2005;**173**:2060–3.

100. Yucel S, De Souza A, Jr, Baskin LS. Neuroanatomy of the human female lower urogenital tract. *J Urol* 2004;**172**:191–5.

101. Martin-Alguacil N, Pfaff DW, Shelley DN, Schober JM. Clitoral sexual arousal: an immunocytochemical and innervation study of the clitoris. *BJU Int* 2008;**101**:1407–13.

102. Vardi Y, Gruenwald I, Sprecher E, Gertman I, Yartnitsky D. Normative values for female genital sensation. *Urology* 2000;**56**:1035–40.

103. Carson C, Kirby R, Goldstein I, eds. *Textbook of erectile dysfunction*. Oxford: Isis Medical Media; 1999.

Approach and evaluation of neurogenic bladder dysfunction

Jalesh N. Panicker, Vinay Kalsi and Marianne de Sèze

Introduction

Lower urinary tract dysfunction (LUTD) can result from a wide range of neurological conditions. The importance of this problem to patients' health, and its negative impact on quality of life and dignity, are now widely recognized. Bladder symptoms often pose a management challenge but in fact these can often be effectively managed.

Neurogenic bladder dysfunction rarely occurs in isolation, bladder complaints often being a component of a pelvic organ symptom complex. Although they may be particularly prominent, a complete assessment of the patient's pelvic function is needed, which invariably requires a multidisciplinary team. The aim of this chapter is to provide the clinician with an approach to neurogenic bladder dysfunction based on the history, physical examination and investigations, in order to optimize patient management and follow-up.

Causes of neurogenic lower urinary tract dysfunction

The lower urinary tract (urinary bladder and outflow tract) has two roles: storage of urine and voiding at appropriate times. To regulate this, a complex neural control system coordinates the reservoir function of the bladder and the sphincteric function of the outflow tract [1–3]. Disruption of the neural pathway anywhere in the peripheral or central nervous system will result in neurogenic LUTD.

The general pattern of LUTD is influenced by the location of the neurological lesion, depending upon whether it is suprapontine, infrapontine-suprasacral or infrasacral (Table 4.1) [4]. However, symptoms may not solely be due to lesions of the neural pathways and can be multifactorial (Table 4.2).

Classification

Classification helps with understanding the functional disturbances occurring in neurogenic LUTD. A perfect classification system does not exist [5], but Madersbacher proposed a very simple classification which focuses on therapeutic consequences [6]. It is based upon the detrusor pressures during the filling phase and urethral sphincter tone during voiding (Fig. 4.1).

Evaluation

Understanding the underlying dysfunction is paramount before starting treatment. Essentially, there are four goals that one would wish to achieve when managing neurogenic bladder dysfunction (Table 4.3) [5]. During the evaluation, non-neurogenic factors that could contribute to LUTD should be excluded.

History

Often, bladder symptoms are overlooked during a neurological consultation. The emphasis of the doctor may be focused on the primary neurological condition and the patient may not realize that their bladder symptoms are a consequence of the neurological condition. It is, however, our experience that neurological patients in the UK and Europe are generally aware of bladder problems in neurological disease, possibly as the result of the efforts of the various societies and disease-specific patient support groups. Though uncommon, lower urinary tract symptoms (LUTS) may be the presenting complaint betraying an underlying neurological diagnosis [7].

Pelvic Organ Dysfunction in Neurological Disease: Clinical Management and Rehabilitation, ed. Clare J. Fowler,
Jalesh N. Panicker & Anton Emmanuel. Published by Cambridge University Press. © Cambridge University Press 2010.

Table 4.1. Neurological disorders causing lower urinary tract dysfunction

Suprapontine causes
Stroke
Traumatic brain injury
Degeneration: Parkinson's disease, multiple system atrophy, Alzheimer's disease, dementia with Lewy bodies
Demyelination: multiple sclerosis, acute disseminated encephalomyelitis
Hydrocephalus, normal pressure hydrocephalus
Cerebral palsy
Neoplasm
Infrapontine-suprasacral causes
Demyelination: multiple sclerosis, transverse myelitis
Traumatic spinal cord injury
Vascular: arteriovenous malformations, spinal cord infarction
Neoplasm: metastasis, primary tumors
Hereditary spastic paraparesis
Infections: tropical spastic paraparesis (HTLV-I), syphilis
Cervical spondylosis
Infrasacral causes
Spina bifida
Intervertebral disc prolapse
Arachnoiditis
Pelvic surgery
Diabetes mellitus and other causes for peripheral neuropathy

Table 4.2. Lower urinary tract symptoms in neurological disease may be multifactorial

- LUTD due to lesions affecting the neurological pathway
- Cognitive or behavioral problems: memory loss, amotivation, apraxia, visuospatial disorientation, language dysfunction
- Urological causes: urinary tract infection, bladder outlet obstruction, genuine stress incontinence, atrophic vaginitis
- Functional incontinence: reduced mobility, general debilitation
- Medications: sedatives, opiates, drugs with anticholinergic properties, diuretics
- Systemic conditions: heart failure, hyperglycemia
- Constipation

History-taking should cover the spectrum of LUTS and should include questions about potential urinary tract complications (e.g. urinary tract infections (UTIs) and stones), fluid intake, factors that exacerbate overactive bladder symptoms (such as caffeine intake, alcohol and fizzy drinks), past urological, gynecological or obstetric history, and present medications. In some conditions, LUTS may occur early in the course of disease, whereas in others it may develop later on and may be confused with age-related LUTD due to non-neurologic origin such as benign prostatic enlargement, stress incontinence or pelvic organ prolapse. History-taking provides a forum to address the current goals and patient's expectations. Bowel and sexual dysfunction often co-exist with neurogenic LUTD and should also be enquired about.

Lower urinary tract symptoms

History-taking should address potential dysfunction in both the storage and voiding phases of micturition. When assessing LUTS, it is relevant to note whether storage or voiding symptoms predominate.

Storage symptoms

Symptoms that suggest storage phase dysfunction include urinary frequency, nocturia, urgency and urgency incontinence [8–10]. In the setting of a neurological disorder, these symptoms usually suggest neurogenic LUTD. Urgency, with or without urgency incontinence, with frequency and nocturia, is called the overactive bladder syndrome, urge syndrome or urgency-frequency syndrome [10]. These symptoms are defined in Table 4.4.

The underlying pathophysiology responsible for these symptoms is detrusor overactivity (DO), reduced bladder compliance and diminished bladder capacity which can have many different neurological causes as described in Chapter 1. However, these symptoms are non-specific and may warrant further evaluations in the appropriate clinical setting (Table 4.4).

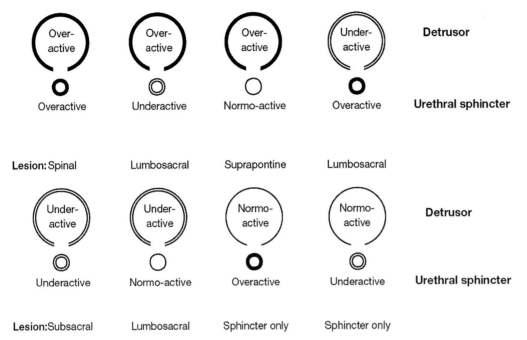

Fig. 4.1. Functional classification of neurogenic lower urinary tract dysfunction based upon the detrusor pressures during the filling phase and urethral sphincter tone during voiding. Adapted from [5, 6].

Table 4.3. Goals to achieve when managing patients with neurogenic LUTD

- Achieve urinary continence
- Improve quality of life
- Prevent urinary tract infections
- Preserve upper urinary tract functions

Nocturia

Nocturia is a non-specific symptom and can be due to a variety of causes [11] (Table 4.5). A bladder diary (see below) is often helpful in evaluating the cause for nocturia. Calculating the nocturia polyuria index and nocturnal bladder capacity index may be helpful in indentifying patients with more than one cause for nocturia (Table 4.6) [12]. Reduced nocturnal bladder capacity is perhaps the most common cause in patients with neurogenic LUTD and occurs due to DO and reduced bladder compliance. Nocturnal polyuria is characterized by overproduction of urine during sleep hours, generally greater than 20% of the 24-hour urine output in the young and 33% in

the elderly. In the setting of neurological disease, it may occur in Parkinson's disease and conditions associated with dysautonomia, though the reasons for this are not exactly known.

Incontinence

Urinary incontinence is the complaint of any involuntary leakage of urine. It is a non-specific complaint that is commonly reported in the general population and can have varying pathophysiology.

In *urgency* urinary incontinence, incontinence is accompanied by or immediately preceded by urgency. In *stress* incontinence, it occurs with effort or exertion, or on sneezing or coughing. Stress urinary incontinence arises if there is any weakness of the striated urethral sphincter or the pelvic floor musculature. This results in urine leak whenever the intra-abdominal pressure rises. However, cough may provoke DO and hence cough-induced incontinence alone may not be specific for stress incontinence. Patients with an open bladder neck may experience urgency and incontinence when in the erect posture [13]. Patients with *mixed* incontinence have features of both urgency and stress

Table 4.4. Definitions of lower urinary tract symptoms* (LUTS) and their possible causes

Lower Urinary Tract Symptom	Definition	Causes
Storage dysfunction		
Daytime frequency (the term pollakisuria is used in some countries)	Complaint of voiding too often during the day	• Overactive bladder syndrome/detrusor overactivity due to the relevant neurological condition • Impaired bladder compliance • Excessive fluid intake • Excessive urine production (polyuria) • Increased bladder sensations • **Urological/urogynecological causes:** prostate enlargement, pelvic organ prolapse, urinary tract infection, bladder tumor, renal tract stones, interstitial cystitis
Nocturia#^	Complaint that the individual has to wake up one or more times to void	
Urgency	Complaint of a sudden compelling desire to void, which is difficult to defer	
Voiding dysfunction		
Slow stream	Individual's perception of reduced urine flow compared to previous performance or in comparison to others	• Detrusor sphincter dyssynergia • Detrusor underactivity • **Urological/urogynecological causes:** bladder outlet obstruction due to prostate enlargement, pelvic organ prolapse, urethral stricture
Intermittent stream	Urine flow which stops and starts on one or more occasions during micturition	
Hesitancy	Difficulty in initiating micturition resulting in a delay in the onset of voiding	
Straining	Muscular effort used to initiate, maintain or improve the urinary stream	
Incomplete bladder emptying	Feeling of bladder fullness after passing urine	

Note: * Definitions as per the standardised terminology proposed by the International Continence Society [10]
Nocturia is the number of voids recorded during a night's sleep. Each void is preceded and followed by sleep
^ Nocturnal polyuria is a related term and is present when an increased proportion of the 24-hour output occurs at night. When measuring the night-time urine output, include the first void of the morning

incontinence. In *overflow* incontinence, involuntary loss of urine occurs due to an overfilled bladder.

The history is often helpful in distinguishing between the various types of incontinence. The volume of urine loss can also provide valuable information as to the nature of incontinence: urgency incontinence is more likely to be associated with a large loss of urine whereas that lost with stress incontinence tends to be small. Nocturnal enuresis is the complaint of loss of urine during sleep.

Table 4.5. The pathophysiological mechanisms behind nocturia and their causes. Adapted from [11, 12]

Due to reduced nocturnal bladder capacity
Detrusor overactivity
Reduced bladder compliance
Prostate enlargement
Malignancy of the lower urinary tract
Bladder calculi
Anxiety disorder
Learned voiding dysfunction
Due to nocturnal polyuria
Congestive cardiac failure
Obstructive sleep apnea
Diabetes mellitus
Peripheral edema
Excessive night-time fluid intake
Parkinson's disease
Due to global polyuria
Diabetes mellitus
Diabetes insipidus
Polydipsia: primary or dipsogenic
Mixed: both reduced nocturnal bladder capacity and nocturnal polyuria

Table 4.6. Formulas for nocturia evaluation. Adapted from [12]

- Nocturia polyuria index (NPi) = nocturnal urine volume ÷ 24-hour urine volume
- Nocturnal bladder capacity index (NBCi) = difference between the actual and predicted number of nightly voids*

Note: * Predicted number of nightly voids = (nocturnal urine volume ÷ maximum voided volume) − 1

Table 4.7. Causes for hematuria and possible sites of bleeding

General/systemic causes: coagulation disorders, anticoagulation therapy (e.g. warfarin), sickle-cell trait or disease, vascular disease, exercise

Kidney: neoplasia, stones, trauma, infection, glomerular disease, renal cystic disease, arteriovenous malformation, renal artery aneurysm, Fabry's disease

Ureter: neoplasia, stones, trauma

Bladder: neoplasia, stones, trauma, infection, foreign body, catheterization, drugs (e.g. cyclophosphamide)

Urethra: prostatic enlargement, neoplasia, catheterization, stone, trauma, infection, foreign body

is due to detrusor sphincter dyssynergia (DSD), characterized by simultaneous contraction of the detrusor muscle and external urethral sphincter, and impaired detrusor contractions. Table 4.4 defines the common symptoms.

Hematuria

Hematuria is defined as the presence of blood in the urine. It can be either macroscopic (gross) when it is visible to the naked eye, or microscopic, if blood is identified only through urine microscopy or dipstick testing. The latter may be found in association with other urological symptoms, such as loin or urethral pain (symptomatic microscopic hematuria), or during a routine medical examination (asymptomatic microscopic hematuria). In the setting of neurogenic LUTD, hematuria may occur due to catheterization, UTIs, stones or rarely bladder cancer (Table 4.7). In patients on oral anticoagulants, hematuria should prompt checking of coagulation parameters. Hematuria should always be fully investigated and all patients with visible hematuria and patients over the age of 50 with microscopic hematuria should be referred for further investigation.

Symptoms of upper urinary tract damage

Upper tract changes may often occur asymptomatically, hence the importance of investigations (see below). However, patients may complain of loin pain, which can arise due to a variety of causes including ascending infection, renal calculi or high detrusor pressures with reflux. Patients who are progressively developing

Voiding symptoms

Symptoms that suggest voiding phase dysfunction are hesitancy, straining for micturition, slow and interrupted urinary stream, sensation of incomplete bladder emptying and double voiding. Patients may notice the need to pass urine again within minutes of having passed urine (double voiding). This most commonly upper tract reflux and dilatation may report recent improvement in incontinence in spite of not receiving any specific treatment.

Symptom scales

Several symptoms scales have been validated for the evaluation of urinary disorders, but none are specific for neurogenic LUTD. Most focus on one type of dysfunction, for example stress urinary incontinence or urge incontinence. However some, like the urinary symptom profile (USP) [8], are more comprehensive and assess symptoms of stress incontinence, overactive bladder and urinary obstruction, in both men and women.

The symptom scores are more likely to be useful in the context of research or a formal treatment protocol. The commonly used scales are International Prostate Symptom Score (IPSS) [14], Urogenital Distress Inventory (UDI-6) [15, 16] and USP [8] (Appendix 1). However, to date, there are no consensual recommendations for a scale for the evaluation and follow-up of neurogenic LUTD.

Quality of life and patient reported outcome measures (PROMs)

In addition to evaluating LUTS, it is important to assess the "bother" or disruption to daily activities or sleep that bladder symptoms cause. Patients with neurological disease face lifestyle restrictions and LUTD can detrimentally affect quality of life (QOL). PROMs are increasingly being used to assess the impact of a disease and, when used in conjunction with objective measures, provide a comprehensive means of assessing the severity of the patient's condition and effectiveness of treatment.

The International Continence Society has recommended the use of LUTS-specific questionnaires that address health-related QOL in clinical trials.

QOL questionnaires can be administered by several means: face-to-face interviews, telephonic or through the internet. This is most effectively achieved by self-completed, validated questionnaires. Amongst the several questionnaires assessing the effects of bladder problems on QOL, only a few have been validated in the neurological population. These include the Incontinence QOL Instrument [17], Urge Incontinence Impact Questionnaire, Urge Urological Distress Inventory [18], Overactive Bladder Questionnaire

Table 4.8. Bladder diaries and what they record: the International Continence Society classification [10, 24]

Micturition time chart: records times of voids in at least 24 hours

Frequency–volume chart: records volumes as well as times of voids for at least 24 hours

Bladder diary: records times of voids and volumes, incontinence episodes, pad usage and other usage including degree of urgency, degree of incontinence and fluid intake

[19], Qualiveen [20, 21] and SF Qualiveen [22] (Appendix 2). While most address incontinence, the Qualiveen questionnaire is distinct amongst these as it addresses the broad range of urinary problems experienced by patients with neurological disorders, such as MS and spinal cord injury, including storage and voiding symptoms, and has been translated into several languages [23].

Bladder diary

Information obtained from history can be supplemented by a bladder diary. This is a useful tool for evaluating neurogenic LUTS and in understanding the extent and severity of symptoms and response to treatment. It is an essential part of the evaluation and follow-up of patients with neurogenic LUTD. Diaries capture the nature of LUTS more accurately as they are completed in the natural environment of the patient. They may also help in identifying causes for LUTS, e.g. increased fluid intake as a cause for urinary frequency. The largest volume of urine voided during a single micturition, the maximum voided volume, provides a rough estimation of the functional bladder capacity. Furthermore, use of the bladder diary allows the patient to actively participate in the management of LUTD.

Different diaries and charts have been described and each varies according to the type of information that can be captured. Bladder diaries record number/time/volume of voids or catheterizations, number/time of incontinent episodes, number/weight of pads, fluid intake and activity related to LUTS. Attention should be paid to any medications taken by the patient. Table 4.8 describes the different tools available and the information they capture [24]. Usually, simpler forms limited to information about voiding and leakages are sufficient and the more comprehensive versions

Day 1		Time / Volume (mL)						Total Fluid intake	Episodes of leakage
Day 1 26/4/20 09	Time	6 AM	10 AM	12:30 PM	3:30 PM	5 PM		1700	4
Time out of bed (am) - 6 AM	Volume	160	120	130	190	140			
	Time	7 PM	8:45 PM	2:30 AM	4 AM				
Time to bed (pm)- 9 PM	Volume	150	170	200	180				
	Time								
	Volume								

Fig. 4.2. Bladder diary over 24 hours demonstrating daytime and night-time frequency, low-volume voids and incontinence. The recorded volumes did not include incontinent episodes. These findings may be seen in patients with detrusor overactivity.

are used in the setting of research protocols (Fig. 4.2). There are no clear guidelines to the number of days that a bladder diary should be maintained to obtain a reliable record, and the duration can range widely from 1 to 14 days. However, 3 to 7 days is generally considered sufficient to assess the frequency of micturition and incontinence [25, 26].

Physical examination

Physical examination should include a neurological, urological, gynecological, abdominal and rectal examination. The neurological examination should aim to identify specific neurological deficits that could point to the possible etiology of bladder disturbances. For example, bladder disturbances have been shown to correlate with lower limb deficits in multiple sclerosis [27] and ADEM [28]. A bed-bound individual with advanced neurological disease may have functional incontinence due to immobility. Findings in the neurological examination may also influence bladder management. For example, the presence of cognitive disturbances would influence the choice of antimuscarinic medications [29] (Chapter 6) and identifying that a patient has impaired manual dexterity would preclude the option of self-catheterization [30]. In a person with unexplained bladder dysfunction, it would be appropriate to examine the integrity of the sacral segments. This would include testing sensations in the sacral dermatomes, rectal examination to assess the resting and voluntary anal tone, and eliciting the bulbocavernous and anal reflexes (S_2–S_4 segments). The urological/gynecological examination includes examination of the external genitalia, vagina and perineum to look for excoriations, masses, pelvic organ prolapse and abnormal perineal sensations. The pelvic floor muscle strength can also be assessed while the examiner is performing a digital vaginal examination. A stress

test can be performed to assess stress incontinence. In this procedure, the patient with a partially full bladder is asked to cough or perform the Valsalva maneuver either in the lithotomy position or when standing, and an immediate loss of urine is consistent with stress incontinence. If there is a significant degree of pelvic organ prolapse, it can cause obstructed voiding which would improve when the prolapse is reduced.

The abdominal examination will reveal scars from previous surgery as well as any organomegaly: a renal mass due to hydronehprosis or a suprapubic swelling due to a palpable bladder. Abdominal striae may be found in association with other markers of abnormal collagen metabolism, prevalent in patients with pelvic organ prolapse and stress incontinence.

"Diagnostic shadowing" should not be allowed to obscure the fact that men with symptoms of poor voiding may have additional outflow obstruction due to prostatic origin. Digital rectal examination may then be a useful examination, though the estimated size may not correlate with luminal encroachment. Palpating a hard gland should raise the possibility of malignancy and should be further evaluated. Fecal impaction and rectal tone can be assessed by rectal examination as well. Pelvic masses of lower gastrointestinal or gynecological origin may also be detected.

Investigations

Investigations help in the evaluation of bladder complaints, to confirm a diagnosis or exclude differential diagnoses.

"Dipstick" urine analysis

This is a quick, simple and inexpensive test that can reveal considerable information about pathology of the urinary tracts. Combined rapid tests of urine using reagent strips for urinalysis, "dipstick" tests, are useful

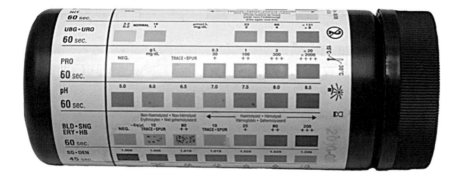

Fig. 4.3. Urine "dipsticks" are a useful screen for urinary tract infections.

to demonstrate the presence of haemoglobin, leucocyte esterase (present in infection), nitrite (present in bacterial infection), protein (present with glomerular disease or infection) and glucose (present in poorly controlled or undiagnosed diabetes) (Fig. 4.3). While the negative predictive value for excluding UTI is excellent (>98%), the positive predictive value for confirming UTI is only 50% and confirmatory tests are required [31]. Abnormalities in urine dipsticks are common in patients doing clean intermittent self-catheterization or with an indwelling catheter and, in the absence of symptoms of UTI, should not be an indication for antibiotics [32].

Mid-stream urine (MSU)

An MSU should be sent for microscopy, culture and sensitivities in the setting of positive dipstick urine analysis. Symptomatic patients with a proven UTI may then be treated with the appropriate antibiotic according to the antibiotic sensitivity.

Urine cytology

In patients with documented hematuria, either gross or on dipstick, urine should be sent for cytology to look for atypical cells. The diagnostic value of cytology is generally poor in the absence of hematuria.

Blood tests

Blood tests of relevance include renal functions (urea, creatinine), electrolytes and hemoglobin.

Most laboratories in the UK now calculate and report an estimated glomerular filtration rate (eGFR) as an indicator of the excretory function of the kidney. The most commonly used formula to calculate eGFR is the 4-variable Modification of Diet in Renal Disease (MDRD) formula and this has been validated in adults (>18 years old) with chronic kidney disease [33] and is also recommended by the National Service Framework in the UK [34]. The formula estimates GFR based on four variables: serum creatinine (μmol/L), age, ethnic origin and gender. An eGFR >90 ml/min/1.73 m^2 is considered normal. Formulas are readily available online; however, eGFR values obtained from the laboratory may be slightly more accurate than these online calculators as their equations take into account local variations in accuracy of creatinine assays. Of relevance to neurology patients, the formula has not been validated in muscle-wasting disease states. Measuring serum cystatin C has been shown to be a more reliable marker of GFR than serum creatinine in spinal cord injured patients and levels are not affected by muscle mass [35].

Men with neurological disease may have lower urinary tract symptoms of prostatic origin and should be evaluated appropriately, including measuring prostate-specific antigen [36]. Performing this screening test for prostate malignancy is controversial because of its unproven benefits and the associated risk for over treatment. Therefore, the patient should be fully counselled and should have consented before this test is carried out.

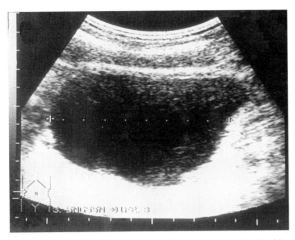

Fig. 4.4. Measuring the post-void residual urine using the bladder scan.

Pad tests

This test is useful if stress incontinence is suspected and also quantifies urine loss. Continence pads are worn for a set period of time and subsequently weighed on their removal for any abnormal increase (>15 g) in pad weight. Though it provides an objective assessment of the degree of stress incontinence, it does not evaluate its impact on QOL. Unlike for LUTD of non-neurogenic origin, where the ICS recommends the use of the pad-weighing test in the pretreatment evaluation of incontinence and at each post-treatment follow-up visit [37], there is no recommendation for its use in neurogenic LUTD.

Bladder scan

The extent of bladder emptying cannot be predicted from the history or clinical examination [38]. The post-void residual volume (PVR) is the volume of urine remaining in the bladder following a void. It is important to recognize persistently elevated PVR as it can predispose to lower urinary tract complications such as urinary tract infections. Elevated PVR results in reduced functional bladder capacity and can trigger reflex detrusor contractions. Both factors result in worsening storage symptoms.

PVR can be measured by microprocessor calculation of bladder volume using a small portable ultrasound device which many specialist nurse continence advisors have access to (Fig. 4.4). An alternative to bladder scan is measuring the residual urine by in-out catheterization, especially in patients who perform intermittent catheterisation. In patients with voiding dysfunction, a PVR of more than 100 ml [32] or more than one-third of bladder capacity is taken as the amount of residual urine that contributes to bladder dysfunction, as bladder capacity is usually also reduced in neurogenic LUTD. However, there is no consensus about the figure of PVR at which intermittent self-catheterization should be initiated. It is recognized that a single measurement of the PVR is not representative and when possible, a series of measurements should be made over the course of one or two weeks [32].

Ultrasound scan

In patients known to be at risk of upper urinary tract disease, surveillance ultrasonography should be performed periodically to evaluate for evidence of damage, such as upper urinary tract dilatation or renal scarring. Ultrasound may also detect complications of neurogenic bladder dysfunction such as calculi, which otherwise would be diagnosed using more expensive and invasive investigations such as CT scan or intravenous pyelography.

Specialist investigations

If the nature of LUTD remains unclear after the initial assessment, a referral to a urologist or uro-gynecologist may be warranted for considering more specialist investigations. Isotope renography using ^{99m}Tc-MAG3 or ^{99m}Tc-DMSA may occasionally be indicated in patients with upper tract disease to assess renal functions or parenchymal scarring. The indications for referring to a specialist service are shown in Table 4.9.

Urodynamics

It is known that history, bladder diary and clinical examination may not always be sufficient for understanding the nature of LUTD. Urodynamic tests involve functional and dynamic assessment of the lower urinary tract and are used to assess detrusor and bladder outlet function. They not only provide information about the nature of LUTD and the effects the neurological disease has on the urinary tract, but also risk factors for urinary tract damage, particularly due to the high detrusor pressure system. In this respect, the main parameters that require special attention in neurogenic patient are high detrusor

Table 4.9. Indications for specialist referral

Frequent urinary tract infections

Hematuria

Evidence of impaired renal function

Pain thought to arise from the upper or lower urinary tract

Suspicion of concomitant urological/uro-gynecological condition, e.g. prostate enlargement, stress incontinence, fistula

Symptoms refractory to medical management

Consideration for intradetrusor injections of botulinum toxin A

Need for suprapubic catheterization

Rare consideration of surgery (e.g. ileocystoplasty, ileal conduit)

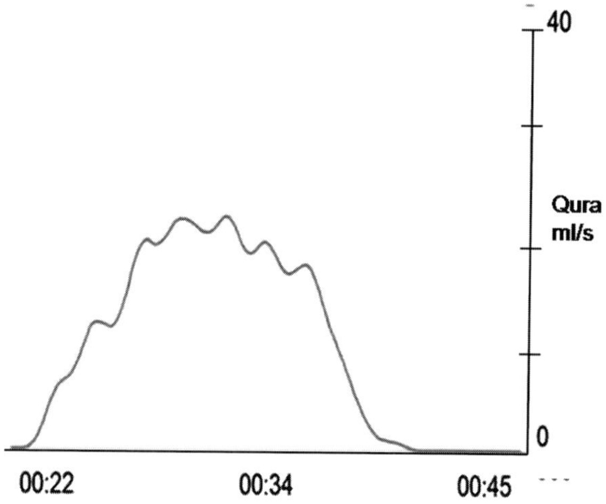

Fig. 4.5. Uroflowmetry, a non-invasive test for voiding functions. This figure demonstrates a normal urinary flow which has a "bell-shape" curve. 320 mL was voided with a maximum flow rate of 21 mL/sec. Qura: urinary flow.

pressure during the filling or storage phase of the bladder and detrusor–external sphincter dyssynergia during micturition [39, 40].

A complete urodynamic study includes non-invasive uroflowmetry and more invasive cystometry. The terminology used and quality of the urodynamic recording and its interpretation are guided by technical recommendations and standards set by the ICS [10, 41]. Ideally, the rectum should be empty before the start of investigation and drugs that influence the LUT should be stopped.

Uroflowmetry

Patients are asked to urinate into a special urinal or toilet with a machine that has a device that measures the urinary flow rate. The results of uroflowmetry provide a fairly accurate assessment of voiding functions [41] (Fig. 4.5). It could be used as a screening test to exclude serious outflow obstruction and, in conjunction with the results of the bladder scan, can provide sufficient information for planning bladder management in most patients with neurological disease. The advantages of this test are that it is simple and non-invasive; however, the utility is limited in patients who are unable to void. Some patients with neurological disease may not be able to void standing and this should also be factored when reviewing the results of uroflowmetry. Urine flow rate is highly dependent on the volume voided and is most

predictable in the volume rage between 200 to 400 ml. Flow rate nomograms have been constructed specifically for age groups and gender and these include the Siroky nomogram (for men <55 years), Bristol nomogram (for men >55 years), and a nomogram for women [42].

Filling cystometry and pressure flow studies

Cystometry evaluates the pressure–volume relationship during non-physiological filling of the bladder and during voiding [41]. Intravesical (P_{ves}) and intra-abdominal pressures (P_{abd}) are recorded using catheters in the bladder and rectum, respectively, that are connected to external pressure transducers. The subtracted pressure (P_{det}) is an estimation of the true detrusor pressure (Fig. 4.6). During the filling phase, saline is infused at a standard rate (usually 50 or 100 ml/min) and the parameters observed include bladder sensations, changes in detrusor pressure and compliance, and maximum cystometric capacity. During voiding, the pressure–flow relationship is studied and parameters observed include detrusor pressures generated and bladder emptying.

A complete urodynamic study provides information about the safety and efficiency of bladder filling and emptying [41]. It is valuable for demonstrating the underlying pathophysiology of LUTD, detecting risk factors for urinary tract damage and planning

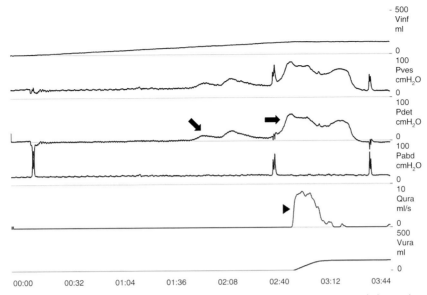

Fig. 4.6. Filling cystometry demonstrating detrusor overactivity. P_{abd} is the intra-abdominal pressure recorded using the rectal catheter. P_{ves} is the intravesical pressure recorded using the bladder catheter. P_{det} is the subtracted detrusor pressure ($P_{ves} - P_{abd}$). V_{inf} and V_{ura} represent volume infused during the test and volume voided, respectively, while Q_{ura} represents urinary flow. Black arrows demonstrate detrusor overactivity and black arrowheads associated incontinence.

management. In addition, a complete urodynamic evaluation may be helpful in identifying concomitant urological conditions such as prostate enlargement or stress incontinence. The necessity to perform a complete urodynamic study in all patients with neurogenic LUTD is the subject of debate. Patients with spinal cord injury, spina bifida and possibly advanced MS should undergo urodynamic studies because of the higher risk for upper tract damage and renal impairment, although ultrasound is a less invasive method for monitoring. Guidelines underlying the key role of urodynamics for baseline evaluation, management and follow-up of neurogenic bladder in these populations have been published [39, 40, 43, 44]. However, in other conditions, such as early MS, stroke and parkinsonism, some authors have recommended to restrict the initial tests to uroflowmetry and measurement of PVR on the basis that the result of these tests determine initial treatment. In early MS, a recent UK consensus paper recommends that urodynamics should be carried out only in those who are refractory to conservative treatment or bothered by their symptoms and wish to undergo further interventions [32]. In the absence of evidence-based data comparing these two models of management, the decision for performing complete baseline urodynamics would depend upon local resources and recommendations.

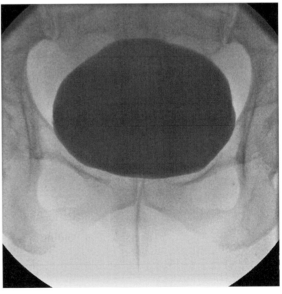

Fig. 4.7. Videourodynamics demonstrating normal bladder outline during the filling phase.

Videourodynamics

Using contrast material rather than saline and simultaneous use of fluoroscopic monitoring during urodynamics allow the relationship between anatomical events, such as bladder neck opening, to be correlated to pressure recordings (Fig. 4.7).

71

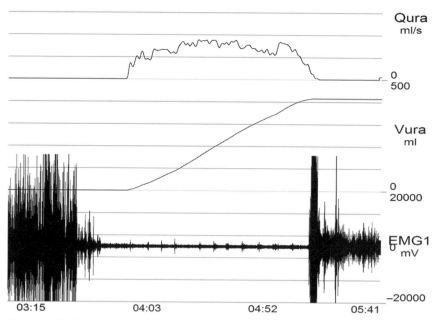

Fig. 4.8. CNE EMG from the urethral sphincter in a man with abnormal voiding. The electrical silence achieved during poor urine flow implicates the bladder neck rather than detrusor-external sphincter dyssynergia as the cause of obstruction.

It is a useful test to demonstrate structural changes resulting from neurogenic LUTD such as diverticuli and vesicoureteral reflux. It is also useful for identifying concomitant urological/urogynecological abnormalities such as bladder outlet obstruction or stress incontinence.

Urethral pressure profile

Urethral pressure profile (UPP) measures the intraluminal pressure within the urethra. It is recorded by withdrawing a catheter which is fitted with pressure sensors along the length of the urethra. The place for UPP in the evaluation of neurogenic LUTD is limited but has proved to be a valuable investigation in women with urinary retention or ineffective voiding (Chapter 19).

Uro-neurophysiology

Electromyography

Electromyography (EMG) is the recording of bioelectrical activity from striated muscles, the waveforms that are recorded reflecting the innervation of muscle fibers as "motor units." The choice of recording device determines the details of what can be recorded, surface electrodes picking up an "envelope" of EMG activity while needle electrodes, specifically concentric needle electrodes (CNEs), allow analysis of individual motor units.

Surface electrodes applied as skin patches or mounted on devices in the urethra or anal canal have been used to record from pelvic floor striated musculature and the sphincters to show the kinesiological activity of the respective muscle. Such recordings have been used to show detrusor sphincter dyssynergia, pelvic floor activation during physiotherapy and for biofeedback muscle training purposes. However, it is difficult to record good-quality EMG from the urethral sphincter with a surface electrode in men attempting to void, and a needle electrode inserted through the perineum is recommended when sphincter dyssynergia is the suspected cause of poor bladder emptying (Fig. 4.8).

Concentric needle electrodes (CNEs) permit accurate placement and allow recordings of the details of motor units to be made. Because of relatively easy access and muscle bulk, CNE EMG of the external anal sphincter muscle is the most often performed uro-neurophysiological investigation and has become established as the preferred method of detecting abnormalities of sacral root innervation [45]. Changes of chronic reinnervation with a reduced interference pattern and enlarged motor units (>1 mv amplitude) can be found in patients with cauda equine syndrome [46] (Chapter 17) whereas the changes of denervation and reinnervation in MSA tend to result in prolonged duration motor units (Chapter 13), presumably because the progressive nature of that disease precludes motor unit "compaction." CNE examination of the urethral sphincter, although much more uncomfortable than anal sphincter EMG, is required in the investigation of urinary retention in women [47] (Chapter 19).

Penilo-cavernosus reflex

The nomenclature of the various reflex responses that can be recorded from pelvic structures in response to electrical stimulation was recently rationalized [48] so that the term used gives an indication as to the site of stimulation and recording. The penilo-cavernosus reflex, formerly known as the "bulbocavernosus" reflex, assesses the sacral root afferent and efferent pathways. The dorsal nerve of the penis (or clitoris) is electrically stimulated and a recording is made from the bulbocavernosus muscle, usually with a CNE. It may be of value in patients with LUTD suspected to be secondary to cauda equina damage, or damage to the LMN pathway. However, a normal value does not exclude the possibility of an axonal lesion.

Pudendal nerve terminal motor latency

The only test of motor conduction from the pelvic floor is pudendal nerve terminal motor latency (PNMTL). The pudendal nerve is stimulated either per rectally or vaginally adjacent to the ischial spine using the St. Mark's electrode, a finger-mounted stimulating device with a surface EMG recording electrode 7 cm proximal located around the base of the finger. This records from the external anal sphincter. Prolongation was initially considered evidence for pudendal nerve damage although a prolonged latency is a poor marker for denervation. Unfortunately this test has not proved contributory in the investigation of pudendal neuralgia (Chapter 18) [49].

Pudendal somatosensory evoked potentials

Pudendal somatosensory evoked potentials can be recorded from the scalp following electrical stimulation of the dorsal nerve of the penis or clitoral nerve [50, 51]. Although this may be abnormal when a spinal cord lesion is the cause of sacral sensory loss or neurogenic DO, such pathology is also usually apparent from the clinical examination [52]. Since better control data exist for the latency of the tibial evoked potentials, measurement of these in a routine clinical neurophysiology laboratory is the recommended investigation.

Approach and management of neurogenic lower urinary tract dysfunction

Approach

The pattern of LUTD depends upon the level of neurological localization, and the expected findings of the diagnostic evaluation are listed in Table 4.10. Suprapontine lesions result in storage dysfunction and patients present with urgency, frequency and urgency incontinence. Urodynamics demonstrate DO. Infrasacral lesions result in detrusor underactivity and voiding dysfunction and patients present with hesitancy, slow and interrupted stream, and a feeling of incomplete emptying, and are often in retention. However, in a subset of patients, there may be DO as a result of "bladder decentralization" due to intact postganglionic neurons (Chapter 1). Infrapontine-suprasacral lesions lead to DO and detrusor sphincter dyssynergia, resulting in both storage and voiding dysfunction [4]. Lower urinary tract symptoms and relevant bedside investigations such as uroflowmetry and bladder scan are therefore useful in the localization of neurological lesions. Variations from the expected pattern of symptoms should warrant a search for additional urological conditions that may occur concomitantly and alter the pattern of lower urinary tract symptoms [53].

Management

The management of neurogenic LUTD must address both voiding and storage dysfunction. An overview to management is provided in Appendix 1. Bladder emptying should be assisted if a post-void residual volume is demonstrated either by in-out catheterization or by ultrasound. A value of 100 ml is commonly taken as the amount of residual urine that contributes to bladder

Table 4.10. Results of the diagnostic evaluation for neurogenic lower urinary tract dysfunction

	Suprapontine lesion eg. stroke, Parkinson's disease	Infrapontine-suprasacral lesion eg. myelopathy	Infrasacral lesion eg. conus medullaris, cauda equina, peripheral nerve
History/bladder diary	Urgency, frequency, urgency incontinence	Urgency, frequency, urgency incontinence, hesitancy, retention	Hesitancy, retention
Post-void residual urine (PVR)	No PVR	± Elevated PVR	PVR > 100 ml
Uroflowmetry	Normal flow	Interrupted flow	Poor/absent flow
Urodynamics	Detrusor overactivity	Detrusor overactivity	Detrusor underactivity
		Detrusor sphincter dyssynergia	Sphincter insufficiency

dysfunction. In most instances, clean intermittent self-catheterization (CISC) is the treatment of choice (Chapter 5).

In the first instance, overactive bladder symptoms may be managed by general measures such as regulating fluid intake and types of fluids, behavioral retraining and pelvic floor exercises if storage dysfunction is mild (Chapter 5). However in most instances, antimuscarinic medications are required (Chapter 6). Often it is a combination of antimuscarinics and CISC that is most effective (Fig. 4.9) [32]. Other treatment options include desmopressin and intradetrusor injections of botulinum toxin (Chapter 6). The treatment options offered to a patient should reflect the severity of LUTD, which generally parallels the extent of neurological disease (Fig. 4.10).

Multidisciplinary approach to lower urinary tract dysfunction

In the field of disability, it is important to consider that the aims of management of the neurogenic bladder are not only to improve continence and minimize the urological disease, but to consider the problems in a holistic sense. The evaluation process should retain this comprehensive approach and encompass the various healthcare professionals involved in bladder care. The approach should promote an interactive consultation between the patient and their home carers, continence advisors, general practitioners, neurologists, members of the rehabilitation team (specialist, physiotherapist, occupational therapist) and urologist (Fig. 4.11). A comprehensive evaluation

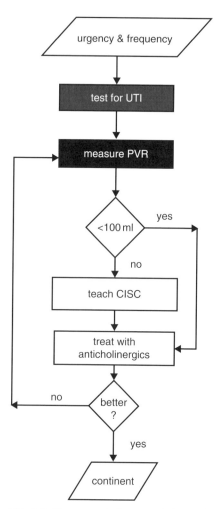

Fig. 4.9. Management of neurogenic lower urinary tract dysfunction. UTI = urinary tract infection; PVR = post-void residual; CISC: clean intermittent self-catheterization. Reproduced from [32] with permission.

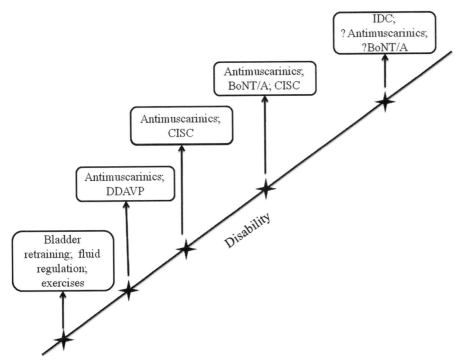

Fig. 4.10. Step-wise approach to neurogenic lower urinary tract dysfunction management. BoNT/A = botulinum toxin A; CISC = clean intermittent self-catheterization, DDAVP = desmopressin, IDC = indwelling catheter, LUTD = lower urinary tract dysfunction.

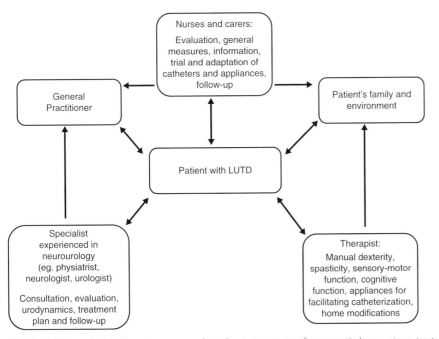

Fig. 4.11. The multidisciplinary team approach to the management of neurogenic lower urinary tract dysfunction (LUTD). With permission from [54].

invoking the ethos of a multidisciplinary approach provides the patient with the most appropriate therapeutic options adapted to the multidimensional needs of the patient.

References

1. de Groat WC, Booth AM. Physiology of the urinary bladder and urethra. *Ann Intern Med* 1980; **92**(Pt 2):312–5.

2. Fowler CJ, Griffiths D, de Groat WC. The neural control of micturition. *Nat Rev Neurosci* 2008; **9**:453–66.

3. Fowler CJ. Integrated control of lower urinary tract – clinical perspective. *Br J Pharmacol* 2006; **147**(Suppl 2):S14–S24.

4. Norris JP, Staskin DR. History, physical examination, and classification of neurogenic voiding dysfunction. *Urol Clin North Am* 1996;**23**:337–43.

5. Stöhrer M, Blok B, Castro-Diaz D, et al. EAU guidelines on neurogenic lower urinary tract dysfunction. *Eur Urol* 2009;**56**:81–8.

6. Madersbacher H. The various types of neurogenic bladder dysfunction: an update of current therapeutic concepts. *Paraplegia* 1990;**28**:217–29.

7. Ahlberg J, Edlund C, Wikkelso C, Rosengren L, Fall M. Neurological signs are common in patients with urodynamically verified "idiopathic" bladder overactivity. *Neurourol Urodyn* 2002;**21**(1):65–70.

8. Haab F, Richard F, Amarenco G, et al. Comprehensive evaluation of bladder and urethral dysfunction symptoms: development and psychometric validation of the Urinary Symptom Profile (USP) questionnaire. *Urology* 2008;**71**:646–56.

9. Andersson KE. The overactive bladder: pharmacologic basis of drug treatment. *Urology* 1997;**50**(6A Suppl):74–84.

10. Abrams P, Cardozo L, Fall M, et al. The standardisation of terminology of lower urinary tract function: report from the Standardisation Sub-committee of the International Continence Society. *Neurourol Urodyn* 2002;**21**:167–78.

11. Van Kerrebroeck P, Abrams P, Chaikin D, et al. The standardization of terminology in nocturia: report from the standardization subcommittee of the International Continence Society. *BJU Int* 2002; **90**(Suppl 3):11–15.

12. Weiss JP. Nocturia: "do the math". *J Urol* 2006; **175**(3 Pt 2):S16–S18.

13. Beck RP, Arnusch D, King C. Results in treating 210 patients with detrusor overactivity incontinence of urine. *Am J Obstet Gynecol* 1976;**125**:593–6.

14. Barry MJ, Fowler FJ, Jr., O'Leary MP, et al. The American Urological Association symptom index for benign prostatic hyperplasia. The Measurement Committee of the American Urological Association. *J Urol* 1992;**148**:1549–57.

15. Uebersax JS, Wyman JF, Shumaker SA, McClish DK, Fantl JA. Short forms to assess life quality and symptom distress for urinary incontinence in women: the Incontinence Impact Questionnaire and the Urogenital Distress Inventory. Continence Program for Women Research Group. *Neurourol Urodyn* 1995;**14**:131–9.

16. Shumaker SA, Wyman JF, Uebersax JS, McClish D, Fantl JA. Health-related quality of life measures for women with urinary incontinence: the Incontinence Impact Questionnaire and the Urogenital Distress Inventory. Continence Program in Women (CPW) Research Group. *Qual Life Res* 1994;**3**:291–306.

17. Schurch B, Denys P, Kozma CM, et al. Reliability and validity of the Incontinence Quality of Life questionnaire in patients with neurogenic urinary incontinence. *Arch Phys Med Rehabil* 2007;**88**:646–52.

18. Lubeck DP, Prebil LA, Peeples P, Brown JS. A health related quality of life measure for use in patients with urge urinary incontinence: a validation study. *Qual Life Res* 1999;**8**:337–44.

19. Coyne K, Revicki D, Hunt T, et al. Psychometric validation of an overactive bladder symptom and health-related quality of life questionnaire: the OAB-q. *Qual Life Res* 2002;**11**:563–74.

20. Costa P, Perrouin-Verbe B, Colvez A, et al. Quality of life in spinal cord injury patients with urinary difficulties. Development and validation of qualiveen. *Eur Urol* 2001;**39**:107–13.

21. Bonniaud V, Bryant D, Parratte B, Gallien P, Guyatt G. Qualiveen: a urinary disorder-specific instrument for use in clinical trials in multiple sclerosis. *Arch Phys Med Rehabil* 2006;**87**:1661–3.

22. Bonniaud V, Bryant D, Parratte B, Guyatt G. Development and validation of the short form of a urinary quality of life questionnaire: SF-Qualiveen. *J Urol* 2008;**180**:2592–8.

23. Acquadro C, Kopp Z, Coyne KS, et al. Translating overactive bladder questionnaires in 14 languages. *Urology* 2006;**67**:536–40.

24. Donovan J, Bosch R, Gotoh M, et al. Symptom and quality of life assessment. In: Abrams P, Cardozo L, Khoury S, Wein A, eds. *Incontinence*. Jersey: Health Publications Ltd; 2005.

25. Homma Y, Ando T, Yoshida M, et al. Voiding and incontinence frequencies: variability of diary data and required diary length. *Neurourol Urodyn* 2002; **21**:204–9.

26. Wyman JF, Choi SC, Harkins SW, Wilson MS, Fantl JA. The urinary diary in evaluation of incontinent women: a test-retest analysis. *Obstet Gynecol* 1988; **71**(6 Pt 1):812–17.

27. Betts CD, D'Mellow MT, Fowler CJ. Urinary symptoms and the neurological features of bladder dysfunction in multiple sclerosis. *J Neurol Neurosurg Psychiatry* 1993;**56**:245–50.

28. Panicker JN, Nagaraja D, Kovoor JM, Nair KP, Subbakrishna DK. Lower urinary tract dysfunction in acute disseminated encephalomyelitis. *Mult Scler* 2009;**15**:1118–22.

29. Staskin DR, Zoltan E. Anticholinergics and central nervous system effects: are we confused? *Rev Urol* 2007;**9**:191–6.

30. Royal College of Nursing. *Catheter Care*. RCN Guidance for Nurses. London: Royal College of Nursing; 2008.

31. Fowlis GA, Waters J, Williams G. The cost effectiveness of combined rapid tests (Multistix) in screening for urinary tract infections. *J R Soc Med* 1994;**87**:681–2.

32. Fowler CJ, Panicker JN, Drake M, et al. A UK consensus on the management of the bladder in multiple sclerosis. *J Neurol Neurosurg Psychiatry* 2009;**80**:470–7.

33. Levey AS, Bosch JP, Lewis JB, et al. A more accurate method to estimate glomerular filtration rate from serum creatinine: a new prediction equation. Modification of Diet in Renal Disease Study Group. *Ann Intern Med* 1999;**130**:461–70.

34. Department of Health. *National service framework for renal services. Part two: chronic kidney disease, acute renal failure and end of life care*. London: Department of Health; 2005.

35. Jenkins MA, Brown DJ, Ierino FL, Ratnaike SI. Cystatin C for estimation of glomerular filtration rate in patients with spinal cord injury. *Ann Clin Biochem* 2003;**40**(Pt 4):364–8.

36. Carroll P, Albertsen P, Greene K, et al. *Prostate-specific antigen best practice statement: 2009 update*. American Urological Association Education and Research, Inc., 2009.

37. Blaivas JG, Appell RA, Fantl JA, et al. Standards of efficacy for evaluation of treatment outcomes in urinary incontinence: recommendations of the Urodynamic Society. *Neurourol Urodyn* 1997; **16**:145–7.

38. Fowler CJ, O'Malley KJ. Investigation and management of neurogenic bladder dysfunction. *J Neurol Neurosurg Psychiatry* 2003; **74**(Suppl 4):iv27–iv31.

39. Stohrer M, Castro-Diaz D, Chartier-Kastler E, et al. Guidelines on neurogenic lower urinary tract dysfunction. *Prog Urol* 2007;**17**:703–55.

40. de Sèze M, Ruffion A, Denys P, Joseph PA, Perrouin-Verbe B. The neurogenic bladder in multiple sclerosis: review of the literature and proposal of management guidelines. *Mult Scler* 2007;**13**:915–28.

41. Schafer W, Abrams P, Liao L, et al. Good urodynamic practices: uroflowmetry, filling cystometry, and pressure-flow studies. *Neurourol Urodyn* 2002;**21**:261–74.

42. Blaivas JG, Groutz A. Bladder outlet obstruction nomogram for women with lower urinary tract symptomatology. *Neurourol Urodyn* 2000;**19**:553–64.

43. Abrams P, Agarwal M, Drake M, et al. A proposed guideline for the urological management of patients with spinal cord injury. *BJU Int* 2008;**101**:989–94.

44. Ruffion A, de Seze M, Denys P, Perrouin-Verbe B, Chartier-Kastler E. Groupe d'Etudes de Neuro-Urologie de Langue Francaise (GENULF) guidelines for the management of spinal cord injury and spina bifida patients. *Prog Urol* 2007;**17**:631–3.

45. Podnar S, Vodusek DB. Standardization of anal sphincter electromyography: utility of motor unit potential parameters. *Muscle Nerve* 2001;**24**:946–51.

46. Podnar S, Trsinar B, Vodusek DB. Bladder dysfunction in patients with cauda equina lesions. *Neurourol Urodyn* 2006;**25**:23–31.

47. Fowler CJ, Christmas TJ, Chapple CR, et al. Abnormal electromyographic activity of the urethral sphincter, voiding dysfunction, and polycystic ovaries: a new syndrome? *BMJ* 1988;**297**:1436–8.

48. Podnar S. Nomenclature of the electrophysiologically tested sacral reflexes. *Neurourol Urodyn* 2006;**25**:95–7.

49. Lefaucheur JP, Labat JJ, Amarenco G, et al. What is the place of electroneuromyographic studies in the diagnosis and management of pudendal neuralgia related to entrapment syndrome? *Neurophysiol Clin* 2007;**37**:223–8.

50. Opsomer RJ, Guerit JM, Wese FX, Van Cangh PJ. Pudendal cortical somatosensory evoked potentials. *J Urol* 1986;**135**:1216–8.

51. Cavalcanti GA, Bruschini H, Manzano GM, et al. Pudendal somatosensory evoked potentials in normal women. *Int Braz J Urol* 2007;**33**:815–21.

52. Delodovici ML, Fowler CJ. Clinical value of the pudendal somatosensory evoked potential. *Electroencephalogr Clin Neurophysiol* 1995;**96**:509–15.

53. Panicker JN, Menon L, Anandkumar A, Sundaram KR, Fowler CJ. Lower urinary tract symptoms following neurological illness may be influenced by multiple factors: observations from a neurorehabilitation service in a developing country. *Neurourol Urodyn* 2010;**29**:378–81.

54. Panicker J, de Sèze M, Fowler C. Neurogenic lower urinary tract dysfunction and its management. *Clin Rehab*. In press.

General measures and non-pharmacological approaches

Jeanette Haslam, Gwen Gonzales and Collette Haslam

Introduction

In a patient with neurological disease, bladder dysfunction is not likely to be an isolated problem and there needs to be realistic treatment and support. Neurological bladder dysfunction can result in both storage and voiding dysfunction and many patients require practical strategies to complement medical management. This chapter gives an overview of the range of non-pharmacological management strategies available for overactive bladder symptoms and voiding dysfunction that are usually offered by nurses and physiotherapists that specialize in continence.

Management of overactive bladder symptoms

Fluid intake

Many patients with neurological bladder dysfunction drink less as their first strategy to reduce their urinary frequency. However, it is generally recommended for the patient to drink 1.5–2 litres in 24 hours, the amount being individualized as appropriate. An assessment of fluid balance using a voiding diary is often helpful (Chapter 4) [1]. Many people report reduction in frequency after reducing caffeine intake [2]. Many patients report worsening bladder symptoms when they are constipated and although there is accumulating scientific evidence about the neural "cross-talk" between the bladder and the bowel, there is little relevant clinical objective measurement of this phenomenon.

Behavioral retraining

Advice on scheduled voiding may be necessary, as patients often go to the toilet not through need but just because a toilet is available – "just in case." This can become a habit and increase voiding frequency. A frequency/voiding chart (Chapter 4) may prove useful in this instance to ascertain over a couple of days the actual fluid intake and any relation to frequency, urgency and incontinence.

Timing toileting and building confidence in the bladder's ability to hold urine can help to alleviate some bladder symptoms such as frequency and urgency. Bladder or behavioral retraining has been shown to be of benefit if the patient is aware of the principle and is committed to the program [3, 4]. However, patients with neurological disease may find this difficult to do because of cognitive impairment or loss of voluntary control. Accurate record keeping, guided education and support from family and medical staff are important for this method to have any success.

Pelvic floor treatments

Initial assessment

A continence assessment should precede any proposed management strategy and this is best carried out by a doctor, nurse or physiotherapist who has an understanding of neurological dysfunction and the possible long-term effect on the patient. This commences with an appropriate individualized assessment of pelvic organ dysfunction and a more in-depth neurological assessment as necessary [5]. The assessment is supplemented by more objective measures of bladder dysfunction such as urodynamics (Chapter 4).

Assessment of any patient commences from first contact, observing mobility, gait and general appearance. Although the referral may be for a neurological

Pelvic Organ Dysfunction in Neurological Disease: Clinical Management and Rehabilitation, ed. Clare J. Fowler,
Jalesh N. Panicker & Anton Emmanuel. Published by Cambridge University Press. © Cambridge University Press 2010.

condition, "life factors" can also affect pelvic organ dysfunction. Pelvic organ dysfunction in a female may be influenced by pregnancy, childbirth, pelvic surgery or hormonal changes in addition to her neurological condition. Similarly, a man may have prostate enlargement or have had surgery or other relevant medical history contributing to his bladder symptoms.

A full medical and surgical history should be taken, including questions regarding bladder and bowel problems or sexual dysfunction. Specific problems can then be discussed in greater detail [6]. Anyone with a neurological condition will require more in-depth questioning regarding their specific condition and a thorough assessment of the relevant dermatomes, myotomes and reflexes (Chapters 4 and 17).

Physical examination

A physical examination of the pelvic floor is necessary if dysfunction is suspected. After informed consent has been given, assistance to disrobe should be offered and a chaperone made available if wanted.

Female examination

External examination can provide information about the condition of the skin and mucosa and to determine any loss of skin sensation, signs of pelvic organ prolapse or atrophic vaginitis, and ability to contract and relax the pelvic floor muscles (PFM). Internal vaginal assessment is essential to determine an appropriate PFM exercise program or other therapy. After separation of the labia, a gloved, lubricated index finger is introduced into the vagina to initially check for any areas of tenderness, pain or reduced/absence of sensations. PFM bulk, resting activity and reaction to cough can all be palpated. Different sections of the PFM can be assessed for quality and duration of response on both sides [6]. Historically, UK physiotherapists and specifically trained nurses have used the modified Oxford grading system, described by Laycock and Jerwood, using a score of 0–5 for voluntary muscle contraction [7]. The International Continence Society has suggested a scale in which voluntary contraction of the PFM be described as absent, weak, normal or strong and voluntary relaxation described as absent, partial or complete [8]; this latter scale is now recommended. In addition to PFM strength, the duration and number of contractions are assessed for an individualized exercise

regimen. Instruction can also be given how to pre-contract and maintain a PFM contraction during a cough or other rises in intra-abdominal pressure, known as teaching "the knack" [9].

Male examination

Male perineal examination involves observing a penile/testicular lift and anal wink, followed by an appropriate anorectal examination. Further description of this may be found in Dorey [10].

Treatment plan

The patient must be informed of what is realistically required of them when planning pelvic floor treatments and a treatment plan agreed, taking full account of home and work life to aid compliance. Written or other forms of instruction should be provided as reference aids; these will include the particular exercise regimen that has been agreed. Discussion also needs to take place regarding any other proposed therapy, realistic expectations, follow-up times and methods of communication.

Treatments

Rationale for PFM training in detrusor overactivity

There are two theories that have good research-based evidence [11] and which underpin PFM training:

- strength training
- precontraction of the PFM prior to any rise in intra-abdominal pressure.

De Ridder et al. [12] showed that pelvic floor training was useful (decreasing frequency and daily incontinence episodes and increasing mean functional bladder capacity) in people with multiple sclerosis having a low Kurtzke score and without pelvic floor spasticity. More recently McClurg et al. [13] also found PFM training effective for those with multiple sclerosis and lower urinary tract dysfunction.

The urgency experienced with an overactive bladder can also be partially or totally suppressed by contracting the PFM, harnessing the "perineo-detrusor inhibitory reflex," as described by Mahoney et al. [14] and investigated further by Shafik and Shafik [15], sometimes also known as the "pro-continence reflex" (see Chapter 1 for the neurological basis). Both PFM training and suppression techniques will require intact neural pathways.

Table 5.1. Suggested parameters for PFM vaginal/anal stimulation

	Frequency	Pulse duration	Intensity	Duty cycle
Stress incontinence	35–40 Hz	0.25 ms	Sufficient to provoke a PFM contraction, e.g. *vaginal*: observed by a deflection of the indicator attached to a Periform (Neen Healthcare, UK)	Determined by strength/endurance of a voluntary contraction. The "off" time is always at least double the "on" time
			anal: sphincter contraction	
Detrusor inhibition	5–10 Hz	0.5–1.0 ms	Maximum current tolerated	Continuous or short rest periods every 10 seconds

Therapeutic electrical stimulation

PFM electrical stimulation techniques are performed with an appropriately designed stimulator and have been used for both stress incontinence and detrusor overactivity. An electrical impulse generator is applied via the vagina, anus, perineal body, penis or clitoris.

Therapists include electrical stimulation as part of therapy for those with symptoms of stress incontinence, or sometimes detrusor overactivity, and it should be considered for:

- initiating a contraction and increasing cortical awareness of the PFM when there is an intact neural pathway but an inability to perform a voluntary contraction. The technique aims to have the patient "joining in" with the electrically induced contractions to gain increased cortical awareness and control. Once this ability has been gained or regained, the aim is to use active exercise appropriate for the individual.

- assisting in normalizing reflex activity for bladder inhibition.

It is thought that the resulting reflex pelvic floor contraction has the same inhibitory effect on detrusor activity as does a voluntary contraction of pelvic floor muscles. Care must be taken during assessment to ascertain that there are no contraindications to stimulation and to determine the correct stimulation parameters (Table 5.1). A study of multiple sclerosis patients showed that the addition of neuromuscular electrical stimulation to a program of pelvic floor muscle training and EMG biofeedback had superior outcomes [16].

Parameters used should be in line with current evidence and should be appropriate for the individual.

Stimulation should be started with shorter time periods to ensure that there are no adverse effects.

Biofeedback

Biofeedback for pelvic floor therapy usually utilizes auditory or visual feedback to enhance a person's knowledge of a particular muscle's activity. McClurg et al. used EMG vaginal or anal biofeedback as part of the PFM training in 37 people with multiple sclerosis and lower urinary tract dysfunction. The positive results in the study led to the conclusion that some form of PFM training should be used as a standard therapy in a rehabilitation program for those with multiple sclerosis and lower urinary tract dysfunction [16].

Recently, Bo and Herbert [17] cautioned against the use of new interventions until their effectiveness had been demonstrated in high-quality randomized clinical trials. However, clinicians may find the use of more recent interventions, such as the use of real-time ultrasound as a method of biofeedback or core stability exercise to initiate PFM contractions, helpful in their practice. Impairment and dysfunction can be multifactorial and the wise therapist keeps an open mind to appropriate therapies whilst heeding and encouraging research. The aim of treatment is to gain control and lessen dysfunction wherever possible, irrespective of the therapeutic method employed.

Posterior tibial nerve stimulation

Posterior tibial nerve stimulation is a minimally invasive treatment option for patients with overactive bladder symptoms. The posterior tibial nerve, a mixed peripheral nerve originating from the same spinal segments as the parasympathetic innervation to the bladder, is stimulated via a needle inserted percutaneously above the medial malleolus. Studies into the treatment of neurogenic detrusor overactivity in patients with multiple sclerosis [18] and Parkinson's disease [19] have shown promising results using posterior tibial nerve stimulation.

Management of voiding dysfunction

Patients with voiding dysfunction complain of hesitancy (difficulty in initiating urinary flow) or difficulty in passing urine. Over time, they often develop their own methods for bladder emptying, such as tapping on the lower abdomen, digital stimulation of the area of the urethral opening (females), rubbing behind the scrotal area (males) and movements such as standing and sitting to induce a detrusor contraction. Many patients use the Credé's maneuver (application of non-forceful, smooth, even pressure from the umbilicus towards the pubis) or hold their breath and bear down (Valsalva maneuver) to aid emptying. There is concern that these can predispose to pelvic organ prolapse and vesicoureteric reflux, and they should not be encouraged [20, 21].

There are little published data on the use of non-invasive aids to enhance voiding in patients with neurogenic bladders. Dasgupta et al. [22] described the use of a small hand-held vibrating device placed on the lower abdomen that helped reduce the post-void residual in a number of MS patients with detrusor hyperreflexia and incomplete emptying who were still relatively mobile and who were able to feel the vibrating stimulus in the suprapubic region. An improvement in flow and reduction in residual volume were seen; however, the mechanism of action is uncertain and results of using this in clinical practice are variable [23].

Bladder emptying should be assisted if a raised post-void residual volume is demonstrated either by in-out catheterization or by ultrasound. A value of 100 ml is commonly taken as the amount of residual urine that contributes to bladder dysfunction, as bladder capacity is usually also reduced by overactivity of the detrusor [24]. It is recognized that a single measurement of the post-void residual volume is not representative and, when possible, a series of measurements should be made over the course of one or two weeks. Often, patients are unaware that they have a large residual volume that may be contributing to their bladder symptoms. In most instances, clean intermittent self-catheterization (CISC) is the treatment of choice for managing a patient who has persistently elevated post-void residual urine. Guidance notes are available for planning and following up patients who require catheters [25].

Intermittent catheterization

CISC was introduced by Lapides et al. [26] and is now a well-accepted technique for the management of both neurogenic and non-neurogenic voiding dysfunction. It greatly reduces the risk of urinary tract infections, and has fewer complications compared to indwelling catheterization [27]. In many cases, the optimal management is a combination of antimuscarinic (anticholinergic) medication with CISC, as this is often the most effective management for neurological bladder dysfunction (Chapter 4 and Appendix 1) [24]. CISC is a simple technique which can transform people's lives. It can give the patient control of bladder emptying, and safeguard their renal function.

The concept of CISC is often quite alien to patients and many nurses are also not familiar with it. To succeed with the technique, the patient should be motivated, with a clear understanding of the reasons for starting CISC and the duration for which it will be required. Good professional instruction, ongoing support and education are necessary to maintain patient compliance [25, 28]. Though the technique may be taught in the hospital setting, it is preferable to follow up the patient in an outpatient clinic or at home.

For women the use of a mirror is usually necessary at the outset to help locate their urethra. However, with experience, it would be hoped that this would no longer be necessary so that CISC could be practised with ease, away from home. The teaching environment should be private and comfortable; privacy and dignity should be maintained at all times [25]. When taught by knowledgeable professionals, patients may require only one teaching session to become competent. However, others may require a few sessions to feel confident about performing the procedure themselves [29]. The frequency of catheterization should be advised at the time of teaching and may range from once a day to once every four hours (during the daytime), depending upon fluid intake and residual volumes.

For patients with neurological disabilities, impaired manual dexterity, visual disturbances, mobility problems and reduced cognition may influence their ability to carry out CISC safely and effectively [25]. Appliances are available that may facilitate CISC

Table 5.2. Details of a selection of single-use intermittent catheters

Name of catheter	Manufacturer	Coating
LoFric	Astra	Hydrophilic
SpeediCath	Coloplast	Hydrophilic
Actreen Glys	B/Braun	Lubricant gel
Advance	Hollister	Lubricant gel

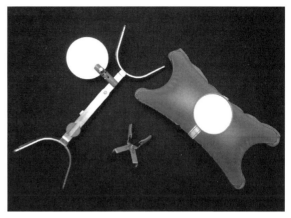

Fig. 5.2. Selection of appliances that may aid leg abduction and labia separation if CISC is difficult owing to hand and leg function.

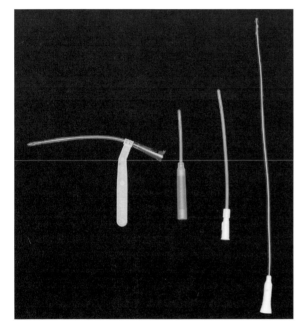

Fig. 5.1. Selection of intermittent catheters (some require lubrication prior to use, others come with a hydrophilic coating or gel).

(Fig. 5.2). In some situations, the technique can be taught to carers if consent is agreed [22]. Diagrams of the lower urinary tract anatomy assist in learning. There are a variety of leaflets, booklets and teaching materials available from the many catheter manufacturers that can assist with teaching of the procedure. Companies provide clinical representatives who often work alongside the continence advisor, the community care worker and patients.

Neurological patients require ongoing support and it is therefore important to give patients and carers the relevant contact numbers and subsequent follow-up appointments where they can discuss their ongoing condition and any concerns.

With a myriad of catheters available in the market, the patient needs guidance as to what is most appropriate for them (Fig. 5.1 and Table 5.2). Most catheters nowadays for CISC are intended to be disposable (single use), though there are a few that are designed to be cleaned and reused. Appliances can help facilitate CISC in patients with neurological disabilities (Fig. 5.2).

Indwelling catheterization

The purpose of indwelling catheters is for short- or long-term urinary drainage when alternative methods of urine drainage are unsuitable or no longer appropriate for the patient. With the progression of some neurological conditions, patients may be unable to intermittently self-catheterize due to their increased disability, worsening detrusor overactivity and declining bladder capacity. If containment methods such as pads and sheaths are not appropriate, indwelling catheterization may have to be considered. Importantly, the patient and carer should not think that the need for catheters represents a failure on their part. The use of an indwelling catheter can be beneficial in reducing the worry of toileting inside and outside the home, and in carrying out day-to-day activities with confidence. However, problems with catheterization such as catheter-associated infection, frequent bladder spasms resulting in urine leakage and/or catheter expulsion (especially noticeable in neurological patients) [30, 31], trauma and recurrent blockage are not uncommon [27].

The common route for urinary catheterization is via the urethra; however, suprapubic catheterization (through an incision in the abdominal wall, just above

Table 5.3. Advantages of suprapubic catheterization

Maintains urethral integrity

Ease of catheter change

Improved perineal hygiene

Permits teaching of CISC per urethra if appropriate

Conducive to sexual activity

Table 5.4. Selection of catheter and duration of use

Catheter material	Maximum duration of use
Uncoated latex	7 days
Plastic or PVC	7 days
Silver alloy hydrogen coated latex	28 days
PTFE (teflon) coated latex	28 days
Hydrogen coated latex	12 weeks
Hydrogen coated silicone	12 weeks
Silicone elastomer coated latex	12 weeks
All silicone	12 weeks

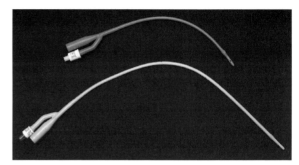

Fig. 5.3. Indwelling catheter – male and female.

the symphysis pubis) is an alternative. Both types of catheter may be associated with urinary tract infections, bypassing (urine leakage around the catheter) and blockage. However, studies have shown that there are benefits of suprapubic over urethral catheterization (Table 5.3) and this should be considered as the favored option for long-term bladder drainage in neurological patients [24, 32]. A note of caution should be sounded here about the insertion of a suprapubic catheter. Whereas this may be a simple procedure in a man with long-standing prostatic outflow obstruction who has a large bladder which has expanded out of the pelvis, patients with advanced neurological disease needing a suprapubic catheter are likely to have a small, contracted bladder which is difficult to locate and there is a risk that attempts to insert the catheter trocar may penetrate overlying bowel loops. Fatalities have been reported in recent years to the National Patient Safety Agency (NPSA) due to fecal peritonitis and there are now stringent national guidelines relating to the procedure (Chapter 7). However, after initial surgery and first catheter change, catheter management can be routinely carried out in the community setting.

Types of indwelling catheters

The self-retaining catheter, introduced by Frederic Foley in the 1930s, remains the most commonly used type of catheter today. Catheters for general use have a double-lumen shaft, one for drainage and the other for inflation or deflation of the retention balloon. To minimize catheter complications, various coatings have been applied to the catheters. Selection of the type of catheter is dependent on the indication, comfort to the patient and presence of any allergies (Table 5.4).

Catheters are made in two lengths: approximately 26 cm for women and 43 cm for men (Fig. 5.3), and in sizes 6–24 Charrière units (Ch) or French gauge (Fg). The diameter in millimeters of the catheter can be determined by dividing the French size by 3, thus an increasing French size corresponds with a larger diameter catheter. Size 12 Ch is usually sufficient for normal urine drainage [33]. The female length catheter should only be used for women as insertion in males can cause severe trauma to the longer male urethra. However, the male length catheter is preferred by some women, in particular those who are obese or who are in wheelchairs, since the longer length allows easier access to the catheter and urine drainage [27].

Urine drainage bags

Various drainage bags are available for use with an indwelling catheter (Fig. 5.4). Drainage bags are available with a range of fluid volume capacities from 350 to 2000 ml. The choice depends on the type of use and fluid volume drained. Bags are usually supplied with leg straps made of Velcro or elastic and, though helpful when ambulant, the straps can cause discomfort if applied too tightly around the leg. Indwelling urethral catheters can cause urethral trauma if there is catheter tension due to excessive filling of the bag, and

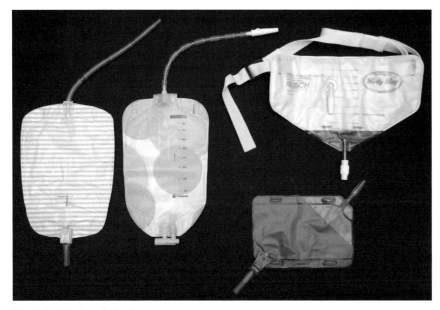

Fig. 5.4. Selection of urine bags.

hence patients are usually advised to empty their bag when it is three-quarters full. Body-worn aids such as net sleeves or waist supports are available for supporting the bag.

The majority of bags are manufactured with a range of inlet lengths from 5 to 40 cm and patients may have a selection of bags depending on their daily activity and preferred clothing. For patients with reduced manual dexterity, the type of drainage outlet tap is very important as some taps are easier to open and close with one hand than others. Bags are usually made of plastic, and some come with a soft material backing for patient comfort. To reduce the risk of ascending infection, a sterile bag with a non-return valve is essential and it is usually advised to be changed weekly [27].

Catheter valves

The introduction of catheter valves (Fig. 5.5) provided an alternative to continuous drainage into a bag for patients with adequate bladder storage capacity. The valve, which is connected to the catheter, allows filling of the bladder and emptying at a convenient time, as would occur with normal bladder function. Use of a catheter valve is suitable for patients who have a stable, reasonable capacity bladder (over 300 ml); volumes less than this would require too frequent

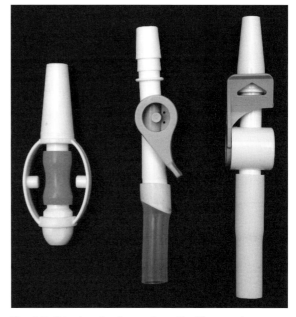

Fig. 5.5. Selection of catheter valves with different outlet mechanisms.

opening of the valve and may increase the risk of contamination and pressure rises. Valves are not recommended for patients with renal impairment. Patients must be able to sense the need to empty the bladder and, as with catheter bags, must be able to

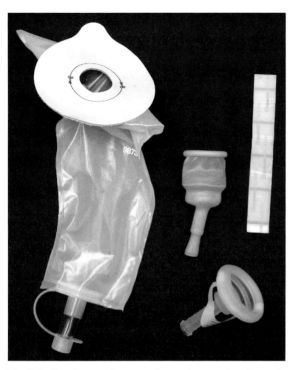

Fig. 5.6. Sheaths: one-piece, two-piece and retracted penis pouch.

manipulate the outlet. Valves are designed to be used for one week or three months, depending on the manufacturer's guidelines. The usual recommendation is to use the valve during the day and attach a drainage bag at night for continuous drainage, although some valves do not have this facility [34].

Appliances to aid continence

At times, patients may require advice on the use of appliances or aids to contain incontinence. It is essential that the appropriate professional (including nurses, physiotherapists and occupational therapists) assesses the patient and works in cooperation with other members of the team to ensure the optimum management plan. Reduced mobility, manual dexterity and cognitive problems must be considered in selecting the most suitable appliance to maintain the patient's dignity and self-esteem when carrying out daily activities. Individual patients may have their own personal requirements as to what they want or require from a product, but in general their first priority is usually containment of any possible leakage. The following subsections discuss appliances that may aid in the management of urine leakage.

Appliances for men

Although intermittent self-catheterization is the method of choice in managing bladder dysfunction in most men, some patients may be unable or unwilling to use a catheter. For men who have urgency/urge incontinence or post-micturition dribbling, a penile sheath system may be the preferred method to contain urine (Fig. 5.6). A penile sheath (also known as a condom urinal, external catheter or incontinence sheath) fits over the penis and is designed to fit onto a non-sterile drainage bag for the collection of urine. It should be changed daily for skin washing and skin inspection. Sheaths vary in size and materials and are unsuitable for men with a small or retracted penis, those who are cognitively impaired and may become confused and pull the device off, and those with reduced manual dexterity. For men who are unable to use the sheath system, an alternative for containment is body-worn urinals. For best compliance, use of the sheath system should be taught to the patient or carer [35].

Absorbent products

The majority of patients with urinary incontinence will have already tried some form of absorbent pad (Fig. 5.7). These are popular with some patients as they are readily available from local shops and they are no longer considered as "taboo" by many people owing to aggressive marketing from companies. Nevertheless there will always be some patients who consider pad usage only as a last resort. There is a wide range of specifically designed pads, and the choice of pad depends on usage, absorbency (amount and type of incontinence) and comfort. Four types of basic design are available:

1. insert pads with waterproof backing – used with net pants for correct fitting
2. insert pads without backing – used with pants that have waterproofing
3. male disposable pouches – used with net pants, Y fronts or pants with waterproof pouches
4. all-in-one disposables – usually used for heavy incontinence.

All products are available in various absorbencies. Some are made of washable materials, and these are becoming more popular for economic and ecological reasons [35].

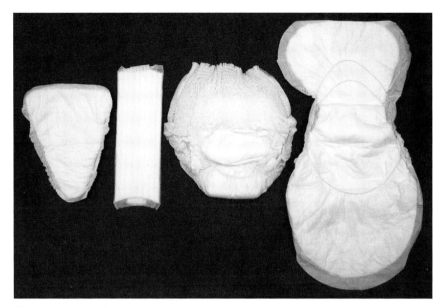

Fig. 5.7. Selection of incontinence pads.

Urinals

A selection of hand-held urinals are available for both male and females. The choice depends on hand function, mobility and carer availability. These are especially useful as they are portable when toilet access is difficult and when detrusor overactivity is the main problem.

Conclusion

Many bladder symptoms can be managed conservatively and it has been shown that successful management with continence products can alleviate the potential detrimental effects on social and working lives and personal relationships [36]. However, for most neurological patients, this must go alongside physical and medical management. Aspects of conservative management should be considered on an individual patient basis. Importantly, neurological deficits can influence toileting and people with neurological conditions are likely to require long-term continence support.

References

1. Hashim H, Abrams P. How should patients with an overactive bladder manipulate their fluid intake? *BJU Int* 2008;**102**:62–6.

2. Bryant CM, Dowell CJ, Fairbrother G. Caffeine reduction education to improve urinary symptoms. *Br J Nurs* 2002;**11**:560–5.

3. Wallace SA, Roe B, Williams K, Palmer M. Bladder training for urinary incontinence in adults. *Cochrane Database Syst Rev* 2004(1):CD001308.

4. Ostaszkiewicz J, Roe B, Johnston L. Effects of timed voiding for the management of urinary incontinence in adults: systematic review. *J Adv Nurs* 2005;**52**:420–31.

5. Lennon S, Stokes M. *Pocketbook of neurological physiotherapy*. Edinburgh: Churchill Livingstone; 2008.

6. Laycock J, Whelan M, Dumoulin C. Patient assessment. In: Haslam J, Laycock J, eds. *Therapeutic management of incontinence and pelvic pain*. London: Springer-Verlag; 2008:57–66.

7. Laycock J, Jerwood D. Pelvic floor assessment; the PERFECT scheme. *Physiotherapy* 2001;**87**:632–42.

8. Messelink B, Benson T, Berghmans B, et al. Standardization of terminology of pelvic floor muscle function and dysfunction: report from the pelvic floor clinical assessment group of the International Continence Society. *Neurourol Urodyn* 2005;**24**:374–80.

9. Miller JM, Ashton-Miller JA, DeLancey JO. A pelvic muscle precontraction can reduce cough-related urine loss in selected women with mild SUI. *J Am Geriatr Soc* 1998;**46**:870–4.

10. Dorey G. The male patient. In: Haslam J, Laycock J, eds. *Therapeutic management of incontinence and pelvic pain*. Second edn. London: Springer-Verlag; 2008:159–62.

11. Bo K. Pelvic floor muscle training is effective in treatment of female stress urinary incontinence, but

how does it work? *Int Urogynecol J Pelvic Floor Dysfunct* 2004;**15**:76–84.

12. De Ridder D, Vermeulen C, Ketelaer P, Van Poppel H, Baert L. Pelvic floor rehabilitation in multiple sclerosis. *Acta Neurol Belg* 1999;**99**:61–4.

13. McClurg D, Lowe-Strong A, Ashe R. Pelvic floor training for lower urinary tract dysfunction in MS. *Nurs Times* 2009;**105**:45–7.

14. Mahony DT, Laferte RO, Blais DJ. Integral storage and voiding reflexes. Neurophysiologic concept of continence and micturition. *Urology* 1977;**9**:95–106.

15. Shafik A, Shafik IA. Overactive bladder inhibition in response to pelvic floor muscle exercises. *World J Urol* 2003;**20**:374–7.

16. McClurg D, Ashe RG, Lowe-Strong AS. Neuromuscular electrical stimulation and the treatment of lower urinary tract dysfunction in multiple sclerosis – a double blind, placebo controlled, randomised clinical trial. *Neurourol Urodyn* 2008;**27**:231–7.

17. Bo K, Herbert R. When and how should new therapies become routine clinical practice?. *Physiotherapy* 2009;**95**:51–7.

18. Kabay SC, Yucel M, Kabay S. Acute effect of posterior tibial nerve stimulation on neurogenic detrusor overactivity in patients with multiple sclerosis: urodynamic study. *Urology* 2008;**71**:641–5.

19. Kabay S, Kabay SC, Yucel M, Ozden H. Acute urodynamic effects of percutaneous posterior tibial nerve stimulation on neurogenic detrusor overactivity in patients with Parkinson's disease. *Neurourol Urodyn* 2009;**28**:62–7.

20. Fader M, Craggs M. Continence problems and neurological disability. In: Getliffe K, Dolman M, eds. *Promoting continence: a clinical and research resource.* London: Baillière Tindall (Elsevier Science); 2003:337–70.

21. Abrams P, Agarwal M, Drake M, et al. A proposed guideline for the urological management of patients with spinal cord injury. *BJU Int* 2008;**101**:989–94.

22. Dasgupta P, Haslam C, Goodwin R, Fowler C. The Queen Square bladder stimulator: a device for assisting emptying of the neurogenic bladder. *Br J Urol* 1997;**80**:234–7.

23. Prasad RS, Smith SJ, Wright H. Lower abdominal pressure versus external bladder stimulation to aid bladder emptying in multiple sclerosis: a randomized controlled study. *Clin Rehabil* 2003;**17**:42–7.

24. Fowler CJ, Panicker JN, Drake M, et al. A UK consensus on the management of the bladder in multiple sclerosis. *J Neurol Neurosurg Psychiatry* 2009;**80**:470–7.

25. Royal College of Nursing. *Catheter Care. RCN Guidance for Nurses.* London: Royal College of Nursing; 2008.

26. Lapides J, Diokno AC, Silber SJ, Lowe BS. Clean, intermittent self-catheterization in the treatment of urinary tract disease. *J Urol* 1972;**107**:458–61.

27. Getliffe K, Fader M. Catheters and containment products. In: Getliffe K, Dolman M, eds. *Promoting continence: a clinical and research resource.* London: Baillière Tindall (Elsevier Science); 2007:159–308.

28. Logan K. Designing a catheter skills training programme. *Nurs Times* 2008;**104**:42–3.

29. Scottish Intercollegiate Guidelines Network. *Management of urinary incontinence in primary care – a national clinical guideline.* Edinburgh: Scottish Intercollegiate Guidelines Network; 2008.

30. Pomfret I. Urinary catheterization: selection and clinical management. *Br J Community Nurs* 2007;**12**:348–54.

31. Pomfret I. Catheter care – trouble shooting. *Journal of Community Nursing* 1991;**13**:20–4.

32. MacDiarmid SA, Arnold EP, Palmer NB, Anthony A. Management of spinal cord injured patients by indwelling suprapubic catheterization. *J Urol* 1995;**154** (2 Pt 1):492–4.

33. Ebner A, Madersbacher H, Schober F, et al. Hydrodynamic properties of Foley catheters and its clinical relevance. *Proceedings of the International Continence Society 15th Meeting.* London: 1985.

34. Disability Equipment Assessment. *Catheter valves – a multi-centre comparative evaluation.* London: Medical Device Agency; 1997.

35. Dasgupta P, Haslam C. Treatment of neurogenic bladder dysfunction. In: Fowler C, ed. *Neurology of bladder, bowel and sexual dysfunction.* Boston: Butterworth Heinemann; 1999:163–83.

36. Paterson J. Stigma associated with post-prostatectomy urinary incontinence. *Journal of Wound, Ostomy and Continence Nursing* 2000;**27**:168–73.

Neurogenic bladder dysfunction: pharmacological interventional approaches

Apostolos Apostolidis, Soumendra Nath Datta, Xavier Gamé and Shahid Khan

Introduction

Neurogenic bladder dysfunction has many different pathogeneses (Chapter 1) and one drug or therapeutic mechanism would be unlikely to be effective for all causes. Dysfunction at various neurological sites results in disturbances in filling or storage of urine with or without abnormalities of voiding and emptying, which in turn contribute to incontinence. The majority of pharmacological interventions are aimed at diminishing neurogenic detrusor overactivity (NDO) and therefore increasing bladder capacity.

Treatment of NDO

Although efficacious, pharmacological interventions frequently have side-effects, which may limit their use. The aim is to obtain symptom relief without interfering with bladder emptying, although rarely is this achieved. However, a proportion of patients taking medication will also need to perform clean intermittent self-catheterization (CISC) already so that further impairment of bladder emptying induced by medication may be manageable.

Antimuscarinic (anticholinergic) drugs
Scientific background – mechanism of action

Antimuscarinic medication has long been the gold standard for treatment of NDO but its exact mechanism of action is still unknown. Until a few years ago the received wisdom was that antimuscarinic drugs act by blocking the detrusor muscarinic receptors which are stimulated by the release of acetylcholine (ACh) from the parasympathetic, cholinergic innervation. However, this traditional view was challenged when, based on the observation that they act mainly

during the storage phase decreasing symptoms of urgency and increasing bladder capacity, it was proposed their action was predominantly on afferents [1]. There is normally no parasympathetic input into the lower urinary tract during the filling phase but there is evidence that antimuscarinics decrease C-fibers and Aδ bladder afferent activity [1, 2]. Animal experiments have shown an efficacy of tolterodine in NDO, but that it is ineffective after treatment with intravesical resiniferatoxin – a capsaicin analogue that induces C-fiber afferent desensitization [3], suggesting that the afferent nerves (Aδ- and C-fibers) are fundamental to its mode of action. Studies measuring afferent nerve activity directly recorded from the pelvic nerves of rats show that both oxybutynin and darifenacin reduce activity in Aδ- and C-fiber afferents [1, 2]. In healthy women, tolterodine has been shown to increase the sensory threshold to electrical stimulation of the bladder, which the authors speculated could be due to tolterodine's effect on the suburothelium [4]. These experimental observations all point to the conclusion that antimuscarinics act on the afferent pathway in the bladder storage phase.

The majority of muscarinic receptors expressed in the detrusor are M2 or M3 but it is the smaller M3 population that mediate detrusor contraction [5]. The main pathway for M3-mediated contraction in the human detrusor is by calcium ion influx via L-type calcium channels and inhibition of myosin light-chain phosphatase through activation of Rho-kinase and protein kinase C, leading to increased sensitivity of the contractile mechanism to the increased calcium ion concentration [6, 7]. The functional role of the M2 receptor has yet to be elucidated; knockout mice studies suggest that M2 receptors indirectly enhance the contractile response

Pelvic Organ Dysfunction in Neurological Disease: Clinical Management and Rehabilitation, ed. Clare J. Fowler, Jalesh N. Panicker & Anton Emmanuel. Published by Cambridge University Press. © Cambridge University Press 2010.

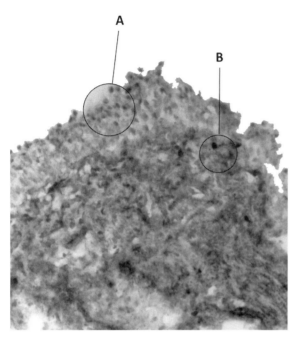

Fig. 6.1. Superficial layers of the bladder labelled with M3 antibody (black). M3 receptors are present (A) in the apical layer of the urothelium and (B) within cell and neuronal structures in the suburothelium.

to M3 receptor activation [8] but there may also be minor M2-mediated direct detrusor contractions. Bladder muscle specimens from patients with NDO have shown that contractions may partially be mediated by the M2 receptors [9].

Muscarinic receptors are found on bladder urothelial and suburothelial cells (Fig. 6.1) but the role for these receptors is yet to be elucidated [10, 11]. A significant increase in suburothelial cell M2 and M3 receptor immunoreactivity has been found in human IDO compared to controls [11]. There is release of ACh from non-neurogenic sources in the urothelium and suburothelium [12, 13] and it has been postulated that it is a combination of ACh and adenosine-5'-triphosphate (ATP) released during the storage phase that has an excitatory effect on nerves in the suburothelium and the detrusor, and which gives rise to bladder afferent activity [14]. Thus it seems likely that the urothelium and suburothelium may be the key therapeutic targets of antimuscarinic drugs.

Importantly, since these drugs work as competitive antagonists, their effects are less significant in the presence of a large concentration of agonist, i.e. ACh as is released during bladder contraction. Although antimuscarinics can cause urinary retention in large doses, the small doses used therapeutically do not cause a reduction in the voiding contraction [16].

Clinical efficacy

All the antimuscarinics with Level 2 or above evidence (Table 6.1) have demonstrated efficacy in the treatment of DO and overactive bladder symptoms. Large-scale, randomized, placebo-controlled studies have shown significant reductions in urinary frequency, urgency episodes and urgency urinary incontinence (UUI) episodes [17, 18]. The currently licensed antimuscarinic drugs in the United Kingdom are listed in Table 6.2.

The clinical relevance of the efficacy of antimuscarinic drugs was questioned by the Herbison's systematic review in 2003, with the conclusion that although they produce statistically significant improvements over placebo, the benefits are of limited clinical significance [18]. Larger, more recent meta-analyses refuted that view by including currently used drugs, showing that this class of drugs are of clinically significant benefit [17, 19, 20]. Chapple et al.'s 2005 systematic review attempted to address the criticisms of Herbison's review by looking at quality-of-life data in included trials and split up the different drugs to assess any variation between them [17]. The conclusions of that review were that antimuscarinics were efficacious, safe and well tolerated, with marked improvements in quality of life. The review criticised the quality of reporting in the selected studies, the limited quality-of-life data and minimal data on older patients. Few trials looked at older patients (>65 years) and at patients with NDO.

An update in 2008 looked at 73 blinded, randomized, placebo- and active-controlled trials of oral and transdermal antimuscarinics to treat overactive bladder (from over 12,000 references) [19]. Antimuscarinics were found to be more effective than placebo, with good tolerability. The mean change with anticholinergic medication was between 0.4 and 1.1 incontinence episodes per day. There were no statistically significant differences for efficacy among treatments in meta-analyses of active controlled trials. All drugs were well tolerated but oxybutynin instant release (IR) was associated with a higher risk of trial withdrawal. Tolterodine 2 mg IR and oxybutynin transdermal system were associated with adverse events similar

Table 6.1 (i) Drugs used in the treatment of detrusor overactivity and the evidence for them from the International Consultation on Incontinence, Paris 2008, reproduced from *Curr Urol* 2009, 19: 38. (ii) International Consultation on Incontinence assessments 2008 using modified Oxford Guidelines

Antimuscarinics	Level of evidence	Grade of recommendation
Tolterodine	1	A
Trospium	1	A
Solefencin	1	A
Darifenacin	1	A
Propantheline	2	B
Atropine, hyoscamine	3	C
Drugs with mixed actions		
Oxybutynin	1	A
Propiverine	1	A
Dicyclomine	3	C
Flavoxate	2	D
Antidepressants		
Imipramine	3	C
Duloxetine	2	C
α-adrenoceptor antagonists		
Alfuzosin	3	C
Doxazosin	3	C
Terazosin	3	C
Tamsulosin	3	C
PDE-5 inhibitors		
Sildenafil, tadalafil, vardenafil	2	B
Toxins		
BoNT (neurogenic)[a]	2	A
BoNT (idiopathic)[a]	3	B
Capsaicin (neurogenic)[b]	2	C
Resiniferatoxin (neurogenic)[b]	2	C
Hormones		
Desmopressin[c]	1	A

Levels of evidence	Grades of recommendation
Level 1 – systematic reviews. Meta-analyses, good-quality RCTs	Grade A – based on level 1 evidence (highly recommended)
Level 2 – RCTs, good-quality prospective cohort studies	Grade B – consistent level 2 or 3 evidence (recommended)
Level 3 – case-control studies, case series	Grade C – level 4 studies or 'majority evidence' (optional)
Level 4 – expert opinion	Grade D – evidence inconsistent/inconclusive (no recommendation possible) or drug not recommended

Notes: [a] Bladder wall
[b] Intravesical
[c] Nocturia (nocturnal polyuria) caution hyponatraemia in the elderly
Assessment based on the Oxford System (modified)
RCT = randomized controlled trial
Oxford Guidelines (modified)

to placebo, while all others (fesoterodine, solifenacin, propiverine IR and extended release (ER), oxybutynin IR and ER, and trospium IR) had an adverse event profile greater than that of placebo. Dry mouth was the most common adverse event, others being constipation, pruritus and headache. The newer drugs allowed dose flexibility and titration of medication depending on efficacy and tolerability. This study again highlighted the limited evidence available in elderly patients with significant co-morbidity. There were very limited data on CNS adverse events, such as memory impairment. The conclusions were that this group of drugs was efficacious, safe and well tolerated, with improved health-related quality of life [19].

Novara et al. reviewed 50 randomized controlled trials and three pooled analyses to evaluate the efficacy and safety of antimuscarinics. They concluded that the trials had good methodological quality to show the efficacy of antimuscarinics, that ER were preferable to IR agents and that the transdermal route of administration did not confer a significant advantage over the oral route due to local site reactions [20]. Few studies did long-term follow-up of patients with

Table 6.2. Currently licensed antimuscarinic medication available in the United Kingdom

Generic name	UK trade name®	Dose (mg)	Frequency	Receptor subtype selectivity	Elimination half life of drug (hours)
Tolterodine tartrate	Detrusitol	2	BD	Non-selective	2.4
Tolterodine tartrate XL	Detrusitol XL	4	OD	Non-selective	8.4
Trospium chloride	Regurin	20	BD	Non-selective	20
Trospium chloride XL	Regurin XL	60	OD	Non-selective	38.5
Oxybutynin chloride		2.5–5	BD–QDS	Non-selective	2.3
Oxybutynin chloride XL	Lyrinel XL	5–30	OD	Non-selective	13.2
Oxybutynin Transdermal	Kentera	3.9/24 hours	Twice weekly	Non-selective	8
Propiverine hydrochloride	Detrunorm	15	OD–QDS	Non-selective	4.1
Darifenacin	Emselex	7.5–15	OD	Selective M3 receptor antagonist	3.1
Solifenacin	Vesicare	5–10	OD	Selective M2/M3 antagonist	40–68
Fesoterodine	Toviaz	4–8	OD	Non-selective	6–9

patient-reported outcomes. The authors point out that the majority of studies were industry-funded trials designed to reflect the needs of the company for registration rather than address the question relevant for clinical practice. However, the resources and cost of any such large-scale trials are beyond the scope of independent researchers.

Efficacy in NDO

Relatively few randomized studies exist looking at the effect in the elderly or patients with NDO. In a randomized controlled trial of 197 cognitively intact elderly women (55–92 years) with DO and urge urinary incontinence, oxybutynin 7.5–15 mg/day was more effective (68.5%) compared to placebo (39.4%) [21]. Placebo-controlled trials also provide evidence for efficacy of trospium, propiverine and tolterodine in improving symptoms of NDO [22]. No data in NDO are available to date for the use of the newer antimuscarinics solifenacin, darifenacin and fesoterodine,

but their efficacy in non-neurogenic overactive bladder has been documented [22].

In 46 patients with dementia and urinary incontinence, urodynamics revealed DO in 58% of Alzheimer's patients and 91% of multi-infarct dementia patients. An open trial of propiverine hydrochloride for two weeks in these same patients, irrespective of DO, found decreased episodes of incontinence in 40% of patients, with both groups of patients responding almost equally [23].

A recent Cochrane review of the use of antimuscarinics in MS patients identified only three randomized controlled trials out of a total 33 studies. Results were considered inadequate to support a recommendation, although this actually shows the real lack of research in this area [24].

Some patients are refractory to antimuscarinic drugs either because of side-effects or insufficient effect with continuing incontinence. A number of studies have looked at the use of high-dose antimuscarinics in neurological patients where there has been no efficacy with the standard licensed dose of antimuscarinic. A small study of 27 patients showed 85% of the patients who previously demonstrated unsatisfactory outcome with dosage-escalated mono-therapy were treated successfully [25]. Five patients (19%) experienced side-effects, with two discontinuing treatment. Another study with MS and spinal cord injury patients showed doubling the licensed dose benefited 16 of 21 patients [26]. Prescribers must be cautious if adopting this approach and be aware that these are unlicensed doses.

Side-effects

Antimuscarinic drugs are widely used for symptoms of urgency and urgency incontinence [27], but they are not organ selective for the bladder. The commonly encountered side-effects that can limit efficacy are dry mouth (mediated by M3 receptors present on the salivary glands), constipation (via M2/M3 receptors on the bowel) and rarely visual disturbances. All antimuscarinics are contraindicated in untreated narrow-angle glaucoma.

Antimuscarinic drugs are divided into tertiary and quaternary amines on the basis of their chemical structure, which significantly impacts on the pharmacokinetics of the molecule. Tertiary amines lack ionic charge, are lipophilic and readily absorbed through the gastrointestinal tract and across the blood–brain barrier. By contrast, positively charged quaternary amines like trospium chloride are hydrophilic, do not easily pass into the brain [28], and have less severe CNS side-effects [29] but still produce peripheral antimuscarinic effects. Tertiary amines undergo significant cytochrome P450 [30] metabolism, creating a greater risk of drug–drug interactions by causing enzyme induction or inhibition, whereas trospium undergoes little enzymatic degradation and is mostly excreted unchanged by renal tubules into the urine, thereby reducing the potential for drug interactions.

Antimuscarinic drugs differ in their ability to penetrate the blood–brain barrier and therefore the concentration present within the CNS. Passive diffusion is greatest for non-polar small molecules with high lipophilicity. Oxybutynin is a relatively small (357 kDa) and highly lipophilic molecule compared to the other antimuscarinics (e.g. tolterodine 475 kDa, solifenacin 480 kDa and darifenacin 507 kDa) [31]. Trospium (428kDa), as a hydrophilic polar quaternary ammonium compound, would be expected to show low penetrative ability (Fig. 6.2).

Attention has recently focused on the clinical impact of using antimuscarinics in neurological patients, because of the theoretical risk that they might exacerbate cognitive impairment. Advancing age appears to be associated with increasing permeability of the blood–brain barrier, which increases susceptibility to CNS effects of medication[32]. Neurological conditions like Alzheimer's disease, stroke, trauma, multiple sclerosis and Parkinson's disease further compromise the integrity of the barrier and increase the risk of cognitive dysfunction [33–36].

All five muscarinic receptors are found in the CNS (Table 6.3) [37] but their roles are not fully understood [38]. Levels of M3 receptors are low but those of M1 receptors are high and widespread (Table 6.3) [37], and M2 receptors are located throughout the brain. M2 receptor knockout mice also show cognitive deficits in behavioral flexibility, working memory and hippocampal plasticity [39, 40], whereas M3 knockout mice show normal cognition and behavior [41]. The M1 receptor has a dominant role in working memory, as demonstrated by severe impairments in knockout mice [42] and M1 receptor agonist therapy reversing impairments in animal models of dementia [43]. Clinical randomized, placebo-controlled studies with an M1/M4 agonist have shown improvements in cognitive function in patients with Alzheimer's disease but with a high incidence of systemic side-effects [44]. These studies suggest that central M1 antagonism could give rise to cognitive impairment and CNS-related side-effects.

Of all the antimuscarinic compounds, darifenacin demonstrates the highest level of M3 receptor selectivity over other subtypes with 16 times more selectivity for M3 compared to M1 receptors, whereas oxybutynin is only 1.8 times more selective [45]. The findings suggest that oxybutynin has the poorest profile for potential negative cognitive effects amongst all the drugs licensed for overactive bladder. A prospective, randomized, double-blind study looking at the effects of oxybutynin against darifenacin in healthy subjects aged 60 or older showed impaired delayed memory recall at three weeks in the oxybutynin group compared to placebo and darifenacin [46]. However, a prospective, randomized, placebo-controlled, double-blind study in 14 children with urgency and urge incontinence evaluating the effects of long-acting oxybutynin and tolterodine on short-term memory and attention in children found no differences [47].

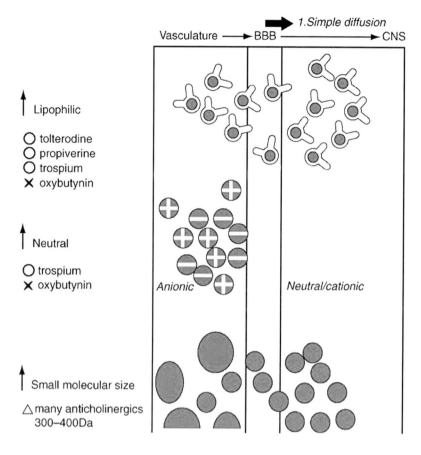

Fig. 6.2. Factors that favor a medication's passive penetration of blood–brain barrier include high lipophilicity (lipid solubility), a neutral charge or low degree of ionization (polarity), and a smaller, less "bulky" molecular size. Given its high lipophilicity, neutrality, and relatively small molecular size, oxybutynin can readily penetrate into the CNS. BBB = blood–brain barrier; CNS = central nervous system; Da = Dalton. Modified from [15].

Diphenhydramine (50 mg) (an anti-histamine with antimuscarinic activity) was compared to oxybutynin IR (5–10 mg) and placebo in older healthy volunteers with a mean age of 69 years in a randomized prospective crossover study, looking at cognitive function. It was found that patients on oxybutynin had similar cognitive dysfunction to patients taking diphenhydramine [48].

A recent cohort study looking at the association of antimuscarinic drugs with cognition in patients with Parkinson's disease examined 235 patients and reassessed them 4 and 8 years later [49]. The results showed that those patients on antimuscarinic drugs had a 6.5 times greater cognitive decline. However, this was a clinical observation study rather than a randomized trial and the group taking antimuscarinics may well have been different at the outset, already being on a steeper trajectory of cognitive decline, due to existing psychopathology or dementia, and more likely to be prescribed non-urological antimuscarinic drugs such as antidepressants. Depression

has previously been shown to be associated with increased cognitive decline [50] and antidepressants were the most commonly used antimuscarinic drugs in this study.

Although there is a potential risk of cognitive impairment from inhibition of muscarinic receptors in the brain [15, 31], apart from oxybutynin, CNS-related side-effects are not commonly found when investigating trial patients on antimuscarinics. There are currently no comparative randomized trials to guide us on the incidence or relative risk of these effects. If there is a particular concern regarding CNS side-effects, practitioners may consider drugs which are least likely to precipitate cognitive dysfunction, i.e. trospium chloride or darifenacin.

Existing recommendations

According to the Guidelines of the European Association of Urology (EAU), there is Level of Evidence 1b and Recommendation Grade A for the use of

Table 6.3. Location of muscarinic receptors in the brain. Reproduced from [37]

Receptor	Location in the brain
M1	Abundant in neocortex, hippocampus and neostriatum
	Pyramidal cells
M2	Throughout brain
	Autoreceptor (inhibitory) in hippocampus and cortex
	Non-cholinergic terminals in hippocampus, cortex and olfactory bulb
	Basal forebrain (e.g. GABAnergic neurons in visual cortex)
	Thalamus
M3	Low levels throughout brain
	Hippocampus
	Thalamus
	Striatal GABAnergic neurons
M4	Abundant in neostriatum; also in the cortex and hippocampus
	Autoreceptor (inhibitory) in striatum
	Striatal medium spiny neurons
M5	Projection neurons of the substantia nigra, pars compacta and ventral tegmental area; also in hippocampus
	Dopaminergic terminals stimulatory in the nucleus accumbens and striatum

oxybutinin, tolterodine, trospium and propiverine in patients with NDO [51]. No studies exist as yet on solifenacin, darifenacin and fesoterodine in NDO patients, so the most recent International Consultation on Incontinence (ICI 2008) could make no specific recommendation, but antimuscarinics as a collective class of drugs have been highly recommended (Grade A) for the treatment of symptoms of NDO [22].

Desmopressin
Scientific background

Desmopressin (also known as antidiuretic hormone) stimulates water reabsorption in the renal medulla via the vasopressin V2 receptor. Vasopressin-receptor

agonists have been used for the treatment of nocturia in patients with overactive bladder symptoms, nocturnal enuresis and neurogenic detrusor overactivity. Desmopressin shows selectivity for its antidiuretic actions over its vasopressor effects and is available in oral, nasal, parenteral and sublingual ("melt") formulations. It is the only currently licensed medication for treating nocturia.

Clinical efficacy

In multiple sclerosis patients, three placebo-controlled, double-blind studies with small patient numbers (16–33 patients total per study) reported a significant reduction of nocturia upon desmopressin administration [52–54]. A further open-labeled study has shown efficacy in the control of abnormal nocturnal polyuria in spinal cord injury patients[55].

Side-effects

Although desmopressin treatment is generally well tolerated, in one study 4 out of 17 patients had to discontinue treatment due to asymptomatic or minimally symptomatic hyponatremia [54]. One study looked at the pooled data from the phase III trials of desmopressin and found 15% of 632 patients developed hyponatremia. Elderly patients (>65 years of age) with a baseline serum sodium concentration below the normal range were reported as being at very high risk (75%) of developing significant hyponatremia [56]. It is recommended to check the serum sodium level 3–7 days after starting therapy and prior to increasing dosage [56].

The manufacturer recommends desmopressin should not be used in patients with hypertension or cardiovascular disease, when used to control nocturia in patients with multiple sclerosis. Desmopressin should also not be prescribed to patients over the age of 65 for the treatment of nocturia associated with multiple sclerosis.

α-adrenoreceptor antagonists (ARs)
Scientific background

The human prostate and the bladder neck contain a dense population of $\alpha_1 AR$ [57] and stimulation of those receptors results in increased smooth muscle tone and increased closure of the urethra. The α_1AR antagonists are effective agents in men with lower urinary tract symptoms such as poor flow, hesitancy, nocturia and frequency.

ARs are G-protein coupled transmembrane receptors that bind the sympathetic neurotransmitter norepinephrine and mediate catecholaminergic actions in the sympathetic nervous system [58]. The AR family consists of α and β subtypes [59], with further subdivision into α_1 and α_2 subtypes [60]. To date, three distinct native members of the α_1AR subfamily (α_{1a}, α_{1b} and α_{1d}) have been identified [61]. In normal human prostatic stroma, α_{1a}ARs overwhelmingly predominate with α_{1d}ARs present to a lesser extent [62, 63]. The predominant subtype in the bladder is α_{1d}, with bladder hypertrophy after bladder outlet obstruction leading to enhanced expression of α_{1d} receptors [64, 65].

Not only may α_1AR antagonists relieve the dynamic component of bladder outflow obstruction but they may also help relieve bladder storage (previously known as irritative) symptoms. The mechanism of this is not clear but it is thought that voiding symptoms may be mediated by α_{1a} receptors in the prostate, while the storage symptoms are mediated by α_{1d} receptors[66]. Supporting evidence comes from trials of tamsulosin (an α_{1a} and α_{1d} adrenoceptor antagonist), which show reduction in storage symptoms in men [67].

A recent study in rats found that tamsulosin, prazosin and silodosin (α_{1a} antagonist) all attenuated DO in a hormone-mediated model of BPH [68]. It seems likely that α_1AR antagonists influence bladder symptoms, in addition to their effects on prostate smooth muscle, and it has been postulated that these agents may act on sensory neurons. α_1ARs have been found to be expressed on sensory neurons and may contribute to signaling of irritative and nociceptive stimuli [69]. Further animal supportive evidence showed that tamsulosin has an inhibitory effect on C-fiber urethral afferents, improving bladder storage function [70]. These data are from animal studies and have to be interpreted with caution with respect to human subjects.

A multicenter, randomized, double-blind placebo-controlled study in 364 women with overactive bladder symptoms showed no efficacy of tamsulosin over placebo [71]. Although these women were not proven to have DO, there was no difference in any of the parameters to indicate clinical efficacy.

Upcoming pharmacological treatments
β-adrenoreceptor agonists
Scientific background

In-vitro studies have shown that non-selective β-adrenoreceptor (βAR) agonists like isoprenaline have a pronounced inhibitory effect on the human bladder, causing increases in bladder capacity [72]. This has not been followed up as a therapeutic option because of probable cardiac side-effects. Subtypes of the βAR have been identified both in the detrusor and in the urothelium [73, 74], with evidence that these are functionally active [75]. RT-PCR experiments have identified β_3AR as being predominantly expressed in the human detrusor [73]. It is thought that β-AR causes relaxation of the detrusor by activation of adenyl cyclase with formation of cAMP together [76]. Animal in-vivo studies have shown that β_3AR agonists increase bladder capacity without affecting voiding parameters [77].

Clinical efficacy

Currently two β_3AR agonists are being evaluated in human studies as possible treatments in DO: solabegron (GW427353) and mirabegron (YM178) [78]. An abstract report showed primary efficacy of significant reduction in mean micturition frequency with mirabegron compared to placebo [79]. Secondary variables included significant improvements in mean volume per micturition, mean number of incontinence episodes, nocturia episodes and urgency incontinence episodes. Commonly reported side-effects included headache and gastrointestinal adverse events. This study demonstrates the proof of the principle of βAR agonists being useful agents in symptoms of overactive bladder and paves the way for further large randomized controlled trials. This group of drugs shows great promise especially if they do not interfere with voiding or affect the residual volume, allowing possible combination with antimuscarinics.

Phosphodiesterase inhibitors
Scientific background

Increasing cGMP through nitric oxide (NO) has been shown to relax the smooth muscle of the bladder outflow tract [80]. Phosphodiesterase (PDE) inhibitors increase both cAMP and cGMP mediated relaxation of the lower urinary tract smooth muscles [81]. There are currently 11 PDE families; most of these families have been demonstrated in different parts of the LUT [81].

Clinical efficacy

Vinpocetine, a low-affinity PDE1 inhibitor, at 20 mg three times a day, was compared in a randomized, double-blind, placebo-controlled study with 62 patients, but failed to show significant effect [82]. Although PDE4 inhibitors have shown promise in various animal models [83, 84], emesis has been observed to be a dose-limiting side-effect in this group of drugs [85].

Numerous randomized controlled trials on PDE5 inhibitors have shown their efficacy in reducing lower urinary tract symptoms in men [86, 87], but so far no studies have looked at this in the context of neurogenic bladder dysfunction. As yet, the mechanism of effect is unknown and may occur in the afferent pathway. Further studies are awaited to determine whether this class of drugs will be useful.

Cannabinoid agonists

The cannabinoid (CB) receptor 2 is distributed on sensory nerves and in the urothelium [88]. The use of selective CB1/CB2 agonists in-vivo in rats and monkeys demonstrated increases in the micturition interval by 46% and threshold pressure by 124%. Further studies have shown mixed CB1/CB2 agonists can suppress normal bladder activity and urinary frequency [89]. Quantitative polymerase chain reaction analysis revealed the expression of CB1 and CB2 receptor mRNA in the bladder, with expression in urothelium approximately two-fold higher than in the detrusor [90]. These findings suggest that the endocannabinoid system has a functional role in the bladder.

Studies using CB agonists have produced encouraging results for potential use in NDO. In patients with advanced MS and LUTS refractory to first-line treatment, sublingual spray containing δ-9-tetrahydrocannabinol (THC) and/or cannabidiol (CBD) significantly reduced urinary urgency, the number and volume of incontinence episodes, daytime frequency and nocturia. [91]. In a large, placebo-controlled study of 647 patients with MS, an oral cannabis extract of δ-9-THC reduced urge incontinence episodes and pad weight significantly more than the placebo drug [92]. A multicenter, double-blind, placebo-controlled trial specifically studying

LUTS in patients with advanced MS used sublingual Sativex, an endocannabinoid modulator comprising THC and CBD in a 1:1 ratio. In the active component, daytime frequency, nocturia and the patient's global impression of change were improved significantly more than in the placebo arm. Reductions were also noted in urgency and urge incontinence episodes, but they were not significantly better than the placebo [93].

Transient receptor potential receptor antagonists

Studies have found that symptoms of sensory urgency are associated with increased TRPV1 expression in the trigonal mucosa [94]. An orally active TRPV1 antagonist has shown the ability to completely prevent bladder reflex overactivity triggered by capsaicin infusion [95].

The TRPV4 cation channel has been found to mediate stretch-evoked Ca2+ influx and ATP release in primary urothelial cell cultures, suggesting this is a sensor molecule in detecting bladder distension [96]. Further evidence that TRPV4 plays a critical role in urothelium-mediated transduction comes from TRPV4-deficient mice, which exhibit a lower frequency of voiding contractions as well as a higher frequency of non-voiding contractions [97]. Stretch-evoked ATP release has been shown to be decreased in isolated whole bladders from TRPV4-deficient mice.

The role of TRPV receptors in normal human physiology and pathophysiology is yet to be determined, but if found to be critical, TRPV antagonists could potentially modulate the sensory transduction process and open up a novel class of drug.

Intravesical treatments

These were developed in an attempt to fill the therapeutic chasm between oral medication and bladder surgery in the management of patients with intractable NDO. Over the past 25 years, we have lived through the disappointments of intravesical installations of lidocaine, oxybutynin, atropine, vanilloids and nociceptin/orphanin, which, despite a sound scientific basis for use, remain unlicensed and of only research value, but are now enjoying the very promising treatment of intravesical injections of botulinum neurotoxin (BoNT). The latter has rapidly evolved from investigational to more widely used off-licence

Source of capsaicin

Source of resiniferatoxin

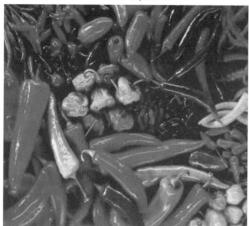
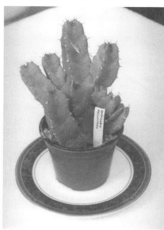

Fig. 6.3. Natural sources of intravesical vanilloids. Capsaicin can be found in red hot chilli peppers (left), whereas resiniferatoxin derives from the cactus Euphorbia resiniferae (right), a species native to Morocco, where it can be found on the slopes of the Atlas Mountains.

second-line treatment of neurogenic incontinence, whilst the results from the global placebo-controlled trials are still awaited.

Various intravesical treatments were based on different rationales. Intravesical lidocaine, vanilloids (capsaicin and resiniferatoxin), nociceptin/orphanin and, partly, oxybutinin were thought to act on the afferent limb of the micturition reflex, whereas the application of atropine, botulinum neurotoxins and, partly, oxybutinin was based on the notion that they would act on the efferent element of the micturition reflex. Novel research findings have enabled a better understanding of the mechanisms of action of intravesical therapies, which in some cases have proven more complicated than initially thought. Intravesically instilled solutions have been shown to exert effects on the urothelial and suburothelial space, but the extent of penetration into the bladder wall has not been elucidated and a direct effect on the efferents is debatable.

Intravesical vanilloids (Fig. 6.3)
Scientific background

The use of intravesical vanilloids in human NDO was based on animal findings suggesting the emergence of an aberrant segmental sacral spinal reflex following spinal lesions [98] (Chapter 1). As the topical application of capsaicin was known to cause prolonged desensitization of capsaicin-sensitive nerve fibers following an initial excitation phase [99], intravesical vanilloids were used in human NDO aiming at desensitization of bladder afferents [100].

The action of vanilloids is mediated by the TRPV1 receptor [101]. Resiniferatoxin (RTX) is 1000 times more potent than capsaicin as a toxin. Consequently, it can be used in lower therapeutic concentrations, thus causing less severe adverse events associated with the excitation phase. Application of RTX to cell lines expressing TRPV1 induced marked changes in structures where TRPV1 was expressed [102, 103] following an increase of intracellular Ca^{++} [104]. Human bladder studies suggested a neurotoxic effect of these compounds on suburothelial afferents [105, 106] (Fig. 6.4), although these findings were not supported by ultrastructural studies in animals [107]. Further to the changes induced in the suburothelial space [108], intravesical vanilloids were shown to have an effect on urothelial cells expressing TRPV1 in neurogenic bladders [109]. It has been suggested that the amount of suburothelial vasculature or degree of vasodilation is implicated in the level of absorption [110].

Clinical efficacy and safety of intravesical vanilloids

A meta-analysis of the literature reported a mean efficacy rate of 84% when using intravesical capsaicin to treat symptoms and/or urodynamic findings of intractable NDO [111]. In randomized trials capsaicin significantly reduced urgency incontinence episodes compared to placebo, primarily in patients with MS [112, 113]. Response rates in open-label studies using RTX in NDO were as high as 92% (range 35–92%) [106, 114],

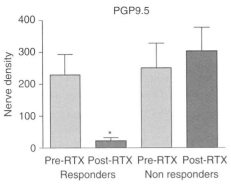

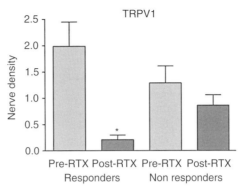

Fig. 6.4. An immunohistochemical study of the human neurogenic overactive bladder showed depletion of TRPV1-immunoreactive suburothelial innervation in patients who benefited from intravesical RTX therapy (right graph), as well as of the total suburothelial nerve fiber count (left graph), supporting a neurotoxic effect of RTX on suburothelial afferents. The graphs show changes in total (immunoreactive to the pan-neuronal marker PGP9.5) and sensory (TRPV1-immunoreactive) suburothelial nerve density following treatment with intravesical RTX. Those who benefited from treatment had significant parallel decreases in both total and sensory nerve density, in contrast to those who did not show symptomatic relief [106].

but randomized and controlled trials failed to support a significant effect, study samples being too small to prove significant differences between groups [117]. Most studies have examined efficacy of both compounds for up to 3 months, but the beneficial effect of capsaicin may exceed 6 months and that of RTX 12 months [112]. Repeat instillations produced sustained effects [118, 119]. Disease severity and duration, degree of disability, type of lesion (spinal versus non-spinal) and the suburothelial vasculature or vasodilation have been postulated to affect the success of intravesical vanilloid therapy, although scientific evidence is lacking [106, 110, 114, 115, 120].

By contrast, what seems to be established is the troublesome clinical profile of intravesical vanilloids. Instillation of the most commonly used doses of capsaicin (100 ml of 1–2 mM capsaicin dissolved in 30% ethanol in saline) was followed by several days of bladder/urethral pain and worsening of overactive bladder symptoms in at least 50% of patients as opposed to 25% of placebo-treated and 12% of RTX-treated, despite similar contact times with the bladder wall (approximately 30 min) [113]. To minimize pungency, glucidic acid was used as a solvent for capsaicin [121] or electromotive drug administration of lidocaine to anesthetize the bladder before capsaicin [108]. Other side-effects include hematuria, autonomic dysreflexia, limb spasms and facial flushing [112, 113, 116]. RTX induced desensitization at lower concentrations (10–100 nM) [114, 120, 122, 123], using a 10% ethanol in saline vehicle, but time-dependent adhesion of the molecule to the polypropylene and PVC-containing

saline bags used during preparation of the drug was then identified as causing poor efficacy [106].

There is little evidence on long-term safety. Repeat capsaicin instillations for up to five years were not associated with any premalignant or malignant lesions [118]. No morphological changes in the bladder mucosa were noted after two instillations of RTX and for a mean period of 26 months [124].

A single study in patients with spinal NDO reported a lack of efficacy of capsaicin, but RTX clearly reduced daily urinary leakage episodes [116]. An earlier non-comparative study had also shown that RTX could be successful where capsaicin had failed to improve patients' symptoms and urodynamic parameters [123]. Another study, however, demonstrated no significant difference in LUTS and urodynamic benefits between the two vanilloid agonists [121].

Botulinum neurotoxin type A (BoNT/A) achieved more significant decreases of incontinence episodes and detrusor pressures than RTX, as well as increases in bladder capacity [119]. In RTX-treated patients, however, post-void residuals did not justify the need for self-catheterizations as opposed to BoNT/A treatment.

Intravesical nociceptin/orphanin FQ, oxybutinin, lidocaine and atropine
Scientific background

Nociceptin/orphanin FQ is thought to act via activation of the opioid-receptor-like OP4, which in animal studies has been shown to inhibit the voiding reflex [125]. Urodynamic studies in humans with neurogenic detrusor overactivity confirm its effect on lower urinary tract function as it was shown to produce an acute increase in bladder cystometric capacity and volume threshold for the appearance of reflex detrusor contraction [126, 127].

Intravesical oxybutynin was initially proposed as alternative to oral oxybutynin in the hope of minimizing the systemic side-effects. However, it was later shown that oxybutynin, as well as other antimuscarinics, has a direct effect on the C-fiber afferents [1], whereas the presumed effect on the detrusor muscle after intravesical instillation was a result of systemic absorption via the blood, the latter achieving serum levels as high as after oral intake! [112] By contrast, the non-selective antimuscarinic atropine has not been found to have systemic side-effects after intravesical instillation. Its short-lived efficacy supports a direct effect on the efferent innervation of the detrusor [112]. Finally, lidocaine is known to have an inhibitory effect on neurite regeneration and synapse formation [128], as well as a local anesthetic effect on the superficial bladder layers. Increases in bladder capacity in patients with DO [129], and a short-lived but significant attenuation of pain and urgency in patients with painful bladder syndrome treated with intravesical instillation of alkalinized lidocaine [130], suggest that lidocaine can modulate already abnormal bladder afferent pathways.

Clinical efficacy

The duration of action ranges from six to eight hours for the antimuscarinics atropine and oxybutynin to a few days for lidocaine [130] and up to two weeks for nociceptin/orphanin FQ [127, 131]. Placebo-controlled studies are available for all treatments but lidocaine, although small in sample size and limited in number (one per treatment). Intravesical oxybutynin is the most studied, with several open-label studies establishing its efficacy and safety in both adults and children with NDO [112]. The use of the treatment is limited by the need to use CISC and the high cost of preparation due to the lack of commercially available solutions. A single study has also shown lidocaine to be effective in children with myelomeningocele [132]. All intravesical treatments increased bladder capacity and improved urodynamic parameters, such as detrusor pressures and volumes at first involuntary detrusor contraction or volume at which first leakage occurred.

Existing recommendations

Based on exhaustive review of the literature, the International Consultation on Incontinence reported only Level of Evidence 3 for the efficacy of intravesical vanilloids. The same committee proposed a low grade of recommendation (C/D) for the use of intravesical vanilloids in intractable NDO, suggesting their use should be limited to clinical trials [133]. The Level of Evidence for efficacy in NDO was evaluated at grade 4 for intravesical oxybutinin as opposed to grade 2 for intravesical atropine and nociceptin/orphanin. However, no recommendation could be made for use of the latter intravesical treatments in intractable NDO by either the ICI or the EAU.

Intravesical injections of Botulinum neurotoxin
Scientific background

Of the seven immunologically distinct serotypes of BoNT (A–F), type A (BoNT/A) is most commonly used in urological applications. The effect of the botulinum toxins is exerted via cleavage of the synaptosomal associated protein SNAP25, one of the proteins of the SNARE complex that are responsible for exocytosis of ACh at the neuromuscular junction [134] (Fig. 6.5). The initial blockade of synaptic transmission from the nerve ending is followed by the emergence of functional nerve sprouts in striated muscle, which eventually regress when functionality returns to the parental nerve terminal (Fig. 6.5) [134, 135].

Worldwide there are four commercial formulations of BoNT – BOTOX (Allergan, Inc., Irvine, CA), Dysport (Ipsen Pharmaceuticals, Slough, UK), Myobloc/Neurobloc (Solstice Neurosciences, Inc., South San Francisco, CA/Solstice Neurosciences Ltd., Dublin, Ireland) and Xeomin (Merz Pharmaceuticals GmbH, Frankfurt, Germany). Three of the four are BoNT/A products (BOTOX, Dysport and Xeomin), and Myobloc is a BoNT serotype B (BoNT/B) product [136].

Lower urinary tract studies have only been reported with Botox and Dysport. Clinical studies have demonstrated clear differences among BoNTs, the formulations being distinct even among the same serotype (BOTOX, Dysport and Xeomin all BoNT/A). The agglutination molecules differ in structure and size and determine properties such as diffusion. Therefore the different BoNT formulations are said

(a)

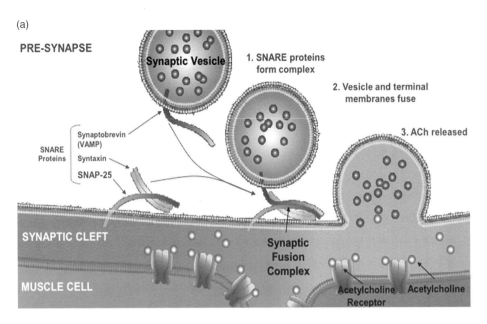

(b)

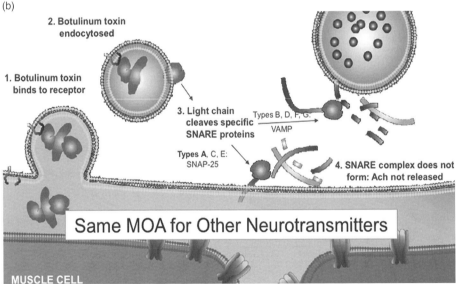

Fig. 6.5. Release of ACh from motor nerve terminals and inhibition of vesicle release by effect of botulinum toxin on SNARE proteins which are necessary for fusion with the postsynaptic membrane. From [134] with permission.

not to be interchangeable and dosage equivalents are somewhat unpredictable. Whether Dysport is associated with a higher risk of drug migration and related side-effects has yet to be proven but reports of distant weakness do seem to be more common with this medication [137].

Twenty years ago, BoNT/A was used in the treatment of detrusor sphincter dyssynergia in spinally injured patients [138], but it was its more recent use in multiple detrusor injections to treat severe NDO that has proved to be so successful. It was given with the intention of paralysing the detrusor smooth muscle by temporarily blocking the release of ACh from the parasympathetic innervation and to date evidence for a direct effect on the detrusor muscle comes from animal studies only [139]. Human and animal data suggest that the mechanism of action of BoNT/A is more complicated and involves a neuromodulatory effect on the afferent bladder pathways [140].

In patients with NDO, BoNT/A injections did not affect the nerve density in the suburothelium or the detrusor, but significantly reduced the levels of suburothelial TRPV1 and $P2X_3$ receptors [141]. These findings may be associated with a post-BoNT/A decrease in the levels of NGF in patients' bladders [142]. In a similar fashion indicating a neuroplastic effect, suburothelial and urothelial levels of muscarinic receptors were restored following successful BoNT/A treatment in patients with NDO [143]. However, BoNT/A did not affect the density of gap junctions in the human overactive bladder wall [144]. In rat bladders, BoNT/A was found to inhibit the abnormal urothelial release of ATP in NDO-simulated conditions [145]. Finally, several studies confirm a post-BoNT/A decrease of neuropeptides involved in neurogenic inflammation (glutamate, SP and CGRP) [146]. On the basis of such observations, it has been hypothesized that BoNT/A injected in the overactive human bladder has a complex inhibitory effect on the release of excitatory neurotransmitters and on the axonal expression of other SNARE complex dependent proteins in the urothelium and suburothelium, which are important in mediation of intrinsic or spinal reflexes thought to cause DO [140] (Fig. 1.6, p. 5).

Procedure

The intradetrusor injection technique has evolved since it was first described [149] and is often now performed as a 10–15 minute minimally invasive day-care or outpatient procedure, performed under local anesthesia [150]. This is a particular advantage considering the need for re-injections in patients with co-morbidities. General anesthesia is used at some centers, and is necessary in patients with spinal cord injury, who are prone to autonomic dysreflexia.

Although there is no good scientific basis for the number of injection sites, wider dispersion of BoNT/A has been reportedly associated with better outcome. The most commonly reported BoNT/A use in literature is 300 U BOTOX [151]. When BOTOX is used, it is recommended to dilute 100 U of the neurotoxin with 10 ml normal saline and inject 1 ml per site [151]. Saline diluent volumes were 3–30 ml for 500 U vials of Dysport, which was injected at 10–30 different sites delivering 16–50 U per site. Most users to

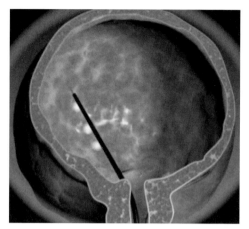

Fig. 6.6. A cartoon representation of a transverse section of the urinary bladder during flexible cystoscopy performed for intravesical injection of botulinum toxin. The highlighted dots represent points of injection of botulinum toxin at a distance of 1 cm between one another and starting almost 2 cm above and lateral to the ureteric orifices, as per the "Dasgupta" minimally invasive injection technique [150].

date have spared the trigone because of the theoretical risk of causing ureteric reflux although this has now been shown not to occur [152]. The proponents favoring trigonal injections support their preference on the grounds of relatively higher nerve density in the trigone.

When using a flexible cystoscope and the minimally invasive technique, first an intra-urethral instillation of lignocaine is given and then the bladder wall inspected. The toxin is injected with an ultrafine injection needle protected in a metal sheath, which passes through the working channel of the cystoscope. A distance of 1 cm is proposed between the injection sites, whilst sparing the bladder trigone (Fig. 6.6). The bladder is emptied after the procedure which has taken approximately 10 minutes; patients are discharged on prophylactic oral antibiotics for 3 days [150]. Pain perception using a visual analogue scale (0–10) revealed an average score of 4 in patients undergoing the procedure under local anesthesia.

The use of an antibiotic prophylaxis remains uncertain as there has been little research of this so far: there has only been one study which looked at the incidence of urinary tract infections (UTI) immediately following detrusor injections of botulinum toxin. The symptomatic rate of UTI was 7.1% and all infections occurred during the first six days. The urinary colonization rate was 31% at day six and 26%

six weeks after the injections, so antibiotic prophylaxis seems to be required [153].

Although a high proportion of spinally injured and multiple sclerosis patients practise CISC, it is important for patients to be told of the need to learn CISC before BoNT therapy as almost all of them will need to rely on CISC to empty their bladders following treatment [154].

Physicians also need to be aware of the contraindications for BoNT therapy which include drugs such as aminoglycosides and anticoagulants. Aminoglycosides enhanced the neuromuscular block caused by BoNT and so should be avoided [155]. Medical conditions including myasthenia gravis, pregnancy and breast-feeding [156] are also contraindications to treatment with BoNT.

Clinical efficacy

Symptoms impressively improve within the first week after treatment [157, 158]. A mean 69% reduction in incontinence episodes has been reported in a review of the published literature, and a mean 57% of patients become fully continent [151]. As a consequence of the relief of symptoms of bladder overactivity, the use of oral antimuscarinics can be reduced or discontinued [159].

Significant improvements are also noted in mean reflex volume, maximum cystometric capacity and in the maximum detrusor pressures, suggesting a protective role for the upper urinary tract [149]. Such efficacy has been demonstrated in both randomized controlled trials [119, 160, 161] and many open-label studies [154, 162–165]. The post-void residual, however, increases following BoNT/A and patients are instructed to start on CISC if there are still bothersome lower urinary tract symptoms with a post-void residual of more than 100–150 ml. It appears that the higher the toxin dose, the greater the chance of needing CISC post-BoNT/A, although a dose reduction appears to reduce the duration of therapeutic effectiveness [166]. Other side-effects included macroscopic hematuria, injection site pain, flu-like symptoms and generalized muscle weakness [162, 167]. Associated hyposthenia and muscle weakness reported mostly with Dysport 1000 U led to researchers using a lesser dose [168].

The duration of effect as a variable is difficult to define clearly due to the absence of an objective measurable definition of response. Reports range from 5–6 months [169–171] to 9–11 months [159, 165, 172, 173], with a mean duration of efficacy in patients with NDO at 8 months [151]. Again the variability of effect has been attributed to the dose of toxin, injection technique, volume of diluent, number of injection sites and the etiology of the neurological bladder dysfunction.

Patients need to be informed in advance that the benefit from the treatment does not last indefinitely [151], but repeat injections can be recommended as there have been several reports confirming the sustained significant improvement after repeat injections of BoNT/A for neurological bladder dysfunction [151]. Importantly, patients' quality of life improves dramatically after each repeat treatment session [174] (see Fig. 14.4, p. 226).

As objective measures are poorly representative or co-related with patient-related outcome measures, validated subjective instruments are highly recommended for addressing the management of overactive bladder symptoms [175]. Observed health-related quality of life improvements were consistent [176] with the first evidence of objective improvement following BoNT/A injections for neurogenic incontinence [160]. Different validated questionnaires have been used as recommended by the International Continence Society.

The impact of BoNT/A injections on symptomatic UTI was assessed and in a study of patients with SCI or MS a reduction in the incidence of symptomatic UTI from 1.77 to 0.2 infections per patient was demonstrated. The suggested mechanism was that this is related to a decrease in bladder pressure [177]. This finding has subsequently been confirmed in two other studies in SCI patients [165, 178].

Existing recommendations

The level of evidence for the use of intradetrusor BoNT/A injections has been ranked highly by a recent panel of European experts as well as by the relevant committee of the International Consultation on Incontinence (ICI) since some, although small, randomized trials show a clear advantage over placebo [160, 161] or other intravesical treatments [119] in improving urodynamic parameters and clinical symptoms. The highest grade of recommendation (Grade A) has been given for its use in patients with intractable spinal NDO [151]. According to the EAU guidelines, NDO should be confirmed by urodynamic studies prior to treatment.

Treatments to overcome external sphincter dyssynergia

Studies assessing medications to decrease urethral resistance are limited and the level of evidence is low. Several treatments have been proposed such as baclofen, dantrolene, α-blockers and NO donors.

Baclofen can be used orally and intrathecally. Orally, a decrease in urethral pressure and in post-void residual volume has been reported but high dosages are required with a significant risk of side-effects [179]. The impact of intrathecal baclofen therapy remains controversial. Moreover, it can induce side-effects on erection and ejaculation [180]. Dantrolene has similar effects as baclofen and high dosages with high risk of side-effects are required [181].

Several α-blockers (indoramine, urapidil and tamsulosin) have been evaluated in clinical trials. Except for indoramine, α-blockers are associated with an improvement of maximum flow rate, an increase of mean voided volume, improved quality of life and a decrease in post-void residual volume, with a decrease in maximum urethral pressure and in maximum urethral closure pressure. Tamsulosin (0.4 and 0.8 mg once daily) in men with spinal cord injury resulted in improvement in 71% of patients (44% slightly and 27% much improved). This treatment was well tolerated and decreased symptoms of autonomic dysreflexia [182] have been reported.

Recently, it has been reported that oral NO donors might be developed as a new pharmacological option to treat DSD in SCI patients [183].

Botulinum neurotoxin A for sphincter

BoNT/A can also be injected in the urethral striated sphincter to treat DSD. It is associated with an increase in urine flow, a decrease in post-void residual volume, a reduction in maximal urethral closure pressure and in voiding P_{detmax}, and an increase in QOL. The improvement rate is between 53% and 100%. Mean duration of effect ranges between one and nine months [151]. Injections are performed via a transurethral, paraurethral or transperineal route with or without electromyogram guidance. However, the effects on urethral sphincter relaxation have not been as sustained, nor are they as reproducible, as the effects of BoNT/A on the detrusor.

Treatments to improve sphincter function

Pharmacotherapy

A variety of drugs have been used with very limited benefit. These include pseudoephedrine and phenyl-propanolamine. These are no longer used to improve bladder emptying. Recently, duloxetine, a selective inhibitor of serotonin and norepinephrine has been shown to increase urethral resistance. Although some studies have shown improvement in continence rates, this is generally limited to mild type. Also, this is compounded by bothersome gastrointestinal side-effects. It has not been specifically tried in neuro-pathic sphincter incontinence.

References

1. De Laet K, De Wachter S, Wyndaele JJ. Systemic oxybutynin decreases afferent activity of the pelvic nerve of the rat: new insights into the working mechanism of antimuscarinics. *Neurourol Urodyn* 2006;**25**:156–61.

2. Iijima K, De Wachter S, Wyndaele JJ. Effects of the M3 receptor selective muscarinic antagonist darifenacin on bladder afferent activity of the rat pelvic nerve. *Eur Urol* 2007;**52**:842–7.

3. Yokoyama O, Yusup A, Miwa Y, et al. Effects of tolterodine on an overactive bladder depend on suppression of C-fiber bladder afferent activity in rats. *J Urol* 2005;**174**:2032–6.

4. Boy S, Schurch B, Mehnert U, et al. The effects of tolterodine on bladder-filling sensations and perception thresholds to intravesical electrical stimulation: method and initial results. *BJU Int* 2007;**100**:574–8.

5. Matsui M, Motomura D, Karasawa H, et al. Multiple functional defects in peripheral autonomic organs in mice lacking muscarinic acetylcholine receptor gene for the M3 subtype. *Proc Natl Acad Sci USA* 2000;**97**:9579–84.

6. Schneider T, Fetscher C, Krege S, Michel MC. Signal transduction underlying carbachol-induced contraction of human urinary bladder. *J Pharmacol Exp Ther* 2004;**309**:1148–53.

7. Takahashi R, Nishimura J, Hirano K, et al. Ca2+ sensitization in contraction of human bladder smooth muscle. *J Urol* 2004;**172**:748–52.

8. Ehlert FJ, Griffin MT, Abe DM, et al. The M2 muscarinic receptor mediates contraction through indirect mechanisms in mouse urinary bladder. *J Pharmacol Exp Ther* 2005;**313**:368–78.

9. Pontari MA, Braverman AS, Ruggieri MR, Sr. The M2 muscarinic receptor mediates in vitro bladder contractions from patients with neurogenic bladder dysfunction. *Am J Physiol Regul Integr Comp Physiol* 2004;**286**:R874–80.

10. Birder LA, de Groat WC. Mechanisms of disease: involvement of the urothelium in bladder dysfunction. *Nat Clin Pract Urol* 2007;**4**:46–54.

11. Mukerji G, Yiangou Y, Grogono J, et al. Localization of M2 and M3 muscarinic receptors in human bladder disorders and their clinical correlations. *J Urol* 2006;**176**:367–73.

12. Yoshida M, Masunaga K, Satoji Y, et al. Basic and clinical aspects of non-neuronal acetylcholine: expression of non-neuronal acetylcholine in urothelium and its clinical significance. *J Pharmacol Sci* 2008;**106**:193–8.

13. Yoshida M, Inadome A, Maeda Y, et al. Non-neuronal cholinergic system in human bladder urothelium. *Urology* 2006;**67**:425–30.

14. Andersson KE, Chapple CR, Cardozo L, et al. Pharmacological treatment of overactive bladder: report from the International Consultation on Incontinence. *Curr Opin Urol* 2009;**19**:380–94.

15. Sakakibara R, Uchiyama T, Yamanishi T, Kishi M. Dementia and lower urinary dysfunction: with a reference to anticholinergic use in elderly population. *Int J Urol* 2008;**15**:778–88.

16. Finney SM, Andersson KE, Gillespie JI, Stewart LH. Antimuscarinic drugs in detrusor overactivity and the overactive bladder syndrome: motor or sensory actions? *BJU Int* 2006;**98**:503–7.

17. Chapple C, Khullar V, Gabriel Z, Dooley JA. The effects of antimuscarinic treatments in overactive bladder: a systematic review and meta-analysis. *Eur Urol* 2005;**48**:5–26.

18. Herbison P, Hay-Smith J, Ellis G, Moore K. Effectiveness of anticholinergic drugs compared with placebo in the treatment of overactive bladder: systematic review. *BMJ* 2003;**326**:841–4.

19. Chapple CR, Khullar V, Gabriel Z, et al. The effects of antimuscarinic treatments in overactive bladder: an update of a systematic review and meta-analysis. *Eur Urol* 2008;**54**:543–62.

20. Novara G, Galfano A, Secco S, et al. A systematic review and meta-analysis of randomized controlled trials with antimuscarinic drugs for overactive bladder. *Eur Urol* 2008;**54**:740–63.

21. Burgio KL, Locher JL, Goode PS, et al. Behavioral vs drug treatment for urge urinary incontinence in older women: a randomized controlled trial. *JAMA* 1998;**280**:1995–2000.

22. Wyndaele JJC, Kovindha A, Madersbacher H, et al. Neurologic urinary and faecal incontinence. In: Abrams P, Cardozo L, Khoury S, Wein A, eds. *Incontinence*. Paris: Health Publication Ltd; 2009: 793–960.

23. Mori S, Kojima M, Sakai Y, Nakajima K. Bladder dysfunction in dementia patients showing urinary incontinence: evaluation with cystometry and treatment with propiverine hydrochloride. *Nippon Ronen Igakkai Zasshi* 1999;**36**:489–94.

24. Nicholas RS, Friede T, Hollis S, Young CA. Anticholinergics for urinary symptoms in multiple sclerosis. *Cochrane Database Syst Rev* 2009:CD004193.

25. Amend B, Hennenlotter J, Schafer T, et al. Effective treatment of neurogenic detrusor dysfunction by combined high-dosed antimuscarinics without increased side-effects. *Eur Urol* 2008;**53**:1021–8.

26. Horstmann M, Schaefer T, Aguilar Y, Stenzl A, Sievert KD. Neurogenic bladder treatment by doubling the recommended antimuscarinic dosage. *Neurourol Urodyn* 2006;**25**:441–5.

27. Andersson KE. Antimuscarinics for treatment of overactive bladder. *Lancet Neurol* 2004;**3**:46–53.

28. Pak RW, Petrou SP, Staskin DR. Trospium chloride: a quaternary amine with unique pharmacologic properties. *Curr Urol Rep* 2003;**4**:436–40.

29. Todorova A, Vonderheid-Guth B, Dimpfel W. Effects of tolterodine, trospium chloride, and oxybutynin on the central nervous system. *J Clin Pharmacol* 2001;**41**:636–44.

30. Guay DR. Clinical pharmacokinetics of drugs used to treat urge incontinence. *Clin Pharmacokinet* 2003;**42**:1243–85.

31. Kay GG, Ebinger U. Preserving cognitive function for patients with overactive bladder: evidence for a differential effect with darifenacin. *Int J Clin Pract* 2008;**62**:1792–800.

32. Kay GG, Abou-Donia MB, Messer WS, Jr., et al. Antimuscarinic drugs for overactive bladder and their potential effects on cognitive function in older patients. *J Am Geriatr Soc* 2005;**53**:2195–201.

33. Kay GG, Granville LJ. Antimuscarinic agents: implications and concerns in the management of overactive bladder in the elderly. *Clin Ther* 2005;**27**:127–38.

34. Bowman GL, Kaye JA, Moore M, et al. Blood-brain barrier impairment in Alzheimer disease: stability and functional significance. *Neurology* 2007;**68**: 1809–14.

35. Pakulski C, Drobnik L, Millo B. Age and sex as factors modifying the function of the blood-cerebrospinal fluid barrier. *Med Sci Monit* 2000;**6**:314–18.

36. Starr JM, Wardlaw J, Ferguson K, et al. Increased blood-brain barrier permeability in type II diabetes demonstrated by gadolinium magnetic resonance imaging. *J Neurol Neurosurg Psychiatry* 2003;**74**:70–6.

37. Abrams P, Andersson KE, Buccafusco JJ, et al. Muscarinic receptors: their distribution and function in body systems, and the implications for treating overactive bladder. *Br J Pharmacol* 2006;**148**:565–78.

38. Volpicelli LA, Levey AI. Muscarinic acetylcholine receptor subtypes in cerebral cortex and hippocampus. *Prog Brain Res* 2004;**145**:59–66.

39. Tzavara ET, Bymaster FP, Felder CC, et al. Dysregulated hippocampal acetylcholine neurotransmission and impaired cognition in M2, M4 and M2/M4 muscarinic receptor knockout mice. *Mol Psychiatry* 2003;**8**:673–9.

40. Seeger T, Fedorova I, Zheng F, et al. M2 muscarinic acetylcholine receptor knock-out mice show deficits in behavioral flexibility, working memory, and hippocampal plasticity. *J Neurosci* 2004;**24**:10117–27.

41. Yamada M, Miyakawa T, Duttaroy A, et al. Mice lacking the M3 muscarinic acetylcholine receptor are hypophagic and lean. *Nature* 2001;**410**:207–12.

42. Anagnostaras SG, Murphy GG, Hamilton SE, et al. Selective cognitive dysfunction in acetylcholine M1 muscarinic receptor mutant mice. *Nat Neurosci* 2003;**6**:51–8.

43. Fisher A. M1 muscarinic agonists target major hallmarks of Alzheimer's disease – the pivotal role of brain M1 receptors. *Neurodegener Dis* 2008;**5**:237–40.

44. Bodick NC, Offen WW, Levey AI, et al. Effects of xanomeline, a selective muscarinic receptor agonist, on cognitive function and behavioral symptoms in Alzheimer disease. *Arch Neurol* 1997;**54**:465–73.

45. Ohtake A, Saitoh C, Yuyama H, et al. Pharmacological characterization of a new antimuscarinic agent, solifenacin succinate, in comparison with other antimuscarinic agents. *Biol Pharm Bull* 2007;**30**:54–8.

46. Kay G, Crook T, Rekeda L, et al. Differential effects of the antimuscarinic agents darifenacin and oxybutynin ER on memory in older subjects. *Eur Urol* 2006;**50**:317–26.

47. Giramonti KM, Kogan BA, Halpern LF. The effects of anticholinergic drugs on attention span and short-term memory skills in children. *Neurourol Urodyn* 2008;**27**:315–18.

48. Katz IR, Sands LP, Bilker W, et al. Identification of medications that cause cognitive impairment in older people: the case of oxybutynin chloride. *J Am Geriatr Soc* 1998;**46**:8–13.

49. Ehrt U, Broich K, Larsen JP, Ballard C, Aarsland D. Use of drugs with anticholinergic effect and impact on cognition in Parkinson's disease: a cohort study. *J Neurol Neurosurg Psychiatry* 2010;**81**:160–5.

50. Starkstein SE, Bolduc PL, Mayberg HS, Preziosi TJ, Robinson RG. Cognitive impairments and depression in Parkinson's disease: a follow up study. *J Neurol Neurosurg Psychiatry* 1990;**53**:597–602.

51. Stöhrer M, Blok B, Castro-Diaz D, et al. EAU guidelines on neurogenic lower urinary tract dysfunction. *Eur Urol* 2009;**56**:81–8.

52. Eckford SD, Swami KS, Jackson SR, Abrams PH. Desmopressin in the treatment of nocturia and enuresis in patients with multiple sclerosis. *Br J Urol* 1994;**74**:733–5.

53. Hilton P, Hertogs K, Stanton SL. The use of desmopressin (DDAVP) for nocturia in women with multiple sclerosis. *J Neurol Neurosurg Psychiatry* 1983;**46**:854–5.

54. Valiquette G, Herbert J, Maede-D'Alisera P. Desmopressin in the management of nocturia in patients with multiple sclerosis. A double-blind, crossover trial. *Arch Neurol* 1996;**53**:1270–5.

55. Zahariou A, Karagiannis G, Papaioannou P, Stathi K, Michail X. The use of desmopressin in the management of nocturnal enuresis in patients with spinal cord injury. *Eura Medicophys* 2007; **43**:333–8.

56. Rembratt A, Riis A, Norgaard JP. Desmopressin treatment in nocturia; an analysis of risk factors for hyponatremia. *Neurourol Urodyn* 2006;**25**:105–9.

57. Caine M, Pfau A, Perlberg S. The use of alpha-adrenergic blockers in benign prostatic obstruction. *Br J Urol* 1976;**48**:255–63.

58. Schwinn DA. The role of alpha1-adrenergic receptor subtypes in lower urinary tract symptoms. *BJU Int* 2001;**88**(Suppl 2):27–34.

59. Ahlquist RP. A study of the adrenotropic receptors. *Am J Physiol* 1948;**153**:586–600.

60. Langer SZ. Presynaptic regulation of catecholamine release. *Biochem Pharmacol* 1974;**23**:1793–800.

61. Andersson KE. Alpha-adrenoceptors and benign prostatic hyperplasia: basic principles for treatment with alpha-adrenoceptor antagonists. *World J Urol* 2002;**19**:390–6.

62. Walden PD, Gerardi C, Lepor H. Localization and expression of the alpha1A-1, alpha1B and alpha1D-adrenoceptors in hyperplastic and non-hyperplastic human prostate. *J Urol* 1999;**161**:635–40.

63. Price DT, Schwinn DA, Lomasney JW, et al. Identification, quantification, and localization of mRNA for three distinct alpha 1 adrenergic receptor subtypes in human prostate. *J Urol* 1993; **150**:546–51.

64. Malloy BJ, Price DT, Price RR, et al. Alpha1-adrenergic receptor subtypes in human detrusor. *J Urol* 1998;**160**:937–43.

65. Hampel C, Dolber PC, Smith MP, et al. Modulation of bladder alpha1-adrenergic receptor subtype expression by bladder outlet obstruction. *J Urol* 2002; **167**:1513–21.

66. Schwinn DA, Price RR. Molecular pharmacology of human alpha1-adrenergic receptors: unique features of the alpha 1a-subtype. *Eur Urol* 1999;**36**(Suppl 1): 7–10.

67. Noble AJ, Chess-Williams R, Couldwell C, et al. The effects of tamsulosin, a high affinity antagonist at functional alpha 1A- and alpha 1D-adrenoceptor subtypes. *Br J Pharmacol* 1997;**120**:231–8.

68. Tatemichi S, Akiyama K, Kobayashi M, et al. A selective alpha1A-adrenoceptor antagonist inhibits detrusor overactivity in a rat model of benign prostatic hyperplasia. *J Urol* 2006;**176**:1236–41.

69. Trevisani M, Campi B, Gatti R, et al. The influence of alpha1-adrenoreceptors on neuropeptide release from primary sensory neurons of the lower urinary tract. *Eur Urol* 2007;**52**:901–8.

70. Yokoyama O, Yusup A, Oyama N, et al. Improvement in bladder storage function by tamsulosin depends on suppression of C-fiber urethral afferent activity in rats. *J Urol* 2007;**177**:771–5.

71. Robinson D, Cardozo L, Terpstra G, Bolodeoku J. A randomized double-blind placebo-controlled multicentre study to explore the efficacy and safety of tamsulosin and tolterodine in women with overactive bladder syndrome. *BJU Int* 2007;**100**:840–5.

72. Anderson KE. Pharmacology of lower urinary tract smooth muscles and penile erectile tissues. *Pharmacol Rev* 1993;**45**:253–308.

73. Michel MC, Vrydag W. Alpha1-, alpha2- and beta-adrenoceptors in the urinary bladder, urethra and prostate. *Br J Pharmacol* 2006;**147**(Suppl 2):S88–119.

74. Otsuka A, Shinbo H, Matsumoto R, Kurita Y, Ozono S. Expression and functional role of beta-adrenoceptors in the human urinary bladder urothelium. *Naunyn Schmiedebergs Arch Pharmacol* 2008;**377**:473–81.

75. Leon LA, Hoffman BE, Gardner SD, et al. Effects of the beta 3-adrenergic receptor agonist disodium 5-[(2R)-2-[[(2R)-2-(3-chlorophenyl)-2-hydroxyethyl]amino] propyl]-1,3-benzo dioxole-2,2-dicarboxylate (CL-316243) on bladder micturition reflex in spontaneously hypertensive rats. *J Pharmacol Exp Ther* 2008;**326**:178–85.

76. Frazier EP, Peters SL, Braverman AS, Ruggieri MR, Sr., Michel MC. Signal transduction underlying the control of urinary bladder smooth muscle tone by muscarinic receptors and beta-adrenoceptors. *Naunyn Schmiedebergs Arch Pharmacol* 2008;**377**:449–62.

77. Kaidoh K, Igawa Y, Takeda H, et al. Effects of selective beta2 and beta3-adrenoceptor agonists on detrusor hyperreflexia in conscious cerebral infarcted rats. *J Urol* 2002;**168**:1247–52.

78. Drake MJ. Emerging drugs for treatment of overactive bladder and detrusor overactivity. *Expert Opin Emerg Drugs* 2008;**13**:431–46.

79. Chapple CR, Yamaguchi O, Ridder A, et al. Clinical proof of concept study (blossom) shows novel β3 adrenoceptor agonist ym178 is effective and well tolerated in the treatment of symptoms of overactive bladder. *European Urol Supplements* 2008;**7**:239.

80. Andersson KE, Arner A. Urinary bladder contraction and relaxation: physiology and pathophysiology. *Physiol Rev* 2004;**84**:935–86.

81. Andersson KE, Uckert S, Stief C, Hedlund P. Phosphodiesterases (PDEs) and PDE inhibitors for treatment of LUTS. *Neurourol Urodyn* 2007;**26**:928–33.

82. Truss MC, Stief CG, Uckert S, et al. Phosphodiesterase 1 inhibition in the treatment of lower urinary tract dysfunction: from bench to bedside. *World J Urol* 2001;**19**:344–50.

83. Kaiho Y, Nishiguchi J, Kwon DD, et al. The effects of a type 4 phosphodiesterase inhibitor and the muscarinic cholinergic antagonist tolterodine tartrate on detrusor overactivity in female rats with bladder outlet obstruction. *BJU Int* 2008;**101**:615–20.

84. Gillespie JI. Phosphodiesterase-linked inhibition of nonmicturition activity in the isolated bladder. *BJU Int* 2004;**93**:1325–32.

85. Giembycz MA. Life after PDE4: overcoming adverse events with dual-specificity phosphodiesterase inhibitors. *Curr Opin Pharmacol* 2005;**5**:238–44.

86. Stief CG, Porst H, Neuser D, Beneke M, Ulbrich E. A randomised, placebo-controlled study to assess the efficacy of twice-daily vardenafil in the treatment of lower urinary tract symptoms secondary to benign prostatic hyperplasia. *Eur Urol* 2008;**53**:1236–44.

87. McVary KT, Roehrborn CG, Kaminetsky JC, et al. Tadalafil relieves lower urinary tract symptoms secondary to benign prostatic hyperplasia. *J Urol* 2007;**177**:1401–7.

88. Gratzke C, Streng T, Park A, et al. Distribution and function of cannabinoid receptors 1 and 2 in the rat, monkey and human bladder. *J Urol* 2009; **181**:1939–48.

89. Hiragata S, Ogawa T, Hayashi Y, et al. Effects of IP-751, ajulemic acid, on bladder overactivity induced by bladder irritation in rats. *Urology* 2007;**70**:202–8.

90. Tyagi V, Philips BJ, Su R, et al. Differential expression of functional cannabinoid receptors in human bladder detrusor and urothelium. *J Urol* 2009;**181**:1932–8.

91. Brady CM, DasGupta R, Dalton C, et al. An open-label pilot study of cannabis-based extracts for bladder dysfunction in advanced multiple sclerosis. *Mult Scler* 2004;**10**:425–33.

92. Freeman RM, Adekanmi O, Waterfield MR, et al. The effect of cannabis on urge incontinence in patients with multiple sclerosis: a multicentre, randomised placebo-controlled trial (CAMS-LUTS). *Int Urogynecol J Pelvic Floor Dysfunct* 2006;**17**:636–41.

93. Kavia R, De Ridder D, Constantinescu S, Fowler CJ. Randomised controlled trial of sativex to treat detrusor over activity in multiple sclerosis. *JNNP* 2010;submitted.

94. Liu L, Mansfield KJ, Kristiana I, et al. The molecular basis of urgency: regional difference of vanilloid receptor expression in the human urinary bladder. *Neurourol Urodyn* 2007;**26**:433–8.

95. Charrua A, Cruz CD, Narayanan S, et al. GRC-6211, a new oral specific TRPV1 antagonist, decreases bladder overactivity and noxious bladder input in cystitis animal models. *J Urol* 2009;**181**:379–86.

96. Mochizuki T, Sokabe T, Araki I, et al. The TRPV4 cation channel mediates stretch-evoked Ca2+ influx and ATP release in primary urothelial cell cultures. *J Biol Chem* 2009;**284**:21257–64.

97. Gevaert T, Vriens J, Segal A, et al. Deletion of the transient receptor potential cation channel TRPV4 impairs murine bladder voiding. *J Clin Invest* 2007;**117**:3453–62.

98. de Groat WC, Kawatani M, Hisamitsu T, et al. Mechanisms underlying the recovery of urinary bladder function following spinal cord injury. *J Auton Nerv Syst* 1990;**30**(Suppl):S71–7.

99. Jancso N, Jancso-Gabor A, Szolcsanyi J. The role of sensory nerve endings in neurogenic inflammation induced in human skin and in the eye and paw of the rat. *Br J Pharmacol Chemother* 1968;**33**:32–41.

100. Fowler CJ, Jewkes D, McDonald WI, Lynn B, de Groat WC. Intravesical capsaicin for neurogenic bladder dysfunction. *Lancet* 1992;**339**:1239.

101. Montell C. Physiology, phylogeny, and functions of the TRP superfamily of cation channels. *Sci STKE* 2001;RE1.

102. Olah Z, Szabo T, Karai L, et al. Ligand-induced dynamic membrane changes and cell deletion conferred by vanilloid receptor 1. *J Biol Chem* 2001;**276**:11021–30.

103. Olah Z, Karai L, Iadarola MJ. Anandamide activates vanilloid receptor 1 (VR1) at acidic pH in dorsal root ganglia neurons and cells ectopically expressing VR1. *J Biol Chem* 2001;**276**:31163–70.

104. Caudle RM, Karai L, Mena N, et al. Resiniferatoxin-induced loss of plasma membrane in vanilloid receptor expressing cells. *Neurotoxicology* 2003;**24**:895–908.

105. Dasgupta P, Chandiramani VA, Beckett A, Scaravilli F, Fowler CJ. The effect of intravesical capsaicin on the suburothelial innervation in patients with detrusor hyper-reflexia. *BJU Int* 2000;**85**:238–45.

106. Brady CM, Apostolidis AN, Harper M, et al. Parallel changes in bladder suburothelial vanilloid receptor TRPV1 and pan-neuronal marker PGP9.5 immunoreactivity in patients with neurogenic detrusor overactivity after intravesical resiniferatoxin treatment. *BJU Int* 2004;**93**:770–6.

107. Avelino A, Cruz F. TRPV1 (vanilloid receptor) in the urinary tract: expression, function and clinical applications. *Naunyn Schmiedebergs Arch Pharmacol* 2006;**373**:287–99.

108. Dasgupta P, Fowler CJ, Stephen RL. Electromotive drug administration of lidocaine to anesthetize the bladder before intravesical capsaicin. *J Urol* 1998;**159**:1857–61.

109. Apostolidis A, Brady CM, Yiangou Y, et al. Capsaicin receptor TRPV1 in urothelium of neurogenic human bladders and effect of intravesical resiniferatoxin. *Urology* 2005;**65**:400–5.

110. Apostolidis A, Yiangou Y, Brady C, et al. Endothelial nitric oxide synthase (eNOS) expression in neurogenic urinary bladders treated with intravesical resiniferatoxin (RTX). *BJU Int* 2004;**93**:336–40.

111. de Seze M, Wiart L, Ferriere J, et al. Intravesical instillation of capsaicin in urology: a review of the literature. *Eur Urol* 1999;**36**:267–77.

112. Reitz A, Schurch B. Intravesical therapy options for neurogenic detrusor overactivity. *Spinal Cord* 2004;**42**:267–72.

113. MacDonald R, Monga M, Fink HA, Wilt TJ. Neurotoxin treatments for urinary incontinence in subjects with spinal cord injury or multiple sclerosis: a systematic review of effectiveness and adverse effects. *J Spinal Cord Med* 2008;**31**:157–65.

114. Silva C, Rio ME, Cruz F. Desensitization of bladder sensory fibers by intravesical resiniferatoxin, a capsaicin analog: long-term results for the treatment of detrusor hyperreflexia. *Eur Urol* 2000;**38**:444–52.

115. Kuo HC. Effectiveness of intravesical resiniferatoxin for anticholinergic treatment refractory detrusor overactivity due to nonspinal cord lesions. *J Urol* 2003;**170**:835–9.

116. Giannantoni A, Di Stasi SM, Stephen RL, et al. Intravesical capsaicin versus resiniferatoxin in

patients with detrusor hyperreflexia: a prospective randomized study. *J Urol* 2002;**167**:1710–14.

117. Kim JH, Rivas DA, Shenot PJ, et al. Intravesical resiniferatoxin for refractory detrusor hyperreflexia: a multicenter, blinded, randomized, placebo-controlled trial. *J Spinal Cord Med* 2003;**26**:358–63.

118. Dasgupta P, Chandiramani V, Parkinson MC, Beckett A, Fowler CJ. Treating the human bladder with capsaicin: is it safe? *Eur Urol* 1998;**33**:28–31.

119. Giannantoni A, Di Stasi SM, Stephen RL, et al. Intravesical resiniferatoxin versus botulinum-A toxin injections for neurogenic detrusor overactivity: a prospective randomized study. *J Urol* 2004;**172**:240–3.

120. De Ridder D, Chandiramani V, Dasgupta P, et al. Intravesical capsaicin as a treatment for refractory detrusor hyperreflexia: a dual center study with long-term follow-up. *J Urol* 1997;**158**:2087–92.

121. de Seze M, Wiart L, de Seze MP, et al. Intravesical capsaicin versus resiniferatoxin for the treatment of detrusor hyperreflexia in spinal cord injured patients: a double-blind, randomized, controlled study. *J Urol* 2004;**171**:251–5.

122. Lazzeri M, Beneforti P, Spinelli M, Zanollo A, Barbagli G, Turini D. Intravesical resiniferatoxin for the treatment of hypersensitive disorder: a randomized placebo controlled study. *J Urol* 2000;**164**:676–9.

123. Lazzeri M, Spinelli M, Beneforti P, Zanollo A, Turini D. Intravesical resiniferatoxin for the treatment of detrusor hyperreflexia refractory to capsaicin in patients with chronic spinal cord diseases. *Scand J Urol Nephrol* 1998;**32**:331–4.

124. Silva C, Avelino A, Souto-Moura C, Cruz F. A light- and electron-microscopic histopathological study of human bladder mucosa after intravesical resiniferatoxin application. *BJU Int* 2001;**88**:355–60.

125. Lecci A, Giuliani S, Meini S, Maggi CA. Nociceptin and the micturition reflex. *Peptides* 2000;**21**:1007–21.

126. Lazzeri M, Calo G, Spinelli M, et al. Urodynamic and clinical evidence of acute inhibitory effects of intravesical nociceptin/orphanin FQ on detrusor overactivity in humans: a pilot study. *J Urol* 2001;**166**:2237–40.

127. Lazzeri M, Calo G, Spinelli M, et al. Urodynamic effects of intravesical nociceptin/orphanin FQ in neurogenic detrusor overactivity: a randomized, placebo-controlled, double-blind study. *Urology* 2003;**61**:946–50.

128. Onizuka S, Takasaki M, Syed NI. Long-term exposure to local but not inhalation anesthetics affects neurite regeneration and synapse formation between identified lymnaea neurons. *Anesthesiology* 2005;**102**:353–63.

129. Higson RH, Smith JC, Hills W. Intravesical lignocaine and detrusor instability. *Br J Urol* 1979;**51**:500–3.

130. Parsons CL. Successful downregulation of bladder sensory nerves with combination of heparin and alkalinized lidocaine in patients with interstitial cystitis. *Urology* 2005;**65**:45–8.

131. Lazzeri M, Calo G, Spinelli M, et al. Daily intravesical instillation of 1 mg nociceptin/orphanin FQ for the control of neurogenic detrusor overactivity: a multicenter, placebo controlled, randomized exploratory study. *J Urol* 2006;**176**:2098–102.

132. Lapointe SP, Wang B, Kennedy WA, Shortliffe LM. The effects of intravesical lidocaine on bladder dynamics of children with myelomeningocele. *J Urol* 2001;**165**:2380–2.

133. Wyndaele JJ, Castro D, Madersbacher H, et al. Neurologic urinary and fecal incontinence. In: Abrams P, Cardozo L, Khoury S, Wein A, eds. *Incontinence*. Paris: Health Publications Ltd; 2004:1059–162.

134. Dolly O. Synaptic transmission: inhibition of neurotransmitter release by botulinum toxins. *Headache* 2003;**43**(Suppl 1):S16–24.

135. de Paiva A, Meunier FA, Molgo J, Aoki KR, Dolly JO. Functional repair of motor endplates after botulinum neurotoxin type A poisoning: biphasic switch of synaptic activity between nerve sprouts and their parent terminals. *Proc Natl Acad Sci USA* 1999;**96**:3200–5.

136. Brashear A. Clinical comparisons of botulinum neurotoxin formulations. *Neurologist* 2008;**14**:289–98.

137. Dmochowski R, Sand PK. Botulinum toxin A in the overactive bladder: current status and future directions. *BJU Int* 2007;**99**:247–62.

138. Dykstra DD, Sidi AA, Scott AB, Pagel JM, Goldish GD. Effects of botulinum A toxin on detrusor-sphincter dyssynergia in spinal cord injury patients. *J Urol* 1988;**139**:919–22.

139. Smith CP, Franks ME, McNeil BK, et al. Effect of botulinum toxin A on the autonomic nervous system of the rat lower urinary tract. *J Urol* 2003;**169**:1896–900.

140. Apostolidis A, Dasgupta P, Fowler CJ. Proposed mechanism for the efficacy of injected botulinum toxin in the treatment of human detrusor overactivity. *Eur Urol* 2006;**49**:644–50.

141. Apostolidis A, Popat R, Yiangou Y, et al. Decreased sensory receptors P2X3 and TRPV1 in suburothelial nerve fibers following intradetrusor injections of botulinum toxin for human detrusor overactivity. *J Urol* 2005;**174**:977–82.

142. Giannantoni A, Di Stasi SM, Nardicchi V, et al. Botulinum-A toxin injections into the detrusor muscle decrease nerve growth factor bladder tissue levels in patients with neurogenic detrusor overactivity. *J Urol* 2006;**175**:2341–4.

143. Datta SN, Popat R, Elneil S, et al. Cholinergic signalling pathways in the superficial layers of the human bladder: Comparing health, disease and the effect of botulinum toxin type A. *J Urol* 2009;**181**:676–7.

144. Roosen A, Datta SN, Chowdhury RA, et al. Suburothelial myofibroblasts in the human overactive bladder and the effect of botulinum neurotoxin type A treatment. *Eur Urol* 2009;**55**:1440–9.

145. Khera M, Somogyi GT, Kiss S, Boone TB, Smith CP. Botulinum toxin A inhibits ATP release from bladder urothelium after chronic spinal cord injury. *Neurochem Int* 2004;**45**:987–93.

146. Welch MJ, Purkiss JR, Foster KA. Sensitivity of embryonic rat dorsal root ganglia neurons to Clostridium botulinum neurotoxins. *Toxicon* 2000;**38**:245–58.

147. Cui M, Khanijou S, Rubino J, Aoki KR. Subcutaneous administration of botulinum toxin A reduces formalin-induced pain. *Pain* 2004;**107**:125–33.

148. Chuang YC, Yoshimura N, Huang CC, Chiang PH, Chancellor MB. Intravesical botulinum toxin a administration produces analgesia against acetic acid induced bladder pain responses in rats. *J Urol* 2004;**172**:1529–32.

149. Schurch B, Stohrer M, Kramer G, Schmid DM, Gaul G, Hauri D. Botulinum-A toxin for treating detrusor hyperreflexia in spinal cord injured patients: a new alternative to anticholinergic drugs? Preliminary results. *J Urol* 2000;**164**:692–7.

150. Harper M, Popat RB, Dasgupta R, Fowler CJ, Dasgupta P. A minimally invasive technique for outpatient local anaesthetic administration of intradetrusor botulinum toxin in intractable detrusor overactivity. *BJU Int* 2003;**92**:325–6.

151. Apostolidis A, Dasgupta P, Denys P, et al. Recommendations on the use of botulinum toxin in the treatment of lower urinary tract disorders and pelvic floor dysfunctions: a European Consensus Report. *Eur Urol* 2009;**51**:100–19.

152. Karsenty G, Elzayat E, Delapparent T, et al. Botulinum toxin type A injections into the trigone to treat idiopathic overactive bladder do not induce vesicoureteral reflux. *J Urol* 2007;**177**:1011–14.

153. Mouttalib S, Castel-Lacanal E, Guillotreau J, et al. Une antibioprophylaxie est-elle nécessaire lors de la réalisation d'injections intradetrusoriennes de toxine botulique A dans le traitement d'une hyperactivite detrusorienne neurogene? *Prog Urol* 2009;**19**:667.

154. Kalsi V, Gonzales G, Popat R, et al. Botulinum injections for the treatment of bladder symptoms of multiple sclerosis. *Ann Neurol* 2007;**62**: 452–7.

155. Molgo J, Lemeignan M, Thesleff S. Aminoglycosides and 3,4-diaminopyridine on neuromuscular block caused by botulinum type A toxin. *Muscle Nerve* 1987;**10**:464–70.

156. Wyndaele JJ, Van Dromme SA. Muscular weakness as side effect of botulinum toxin injection for neurogenic detrusor overactivity. *Spinal Cord* 2002;**40**:599–600.

157. Kalsi V, Apostolidis A, Gonzales G, et al. Early effect on the overactive bladder symptoms following botulinum neurotoxin type A injections for detrusor overactivity. *Eur Urol* 2008;**54**:181–7.

158. Rapp DE, Lucioni A, Katz EE, et al. Use of botulinum-A toxin for the treatment of refractory overactive bladder symptoms: an initial experience. *Urology* 2004;**63**:1071–5.

159. Reitz A, Stohrer M, Kramer G, et al. European experience of 200 cases treated with botulinum-A toxin injections into the detrusor muscle for urinary incontinence due to neurogenic detrusor overactivity. *Eur Urol* 2004;**45**:510–15.

160. Schurch B, de Sèze M, Denys P, et al. Botulinum toxin type A is a safe and effective treatment for neurogenic urinary incontinence: results of a single treatment, randomized, placebo controlled 6-month study. *J Urol* 2005;**174**:196–200.

161. Ehren I, Volz D, Farrelly E, et al. Efficacy and impact of botulinum toxin A on quality of life in patients with neurogenic detrusor overactivity: a randomised, placebo-controlled, double-blind study. *Scand J Urol Nephrol* 2007;**41**:335–40.

162. Popat R, Apostolidis A, Kalsi V, et al. A comparison between the response of patients with idiopathic detrusor overactivity and neurogenic detrusor overactivity to the first intradetrusor injection of botulinum-A toxin. *J Urol* 2005;**174**:984–8.

163. Del Popolo G, Filocamo MT, Li Marzi V, et al. Neurogenic detrusor overactivity treated with English botulinum toxin A: 8-year experience of one single centre. *Eur Urol* 2008;**53**:1013–20.

164. Schulte-Baukloh H, Knispel HH, Stolze T, et al. Repeated botulinum-A toxin injections in treatment of children with neurogenic detrusor overactivity. *Urology* 2005;**66**:865–70.

165. Giannantoni A, Mearini E, Del Zingaro M, Porena M. Six-year follow-up of botulinum toxin A intradetrusorial injections in patients with

refractory neurogenic detrusor overactivity: clinical and urodynamic results. *Eur Urol* 2009;**55**:705–11.

166. Kuo HC. Will suburothelial injection of small dose of botulinum A toxin have similar therapeutic effects and less adverse events for refractory detrusor overactivity? *Urology* 2006;**68**:993–7.

167. Ruffion A, Capelle O, Paparel P, et al. What is the optimum dose of type A botulinum toxin for treating neurogenic bladder overactivity? *BJU Int* 2006;**97**:1030–4.

168. Del Popolo G. *Botulinum-A toxin in the treatment of detrusor hyperreflexia*. 31st Annual Meeting of the International Continence Society, Seoul, Korea, 2001: Abstract 2001.

169. Kessler TM, Danuser H, Schumacher M, Studer UE, Burkhard FC. Botulinum A toxin injections into the detrusor: an effective treatment in idiopathic and neurogenic detrusor overactivity? *Neurourol Urodyn* 2005;**24**:231–6.

170. Kuo HC. Urodynamic evidence of effectiveness of botulinum A toxin injection in treatment of detrusor overactivity refractory to anticholinergic agents. *Urology* 2004;**63**:868–72.

171. Schulte-Baukloh H, Schobert J, Stolze T, et al. Efficacy of botulinum-A toxin bladder injections for the treatment of neurogenic detrusor overactivity in multiple sclerosis patients: an objective and subjective analysis. *Neurourol Urodyn* 2006;**25**:110–15.

172. Grosse J, Kramer G, Stohrer M. Success of repeat detrusor injections of botulinum A toxin in patients with severe neurogenic detrusor overactivity and incontinence. *Eur Urol* 2005;**47**:653–9.

173. Kalsi V, Popat RB, Apostolidis A, et al. Cost-consequence analysis evaluating the use of botulinum neurotoxin-A in patients with detrusor overactivity based on clinical outcomes observed at a single UK centre. *Eur Urol* 2006;**49**:519–27.

174. Khan S, Kessler TM, Panicker J, et al. Sustained and significant quality of life improvement after intra-detrusor botulinum toxin type A injections for

neurogenic detrusor overactivity secondary to multiple sclerosis. *Br J Urol* 2009;**103**:37.

175. Abrams P, Artibani W, Gajewski JB, Hussain I. Assessment of treatment outcomes in patients with overactive bladder: importance of objective and subjective measures. *Urology* 2006;**68**:17–28.

176. Schurch B, Denys P, Kozma CM, et al. Botulinum toxin A improves the quality of life of patients with neurogenic urinary incontinence. *Eur Urol* 2007;**52**:850–8.

177. Game X, Castel-Lacanal E, Bentaleb Y, et al. Botulinum toxin A detrusor injections in patients with neurogenic detrusor overactivity significantly decrease the incidence of symptomatic urinary tract infections. *Eur Urol* 2008;**53**:613–18.

178. Wefer B, Ehlken B, Bremer J, et al. Treatment outcomes and resource use of patients with neurogenic detrusor overactivity receiving botulinum toxin A (BOTOX®) therapy in Germany. *World J Urol*; DOI 10.1007/s00345-009-0466-1 (not yet published in journal).

179. Leyson JF, Martin BF, Sporer A. Baclofen in the treatment of detrusor-sphincter dyssynergia in spinal cord injury patients. *J Urol* 1980;**124**:82–4.

180. Denys P, Mane M, Azouvi P, et al. Side effects of chronic intrathecal baclofen on erection and ejaculation in patients with spinal cord lesions. *Arch Phys Med Rehabil* 1998;**79**:494–6.

181. Murdock MM, Sax D, Krane RJ. Use of dantrolene sodium in external sphincter spasm. *Urology* 1976;**8**:133–7.

182. Abrams P, Amarenco G, Bakke A, et al. Tamsulosin: efficacy and safety in patients with neurogenic lower urinary tract dysfunction due to suprasacral spinal cord injury. *J Urol* 2003;**170**:1242–51.

183. Reitz A, Knapp PA, Muntener M, Schurch B. Oral nitric oxide donors: a new pharmacological approach to detrusor-sphincter dyssynergia in spinal cord injured patients? *Eur Urol* 2004;**45**:516–20.

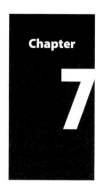

Neurogenic bladder dysfunction: surgical interventional approaches

Xavier Gamé, Thomas M. Kessler, Sohier Elneil and Rizwan Hamid

Introduction

The first-line management of neurogenic bladder dysfunction is based on conservative treatments, such as general measures, non-pharmacological approaches and pharmacological treatment. However, when these measures fail, are not well tolerated or the patient has complications, such as renal impairment or low bladder compliance, surgical treatment may be indicated. There are several different procedures which can be considered including electrical stimulation, bladder and urethral reconstructive surgery, bladder outlet obstruction management and the treatment of stress urinary incontinence. The choice of surgical treatment is based on a multidisciplinary assessment involving urologists, rehabilitation physicians, physiotherapists, specialist nurses and often neurologists, neurosurgeons and gastroenterologists and must be appropriate for the patient's disability, cognitive functions and hand functions.

The goals of surgical management of the neurogenic bladder are to preserve the upper urinary tract and renal function, to avoid urological complications and to improve quality of life by restoring continence and independence. Surgery is not commonly performed in patients with progressive neurological disease and bladder dysfunction, but may be the best option for those who have had a spinal cord injury (SCI), those with myelomeningocele and occasionally patients with multiple sclerosis. In those with non-progressive disease, surgery for neurogenic bladder disorders is often performed in young people with an otherwise near normal life expectancy and hence its benefits must be durable.

This chapter describes the different surgical procedures for managing neurogenic bladder.

Electrical stimulation

Electrical stimulation to manage bladder dysfunction in patients with neurological disorders has been used since the 1950s. Nowadays, electrical stimulation therapies include intravesical electrostimulation, sacral neuromodulation and sacral anterior root stimulation with selective sacral rhizotomy.

Intravesical electrostimulation

Intravesical electrostimulation was first described by Saxtorph in 1887 but reintroduced by Katona in 1959 [1, 2]. The bladder is filled with saline, a monopolar electrode (cathode) is inserted urethrally into the bladder and a second one attached to the abdominal wall (anode). Electrical stimulation is given for between 60 and 90 minutes for 5 days per week, usually using an intensity between 1 and 10 mA, a rate of 20 Hz and a pulse duration of 2 ms.

It is thought that this acts primarily by stimulating Aδ mechanoreceptor afferents [3] inducing bladder sensation and the urge to void, and consequently increasing the efferent output, with improvement of micturition and conscious control. Thus, patients with a hyposensitive and underactive detrusor may be offered intravesical electrostimulation [4, 5], especially in combination with intermittent self-catheterization, before invasive surgical procedures are considered. However, it should only be used in patients with at least some sensation in the sacral dermatomes indicating functioning afferent fibers and if the detrusor muscle is still able to contract.

This therapy has been used mainly in children with myelomeningocele but clinical studies have been limited and results remain controversial. The only

Pelvic Organ Dysfunction in Neurological Disease: Clinical Management and Rehabilitation, ed. Clare J. Fowler, Jalesh N. Panicker & Anton Emmanuel. Published by Cambridge University Press. © Cambridge University Press 2010.

randomized, sham-controlled and blinded clinical study in fact failed to reveal any improvement in bladder capacity, development of detrusor contractions, improvement in detrusor compliance or acquisition of bladder sensation in the active treatment group [6].

Sacral neuromodulation

Sacral neuromodulation (SNM) was developed in the 1980s by Tanagho and Schmidt and it has now come to occupy the position of a second-line treatment for refractory non-neurogenic voiding dysfunctions such as urgency-frequency syndrome, urgency incontinence and non-obstructive chronic urinary retention [7].

The first use of neuromodulation on neurogenic voiding dysfunction was reported by Bosch and colleagues in 1996 [8] and since then a number of other studies have been reported [9–15]. There is now some evidence that sacral neuromodulation may have a place in treating bladder dysfunction in incomplete SCI, multiple sclerosis, cerebrovascular disease or myelomeningocele.

The exact mechanism of action of SNM is still not fully understood but in non-neurological patients it has been suggested that by using a continuous or cycling mode of electrical pulses, SNM stimulates sacral afferent nerves. In conditions of detrusor over-activity these may have an inhibitory effect on sacral efferent activity whereas in some causes of retention the afferent activity "re-informs the midbrain" (see Chapter 19). So in both types of disorder, SNM is effective by modulation of spinal cord reflexes or brain networks, rather than direct stimulation of the motor response of the detrusor or urethral sphincter [16–18]. The same inhibitory effect may operate in neurogenic DO although SNM has not been found to be very effective in neurogenic retention or incomplete bladder emptying.

Surgical technique

The technique for SNM has undergone several modifications since its first introduction. The technique has always involved two steps, a test stimulation and a permanent implant, the test stimulation providing an opportunity to evaluate the possible outcome of the final implant. Nowadays, a two-staged percutaneous technique is carried out using the tined lead developed by Spinelli in 2003 [19]. Under fluoroscopic guidance, and local or general anesthesia,

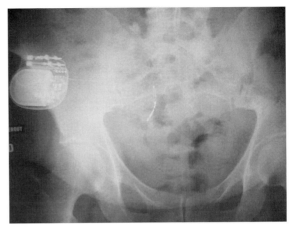

Fig. 7.1. Pelvic x-ray showing a tined lead connected to a permanent implanted pulse generator.

the tined lead is implanted and attached to an external stimulator for up to a month, allowing a prolonged period of testing. If the first stage fails, the electrode can be removed. If the patient responds, a permanent implantable pulse generator (IPG) is implanted in the upper buttock region (Interstim® model) (Fig. 7.1) and connected to the tined lead already *in situ*. Buttock placement of the battery has been shown to decrease the incidence of postoperative and position-related pain, and infection [20]. The average battery life with Interstim® and Interstim II® is around seven and five years, respectively, but this varies with the settings used [21].

Results

Bosch reported the results of SNM in 6 patients with refractory urgency incontinence secondary to multiple sclerosis and, at a mean follow-up of 35 months, showed a reduction in incontinence episodes from 4 to 0.3 per day [8]. Chartier-Kastler then confirmed these findings in 9 women, including 4 from Bosch's series and 5 others with traumatic SCI or myelitis, and showed that the results remained stable with a long-term follow-up (43.6 months) [10]. By contrast, Hohenfellner reported that SNM was effective in 8 patients with neurogenic bladder dysfunction but for less than 54 months, after which all implants became ineffective [11]. No patients with MS were included in that series, which consisted of incomplete SCI, disc prolapse or surgical pelvic nerve damage.

The two largest series of SNM in neurogenic bladder disorders have been reported by Wallace and Lombardi respectively and demonstrated a degree of efficiency [14, 15]. In a retrospective series of 33 patients with neurologic disease, Wallace reported that 28 patients (85%) underwent implantation. Thirteen of the 16 patients with MS, 4 of 6 with Parkinson disease and all 11 of those with various other neurologic disorders received a permanent implant. Incontinence episodes decreased by 68%, number of voids by 43%, nocturia by 70% and there was a 58% reduction in intermittent self-catheterization per 24 hours [15]. Lombardi reported on the outcome of 24 incomplete SCI patients with a follow-up of 61 months. He found that all subjects maintained a clinical improvement of more than 50% compared with baseline, although 4 subjects with urinary retention needed a new implant at the contralateral S_3 because of loss of efficacy [14].

In children, Guys reported a prospective, randomized, controlled study of 42 patients with neurological disease (mean age 11.9 years) including 33 with spina bifida [13]. Patients were randomized into the control group treated conventionally and an implant group treated with SNM. Some improvement was noted in the SNM group but the differences compared with the control group were not significant and furthermore it was observed that it could be difficult to identify the relevant sacral roots and place leads accordingly in some of the patients with spina bifida.

In two separate studies, Scheepens and Amundsen reported that a neurologic condition is associated with a reduced improvement rate in comparison to non-neurogenic patients [9, 12]. Furthermore, it appears to be less effective in improving urinary retention than reducing detrusor overactivity.

Recently, Van Rey has reported in a selected MS patient population that despite a 61% positive response rate to the first stage, at two years of follow-up neuromodulation remained efficient in only 18% of the implanted patients, the efficacy being lost with progression of the neurological disease in all cases [22]. The conclusion from this study therefore is that this costly intervention should probably not be undertaken in patients with MS. However the advent of effective disease-modifying drugs which slow or even halt the progression of MS may significantly alter the situation in the near future.

The impact of neuromodulation on DSD is not yet defined and currently neuromodulation should be proposed only in patients without DSD and with incomplete SCI. It appears that prospective studies are needed to determine the place of SNM as a treatment of neurogenic voiding dysfunction in children and adults.

Very recently, sacral neuromodulation has been used in the acute SCI setting, i.e. in the state of spinal shock, and been shown to prevent the development of neurogenic detrusor overactivity, reducing urinary infections as well as improving bowel function. Continence is maintained by clean intermittent self-catheterization (CISC). So far the benefit has been sustained for more than two years [23] and if this effect can be confirmed in a large scale trial, SNM may well transform the management of NDO in SCI patients.

Complications

SNM is not without a significant complication rate and need for revision surgery. Complications include lead migration, pain at the IPG site, leg pain, infection and failure of the device over time. The reported incidence of lead migration and lead breakages is 11% and 20% respectively [21, 24]. Siegel summarized the adverse events in 219 patients who underwent implantation of the Interstim® IPG and the most common complaint was pain at the IPG site in 15.3% of patients [25]. The surgical revision rate was 33%. Everaert reported a 34% device-related pain rate, with a 23% surgical revision rate [26]. Grunewald reported a revision rate of 30% over four years. Lead migration was noted as 5.4% and IPG site pain as 8.1% [27]. Recently authors have reported much higher long-term revision rates at 54% [28], 48.3% [21] and 43.9% [29] excluding battery changes. Similar results were obtained in a worldwide SNM clinical study in non-neurological voiding dysfunction, carried out by Van Kerrebroeck [30].

It is important that patients are counselled regarding the possible failure of the procedure and the significant revision rate.

Sacral anterior root stimulation with sacral deafferentation

Sacral anterior root stimulation with sacral deafferentation was introduced by Brindley in 1970s [31]. Essentially this procedure involved section of the dorsal sacral roots to abolish detrusor overactivity and stimulation of the sacral anterior roots (S_2, S_3 and S_4) to produce detrusor contraction and bladder emptying. After a laminectomy to expose the nerve roots, the anterior roots were placed in special stimulating electrodes and were tunneled to connect to a subcutaneous radio receiver positioned over the lower anterior chest wall. The patient placed a radio transmitter over the receiver and activated the device with settings as required for micturition, defecation and even erection. Bladder emptying was accomplished usually by stimulation of S_3 with a bladder emptying success rate of 70% [32].

This device could only be used in individuals with complete suprasacral SCI because those with incomplete lesions found even efferent root stimulation painful. But because of the posterior rhizotomy which was required to abolish detrusor overactivity, men lost reflex erections and it is probably because of this destructive component that this intervention is now little used.

Surgical technique

Two approaches have been described, the intradural and the extradural approaches, and a specific electrode has been developed for each [33].

The surgical technique for intrathecal implantation developed by Brindley [34] involves laminectomy of the fourth and fifth lumbar vertebrae and the first two segments of the sacrum, exposing 10–12 cm of dura. The dura and arachnoid are opened in the midline to expose the roots, the roots identified by their size, situation and by perioperative stimulation during which the bladder pressure is recorded and skeletal muscle responses observed. Stimulation of the S_2 anterior roots contracts the triceps surae, the glutei, and the biceps femoris, S_3 anterior roots the pelvic floor and the toe flexors, and S_4 anterior roots the pelvic floor. The sphincters (anorectal and urethral) are innervated predominantly by S_4 and to a lesser degree by S_3 and S_2. A detrusor response can almost always be obtained by stimulation of S_3 and S_4, and sometimes S_2. The roots need to be split into the anterior and posterior components and when the posterior roots are confirmed by an absence of a motor response to electrical stimulation, a segment measuring about 20–40 mm in length is removed. When the S_5 root is identified, it is resected if no bladder response is obtained.

The surgical technique for extradural implantation involves laminectomy of the first three segments of the sacrum. It may also involve laminectomy of the L_5 vertebra, depending on whether electrodes are to be placed on S_2 roots. A posterior rhizotomy is done at the level of the conus medullaris at the same operation through laminectomy of T_{12}, L_1 and, sometimes, L_2. At this stage it is straightforward to identify and to cut all posterior roots that enter the last 30 mm at both sides of the spinal cord.

Once the rhizotomy has been performed, electrodes are put on the motor fibers and a sleeve is fixed over the cables to prevent leakage of cerebrospinal fluid. After closure of the dura, the cables are tunneled to a subcutaneous pocket on the lower part of the thorax or on the abdominal wall and connected to the radio receiver block. Stimulation is started between days 8 and 14 after surgery according to the level of the spinal cord lesion.

Results

The results of implanting the Brindley stimulator are summarized in Table 7.1 [35–44]. Postoperative continence is achieved in between 80% and 90% of the cases. The goal of the posterior rhizotomy is to abolish detrusor activity and to normalize bladder compliance. Continuing urinary incontinence is related either to an incomplete rhizotomy or to sphincter incompetence. Bladder capacity increases and reaches more than 400 ml in all cases although it is recommended that bladder volumes be kept to less than 600 ml. Bladder emptying is complete in 69–100% of the cases. Use of the stimulator is associated with a decrease in complications, such as symptomatic urinary tract infections, vesico-ureteric reflux and autonomic dysreflexia.

Follow-up

Urodynamic studies are needed one month after the surgery to check electrical stimulation produces an efficient bladder contraction and thereafter at four months and one year, then every 2–3 years subsequently.

Urinary tract reconstructive surgery

The goal of urinary tract reconstructive surgery in neurological patients is to create a low-pressure urinary tract, to preserve the upper urinary tract and renal function and to improve patients' quality of life by restoring continence and independence.

The various urinary tract reconstructive operations for patients with neurogenic bladder dysfunction include bladder augmentation, cutaneous continent diversion and an ileal conduit.

Surgery should be performed in departments which are used to managing neurological patients.

Table 7.1. Results of sacral anterior root stimulation and sacral posterior rhizotomy in complete spinal cord injured patients

| Authors (year) | n | Sex | | Mean follow-up (years) | Continence | | Mean bladder capacity | | Post-void residual volume < 50 ml (%) | AD | | UTI | |
		Men	Women		Preop (%)	Postop (%)	Preop (ml)	Postop (ml)		Preop (%)	Postop (%)	Preop (%)	Postop (%)
Barat (1993) [35]	40	26	14	2.5	2.5	90	210	463	82	–	–	100	30
Brindley (1994) [36]	500	271	229	4	–	–	–	–	82	–	–	–	–
Van Kerrebroeck (1996) [37]	52	29	23	3.5	–	81	285	592	87	14	4	4.2/an	1.4/an
Schurch (1997) [38]	10	3	7	3.4	0	80	160	>500	100	60	60	80	30
Egon (1998) [39]	96	68	28	5.5	1	88	200	565	89	22	0	100	32
Van der Aa (1999) [40]	37	33	4	6	–	84	75% <400	95% >400	91	–	–	–	–
Creasey (2001) [41]	23	16	7	1	65	87	243	>400	69	35	7	82	78
Bauchet (2001) [42]	20	6	14	4.5	0	90	190	460	90	15	0	100	–
Vignes (2001) [43]	32	–	–	8	0	90	220	550	80	18	2	100	30
Kutzenberger (2005) [44]	464	224	220	6.6	–	83	173	470	81	–	–	6.3/an	1.2/an

Preop = preoperative; Postop = postoperative; AD = autonomic dysreflexia; UTI = urinary tract infections

There should be suitable infrastructure and environment including adapted patients' alarms, beds, toilets and bathrooms and an adequate number of specially trained nurses [45].

Bladder augmentation

Detrusor myectomy

Detrusorotomy was proposed by Mahony and Laferte, in the 1970s, as an alternative to enterocystoplasty [46], the technique being subsequently modified by Cartwright and Snow who proposed a partial detrusor excision [47]. These procedures have been used mainly in children.

Surgical technique

The principle of detrusor myectomy is to excise detrusor muscle over the entire dome of the bladder, leaving the urothelium intact. Bladder pressure gradually dilates the excised area and a large diverticulum appears. It was initially performed using an open approach, but nowadays it can be performed laparoscopically or with robotic assistance [48, 49].

Results

The level of evidence for efficacy for either procedure is low. Most series report poor results and failure of this technique with time [50–53]. Bladder volume increases in most of the cases but it may take 3–12 months to reach full capacity and then a secondary retraction frequently occurs. Furthermore, detrusor overactivity often persists so that the improvement in symptoms may be small. Kumar reported a failure rate of 83% with a mean follow-up of 79 months. A retrospective study comparing detrusor myectomy and enterocystoplasty found enterocystoplasty to be more effective [54]: whereas urodynamic improvement was 50% in detrusor myectomy, it was 100% in enterocystoplasty and symptom improvement was 42% vs 94%, respectively. However, detrusor myectomy avoids the digestive complications which may occur following enterocystoplasty (20% vs 3%, respectively). Bladder autoaugmentation by detrusor myectomy is rarely carried out now.

Bladder augmentation enterocystoplasty

Bladder augmentation enterocystoplasty was first performed by Von Mickulicz in 1889 [55] to manage chronic tuberculosis cystitis. Nowadays, bladder augmentation is mainly for SCI patients and patients with myelomeningocele who have low bladder capacity, a reduced bladder compliance and detrusor overactivity which is resistant to all conservative treatments including oral antimuscarinics, intradetrusor botulinum toxin injections and possibly sacral neuromodulation. Bladder augmentation is contraindicated in severe inflammatory bowel disease such as Crohn's disease, hemorrhagic colitis, irradiation related bowel damage, short bowel syndrome, compromised renal function, and in patients who refuse to perform CISC.

Surgical technique

Before performing a bladder augmentation enterocystoplasty, the patient is cystoscoped to exclude bladder cancer, kidney function is checked and gastrointestinal tract function evaluated. The patient must be able and willing to perform CISC [56].

Several techniques have been proposed according to the type of bowel segment to be used and the state of the bladder. The principal two methods of bladder augmentation are bivalving the bladder and performing a subtrigonal cystectomy. The choice is generally based on the bladder wall thickness. Hence, if there is significant loss of viscero-elastic properties, it is better to perform a subtrigonal cystectomy. Nowadays, it constitutes the most frequent condition because reduced bladder compliance without bladder wall fibrosis is most often managed with botulinum toxin injections.

Several intestinal segments such as colon, ileum or stomach can be used, most commonly the ileum. After preparation of the bladder or a supratrigonal cystectomy, a 15–45 cm detubularized intestine segment is isolated and stitched in the defect (Fig. 7.2). Several approaches have been reported including open (Pfannenstiel or midline incision), laparoscopic and robotic. If the patient has difficulty performing CISC via the urethra, a cutaneous diversion can be fashioned at the same time (see below) [57, 58]. Usually, no ureteric reimplantation is required as even in the case of vesico-ureteric reflux before surgery, this is corrected in more than 90% of cases by the decrease in pressure associated with the bladder augmentation.

An indwelling catheter is left *in situ* following surgery and 10 days later a check cystogram is

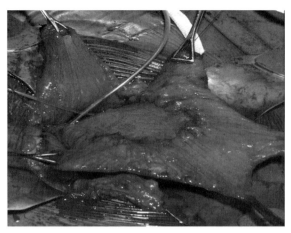

Fig. 7.2. Bivalved bladder with intestinal segment stitched to the posterior wall.

performed and the catheter removed. The patient then starts CISC and, for the first few months, catheterizes three-hourly. The bladder usually reaches its definitive capacity about three months after the surgery and patients then catheterize every four hours at daytime and every eight hours during the night.

Results

The perioperative mortality rate is between 0 and 3.2%. The early post-operative morbidity rate is between 3% and 28%. Ileus is the most frequent complication with a rate up to 11.7%. Late morbidity is mainly related to the type of intestinal segment used and includes mucus production, stones (10–50%), persistent asymptomatic or symptomatic bacteriuria (up to 70%), hyperchloremic metabolic acidosis (0–15%), deterioration of renal function, bowel disturbances and bowel patch cancer (1%) [59–64]. However, the most serious complication is the spontaneous rupture which occurs in 5–13% of patients and requires emergency surgery [65]. It is usually related to bladder overdistension but sometimes to a traumatic catheterization.

The long-term results are very good with excellent control of overactivity and incontinence [66]. Furthermore, quality-of-life studies report an improvement of over 90% [66]. Continence is achieved in more than 90% for night-time and between 91% and 100% during the day [59, 60, 67]. If incontinence remains, intradetrusor botulinum toxin injections to treat persistent detrusor overactivity can be

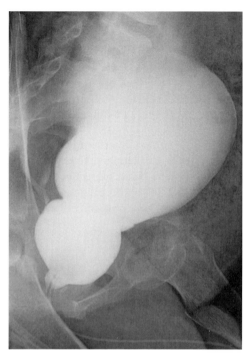

Fig. 7.3. Sagittal view of a cystogram performed one year after subtrigonal cystectomy and enterocystoplasty in a T12 ASIA A paraplegic patient.

performed or an artificial urinary sphincter or sling can be placed in case of sphincter incompetence.

Follow-up

The follow-up of patients who have had a "clam" cystoplasty should be life-long, as a variety of problems can develop (see above). Kidney and bladder ultrasound and renal function assessment should be performed at one and six months after the surgery and yearly thereafter. Cystogram (Fig. 7.3), cystoscopy and urodynamics are usually performed one year after the surgery and then on an as-required basis.

Future possibilities

New bladder augmentation techniques have been proposed which may be developed in the future, using biomaterials such as extracellular matrix of the small intestinal submucosa (SIS, Cook®) [68] or porcine xenograft acellular matrix (Pelvicol, Bard®) [69] for "clam" cystoplasty. An alternative approach may be to use tissue that has been engineered using selective cell transplantation [70].

Cutaneous urinary diversions

Cutaneous continent diversion

Cutaneous continent diversions may be performed in neurological patients, mainly in the young myelomeningocele patient or those with SCI who cannot perform CISC via the urethra because of congenital abnormalities, urethral pain, obesity, strictures or poor hand mobility. Cutaneous continent diversions are contraindicated in patients who simply refuse to perform CISC, have permanent severe cognition dysfunction (brain injury) or have severely limited manual dexterity through a quadriplegic injury. However, a tendon transfer, such as extensor carpi radialis longus to flexor digitorum profundus, facilitates apposition of the thumb and first finger and so enables such a patient to perform CISC.

The principle is to fashion a drainage channel between bladder and umbilicus or lower abdominal wall, through which the patient can completely empty their bladder.

Surgical techniques

Nowadays, two procedures are used. The first, which uses the appendix, is called a Mitrofanoff procedure [71], and the second, which uses the ileum, is known as a Yang-Monti procedure [58]. If the appendix is available, it is preferable to use this, so that the Yang-Monti procedure is reserved for the patients in whom an appendectomy has previously been performed or those in whom the appendix does not look suitable or is already in use [72]. The fashioned tube is inserted into the bladder wall via an at least 4 cm submucosal tunnel [73].

In case of reduced bladder compliance or neurogenic detrusor overactivity, a bladder augmentation is usually performed at the same time. Usually, the bladder neck is left open as a "safety mechanism." If the native bladder cannot be preserved, for example because of bladder cancer, a substitution cystoplasty using ileum or colon can be performed with the complications the same as those described above for cystoplasty. Nowadays, the most popular substitution cystoplasty performed is the "Florida pouch" which uses a low-pressure detubularized colonic reservoir with a tapered ileum and a purse string suture around the ileocecal valve as its continent mechanism [74].

During the surgery, an indwelling catheter is left through the native urethra and another into the stoma. These are usually removed 21 days after performing a cystogram, and the patient then starts CISC. For the first months, patients have to catheterize themselves every three hours in daytime and at night. About three months after the surgery, the bladder reaches its definitive capacity and patients catheterize every four hours during the day and eight-hourly during nights.

Results

Morbidity and mortality are comparable to those reported above for bladder augmentation enterocystoplasty. However, specific stoma complications occur in 16–60% with a follow-up between 30 and 240 months. The main complication, which has an incidence of 3.5–45%, is stomal stricture preventing catheterization attempts. Other complications include tube necrosis, diverticulae, tube traumatism and mucosa prolapse. Stoma complications require a second intervention in 5–38% of cases [75].

Continence is achieved in 70–98% of the patients. Furthermore, an improvement of the quality of life has also been reported, as a result of better patient independence, continence and sex life [76].

Follow-up

Follow-up must be similar to that of patients with bladder augmentation enterocystoplasty (see above).

Ileal conduit

An ileal conduit is a non-continent diversion, performed for patients with severe motor or cognitive disability or with urological complications such as deteriorating renal function, usually in the context of advanced MS or complicated myelomeningocele or SCI. The procedure is regarded as an "end of line" management option for the neurogenic bladder. A cystectomy may be performed simultaneously, although adding to postoperative morbidity, as there is a risk of bladder cancer or pyocystis if the defunctioning bladder remains.

Surgical techniques

After removing the bladder, a segment of ileum is anastomosed to the ureters at the proximal end, the distal end being inserted through the right side of the abdominal wall. Two ureteral stents are left for several days and then removed. An ileal conduit can be performed using an open, laparoscopic (Fig. 7.4) or robotic approach [77–79].

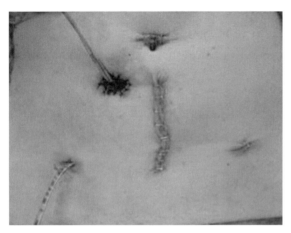

Fig. 7.4. Post-operative view of an MS patient managed with a laparoscopic assisted ileal conduit (the upper stents are ureteral).

The role of the ileum segment is to conduct, not to collect, urine through the abdominal wall into a bag attached to the skin. An important point is the localization of the stoma, which must be determined before the surgery and adapted to the patient's anatomy and disability. In a wheelchair-bound patient, the stoma should be placed higher on the abdomen than in someone who is ambulant.

Results

The perioperative mortality rate is between 1.3% and 3.1%. The early postoperative morbidity rate is between 3.8% and 33.4%, related mainly to the development of an ileus or transient impairment of respiratory function in a very disabled patient [78, 80, 81]. Late complications are mainly related to uretero-ileal anastomosis (stenosis: 2–7.8%), stomal hernia and pyelonephritis (6–32%) [81, 82]. Long-term renal function in patients with ileal conduit has been studied in children and although this may remain stable for the first few years it may subsequently deteriorate [81].

Nevertheless an ileal conduit may be a means of preventing urinary tract damage and infections, or preventing progressive renal function impairment, and may be able to improve patients' quality of life [83].

Sphincter surgery

The aim of sphincter surgery is to relieve bladder outlet obstruction due to external urethral sphincter contraction. It can be performed only in men because patients become incontinent and need a condom to collect urine. In men who cannot perform self-catheterization and who have no detrusor contractility impairment, especially quadriplegics or men with advanced MS, it can improve bladder management considerably. Several procedures have been proposed such as sphincterotomy or urethral stenting.

Sphincterotomy

Endoscopic sphincterotomy was developed for the treatment of DSD in the 1950s. It has been demonstrated to be effective for both the treatment and the prevention of genitourinary complications. However, this technique is associated with a failure rate of 15–50%, erectile dysfunction in 4–40% of cases, perioperative complications such as septicemia and hemorrhage in 5% of cases, and is irreversible [84]. Balloon dilatation of the striated sphincter was also described, but subsequently abandoned owing to the high failure rate.

Stents

Urethral sphincter stents were developed in the 1990s. There are two types: temporary (Memokath®, Diabolo®) or permanent (Urolume®, Memotherm®) (Fig. 7.5). Temporary stents can be used as a therapeutic test to ensure adequate continence control in combination with a condom catheter, to check that a stent does not induce troublesome autonomic dysreflexia, to assess acceptability of the bladder drainage method, to verify bladder emptying will be achieved, to study bladder emptying in the sitting position, to improve the patient's independence and give the patient time to think about a definitive management strategy. Temporary stents can also be used as a reversible treatment in patients with transient problems or who cannot do CISC or in patients during the initial period following the injury whilst awaiting recovery or rehabilitation of the upper limbs. In neurological patients, temporary stents can be used to help determine whether or not urinary symptoms are related to benign prostatic hyperplasia (BPH): if urinary symptoms mimicking BPH are relieved by placing a stent in the prostatic part of the urethra, prostate surgery should be considered [85].

After a temporary urethral sphincter stent, 70% of patients choose a permanent one as the preferred management of their bladder dysfunction [86]. Complications with temporary stents include a higher rate

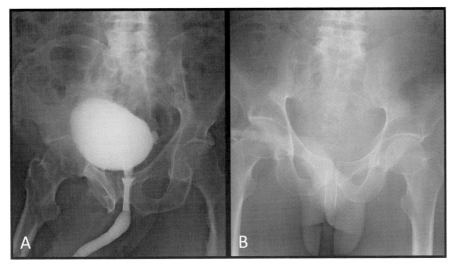

Fig. 7.5. Quadriplegia patients with a temporary urethral sphincter stent (A) and a permanent urethral sphincter stent (B).

of stent migration, stent blockage with stone or calcification, and recurrent urinary tract infections [87].

Temporary and permanent stents may ensure effective bladder emptying and lower bladder voiding pressure, thus reducing autonomic and infectious complications and minimizing the risk of renal damage [88]. Rivas found no significant differences in terms of efficacy between urethral stents and endoscopic sphincterotomy, but stents were associated with less blood loss and earlier discharge from the hospital [89]. The long-term complications with permanent stents are stent encrustation, migration, bladder neck obstruction and, if required, difficult stent removal [90].

Stress urinary incontinence management

Urinary incontinence in neurological patients is mainly due to detrusor overactivity but in some cases coincidental striated sphincter incompetence, or urethral hypermobility in women, can lead to stress urinary incontinence.

Slings

Slings are mainly used in women and are made either from autologous tissue (rectus fascia) or synthetic material (polypropylene mesh). The sling is placed vaginally under the mid urethra or under the bladder neck. With a follow-up of 27 months, an efficacy of

up to 83% has been reported [91]. In neurological patients who are already performing CISC (SCI or MS patients or patients with peripheral neuropathy causing impaired detrusor contractility), the sling can be placed somewhat more tightly to increase the chance of achieving continence. However, in women who void spontaneously, preoperative urodynamics are mandatory to check bladder contractility since urinary retention after sling surgery requiring CISC may be due to detrusor hypocontractility. Apart from urinary retention, complications include urethral and bladder erosion, difficulty in self-catheterization and development of de novo detrusor overactivity.

Slings have been used in boys with spina bifida when they have been placed around the bladder neck using either an abdominal or abdomino-perineal approach. The success rate of slings in spina bifida boys is up to 75% [92] with complications similar to those in women.

Adjustable continence therapy (ACT)

ACT was developed for the treatment of post-prostatectomy incontinence, and in men and women for recurrent stress urinary incontinence resulting from sphincter incompetence. Two balloons are implanted under the bladder neck or close to the prostatic apex in men and attached to an injectable port which is located in the scrotum in men and in the labia majora in women. The port allows postoperative adjustment of balloon pressure and volume.

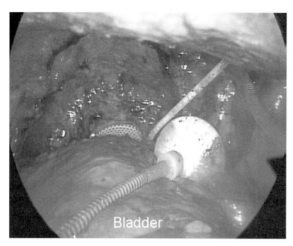

Fig. 7.6. Laparoscopic view of the retropubic space showing the anterior part of cuff around prostate and the reservoir in laterovesical position.

Bastien has suggested this may be a new alternative treatment option for managing stress urinary incontinence in neurological patients [93]. This procedure appears to be safe and completely reversible but in patients performing CISC, ACT was associated with high rate of urethral erosion.

Bulking agents

The injection of bulking agents to increase urethral resistance and leak point pressures is a minimally invasive endoscopic technique. Initially collagen-based beads were implanted but these were found to degrade over time so that now, silicone-based substances (Macroplastique-polydimethylsiloxane) are used. In non-neurological patients, they are effective in 60–80% of cases although the effects last for only about two years or so and quite often more than one injection is required to achieve the desired results. Importantly, their use does not preclude any further treatment. In neurological patients, studies are limited but it is known that this intervention is contraindicated in patients performing CISC.

Artificial urinary sphincter (AUS)

The AUS is an excellent device for achieving continence. Although more commonly used in men, it can be used in both sexes. However, the results in neurogenic patients are not as satisfactory as in the non-neurogenic group. The reason for this is not known but pressure on the perineum sustained from sitting

in a wheelchair and self-catheterization may be contributing factors.

The device has three components, a cuff which is placed around the bulbar urethra or prostate, a balloon which is placed in the prevesical space and a pump which is located in the scrotum. In women, the cuff is placed around the bladder neck and the pump is installed in the labia. Its use in patients with neurological disorders has mainly been in those with SCI, myelomeningocele or cauda equina damage.

The early postoperative morbidity rate is 25% but at 10 years the success rate is up to 82%, although the average AUS life is 8 years. Late complications include mechanical failure, erosion of the cuff or infection requiring removal of the implant. It is claimed that the incidence erosion is less with bladder neck cuff placement than with bulbar urethra in men [94]. The AUS can be placed using an open, laparoscopic or robotic approach (Fig. 7.6) [95].

Suprapubic catheter (SPC)

An indwelling catheter use should be limited for patients without a long life expectancy and as an "end-line" treatment. An SPC is generally considered the preferred management option in advanced MS, disabled patients with MSA or quadriplegics who become unable to perform CISC. An SPC is preferred to a urethral catheter as the latter can cause pressure necrosis with cleavage of the urethra in males and that of bladder neck in females and is also hygienically superior.

An SPC is placed percutaneously directly into the bladder through the abdominal wall. Because of the small bladder size and thickness of the wall of neurogenic bladders, its placement in neurological patients requires endoscopic control and sometimes a short general anesthetic. A relative contraindication is severe abdominal adhesions from previous surgery. Precautions are necessary to prevent complications such as bowel perforation or epigastric artery injury. In the UK between September 1, 2005 and June 30, 2009, 259 incidents were reported to the National Patient Safety Agency's Reporting and Learning System relating to the insertion and management of SPCs. Of these, nine were the result of bowel perforation – three deaths and six cases of severe harm.

The specific problems of long-term catheters are:

- recurrent urinary tract infections: a foreign body is frequently colonized with bacteria

- blockage of catheters: the catheters become blocked by matrix-crystal complex formed by the interaction of bacterial biofilms with magnesium and phosphate crystals, leading to incontinence. However, if the catheter blocks and there is outlet resistance, the bladder can distend and lead to autonomic dysreflexia in those with SCI. Indeed, catheter blockage is one of the most common causes of autonomic dysreflexia. Some patients require regular bladder washouts and frequent catheter changes and an increase in size of the catheter may be helpful. It is also thought that cycling the bladder with a flip flow value helps preserve the bladder capacity and decreases the chances of catheter blockages
- bladder stones: about 25% of patients with long-term catheters will form stones. The mechanism is thought to be an extension of the one described above for catheter blockages
- bladder cancer: the chronic inflammatory process can lead to squamous metaplasia leading to cancer. This is generally a squamous cell carcinoma with a poor prognosis and is thought to occur in 8% of those with a long-term catheter.

References

1. Saxtorph M. Stricture urethrae, fistula perinee, retentio urinae. *Clinisk Chirurgi Copenhagen Gyldenldalske Fortlag* 1887:265–80.

2. Katona F, Benyo I, Lang I. Uber intraluminare Elektrotherapie von verschiedenen paralytischen Zustanden des Gastroinestinalen Traktes mit Quadrangularstrom. *Zentralbl Chir* 1959;**84**:929–33.

3. Ebner A, Jiang C, Lindstrom S. Intravesical electrical stimulation – an experimental analysis of the mechanism of action. *J Urol* 1992;**148**:920–4.

4. Gladh G, Mattsson S, Lindstrom S. Intravesical electrical stimulation in the treatment of micturition dysfunction in children. *Neurourol Urodyn* 2003;**22**:233–42.

5. Madersbacher H. Intravesical electrical stimulation for the rehabilitation of the neuropathic bladder. *Paraplegia* 1990;**28**:349–52.

6. Boone TB, Roehrborn CG, Hurt G. Transurethral intravesical electrotherapy for neurogenic bladder dysfunction in children with myelodysplasia: a prospective, randomized clinical trial. *J Urol* 1992;**148** (2 Pt 2):550–4.

7. Tanagho EA, Schmidt RA. Electrical stimulation in the clinical management of the neurogenic bladder. *J Urol* 1988;**140**:1331–9.

8. Ruud Bosch JL, Groen J. Treatment of refractory urge urinary incontinence with sacral spinal nerve stimulation in multiple sclerosis patients. *Lancet* 1996;**348**:717–19.

9. Amundsen CL, Romero AA, Jamison MG, Webster GD. Sacral neuromodulation for intractable urge incontinence: are there factors associated with cure? *Urology* 2005;**66**:746–50.

10. Chartier-Kastler EJ, Ruud Bosch JL, Perrigot M, et al. Long-term results of sacral nerve stimulation (S3) for the treatment of neurogenic refractory urge incontinence related to detrusor hyperreflexia. *J Urol* 2000;**164**:1476–80.

11. Hohenfellner M, Humke J, Hampel C, et al. Chronic sacral neuromodulation for treatment of neurogenic bladder dysfunction: long-term results with unilateral implants. *Urology* 2001;**58**:887–92.

12. Scheepens WA, Jongen MM, Nieman FH, et al. Predictive factors for sacral neuromodulation in chronic lower urinary tract dysfunction. *Urology* 2002;**60**:598–602.

13. Guys JM, Haddad M, Planche D, et al. Sacral neuromodulation for neurogenic bladder dysfunction in children. *J Urol* 2004;**172**(4 Pt 2):1673–6.

14. Lombardi G, Del Popolo G. Clinical outcome of sacral neuromodulation in incomplete spinal cord injured patients suffering from neurogenic lower urinary tract symptoms. *Spinal Cord* 2009;**47**:486–91.

15. Wallace PA, Lane FL, Noblett KL. Sacral nerve neuromodulation in patients with underlying neurologic disease. *Am J Obstet Gynecol* 2007;**197**:96.e1–5.

16. Fowler CJ, Swinn MJ, Goodwin RJ, Oliver S, Craggs M. Studies of the latency of pelvic floor contraction during peripheral nerve evaluation show that the muscle response is reflexly mediated. *J Urol* 2000;**163**:881–3.

17. Schurch B, Reilly I, Reitz A, Curt A. Electrophysiological recordings during the peripheral nerve evaluation (PNE) test in complete spinal cord injury patients. *World J Urol* 2003;**20**:319–22.

18. Dasgupta R, Critchley HD, Dolan RJ, Fowler CJ. Changes in brain activity following sacral neuromodulation for urinary retention. *J Urol* 2005;**174**:2268–72.

19. Spinelli M, Giardiello G, Arduini A, van den Hombergh U. New percutaneous technique of sacral nerve stimulation has high initial success rate: preliminary results. *Eur Urol* 2003;**43**:70–4.

20. Scheepens WA, Weil EH, van Koeveringe GA, et al. Buttock placement of the implantable pulse generator: a new implantation technique for sacral neuromodulation – a multicenter study. *Eur Urol* 2001;**40**:434–8.

21. van Voskuilen AC, Oerlemans DJ, Weil EH, de Bie RA, van Kerrebroeck PE. Long term results of neuromodulation by sacral nerve stimulation for lower urinary tract symptoms: a retrospective single center study. *Eur Urol* 2006;**49**:366–72.

22. Van Rey F, Jongen PJH, Heesakkers J. Treatment of voiding dysfunction by neuromodulation in a selected MS patient population. *Eur Urol* 2009;**8**:241.

23. Sievert KD, Amend B, Gakis G, et al. Early sacral neuromodulation prevents urinary incontinence after complete spinal cord injury. *Ann Neurol* 2010;**67**:74–84.

24. Bosch JL, Groen J. Sacral nerve neuromodulation in the treatment of patients with refractory motor urge incontinence: long-term results of a prospective longitudinal study. *J Urol* 2000;**163**:1219–22.

25. Siegel SW, Catanzaro F, Dijkema HE, et al. Long-term results of a multicenter study on sacral nerve stimulation for treatment of urinary urge incontinence, urgency-frequency, and retention. *Urology* 2000;**56**(6 Suppl 1):87–91.

26. Everaert K, De Ridder D, Baert L, Oosterlinck W, Wyndaele JJ. Patient satisfaction and complications following sacral nerve stimulation for urinary retention, urge incontinence and perineal pain: a multicenter evaluation. *Int Urogynecol J Pelvic Floor Dysfunct* 2000;**11**:231–5.

27. Grunewald V, Hofner K, Thon WF, Kuczyk MA, Jonas U. Sacral electrical neuromodulation as an alternative treatment option for lower urinary tract dysfunction. *Restor Neurol Neurosci* 1999;**14**:189–93.

28. Dasgupta R, Wiseman OJ, Kitchen N, Fowler CJ. Long-term results of sacral neuromodulation for women with urinary retention. *BJU Int* 2004;**94**:335–7.

29. Elhilali MM, Khaled SM, Kashiwabara T, Elzayat E, Corcos J. Sacral neuromodulation: long-term experience of one center. *Urology* 2005;**65**:1114–17.

30. van Kerrebroeck PE, van Voskuilen AC, Heesakkers JP, et al. Results of sacral neuromodulation therapy for urinary voiding dysfunction: outcomes of a prospective, worldwide clinical study. *J Urol* 2007;**178**:2029–34.

31. Brindley GS. An implant to empty the bladder or close the urethra. *J Neurol Neurosurg Psychiatry* 1977;**40**:358–69.

32. Brindley GS. The actions of parasympathetic and sympathetic nerves in human micturition, erection and seminal emission, and their restoration in paraplegic patients by implanted electrical stimulators. *Proc R Soc Lond* 1988;**235**:111–20.

33. Egon G, Chartier-Kastler E, Denys P, Ruffion A. Traumatise medullaire et neuro-stimulation de Brindley. *Prog Urol* 2007;**1**:535–9.

34. Brindley GS, Polkey CE, Rushton DN. Sacral anterior root stimulators for bladder control in paraplegia. *Paraplegia* 1982;**20**:365–81.

35. Barat M, Egon G, Daverat P, et al. L'electrostimulation des racines sacrees anterieures dans le traitement des neurovessies centrales. *J Urol (Paris)* 1993;**99**:3–7.

36. Brindley GS. The first 500 patients with sacral anterior root stimulator implants: general description. *Paraplegia* 1994;**32**:795–805.

37. Van Kerrebroeck PE, Koldewijn EL, Rosier PF, Wijkstra H, Debruyne FM. Results of the treatment of neurogenic bladder dysfunction in spinal cord injury by sacral posterior root rhizotomy and anterior sacral root stimulation. *J Urol* 1996;**155**:1378–81.

38. Schurch B, Rodic B, Jeanmonod D. Posterior sacral rhizotomy and intradural anterior sacral root stimulation for treatment of the spastic bladder in spinal cord injured patients. *J Urol* 1997;**157**:610–14.

39. Egon G, Barat M, Colombel P, et al. Implantation of anterior sacral root stimulators combined with posterior sacral rhizotomy in spinal injury patients. *World J Urol* 1998;**16**:342–9.

40. van der Aa HE, Alleman E, Nene A, Snoek G. Sacral anterior root stimulation for bladder control: clinical results. *Arch Physiol Biochem* 1999;**107**:248–56.

41. Creasey GH, Grill JH, Korsten M, et al. An implantable neuroprosthesis for restoring bladder and bowel control to patients with spinal cord injuries: a multicenter trial. *Arch Phys Med Rehabil* 2001;**82**:1512–19.

42. Bauchet L, Segnarbieux F, Martinazzo G, Frerebeau P, Ohanna F. Traitement neurochirurgical de la vessie hyperactive chez le blesse medullaire. *Neurochirurgie* 2001;**47**:13–24.

43. Vignes JR, Liguoro D, Sesay M, Barat M, Guerin J. Dorsal rhizotomy with anterior sacral root stimulation for neurogenic bladder. *Stereotact Funct Neurosurg* 2001;**76**:243–5.

44. Kutzenberger J, Domurath B, Sauerwein D. Spastic bladder and spinal cord injury: seventeen years of experience with sacral deafferentation and implantation of an anterior root stimulator. *Artif Organs* 2005;**29**:239–41.

45. Game X, Castel-Lacanal E, Bastie JP, et al. Évaluation de la charge en soins paramédicaux des patients

neurologiques dans un service d'urologie. *Prog Urol* 2009;**19**:122–6.

46. Mahony DT, Laferte RO. Studis of enuresis. IV. Multiple detrusor myotomy: a new operation for the rehabilitation of severe detrusor hypertrophy and hypercontractility. *J Urol* 1972;**107**:1064–7.

47. Cartwright PC, Snow BW. Bladder autoaugmentation: early clinical experience. *J Urol* 1989;**142**(2 Pt 2):505–8.

48. Ehrlich RM, Gershman A. Laparoscopic seromyotomy (auto-augmentation) for non-neurogenic neurogenic bladder in a child: initial case report. *Urology* 1993;**42**:175–8.

49. Mammen T, Balaji KC. Robotic transperitoneal detrusor myotomy: description of a novel technique. *J Endourol* 2005;**19**:476–9.

50. Kumar SP, Abrams PH. Detrusor myectomy: long-term results with a minimum follow-up of 2 years. *BJU Int* 2005;**96**:341–4.

51. MacNeily AE, Afshar K, Coleman GU, Johnson HW. Autoaugmentation by detrusor myotomy: its lack of effectiveness in the management of congenital neuropathic bladder. *J Urol* 2003;**170**(4 Pt 2):1643–6.

52. Potter JM, Duffy PG, Gordon EM, Malone PR. Detrusor myotomy: a 5-year review in unstable and non-compliant bladders. *BJU Int* 2002;**89**:932–5.

53. Marte A, Di Meglio D, Cotrufo AM, et al. A long-term follow-up of autoaugmentation in myelodysplastic children. *BJU Int* 2002;**89**:928–31.

54. Leng WW, Blalock HJ, Fredriksson WH, English SF, McGuire EJ. Enterocystoplasty or detrusor myectomy? Comparison of indications and outcomes for bladder augmentation. *J Urol* 1999;**161**:758–63.

55. Von Mikulicz J. Zur operation der angerborenen blasensplate. *Zentralbl Chir* 1889;**26**:641–3.

56. Rink RC. Bladder augmentation. Options, outcomes, future. *Urol Clin North Am* 1999;**26**:111–23.

57. Liard A, Seguier-Lipszyc E, Mathiot A, Mitrofanoff P. The Mitrofanoff procedure: 20 years later. *J Urol* 2001;**165**(6 Pt 2):2394–8.

58. Monti PR, de Carvalho JR. Tubulisation transversale de segments intestinaux: un conduit catheterisable alternatif au procede de Mitrofanoff. *Prog Urol* 2001;**11**:382–4.

59. Game X, Karsenty G, Chartier-Kastler E, Ruffion A. Traitement de l'hyperactivite detrusorienne neurologique: enterocystoplasties. *Prog Urol* 2007;**17**:584–96.

60. Chartier-Kastler EJ, Mongiat-Artus P, Bitker MO, et al. Long-term results of augmentation cystoplasty in spinal cord injury patients. *Spinal Cord* 2000;**38**:490–4.

61. Greenwell TJ, Venn SN, Mundy AR. Augmentation cystoplasty. *BJU Int* 2001;**88**:511–25.

62. Khoury AE, Salomon M, Doche R, et al. Stone formation after augmentation cystoplasty: the role of intestinal mucus. *J Urol* 1997;**158**(3 Pt 2):1133–7.

63. Nurse DE, McInerney PD, Thomas PJ, Mundy AR. Stones in enterocystoplasties. *Br J Urol* 1996;**77**:684–7.

64. Shaw J, Lewis MA. Bladder augmentation surgery – what about the malignant risk? *Eur J Pediatr Surg* 1999;**9**(Suppl 1):39–40.

65. Shekarriz B, Upadhyay J, Demirbilek S, Barthold JS, Gonzalez R. Surgical complications of bladder augmentation: comparison between various enterocystoplasties in 133 patients. *Urology* 2000;**55**:123–8.

66. Khastgir J, Hamid R, Arya M, Shah N, Shah PJ. Surgical and patient reported outcomes of "clam" augmentation ileocystoplasty in spinal cord injured patients. *Eur Urol* 2003;**43**:263–9.

67. Mundy AR, Stephenson TP. "Clam" ileocystoplasty for the treatment of refractory urge incontinence. *Br J Urol* 1985;**57**:641–6.

68. Caione P, Capozza N, Zavaglia D, Palombaro G, Boldrini R. In vivo bladder regeneration using small intestinal submucosa: experimental study. *Pediatr Surg Int* 2006;**22**:593–9.

69. Barrington JW, Dyer R, Bano F. Bladder augmentation using Pelvicol implant for intractable overactive bladder syndrome. *Int Urogynecol J Pelvic Floor Dysfunct* 2006;**17**:50–3.

70. Atala A. Tissue engineering of artificial organs. *J Endourol* 2000;**14**:49–57.

71. Mitrofanoff P. Cystostomie continente transappendiculaire dans le traitement des vessies neurologiques. *Chir Pediatr* 1980;**21**:297–305.

72. Lemelle JL, Simo AK, Schmitt M. Comparative study of the Yang-Monti channel and appendix for continent diversion in the Mitrofanoff and Malone principles. *J Urol* 2004;**172**(5 Pt 1):1907–10.

73. Karsenty G, Chartier-Kastler E, Mozer P, et al. A novel technique to achieve cutaneous continent urinary diversion in spinal cord-injured patients unable to catheterize through native urethra. *Spinal Cord* 2008;**46**:305–10.

74. Salom EM, Mendez LE, Schey D, et al. Continent ileocolonic urinary reservoir (Miami pouch): the University of Miami experience over 15 years. *Am J Obstet Gynecol* 2004;**190**:994–1003.

75. Karsenty G, Vidal F, Ruffion A, Chartier-Kastler E. Derivation cutanee continente en neuro-urologie. *Prog Urol* 2007;**17**:542–51.

76. Moreno JG, Chancellor MB, Karasick S, et al. Improved quality of life and sexuality with continent urinary diversion in quadriplegic women with umbilical stoma. *Arch Phys Med Rehabil* 1995;**76**:758–62.

77. Game X, Mallet R, Guillotreau J, et al. Uterus, fallopian tube, ovary and vagina-sparing laparoscopic cystectomy: technical description and results. *Eur Urol* 2007;**51**:441–6.

78. Chartier-Kastler EJ, Mozer P, Denys P, et al. Neurogenic bladder management and cutaneous non-continent ileal conduit. *Spinal Cord* 2002;**40**:443–8.

79. Hubert J, Chammas M, Larre S, et al. Initial experience with successful totally robotic laparoscopic cystoprostatectomy and ileal conduit construction in tetraplegic patients: report of two cases. *J Endourol* 2006;**20**:139–43.

80. Guillotreau J, Game X, Castel-Lacanal E, et al. Cystectomie laparoscopique et ureterostomie trans-ileale pour troubles vesico-sphincteriens d'origine neurologique. Evaluation de la morbidite. *Prog Urol* 2007;**17**:208–12.

81. Bart S, Game X, Mozer P, Ruffion A, Chartier-Kastler E. Derivation cutanee non continente en neuro-urologie. *Prog Urol* 2007;**17**:552–8.

82. McDougal WS. Use of intestinal segments and urinary diversion. In: Walsh PC, Retik AB, Kavoussi LR, et al, eds. *Campbell's urology*. Philadelphia: WB Saunders; 2002.

83. Herschorn S, Rangaswamy S, Radomski SB. Urinary undiversion in adults with myelodysplasia: long-term followup. *J Urol* 1994;**152**(2 Pt 1):329–33.

84. Fontaine E, Hajri M, Rhein F, et al. Reappraisal of endoscopic sphincterotomy for post-traumatic neurogenic bladder: a prospective study. *J Urol* 1996;**155**:277–80.

85. Chartier-Kastler E, Mozer P, Ayoub N, Richard F, Ruffion A. Hypertrophie benigne de la prostate et neuro-urologie. *Prog Urol* 2007;**17**:529–34.

86. Game X, Chartier-Kastler E, Ayoub N, et al. Outcome after treatment of detrusor-sphincter dyssynergia by temporary stent. *Spinal Cord* 2008;**46**:74–7.

87. Low AI, McRae PJ. Use of the Memokath for detrusor-sphincter dyssynergia after spinal cord injury – a cautionary tale. *Spinal Cord* 1998;**36**:39–44.

88. Denys P, Thiry-Escudie I, Ayoub N, et al. Urethral stent for the treatment of detrusor-sphincter dyssynergia: evaluation of the clinical, urodynamic, endoscopic and radiological efficacy after more than 1 year. *J Urol* 2004;**172**:605–7.

89. Rivas DA, Chancellor MB, Bagley D. Prospective comparison of external sphincter prosthesis placement and external sphincterotomy in men with spinal cord injury. *J Endourol* 1994;**8**:89–93.

90. Chancellor MB, Gajewski J, Ackman CF, et al. Long-term followup of the North American multicenter UroLume trial for the treatment of external detrusor-sphincter dyssynergia. *J Urol* 1999;**161**:1545–50.

91. Hamid R, Khastgir J, Arya M, Patel HR, Shah PJ. Experience of tension-free vaginal tape for the treatment of stress incontinence in females with neuropathic bladders. *Spinal Cord* 2003;**41**:118–21.

92. Perez LM, Smith EA, Broecker BH, et al. Outcome of sling cystourethropexy in the pediatric population: a critical review. *J Urol* 1996;**156**(2 Pt 2):642–6.

93. Bastien L, Bart S, Vidart A, et al. Traitement de l'incontinence urinaire par insuffisance sphinctérienne neurologique à l'aide des ballons ACT™ (femme) et Pro-ACT™ (homme): résultats à 2 ans. *Prog Urol* 2008;**18**(Suppl 6):O87.

94. Ruffion A, Genevois S, Game X, et al. Peri-prostatic artificial urinary sphincter AMS 800 in adult neurogenic patients: a multi-centric study. *Eur Urol* 2009;**8**:244.

95. Game X, Bram R, Abu Anz S, et al. Laparoscopic insertion of artificial periprostatic urinary sphincter. *Urology* 2009;**73**:442 e1–3.

Chapter

8

Approach and evaluation of neurogenic bowel dysfunction

Klaus Krogh

Introduction

Symptoms of colorectal and anal sphincter dysfunction are common in patients with neurological disorders. Until recently, symptoms were underrecognized and the pathophysiology of neurogenic bowel dysfunction (NBD) was poorly understood. This is unfortunate as NBD often has a profound impact on quality of life (QOL) and newer treatment modalities are being introduced.

Prevalence

Previous studies amongst subjects with spinal cord injury (SCI) showed that 42–95% have constipation [1–5], 65% have to perform digital stimulation or evacuation of the rectum [2], 75% have fecal incontinence at least once per year and 20% at least once per month [2]. In patients with multiple sclerosis, 36–43% suffer from constipation and 20–30% are incontinent at least once per week [6, 7]. Amongst children with myelomeningocele, 79% have constipation or fecal incontinence [8] and even though symptoms become less frequent with age, QOL continues to be impaired [9]. Amongst persons surviving stroke, 9–15% will have persisting fecal incontinence and 23% constipation at follow-up [10, 11]. Changes in bowel function in Parkinson's disease are due to delayed colon transit and impaired anorectal muscle coordination [12] and may be mediated by central and peripheral mechanisms, e.g. loss of dopamine in the enteric nerve system. The most common symptoms are unsuccessful attempts at defecation in 37% and bowel movements less than every second day in 27% [13].

Evaluation of bowel function in patients with neurological disorders has to be individualized and focused on parameters that have a clinical consequence.

However, evaluation of NBD often includes the following steps: history taking, standard physical examination, determination of colorectal transit time and, in some patients, anorectal physiology tests. In some patients, endoscopy is indicated.

Evaluation

The most frequent symptoms of NBD are constipation, fecal incontinence and abdominal pain. As only few objective tests are available for routine clinical evaluation of patients with NBD, history taking is important to capture the spectrum of bowel symptoms and their impact on QOL. In SCI patients, constipation and abdominal pain become more common with time [14, 15] and in patients with multiple sclerosis or Parkinson's disease, bowel symptoms become more severe as the disease progresses [13]. Therefore, bowel functions may have to be re-evaluated at follow-up visits.

Both evaluation and treatment [16] of NBD will remain to be empirical until large, well-designed studies have been performed. The evaluation of bowel functions has received much more attention in patients with SCI compared to other patient groups and most of the effort has been through the international cooperation between the International Spinal Cord Society (ISCoS) and the American Spinal Cord Injury Association (ASIA). Recently, international standards for *classification* of autonomic function after SCI have been published [17], an attempt has been made to develop an *NBD score* specific for subjects with SCI [18], international bowel function SCI data sets for *documentation* of bowel function in clinic and research have been developed [19, 20], and recommendations for *outcome measures*, including bowel function, have been published [21]. The reproducibility and validity of the most commonly

Pelvic Organ Dysfunction in Neurological Disease: Clinical Management and Rehabilitation, ed. Clare J. Fowler, Jalesh N. Panicker & Anton Emmanuel. Published by Cambridge University Press. © Cambridge University Press 2010.

used method for objective assessment of colonic function, radiographically determined *colorectal transit time*, have been described [22, 23], and the usefulness of *anorectal physiology tests* in predicting the outcome of treatment has been discussed [24, 25].

International standards to document remaining autonomic function after SCI

Bowel dysfunction should be viewed in relation to other complications following SCI. The commonly used classification of SCIs from the International Standards for the Neurological Classification of SCI [26] involves assessing motor and sensory functions but does not include autonomic dysfunction. The Autonomic Standards Assessment Form developed by an international group of experts commissioned by the ISCoS and ASIA provides only indirect and very limited information about neurogenic bowel function [17, 21].

Symptom-based scores for neurogenic bowel dysfunction

A number of scores for fecal incontinence and constipation exist. The most commonly used are the Wexner [27] and St. Mark's [28] scores for fecal incontinence and the Cleveland Constipation score [29]. All have been extensively used in clinical studies of other patient groups and in a randomized trial among SCI patients they were useful for evaluation of treatment of NBD [30]. However, a limitation is that they cover either constipation or fecal incontinence, whereas most patients have combinations of both symptom complexes. The scores have not been developed specifically for individuals with neurological disease and their validity and reproducibility in that group needs to be studied.

The NBD score was constructed to overcome these limitations in the evaluation of bowel symptoms in SCI patients. It is based upon a mailed questionnaire that includes questions on fecal incontinence (10 items), constipation (10 items), difficult rectal evacuation (8 items) and self-assessed impact on QOL (three items) that was sent out to 424 adult Danish SCI patients. The reproducibility and validity of each item was tested in 20 randomly chosen respondents and only items in which reproducibility and validity were fair, good or very good (kappa coefficient >0.40) were considered for inclusion in the NBD score. A multivariate logistic regression analysis was made with colorectal symptoms as independent variables and self-assessed impact on QOL as the dependent variable. Ten variables were significantly ($p < 0.05$) associated with self-reported impact on QOL and were therefore included in the NBD score. Not all items had the same risk of affecting QOL and the number of points given to each of the 10 items depended on that item's odds ratio (OR) of having some or major impact on QOL. The NBD score is shown in Appendix 2. It has been translated to and used in English, German, Italian, Swedish and Danish [24, 30]. However, further validity studies are needed and future modifications are likely.

Some basic relevant clinical lessons can be drawn from the NBD score. The item having the greatest impact on QOL was fecal incontinence. Patients having fecal incontinence once or more per day had 13 times greater risk (OR=13) for having impaired QOL. Fecal incontinence occurring less than once a month apparently does not impair QOL. The other symptoms most commonly impairing QOL are frequency of defecation less than once per week (OR = 6), prolonged time required for each bowel opening more than an hour (OR = 7), and the need for digital stimulation or evacuation of the anorectum one or more times per week (OR = 6).

The NBD score has been evaluated in children with myelomeningocele and in adults with Parkinson's disease. However it was not found to be valid in those populations [9, 13].

International bowel function spinal cord injury data sets

The international bowel function SCI data sets were developed to collect data on bowel symptoms after SCI in a common format. It is hoped that this will facilitate comparison of symptoms, treatment modalities and outcomes between various centres and countries. The process was supported by the ISCoS and ASIA. An international working team developed the basic SCI data set for clinical use [19] and an extended SCI data set is available for research purposes [20]. Other groups have developed data sets for various complications of SCI (i.e. upper and lower urinary tract dysfunction, spasticity, pain and sexual dysfunction). Information from these data sets should usually be used with the background information from the International SCI core data set [31].

The 12 items of the international bowel function basic SCI data set are shown in Table 8.1. This is

Table 8.1. International SCI bowel function basic data set

Date performed: YYYYMMDD ☐ Unknown

Gastrointestinal or anal sphincter dysfunction unrelated to the spinal cord lesion:

☐ No ☐ Yes, specify_____ ☐ Unknown

Surgical procedures on the gastrointestinal tract:

☐ No ☐ Appendicectomy, date performed YYYYMMDD

☐ Cholecystectomy, date performed YYYYMMDD

☐ Colostomy, date last performed YYYYMMDD

☐ Ileostomy, date last performed YYYYMMDD

☐ Other, specify: _____, date last performed YYYYMMDD

☐ Unknown

Awareness of the need to defecate (within the last four weeks):

☐ Normal (direct)

☐ Indirect (For example: Abdominal cramping or discomfort – Abdominal muscle spasms – Spasms of lower extremities – Perspiration – Piloerection – Headache – Chills)

☐ None

☐ Unknown

Defecation method and bowel care procedures (within the last four weeks):

	Main	Supplementary
Normal defecation	☐	☐
Straining/bearing down to empty	☐	☐
Digital anorectal stimulation	☐	☐
Suppositories	☐	☐
Digital evacuation	☐	☐
Mini enema (Clysma ≤150 ml)	☐	☐
Enema (≥150 ml)	☐	☐
Colostomy	☐	
Sacral anterior root stimulation	☐	☐
Other method, specify_____	☐	☐

☐ Unknown

Average time required for defecation (within the last four weeks):

☐ 0–5 minutes ☐ 6–10 minutes ☐ 11–20 minutes ☐ 21–30 minutes

☐ 31–60 minutes ☐ More than 60 minutes ☐ Unknown

Frequency of defecation (within the last four weeks):

☐ Three times or more per day ☐ Twice daily ☐ Once daily

☐ Not daily but more than twice every week

☐ Twice every week ☐ Once every week

Table 8.1. (*cont.*)

☐ Less than once every week, but at least once within the last four weeks

☐ No defecation within the last four weeks

☐ Not applicable   ☐ Unknown

Frequency of fecal incontinence (within the last three months):

☐ Two or more episodes per day   ☐ One episode per day

☐ Not every day but at least once per week

☐ Not every week but at least once per month

☐ Once every month   ☐ Less than once per month   ☐ Never

☐ Unknown

Need to wear pad or plug (within the last three months):

☐ Daily use   ☐ Not every day but at least once per week

☐ Not every week but at least once per month

☐ Less than once per month   ☐ Never

☐ Unknown

Medication affecting bowel function/constipating agents (within the last four weeks):

☐ No   ☐ Yes, anticholinergics

          ☐ Yes, narcotics

☐ Yes, other, specify: _____

☐ Unknown

Oral laxatives (within the last four weeks):

☐ No   ☐ Yes, osmotic laxatives (drops)

          ☐ Yes, osmotic or bulking laxatives (tablets or granulates)

          ☐ Yes, irritant laxatives (drops)

          ☐ Yes, irritant laxatives (tablets)

          ☐ Yes, prokinetics

          ☐ Yes, other, specify:_____

☐ Unknown

Perianal problems (within the last year):

☐ None   ☐ Haemorrhoids   ☐ Perianal sores   ☐ Fissures   ☐ Rectal prolapse

☐ Other, specify_____   ☐ Unknown

considered the minimal amount of information on bowel function to be obtained in clinical practice (i.e. at control visits) and is based on patient history. Medications may alter gastrointestinal function and should be noted when filling in the basic data set. The 32 items of the international bowel function extended SCI data set shown in Table 8.2 are intended for epidemiological studies and clinical trials. The items are obtained through patient history, digital anorectal examination and radiographically determined colorectal transit time. The most commonly used scores (Wexner, St. Mark's, Cleveland constipation and NBD) can be derived by combining the information from the basic and

Table 8.2. International SCI bowel function extended data set

Date of data collection: YYYYMMDD   ☐ Unknown

Duration of constipation:

☐ Less than a year	☐ 1–5 years	☐ 6–10 years	☐ 11–20 years
☐ More than 20 years	☐ Not applicable	☐ Unknown	

Unsuccessful attempts at defecation (within the last three months):

☐ Never	☐ Less than once per month	☐ Less than once per week but at least once per month	☐ Once or more per week but not every day
☐ 1–3 per day	☐ 4–6 per day	☐ 7–9 per day	☐ 10 times or more per day
☐ Not applicable	☐ Unknown		

Incomplete rectal emptying after defecation (within the last three months):

☐ Daily   ☐ Not every day but at least once per week

☐ Not every week but at least once per month

☐ Less than once per month	☐ Never	☐ Not applicable	☐ Unknown

Abdominal bloating (within the last three months):

☐ Daily   ☐ Not every day but at least once per week

☐ Not every week but at least once per month

☐ Less than once per month	☐ Never	☐ Unknown

Abdominal pain/discomfort (within the last three months):

☐ Daily   ☐ Not every day but at least once per week

☐ Not every week but at least once per month

☐ Less than once per month	☐ Never	☐ Unknown

Any respiratory discomfort (shortness of breath/difficulty in taking a deep breath) considered to be entirely or partly due to a distended abdomen (within the last three months):

☐ Daily   ☐ Not every day but at least once per week

☐ Not every week but at least once per month

☐ Less than once per month	☐ Never	☐ Not applicable	☐ Unknown

Perianal pain during defecation (within the last three months):

☐ Daily   ☐ Not every day but at least once per week

☐ Not every week but at least once per month

☐ Less than once per month	☐ Never	☐ Not applicable	☐ Unknown

Frequency of flatus incontinence (within the last three months):

☐ Daily   ☐ Not every day but at least once per week

☐ Not every week but more than once per month

Table 8.2. (*cont.*)

□ Once per month	□ Less than once per month	□ Never
□ Not applicable	□ Unknown	

Frequency of incontinence to *liquid* stools (within the last three months):

□ Two or more episodes per day   □ Once daily

□ Not every day but at least once per week

□ Not every week but more than once per month

□ Once per month	□ Less than once per month	□ Never
□ Not applicable	□ Unknown	

Frequency of incontinence to *solid* stools (within the last three months):

□ Two or more episodes per day   □ Once daily

□ Not every day but at least once per week

□ Not every week but more than once per month

□ Once per month	□ Less than once per month	□ Never
□ Not applicable	□ Unknown	

Ability to defer defecation for 15 minutes or more (within the last three months):

□ Yes	□ No	□ Not applicable	□ Unknown

Position for bowel care (within the last three months):

□ Bed	□ Toilet chair/commode	□ Raised toilet seat
□ Conventional toilet	□ Other, specify_____	□ Unknown

Degree of independency during bowel management (within the last three months):

□ Requires total assistance   □ Requires partial assistance; does not clean self

□ Requires partial assistance; cleans self independently

□ Uses toilet independently in all tasks but needs adaptive devices or special setting (e.g. bars)

□ Uses toilet independently; does not need adaptive devices or special setting

□ Unknown

Bowel care facilitators (within the last three months):

□ Digital stimulation or evacuation	□ Abdominal massage
□ Gastrocolonic response	□ Other, specify:_____
□ None	□ Unknown

Events and intervals of defecation (1): average time from initiation of bowel care to stool comes out (within the last three months):

_____minute(s)

□ Not applicable   □ Unknown

Events and intervals of defecation (2): average time during bowel movement that stool intermittently or continuously comes out with or without assistance (within the last three months):

_____minute(s)

Table 8.2. (cont.)

□ Not applicable   □ Unknown

Events and intervals of defecation (3): average time spent waiting after last stool passes before ending bowel care (within the last three months):

_____minute(s)

□ Not applicable   □ Unknown

Lifestyle alteration due to *anal incontinence* (within the last three months):

□ Lifestyle altered each day   □ Lifestyle altered at least once per week but not every day

□ Lifestyle altered more than once per month but not every week

□ Lifestyle altered once per month   □ Lifestyle altered less than once per month

□ Lifestyle not altered   □ Not applicable   □ Unknown

Lifestyle alteration due to *constipation* (within the last three months):

□ Lifestyle altered each day   □ Lifestyle altered at least once per week but not every day

□ Lifestyle altered more than once per month but not every week

□ Lifestyle altered once per month   □ Lifestyle altered less than once per month

□ Lifestyle not altered   □ Not applicable   □ Unknown

Self-reported impact on quality of life due to bowel dysfunction:

□ Major impact   □ Some impact   □ Little impact   □ No impact

□ Unknown

To be collected after physical examination:

Anal tone:

□ Normal   □ Reduced   □ Excessive   □ Not tested   □ Not applicable

Voluntary contraction of the anal canal:

□ Yes   □ No   □ Not tested   □ Not applicable

To be collected after x-ray investigation:

Total gastrointestinal or colonic transit time:

_____days _____ hours   □ Not tested

Right colonic transit time:

_____days _____ hours   □ Not tested

Left colonic transit time:

_____days _____ hours   □ Not tested

extended data sets. It is appreciated that not all parameters from the data sets will be appropriate in every study and researchers are free to choose items.

The international bowel function SCI data sets are based on the opinions of the expert group and therefore represent a low level of evidence. However, during the process of creating the data sets, a large number of relevant scientific and professional organisations and societies (approximately 40) and individuals with special interest were involved. Furthermore, the data sets were posted on the ISCoS and ASIA websites for three months to allow comments and suggestions. The validity and reproducibility of the data sets need to be studied. As the data sets are intended for international use, their validity will have to be tested in several cultures and countries. A thorough description of each item of the data sets is beyond the scope of the present chapter but can be found in the cited publications [19, 20] and on the ISCoS and ASIA websites.

Outcome measures for bowel function in spinal cord injury

Over the years, a number of parameters have been used to describe bowel function in SCI. Some of these have been reviewed as part of the international spinal cord outcomes partnership endeavour (SCOPE). SCOPE is a broad-based consortium of scientists and researchers representing academic institutions, industry, government agencies, user organizations and foundations [21]. It was concluded that most previously used outcome measures were useful in specific research projects only and that their clinical applications were limited. The most useful – radiographically determined colorectal transit times and the NBD score – need further validation.

Investigations
Colorectal transit times

Most clinicians prefer to support the history with more objective investigations. The technique most often used to study colorectal functions in patients with neurological diseases is radiographically determined colorectal transit time (CTT). This can be carried out in various ways: single intake of markers followed by a single abdominal x-ray after a specific time interval, single intake of markers followed by multiple x-rays after specific time intervals, or multiple intake of markers at specific time intervals followed by a single abdominal x-ray. The advantage of the first method is that it is easy to perform and only one dose of marker has to be taken. Compliance is high and radiation dose is low. The disadvantage is that it does not provide any quantitative assessment of CTT (i.e. in days or hours) but only

information as to whether it is prolonged or not and whether this is mainly due to generalized or left-sided prolonged transit. However, in most clinical situations, this information is sufficient and the single intake–single x-ray method is most commonly used. The second method allows quantitative description of CTT [32], but it may be cumbersome as it requires x-rays to be taken on two or more days and hence the radiation dose is higher. The third method, multiple markers–single x-ray, also allows quantitative description of CTT and the radiation dose is low. However, compliance may be a problem as patients have to remember to take markers on several days (usually six). Furthermore, it is valid only if the CTT is less than the number of days the markers have been ingested. The last method has been used most often in studies of CTT in neurological disorders [33, 34, 35] and it is also used clinically at some centers. An example of radiographically determined CTT is shown in Fig. 8.1.

Correlations between CTT and colorectal symptoms have been the subject of two studies among patients with SCI [22, 23]. In one study, prolonged left CTT was associated with a subjective feeling of unsuccessful rectal emptying [22]. Neither total nor left-sided transit time was associated with time required for bowel care or with bloating. In another study total CTT, but not segmental CTT, had acceptable reproducibility but neither was significantly associated with scores of colorectal symptoms or individual symptoms [23]. Due to the poor correlation between CTT and symptoms, the use of CTT in subjects with SCI has been questioned [22]. Information about the value of CTT in selection of patients for treatment or for selection of treatment modality is extremely scarce. However, in a study of long-term outcomes of transanal colonic irrigation in 211 patients with NBD, successful outcome was associated with prolonged CTT before treatment [25].

Scintigraphy has been used in order to describe intestinal and colorectal transit in SCI patients [36, 37]. It is superior to radio-opaque markers in the evaluation of small intestinal transit but not in the clinically more important evaluation of CTT. The radiation dose of scintigraphic transit studies is much higher than when using radio-opaque markers and it is also more expensive. Therefore, scintigraphic assessment of colorectal transit is only used in the research setting. Scintigraphy has also been used to

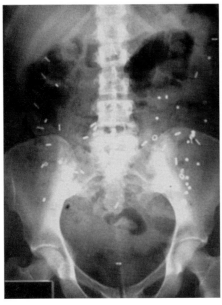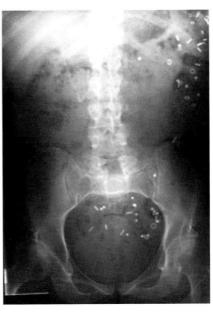

Fig. 8.1. Radiographically determined colorectal transit time. A capsule containing 10 markers was taken on 6 consecutive days and a plain abdominal x-ray was taken on day 7. Examples from a patient with generalized prolonged colonic transit time due to supraconal spinal cord injury (left) and from a patient with left colonic and rectal dysfunction due to low spinal cord injury (right). In healthy males the upper normal limit is 23 markers corresponding to 2.8 days.

evaluate reduced colorectal emptying at defecation in patients with low SCI [38]. Defecation scintigraphy is used only for research purposes as well.

Anorectal physiology

A number of tests have been developed to study anorectal function. Intersubject variations are very large and there is overlap between values found in patients and healthy subjects. Therefore, all anorectal physiology tests should be interpreted with caution and always in the light of the patient's symptoms. The tests used in most anorectal physiology laboratories include those listed in Table 8.3.

The tests listed in Table 8.3 are useful in patients with NBD especially when considering treatment options beyond standard laxatives, suppositories or digital evacuation. Patients with SCI, myelomeningocele or multiple sclerosis may have normal anal resting pressure (internal anal sphincter consisting of smooth muscle cells) but reduced anal squeeze pressure (external anal sphincter consisting of striated muscle cells). Rectal and anal sensibility may be reduced or lost as well. Patients with Parkinson's disease may typically show impaired muscle coordination and the external anal sphincter may be

Table 8.3. Commonly performed anorectal investigations

1. Anal manometry: with determination of anal resting pressure (reflecting the function of the internal anal sphincter muscle) and anal squeeze pressure (reflecting the function of the external anal sphincter muscle)

2. Rectal balloon distension: to evaluate rectal sensations and rectal wall compliance

3. Electrophysiology test: to determine pudendal nerve terminal motor latency

4. Electrical stimulation: anal mucosa stimulation to evaluate anal sensibility

5. Transanal ultrasonography: to detect tears of the internal or anal sphincter muscle

6. Defecography: radiography after rectal installation of contrast may be performed in select patients

shown to be in contraction during attempted defecation [12]. It, however, still remains to be shown that anorectal physiology tests contribute to better selection of NBD patients for specific treatment modalities [24].

Physical evaluation

Physical evaluation should be performed in all patients. Perianal inspection should be performed to detect pressure sores, hemorrhoids, anal fissures, rectal prolapse or signs of soiling. Anorectal digitation should be performed to assess anorectal sensibility, anal tone and voluntary contraction.

Colonoscopy is generally recommended in persons over 40 with alarm symptoms including blood in stools, unexplained changes in bowel habits, newly developed abdominal pain, weight loss and anaemia. Most patients with NBD will be constipated and have abdominal pain or discomfort. Furthermore, hemorrhoids are common due to straining at defecation, and anorectal bleeding is more frequent due to digital stimulation and use of suppositories or enemas. In many patients with NBD, bowel cleansing before endoscopy is difficult due to constipation and can be unpleasant as it may result in watery stools and fecal incontinence. For these reasons, it is likely that many patients with neurological disorders do not have colonoscopy performed in spite of what would otherwise be termed alarm symptoms. This clinically relevant problem needs further study.

Other causes of secondary constipation should be considered and evaluating for these causes may be performed if clinically appropriate.

References

1. Glickmann S, Kamm MA. Bowel dysfunction in spinal-cord-injury patients. *Lancet* 1996; 347:1651–3.

2. Krogh K, Nielsen J, Djurhuus JC, et al. Colorectal function in patients with spinal cord lesions. *Dis Colon Rectum* 1997;**40**:1233–9.

3. Stone JM, Nino-Murcia M, Wolfe VA, Perkash I. Chronic gastrointestinal problems in spinal cord injury patients: a prospective analysis. *Am J Gastroenterol* 1990;**85**:1114–19.

4. Lynch AC, Wong C, Anthony A, Dobbs BR, Frizelle FA. Bowel dysfunction following spinal cord injury: a description of bowel function in a spinal cord-injured population and comparison with age and gender matched controls. *Spinal Cord* 2000;**38**:717–23.

5. Menter R, Weitzenkamp D, Cooper D, et al. Bowel management outcomes in individuals with long-term spinal cord injuries. *Spinal Cord* 1997;**35**:608–612.

6. Hinds JP, Eidelman BH, Wald A. Prevalence of bowel dysfunction in multiple sclerosis. A population survey. *Gastroenterology* 1990;**98**:1538–42.

7. Chia YW, Fowler CJ, Kamm MA, et al. Prevalence of bowel dysfunction in patients with multiple sclerosis and bladder dysfunction. *J Neurol* 1995; **242**:105–8.

8. Lie HR, Lagergren J, Rasmussen F, et al. Bowel and bladder control of children with myelomeningocele: a Nordic study. *Dev Med Child Neurol* 1991; **33**:1053–61.

9. Krogh K, Lie HR, Bilenberg N, Laurberg S. Bowel function in Danish children with myelomeningocele. *APMIS* 2003(Suppl 109):81–85.

10. Su Y, Zhang X, Zeng J, et al. New-onset constipation at acute stage after first stroke: incidence, risk factors and impact on stroke outcome. *Stroke* 2009;4:1304–9.

11. Bracci F, Badiali D, Pezzotti P, et al. Chronic constipation in hemiplegic patients. *World J Gastroenterol* 2007;**13**:3967–72.

12. Edwards LL, Quigley EMM, Pfeier RF. Gastrointestinal dysfunction in Parkinson's disease: frequency and pathophysiology. *Neurology* 1992;**42**:726–32.

13. Krogh K, Ostergaard K, Sabroe S, Laurberg S. Clinical aspects of bowel symptoms in Parkinson's disease. *Acta Neurol Scand* 2008;**117**:60–4.

14. Faaborg PM, Christensen P, Finnerup N, Laurberg S, Krogh K. The pattern of colorectal dysfunction changes with time since spinal cord injury. *Spinal Cord* 2008;**46**:234–8.

15. Finnerup NB, Faaborg PM, Krogh K, Jensen TS. Abdominal pain in long-term spinal cord injury. *Spinal Cord* 2008;**46**:198–203.

16. Wiesel PH, Norton C, Brazzelli M. Management of faecal incontinence and constipation in adults with central neurological diseases. *Cochrane Database Syst Rev* 2001;4:CD002115.

17. Alexander MS, Biering-Sorensen F, Bodner D et al. International standards to document remaining autonomic function after spinal cord injury. *Spinal Cord* 2009;**47**:36–43.

18. Krogh K, Christensen P, Sabroe S, Laurberg S. Neurogenic bowel dysfunction score. *Spinal Cord* 2006;**44**:625–631.

19. Krogh K, Perkash I, Stiens S, Biering-Sorensen F. International bowel function basic spinal cord injury data set. *Spinal Cord* 2009;**47**:230–4.

20. Krogh K, Perkash I, Stiens S, Biering-Sorensen F. International bowel function extended spinal cord injury data set. *Spinal Cord* 2009;**47**:235–41.

21. Alexander MS, Anderson KD, Biering-Sorensen F et al. Outcome measures in spinal cord injury: recent assessments and recommendations for future directions. *Spinal Cord* 2009;**47**:582–91.

22. Leduc BE, Spacek E, Lepage Y. Colonic transit after spinal cord injury: any clinical significance? *J Spinal Cord Med* 2002;**25**:161–6.

23. Media S, Christensen P, Lauge I, et al. Reprodicibility and validity of radiographically determined gastrointestinal and segmental colonic transit times in spinal cord-injured patients. *Spinal Cord* 2009;**47**:72–5.

24. Christensen P, Bazzocchi G, Coggrave M, et al. Outcome of transanal irrigation for bowel dysfunction in patients with spinal cord injury. *J Spinal Cord Med* 2008;**31**:560–7.

25. Faaborg PM, Christensen P, Kvitsau B, et al. Long-term outcome and safety of transanal irrigation for neurogenic bowel dysfunction. *Spinal Cord* 2009;**47**:545–9.

26. Marino R, Barros T, Biering-Sorensen F, et al. International standards for neurological classification of spinal cord injury. *J Spinal Cord Med* 2003; **26**(Suppl 1):S50–6.

27. Jorge JMN, Wexner SD. Etiology and management of faecal incontinence. *Dis Colon Rectum* 1993;**36**:77–97.

28. Vaizey CJ, Carapeti E, Cahill CA, Kamm MA. Prospective comparison of faecal incontinence grading systems. *Gut* 1999;**44**:77–80.

29. Agachan F, Chen T, Pfeiffer J, Reisman P, Wexner S D. A constipation scoring system to simplify evaluation and management of constipated patients. *Dis Colon Rectum* 1996;**39**:681–5.

30. Christensen P, Bazzocchi G, Coggrave M, et al. A randomized controlled trial of transanal irrigation versus conservative bowel management in spinal cord-injured patients. *Gastroenterology* 2006;**131**:738–47.

31. DeVivo M, Biering-Sorensen F, Charlifue S, et al. International spinal cord injury core data set. *Spinal Cord* 2006;**44**:535–40.

32. Menardo G, Bausano G, Corazziari E, et al. Large-bowel transit in paraplegic patients. *Dis Colon Rectum* 1987;**30**:924–8.

33. Nino-Murcia M, Stone J, Chang P, Perkash I. Colonic transit in spinal cord-injured patients. *Invest Radiol* 1990;**25**:109–12.

34. Krogh K, Mosdal C, Laurberg S. Gastrointestinal and segmental transit times in patients with acute and chronic spinal cord injury. *Spinal Cord* 2000; **38**:615–21.

35. Krogh K, Bach Jensen M, Gandrup P, et al. Efficacy and tolerability of Prucalopride in patients with constipation due to spinal cord injury. *Scand J Gastroenterology* 2002;**37**:431–6.

36. Keshavavarzian A, Barnes WE, Bruninga K, et al. Delayed colonic transit in spinal cord-injured patients measured by Indium 111 Amberlite scintigraphy. *Am J Gastroenterol* 1995;**90**:1295–300.

37. Freedman PN, Goldberg PA, Fataar AB, Mann MM. Comparison of methods of assessment of scintigraphic colonic transit. *J Nuc Med Tech* 2006;**34**:76–81.

38. Krogh K, Olsen N, Christensen P, Madsen JL, Laurberg S. Colorectal transport during defecation in patients with lesions of the sacral spinal cord. *Neurogastroenterol Motil* 2003;**15**:25–31.

Neurogenic bowel management

Maureen Coggrave and Anton Emmanuel

Introduction

Evidence to support management of neurogenic bowel dysfunction remains sparse in comparison to other areas of care; such evidence as is available arises mostly from the spinal cord injury arena. Neurogenic bowel dysfunction is almost ubiquitous amongst individuals with spinal cord injury; only 6% of these individuals report no need for intervention, and around a third need the assistance of a carer to manage bowel dysfunction [1]. Among individuals with other central neurological conditions, the prevalence of fecal incontinence and constipation and related dependency varies, but is always greater than in the general population [2–11].

The risk of fecal incontinence and constipation, often both in the same individual, is frequently accompanied by abdominal pain, bloating, fecal impaction and hemorrhoids. In the longer term, rectal prolapse, fissures, rectal abscesses, solitary rectal ulcer and prolonged duration of bowel evacuation are common [12–17]. While these conditions are not usually life-threatening, they contribute significantly to reduced quality of life. As the life-span of some groups has increased, chronic problems have become more apparent, raising the question of whether such problems are related to the duration of injury or the methods employed to manage them [1, 18]. In individuals with spinal cord injury at or above the sixth thoracic vertebra, autonomic dysreflexia is an additional risk. The bowel is a common stimulus for this abnormal sympathetic nervous system response to a noxious stimulus below the level of cord damage, which results in rapidly rising blood pressure with accompanying risk of brain hemorrhage and death [19, 20]. Immediate removal of the acute stimulus, cessation of bowel interventions for instance, will result in rapid resolution of symptoms.

However, urgent review and appropriate modification of the bowel program are essential in preventing further episodes; repeated episodes of autonomic dysreflexia increase susceptibility to the condition. Bowel distension caused by impaction, rectal stimulation, suppository insertion and enemas have all been reported as triggers [21] for autonomic dysreflexia in the literature. All of these plus constipation, prolonged bowel evacuation and presence of anal fissure, or prominent or inflamed hemorrhoids, can provoke non-acute autonomic nervous system responses such as profuse sweating and feelings of exhaustion [22]. Autonomic symptoms may last for many hours after bowel management is completed, limiting ability or willingness to engage in normal daily activities, and can be a major factor in reduced quality of life.

Impact on quality of life

Dysfunction of the bowel, such a personally and socially unacceptable aspect of bodily function, has considerable implications for quality of life. Most people find bowel function a difficult area for discussion; once voluntary control is established in young children, the subject of bowel evacuation is very rarely raised again. Embarrassment and lack of an appropriate vocabulary hinder communication. The impact of poorly managed bowel dysfunction can pervade every aspect of life, interfering with "physical, psychological, social, recreational, and sexual function" [23].

If the individual is to maintain, or return to, an active role in the community – to attend work, school or college, to resume or maintain their role as parent or partner – a bowel management program that is effective, timely and sustainable is essential. An effective program may require considerable resources in terms of time, effort and self-discipline and for some

Pelvic Organ Dysfunction in Neurological Disease: Clinical Management and Rehabilitation, ed. Clare J. Fowler, Jalesh N. Panicker & Anton Emmanuel. Published by Cambridge University Press. © Cambridge University Press 2010.

people the input of a carer; for many individuals the fear of fecal incontinence is an ever-present anxiety. In addition, the time spent on bowel care is a significant factor in reduced quality of life; prolonged bowel care is associated with anxiety and dissatisfaction [1, 24, 25]. Difficulty in obtaining appropriate care in the community and in non-specialist inpatient care settings also contributes to anxiety around bowel management for dependent individuals. Among individuals choosing colostomy as a method of dealing with bowel management problems, 14% cite difficulties with obtaining bowel care in the community as a reason for deciding on a stoma [26]. Community nursing staff are often reluctant to agree to the regular and ongoing commitment of resources required to support dependent individuals with neurogenic bowel dysfunction. Non-professional carers are seldom trained and supported in this care by their employing agency. Individuals able to employ personal assistants are usually able to receive bowel care in the manner and at a time of their choosing, but individuals in this position are in a very small minority. For a proportion of individuals, bowel care is not effective and management may dominate day-to-day life, severely curtailing community reintegration [13].

The impact of bowel dysfunction is as significant to individuals with chronic spinal cord injury as loss of mobility [1, 25], and is the worst aspect of spinal cord injury for the newly injured [27]. The management of bowel dysfunction amongst these patients has received scant attention over the years. However, in discussions regarding priorities for research and development, this is an area of care which is very high on the agenda of patients [28] and the negative effects of neurogenic bowel on the quality of life in this population are now widely acknowledged [1, 12, 24, 29–32].

Clinical assessment for bowel management

Assessment of an individual for neurogenic bowel management is a multidisciplinary activity, focused on the needs of the patient [33]. Eliciting and understanding the main concerns of the patient and early identification of their objectives is essential. The objectives of an older person with Parkinson's disease, a mother with multiple sclerosis and a young spinal cord injured individual with relatively stable bowel function wishing to return to work or college are likely to be very different.

Assessment for bowel management occurs in the context of other, often complex, impairments which may include paralysis, spasticity, weakness and fatigue, loss of balance, reduced mobility, impaired manual dexterity and psychosocial dislocation. Medical assessment will identify the neurological deficit and remaining function. Input from occupational therapists and physiotherapists will optimise remaining function and promote appropriate adaptation to achieve maximum independence. Emotional and psychological issues may require the input of psychologists. Nursing contributes practical management during acute illness and rehabilitation of individuals with regard to their altered bowel function. A bowel management program is developed in collaboration with the individual, and their carers where possible; education of all parties is a significant part of this process [33]. In individuals with stroke, education by a specialist nurse has been found to improve bowel management, maintained up to a year later [34]. Patients may undergo bowel assessment in a range of contexts: individuals undergoing rehabilitation following acute spinal cord injury or stroke, individuals with gradually deteriorating or fluctuating function due to multiple sclerosis, and young people with spina bifida in transition from parental care to self-care.

Bowel habit prior to neurological impairment and previous bowel-related medical history should be explored. Aligning the bowel management routine with bowel habit prior to onset of the neurological condition may assist in establishing a routine. Existing conditions such as irritable bowel syndrome or inflammatory bowel conditions will need to be considered in planning bowel management. Obstetric history may reveal birth-related trauma to the anal canal or pelvic floor which again may complicate neurogenic bowel management. Medications may have a significant impact on bowel function and current medication should be established. Polypharmacy is associated with bowel problems and many individuals with neurological disease or trauma will be taking medication to manage pain, spasticity and bladder dysfunction, all of which may individually influence bowel function [15]. In addition, antibiotics, antidepressants, anti-Parkinson drugs, antihistamines, diuretics, aluminium-based antacids, anti-hypertensives, statins and drugs to control diabetes all influence bowel function.

Current management of the bowel should be recorded, including the physical interventions employed, oral laxatives, rectal stimulants, diet in regard to fiber intake and any manipulation of the diet, timing of bowel evacuation, where and by whom bowel care is conducted and how long it takes. Most of these items can usefully be recorded for one to two weeks by the patient in a bowel diary and brought to the assessment. A record of bowel management over an extended period may give a more accurate impression of the issues than a history alone. A separate food diary can also be used to assess content and regularity of food intake; ability to take a full diet may need to be considered for some individuals. Pain, abdominal distension or bloating, and rectal bleeding should be explored carefully to avoid diagnostic overshadowing. Individuals with neurogenic bowel dysfunction are as much at risk (but not more so) of cancer, diverticulitis and inflammatory diseases as the wider population, and accurate diagnosis can be difficult in the absence of the usual clues. Prompt onward referral for further diagnostic tests or medical intervention should be available. The outcomes of management should be recorded. A tool such as the Neurogenic Bowel Dysfunction Score [35] can be useful, along with simple, locally developed scales to assess patient satisfaction with management. Objective outcome measures will include duration of bowel care, stool form, frequency of bowel management episodes where no stool was passed and frequency of fecal incontinence. The Bristol Stool Form Scale provides descriptors for stool form which allow objective description and so better communication regarding stool form [36]. The scale has been shown to correlate well with transit times [37].

The level of physical activity undertaken by the individual should be noted; general self-care activities, sports participation, use of a standing frame and passive movements can all contribute to optimal bowel function [38].

Cognitive ability is important in enabling the individual to understand his or her bowel dysfunction and to implement management strategies. This encompasses the ability to communicate needs and instructions to carers. Psychological and emotional factors must also be assessed. Readiness to learn about bowel care and to take responsibility for that care will vary amongst individuals, and in different care settings.

An assessment of the home environment, conducted by community or outreach occupational therapists, to facilitate independent management or the intervention of carers is essential. Easy access to a toilet can make the difference between continence and incontinence. A well laid out bathroom with an appropriate hoist or shower chair which can also be wheeled over the toilet can facilitate bowel care over the toilet rather than on the bed. Assessment of activities of daily living will identify the need for adapted clothing, suppository inserters and other aids to independence [33].

Lifestyle goals related to employment, study and family commitments and the availability of appropriate carers will inform the development of a workable bowel management routine. Where an individual is independent, fitting bowel management around other life activities may be straightforward. Where the input of a carer is required, consideration must be give to a number of issues, not least who will provide the care and when. The involvement of spouses and partners in this aspect of care is discouraged as it is thought that involvement is deleterious to this kind of relationship. Parents may be involved in bowel management for their offspring; eventually this becomes inappropriate, due to maturation of the child or aging of the parent. Finding appropriate carers to deliver bowel care in the community is challenging; owing to limited resources, community nursing services may be unable to commit to a regular time for bowel care and often have other priorities which means that bowel care cannot be delivered regularly at a time that is conducive to the goals of the individuals, for work or other activities. Local nursing work practices or protocols may also prevent the delivery of bowel care as established by specialist centers, for instance delivery of rectal interventions with the individual over the toilet. Spouses or partners may take on responsibility for bowel care to allow the individual and their family greater control over the situation; a parent may continue to give bowel care well beyond what is appropriate.

A physical examination should be conducted as part of the assessment to establish the condition of the anal and perianal area and the presence of hemorrhoids or other abnormalities. Bowel function can be objectively assessed through a digital rectal examination by a doctor or a suitably qualified and experienced nurse [39].

Investigational assessment for bowel management

Anorectal manometry tests can be used to quantify more precisely the functional status of the anorectum [40]. Colonic transit time studies can identify whether stool transit time is normal or, if not normal, where delays occur. Such studies require the ingestion of radio-opaque markers over a number of days and usually a single abdominal x-ray to assess how many markers remain and their distribution through the colon. A plain abdominal x-ray may illustrate the current status of the colon with regard to stool load or distension by flatus and exclude other complications. Delayed colonic transit is common in many individuals with neurogenic bowel dysfunction, resulting in an increased risk of constipation. Individuals with lower motor neuron damage often demonstrate delay in the anorectum and sigmoid colon, while those with upper motor neuron damage may have pan-colonic delay. In some conditions, such as multiple sclerosis, the degree of impairment may fluctuate resulting in varying dysfunction, while in others such as spinal cord injury, the impairment is determined at the point of injury. However, in all central neurological conditions, changes in levels of function and independence related to concomitant health conditions, aging, increasing duration of the condition or changing neurology will have an impact on bowel management and should trigger reassessment.

Assessment for neurogenic bowel management includes identification of the underlying disease or trauma of the central nervous system and the resulting impairment of bowel control or function. In some neurological conditions, the nature of the resulting bowel dysfunction is very clearly defined. For instance, following an upper motor neuron injury of the spinal cord, in the thoracic or cervical spine, whilst sensation and voluntary control of the bowel are abolished, the reflex arcs between the anorectum and sacral cord remain intact. These reflex arcs can be stimulated to produce reflex or automatic emptying of the rectum. In individuals with trauma or disease of the lower motor neurons, as in cauda equina syndrome, sensation and voluntary control over anorectal function are again lost, but the reflex arcs connecting the sacral cord and lower bowel are also damaged. Reflex activity is absent from the anus and rectum; the anal canal is relaxed or flaccid. No reflex evacuation can be produced. In other conditions, such as multiple sclerosis, or in individuals with incomplete spinal cord damage or conus injuries, the impairment may be less clear cut. In such individuals, use of anorectal manometry and electrosensory testing can give a clearer understanding of remaining function and control. Establishing the presence or absence of sensation, voluntary control and reflex function is important as this will indicate the interventions which may be suitable, and the appropriate stool consistency to be aimed for.

Management of fecal impaction

Fecal impaction is a relatively common occurrence in individuals with neurogenic bowel dysfunction; an incidence of around 13% has been reported [14, 41]. In individuals with neurogenic bowel dysfunction, lack of, or ineffective, routine bowel management is a very common cause. Prior to establishing any sort of bowel routine, however, impaction needs to be sought and dealt with.

There is no universally agreed definition of fecal impaction; however, presence of copious formed stool in the colon (not only the rectum) which is not progressing through the colon or which cannot be expelled from the rectum is a salient symptom. A number of factors contribute to this slow colonic transit: altered neural connections to the gut, reduced mobility associated with many disabling central neurological conditions, poor intake of dietary fiber and fluids, co-prescription of constipating drugs and polypharmacy, depression, metabolic imbalances including hypercalcemia and hypokalemia, and hypothyroidism [42]. It is more common in the elderly [43].

Symptoms may include absent or reduced passage of stool for a period which is significantly longer than usual for that individual, bloating, distension, nausea and pain. Frequently, however, patients may not report any of these symptoms except in retrospect. Impaction may be accompanied by "spurious" or "overflow" diarrhea, where the impacted fecal mass remains unmoved, but wetter, thinner stool leaks around it; this is typically associated with fecal soiling. Fecal impaction in individuals with compromised respiratory function, such as those with high-level spinal cord injuries, may result in breathlessness due to reduced diaphragmatic excursion. While any stool passed will usually be hard and dry (Bristol Stool Form Scale 1–2; Fig. 9.1), "soft impaction" with putty-like stool is possible, and is associated with a high-fiber diet or bulk-forming laxative use in immobile individuals. Individuals with spinal cord injury at or above the sixth thoracic segment may demonstrate subacute symptoms of autonomic dysreflexia while impacted (headache, sweating, goose bumps).

Bristol Stool Chart

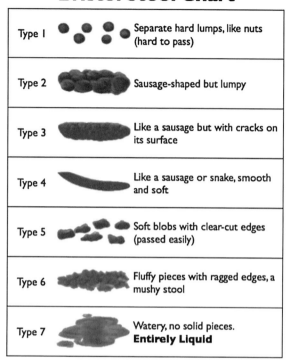

Type 1		Separate hard lumps, like nuts (hard to pass)
Type 2		Sausage-shaped but lumpy
Type 3		Like a sausage but with cracks on its surface
Type 4		Like a sausage or snake, smooth and soft
Type 5		Soft blobs with clear-cut edges (passed easily)
Type 6		Fluffy pieces with ragged edges, a mushy stool
Type 7		Watery, no solid pieces. **Entirely Liquid**

Fig. 9.1. The Bristol stool form scale illustrating stool type from most to least formed. Type 1 stools are associated with slowest whole gut transit and Type 7 with most rapid transit. Reproduced with permission.

Acute autonomic dysreflexia (rapid development of severe headache, bradycardia and hypertension) may also occur in response to impaction, particularly during digital rectal interventions or upon administration of an enema, or during reflex or volitional evacuation. The dysreflexic response to rectal interventions can be minimized by use of 2% gel applied to the anorectal area 3–5 minutes prior to planned intervention [44, 45].

A careful history and radiographic confirmation of fecal loading should be undertaken to confirm fecal impaction and to exclude intestinal perforation or obstruction. It is vital that the cause of the episode of impaction is identified if possible so that subsequent management can be adapted to avoid repeated episodes.

Evidence for management of impaction remains scanty. Few compounds have been formally studied in the setting of impaction rather than just constipation. An exception is Movicol (Norgine Ltd), which is licensed for this purpose and can be combined with rectal interventions if necessary. Eight sachets of

Movicol should be consumed over a six-hour period; this may be repeated for three consecutive days [46]. A large-volume (118 ml) phosphate enema will moisten any stool retained in the rectum and facilitate volitional or reflex evacuation of stool. Digital removal of stool may also be required. Maintenance of a regular routine of rectal intervention while treating the impaction is essential.

The process of eradication of fecal impaction can result in considerable practical difficulties for physically disabled individuals. If the individual is unable to manage independently or if suitable assistance is unavailable in the community, admission for inpatient care may be appropriate. In the case of frail or "sick" individuals, inpatient management is mandatory. Wherever it is conducted, successful clearance of impaction must be followed immediately by re-evaluation of the individual with regard to their bowel function and management needs, and instigation and evaluation of an effective management routine.

Specific management of neurogenic bowel dysfunction

Where control of fecal continence is compromised, the primary aim of bowel management is to provide the individual with managed continence. In individuals where the main problem is constipation, promotion of stool transit and effective regular evacuation are the focus. The bowel program should promote quality of life by minimizing the impact of bowel management and promote the independence and autonomy of the individual. Education of the individual and their carer is an essential part of developing an effective program.

Most individuals will use a conservative preemptive approach to management which may include establishment of a routine, dietary manipulation, use of laxatives, rectal stimulation and digital interventions. Assistive techniques such as abdominal massage and stimulation of the gastrocolic reflex may also be employed. Where this approach is ineffective, the choices are limited but may include biofeedback, transanal irrigation, sacral anterior root stimulation, sacral nerve stimulation, antegrade continence enema, percutaneous endoscopic colostomy and stoma formation.

The conservative bowel management program is designed to ensure bowel evacuation at a chosen time when the individual and their carer, if required, are prepared and available. This pre-emptive approach entails a two-part process; promoting the arrival of stool of an appropriate consistency in the rectum at the right time for effective evacuation; and facilitating that evacuation. In the absence of evidence to support any single regimen, trial and error are required to find the most effective combination of interventions, which are discussed below [47].

Establishment of a routine

A well-established routine of regular evacuation is fundamental to bowel management. Irregular or too infrequent management is associated with incontinence and constipation [1]. Management must be frequent enough to avoid incontinence and constipation, but should not be more frequent than necessary, as increasing time spent on bowel care reduces quality of life [1, 25]. Individuals with flaccid bowel function and reduced anal sphincter tone are at high risk of fecal incontinence and usually need to evacuate the rectum on a daily or twice-daily routine. Those with reflex function may evacuate on a daily or alternate day routine. While a regular routine is essential, individuals should be encouraged to retain some flexibility as those who do not regard their management program as flexible are more likely to report greater impact on quality of life [1]. The routine should be timed to fit in with the individual's intended lifestyle and daily activities, and with availability of care; the actual time of day is not otherwise significant.

Diet

While diet is thought to be important in bowel management, there is no sound evidence to support any particular approach or strategy. Despite this, dietary manipulation is common [1, 25, 48]. Bearing in mind the well-evidenced benefits, five portions of fruit and vegetables and two portions of whole grain foods, such as wholemeal bread or unrefined cereals, a day should be encouraged, in accordance with the UK government "five a day" strategy [49]. Intake of these foods should be increased gradually. Stool consistency can then be assessed and the diet adjusted accordingly to achieve an appropriate stool consistency. Individuals with reflex bowel function are encouraged to aim for a soft-formed stool consistency (Bristol Scale 4), while those with flaccid bowel function are more likely to avoid fecal incontinence if they aim for

firmer stools (Bristol Scale 3). Digital evacuation of stool is also facilitated by a firmer stool consistency. In some individuals, a diet with increased fiber may result in increased flatus and feelings of abdominal bloating and discomfort; these symptoms often settle down over one or two weeks, but if not, the diet should be adjusted to relieve them.

Generally, between 1.5 and 2.5 l of fluid daily is adequate for the general adult population, depending on level of activity and prevailing weather conditions [50]. Urine color is correlated with the concentration of urine; urine of a "pale straw color" indicates adequate hydration [50] and is a simple "rule of thumb" which is useful to patients. Fluid intake may be limited by specific bladder management approaches, such as intermittent catheterization; excessive fluid intake does not improve constipation in normally hydrated individuals [51].

Gastrocolic reflex

The gastrocolic reflex is a reflexic response to the introduction of food or drink into the stomach, resulting in an increase in propulsive muscular activity throughout the gut [34] which can result in movement of stool into the rectum ready for evacuation. The response may be reduced or absent in some neurological conditions [52–54]. However, it is a non-invasive adjunctive intervention that appears to assist with management in many individuals [15, 55]. The individual is advised to take some food or drink 15–20 minutes prior to commencing other bowel management activities and the response is thought to be strongest after the first meal of the day.

Abdominal massage

Massage is applied to the abdomen following the supposed lie of the colon in a clockwise direction; using the back or heel of the hand or a tennis ball or similar, pressure is applied and released firmly but gently in a continuous progression around the abdomen, starting in the right lower quadrant. Lighter stroking movements over the same areas may also be used, which may trigger somato-visceral reflexes. Massage may be used prior to and during bowel evacuation to promote stool transit.

The use of abdominal massage has been reported in 22–30% of individuals with neurogenic bowel dysfunction [1, 14]. Several small studies have suggested that it is beneficial in some patient groups [38, 56, 57] while a study of massage in constipated elderly individuals found no effect [58]. Recent physiological studies have demonstrated that massage produces a measurable response in the rectum and anus [59].

Digital rectal stimulation

In individuals where voluntary ability to initiate expulsion of stool has been lost, digital rectal stimulation can be used to prompt reflex evacuation. This is a technique which increases reflex muscular activity in the rectum, raising rectal pressure to aid in expelling stool, and relaxes the external anal sphincter, reducing outlet resistance [60, 61]. It is used to stimulate the movement of stool into the rectum and to initiate defecation at a chosen time. It relies upon intact reflexes and so is only effective in individuals with spinal cord lesions above the sacral segments and functioning sacral reflex arcs. Use of digital stimulation is reported in 35–50% of individuals with neurogenic bowel dysfunction [1, 12, 14, 41] and is most commonly used by those with spinal cord injury. In some individuals digital rectal stimulation can replace the use of pharmacological rectal stimulants but for most individuals it is combined with the use of suppositories or enemas. The technique may not be as effective in all individuals with reflex bowel function and may be associated with longer duration of bowel management [59]; thorough assessment of effectiveness is therefore essential. Digital stimulation is performed by inserting a gloved, lubricated finger gently through the anal canal into the rectum and slowly rotating the finger in a circular movement, maintaining contact with rectal mucosa [60, 62] and gently stretching the anal canal. Stimulation is continued until relaxation of the external sphincter is felt, flatus or stool pass, or the internal sphincter contracts (a sign of colonic activity) and is seldom required for more than 15–20 seconds; longer than one minute is rarely necessary [32]. The stimulation may be repeated when the response has subsided, approximately every 5–10 minutes. The number of times this intervention can be used within one bowel management episode is debatable; there is no evidence on which to base a recommendation and experience suggests that there is considerable variation between individuals as to what is required. Therefore the needs of the individual should be the prime consideration; digital stimulation should be repeated until reflex evacuation is complete and there is no more stool in the rectum or until it is evident that the reflex has "tired" and is not effective in prompting reflex evacuation of stool present in the rectum or until the individual wishes to finish bowel management. Digital evacuation of stool should be employed to ensure that the rectum is empty if required, to avoid fecal incontinence or discomfort. For optimal digital rectal stimulation, a bulky, soft-formed stool is preferable [Bristol Scale 4]; looser stool and constipated stool both result in less effective responses. Digital rectal stimulation may be performed sitting (over the toilet, shower chair or commode) or lying by a carer or by the patient. There is no evidence to suggest that stimulation in either position is more harmful than another, and practice should be individualized depending on response to interventions and an appropriate risk assessment.

Both digital stimulation of the rectum and digital evacuation of stool may be associated with autonomic dysreflexic symptoms in individuals with spinal cord injury at or above the sixth thoracic vertebra; 36% report dysreflexic symptoms occasionally and 9% always when they conduct bowel management [1]. Raised blood pressure during bowel management even in the absence of symptoms has been recorded [44, 48] but it is not clear that any treatment is required in the absence of symptoms [48]. The patient should be observed for symptoms of autonomic dysreflexia which include flushing, sweating and blotchiness above the lesion, chills, nasal congestion and headache; some susceptible individuals experience some of these symptoms mildly whenever they undertake bowel management. Less frequently, where the bowel is loaded with constipated stool or where severe hemorrhoids or anal fissure are present, acute autonomic dysreflexia may occur in response to bowel evacuation, including digital interventions. The principal sign of acute autonomic dysreflexia is a rapidly developing severe headache [19, 20]. In this instance bowel management should be stopped and a medical assessment undertaken. If acute autonomic dysreflexia persists after stopping the procedure, this should be treated promptly. Autonomic dysreflexia is most likely to occur in response to ineffective bowel care due to withholding of essential interventions, so prevention through good bowel management is the best approach. Existing anorectal problems, fecal loading and constipation should be treated appropriately and the bowel care program reviewed to ensure effectiveness and prevent recurrence. Even in the presence of dysreflexic symptoms, bowel management must still be conducted; local anaesthetic gel, applied rectally prior to digital interventions, may reduce or eradicate autonomic dysreflexia during bowel care [44, 45] but should only be used in the short term. If significant autonomic dysreflexia persists despite effective bowel care, further investigation of the bowel should be undertaken; assessment of autonomic nervous system function may also be helpful.

Digital evacuation of feces

This intervention involves the insertion of a single, gloved, lubricated finger into the rectum to break up or remove stool [63]. It is a commonly used intervention in the neurogenic dysfunction population, reported by more than half of individuals in a recent study [1]. It is associated with shorter duration of bowel care and fewer episodes of fecal incontinence [1, 64]. Manual evacuation is recommended in the early acute phase after spinal cord injury to remove stool from the areflexic rectum to prevent overdistension with consequent damage to later reflex rectal function [60, 65]. It is the method of choice for long-term bowel management in individuals with flaccid bowel dysfunction [32], and is used to remove stool prior to placing suppositories in individuals with reflex bowel or to complete evacuation where reflex activity alone is insufficient to empty the bowel. If properly conducted, digital evacuation of stool is a safe intervention; a firm stool (Bristol Stool Form Scale 3) should be encouraged to facilitate this technique, but excessively constipated stools should be discouraged to avoid trauma during evacuation. Individuals who have begun to use this technique through their own "trial and error" should be reassured that they are not doing anything wrong, and given advice to ensure they are conducting the intervention appropriately; those with an acute onset to their bowel dysfunction will be taught appropriately during rehabilitation. Digital evacuation may be conducted by the individual on the bed or over the toilet, or by a carer usually on the bed to facilitate safety. Carers need to be taught how to undertake this intervention and may need reassurance regarding its use; digital evacuation should always be seen as part of an effective holistic bowel management program with significant outcomes for the quality of life of the individual.

Suppositories and enemas

In individuals without voluntary control over evacuation, rectal stimulants such as suppositories or enemas are used to trigger reflex evacuation of the bowel at a chosen time, giving control over evacuation. They may also be used to facilitate evacuation in constipated individuals. Suppositories of some kind are reported to be used by 60–71% of spinal cord injured individuals [1, 41] and glycerine suppositories by 32–47% [1, 12].

Glycerin suppositories are the mildest and most commonly used type, providing mild local stimulation and lubrication to the rectum, and are expected to stimulate a response in approximately 15–20 minutes. Sodium bicarbonate suppositories (Lecicarbon E) release carbon dioxide which stimulates rectal reflex activity within 15–20 minutes. Bisacodyl suppositories deliver a stimulant laxative resulting in increased gut motility. Response time is longer, approximately 30–40 minutes, as the hard fat excipient must melt prior to absorption of the drug. Bisacodyl suppositories with a polyethylene glycol base are reported to act more rapidly than those with a hydrogenated vegetable oil base [66, 67] but are currently not available on prescription in the UK.

An enema is a method of delivering a volume of fluid, with or without a drug, to the rectum. Generally, large-volume enemas are not used in neurogenic bowel management as individuals may be unable to retain the fluid, overdistension may occur or trauma may be caused to the rectal mucosa [32, 68]. Large-volume enemas may cause electrolyte imbalance, onset of action may be unpredictable, irritation of the rectal mucosa may occur and they may cause watery stools and abdominal cramping [62]. Practically, such enemas must be administered in a side-lying position, and may be expelled during transfer from bed to toilet, so for many individuals their use means that bowel evacuation must be managed on the bed, limiting the potential for the normalcy of toilet use and independence. However, small-volume enemas are more likely to be retained and can be administered in a side-lying position or when seated on a toilet or commode. Docusate enemas have been reported to be safe and effective [69], and more effective than either glycerine or bisacodyl suppositories [70], acting within 5–20 minutes. Small-volume sodium citrate/sorbitol enemas can also be administered in the lying or sitting position and act in around

15 minutes. Both of these may result in abdominal cramps, pain and discomfort.

There are few studies of efficacy of suppositories and enemas in individuals with neurogenic bowel dysfunction and their samples are small. It is sensible to initially use milder rectal stimulants, increasing potency if required, bearing in mind duration of bowel care, completeness of evacuation and the risk of continuing response to stimulation resulting in fecal incontinence. Rectal stimulants alone are seldom sufficient to prompt complete evacuation; most individuals also require digital stimulation or digital evacuation of stool or both [1].

Laxatives

Use of oral laxatives is not essential for all individuals with neurogenic bowel dysfunction. They are associated with fecal incontinence and may cause bloating, abdominal cramps and pain; they should only be used following individual assessment and with a clear understanding of the intended outcome. Use of oral laxatives is, however, very common, reported in up to 60% of spinal cord injured individuals [1, 16, 25], even though little research has been conducted to evaluate the efficacy of laxatives in neurogenic bowel management.

Commonly used laxatives include stimulants (e.g. senna, bisacodyl), softeners (e.g. dioctyl), bulkers (e.g. ispaghula husk) and osmotics (e.g. polyethylene glycol, lactulose). Laxatives aimed at modulating stool form, (softeners, bulkers and osmotics) should be taken regularly to maintain a predictable stool consistency of the type appropriate to the individual's bowel dysfunction. Experience suggests that polyethylene glycol can be used to successfully modulate stool consistency if carefully titrated; if given in doses sufficient to stimulate evacuation it often results in incontinence in this group of patients. Bulk formers can be beneficial when used to supplement a diet low in natural fiber, but excessive use can result in overloading of the colon with putty-like stool, sometimes called "soft impaction," particularly in individuals with limited mobility. They should be taken with food and an ample fluid intake. Stimulant laxatives, which prompt increased bowel activity resulting in the movement of stool into the sigmoid colon and rectum, should be taken 8–12 hours prior to planned evacuation of stool only, and the timing and size of the dose adjusted to optimize evacuation. In individuals without voluntary control over defecation, the use of laxatives must be accompanied by planned defecation using rectal stimulants or digital interventions; failure to do so is likely to result in fecal incontinence.

Antidiarrheal agents

Occasionally, individuals with neurogenic bowel dysfunction will present with stool that is too soft or loose (Bristol Stool Form Scale 5–7). Soft stool increases the risk of fecal incontinence, is more difficult for the bowel to expel and more difficult to remove by digital evacuation. Dietary factors should be explored, medications including laxatives reviewed and alternatives tried if appropriate, and other possible non-neurogenic causes excluded. Loperamide can be used to reduce the speed of colonic transit allowing greater absorption of fluid from the stool and formation of a firmer, more manageable stool [71]. Loperamide syrup 1 mg in 5 ml is the formulation of choice, as this allows finer titration to control symptoms without causing constipation. Treatment is commenced on a very low dose and increased until the optimal stool consistency is achieved. Doses of 0.5–16 mg per day can be used as required by the individual and adjusted by them as required to manage symptoms. If loperamide is not well tolerated, codeine phosphate or co-phenotrope may be tried.

Putting a bowel management program together

A bowel management program is developed in discussion with the individual and their carers. While the program must be achievable in the real world and must therefore reflect the availability of carers and the setting of care, it should primarily reflect the wishes of the individual and their needs, promoting autonomy, independence and control in this very personal area of care [33].

The program will specify the frequency, timing and location of management, the interventions and equipment to be used, and by whom care is to be given if the individual is not independent. For instance, for an individual with reflex bowel dysfunction following complete spinal cord injury, without sensation or voluntary control of the anorectum but independent in self-care, bowel management might be planned for alternate days at 8 a.m. following breakfast to prompt the gastrocolic reflex. If stimulant laxatives were required, they would be taken 8–12 hours prior to commencing the routine. Insertion of two glycerin suppositories sitting on the toilet is followed by abdominal massage. Following partial reflex evacuation in response to the suppositories, digital rectal stimulation is used to stimulate further evacuation, followed by brief digital evacuation of remaining stool. Abdominal massage can be used between the other interventions. When no more stool presents in the rectum, a period of around five minutes is allowed with no intervention and a gentle digital check is performed to ensure that no more stool is present. Management is then complete. The duration of this period of waiting is individual; people who lack "normal" sensation in the anorectum may come to be able to judge very accurately whether their evacuation is complete or not based on other sensations they learn to interpret over time.

The majority of individuals with neurogenic bowel dysfunction will use the conservative methods described to manage their bowel dysfunction. For those individuals in whom conservative methods are not effective, there are a few options which are discussed below.

Biofeedback

Biofeedback may include a number of the interventions discussed above. It is an approach which includes sphincter exercises, bowel habit retraining, counselling, health education and the use of medications [72]. Biofeedback may be beneficial to individuals with mild to moderate multiple sclerosis but there is no evidence that it demonstrates greater effectiveness compared to conservative management in this or any other neurogenic patient group [73].

Transanal irrigation

Transanal irrigation of the bowel can be defined as a process of facilitating evacuation of feces from the bowel by passing water (or other liquids) into the bowel via the anus in a quantity sufficient to reach beyond the rectum. This technique is well established in children with spina bifida [74] and has been found to improve fecal incontinence, constipation, duration of bowel care and symptom-related quality of life in adults with problematic bowel management [75–77]. Overall it may be a cost-effective choice [78], and the need for digital interventions, such as rectal stimulation and digital evacuation of stool, is greatly reduced. Around 60% of individuals with neurogenic dysfunction who instigate irrigation continue with it [75]; criteria to allow more appropriate patient selection are yet to be identified [79]. Irrigation is conducted over a toilet or commode for practical reasons and can be self-administered or administered by an appropriately trained carer. Transanal irrigation may be considered for individuals who experience fecal incontinence, constipation, abdominal pain associated with evacuation, bloating or prolonged duration of bowel evacuation, or simply at the preference of the individual. However, autonomic dysreflexia is a risk and bowel perforation is a rare complication already reported in the literature [80]. Individuals using the system should be assessed, taught and monitored by nurses with appropriate expertise. The Peristeen® system is licensed in Europe for the management of neurogenic bowel dysfunction (Fig. 9.2). Thought must be given to who will undertake the irrigation where assistance is required. Community nurses may be reluctant to commit the time required on a regular and ongoing basis, but non-professional carers have been taught successfully, some individuals teaching their own carers once they themselves have received instruction. Transanal irrigation provides a "step up" from conservative care, which for appropriate patients should be evaluated prior to considering other more invasive approaches.

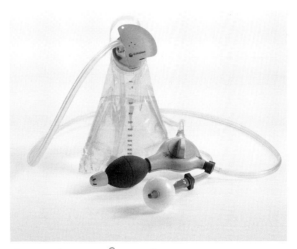

Fig. 9.2. The Peristeen® transanal irrigation system comprising, from back to front, the water reservoir with tubing, the hand pump with adjustable valve system and the catheter with inflated rectal balloon. Reproduced with permission.

Surgical interventions

A small number of surgical interventions have been developed to facilitate management of neurogenic bowel dysfunction. These are usually considered when conservative measures and transanal irrigation, if appropriate, have failed.

Antegrade continence enema (ACE)

The ACE is a continent catheterizable stoma formed from the appendix or cecum, giving access to the colon to allow administration of irrigation for bowel management. The ACE procedure may reduce the duration of bowel care and incidence of fecal incontinence [82–86]; autonomic dysreflexia was eradicated in one case study [82]. While common in children with spina bifida, relatively few ACEs have been reported in adults with neurogenic bowel dysfunction and the failure rate in some studies is high [84]. Little is known about continued efficacy of the ACE as children with neurogenic bowel dysfunction grow into adulthood.

Percutaneous endoscopic colostomy (PEC)

In this procedure a tube is placed into the descending colon via a colonoscope and then pulled through the colon and abdomen and attached to the external wall of the abdomen. Irrigation of the descending colon and rectum can then be undertaken. In adults it is most commonly undertaken to treat recurrent sigmoid volvulus and acute colonic pseudo-obstruction but it may also be used to treat fecal incontinence and constipation where other strategies have failed [87]. However, PEC may be less effective for constipation and continence issues than for sigmoid volvulus, the surgical procedure has a high infection rate and it should only be used in carefully selected cases [88]. The number of these procedures undertaken for neurogenic bowel dysfunction is unknown but experience suggests they are rare.

Stoma formation

The formation of a colostomy has been seen until recently as a last resort when dealing with neurogenic bowel dysfunction, and even as a failure of rehabilitation services. Consequently, colostomy has often not been conducted until an individual has suffered many years of problematic neurogenic bowel management, often with immense impact on quality of life. Around 2.4% of spinal cord injured individuals in the UK have a colostomy formed for problems such as excessive duration of bowel management, fecal incontinence, constipation and difficulties with obtaining bowel care [1, 26]. The formation of a stoma can greatly improve quality of life for such individuals. It results in a significant reduction in time spent on bowel management [26, 89] and, because the stoma is on the front of the body and more accessible, independence is often enhanced [90]. Even where help is still required, the type of assistance required is more readily obtained in the community setting. Despite largely positive outcomes, stomas are not without complications. These include paralytic ileus and bowel obstruction postoperatively, peristomal hernia, diversion colitis (inflammatory changes in the redundant section of bowel) and skin rashes around the stoma causing problems with collection devices. The discharge of mucus from the remaining defunctioned rectum can also be problematic, necessitating the use of pads [90, 91]. If the colostomy is to be undertaken to address constipation, the location of the stoma along the length of the colon needs careful consideration; around 40% of individuals with spinal cord injury and stoma continue to use laxatives after surgery. In individuals with long-established neurogenic bowel dysfunction, megacolon and pan-colonic slow transit are not uncommon; an ileostomy may sometimes be a better option than colostomy.

Sacral anterior root stimulator (SARS)

Insertion of an SARS involves cutting the sensory nerves to the bladder and anorectum; sensation and reflex function, including reflexogenic erections, are abolished. Electrodes are implanted on the second, third and fourth sacral anterior nerve roots and connected to a subcutaneously sited receiver-stimulator. An external hand-held controller allows high-voltage, short-lived stimulation to be applied several times daily to empty the bladder; the colon is also stimulated simultaneously, resulting in increased colonic activity, reduced constipation and sometimes defecation during stimulation [92]. The SARS has been available for several decades and, though usually implanted primarily for bladder management problems after spinal cord injury, it has been reported to have a very beneficial effect on bowel management for many individuals, reducing constipation and duration of bowel care and increasing satisfaction [93–95]. However, implantation of SARSs remains rare; just 7 of more than 1330 respondents to a postal questionnaire reported using an SARS for bowel management [1]. An even more rarely performed surgical variant is the sacral anterior and posterior root stimulator (SPARS) in which electrodes are placed on posterior roots as well as the anterior ones; this has the advantage of obviating the need for sacrifice of the posterior nerve roots (rhizotomy).

Sacral nerve stimulation (SNS)

SNS is used to treat both fecal incontinence and constipation. It is similar to the SARS but uses lower-amplitude, continuous stimulation of the sacral plexus [96] which is interrupted using an external magnet to allow defecation. An intact sphincter and sacral nerves are required, and SNS is not effective in individuals with complete spinal cord injury [97]; the benefits of this technique for individuals with neurogenic bowel dysfunction, who have often been excluded from SNS studies, remain to be clarified [97].

Conclusion

Neurogenic bowel dysfunction and its management have a significant negative impact on the quality of life of individuals with central neurological conditions. Until recently this area has received little clinical attention even in neuroscience specialties and little research effort has been expended on developing new solutions for this intractable problem. The importance of this highly stigmatized impairment to the individuals who suffer it is now more widely recognized and innovative approaches are beginning to emerge.

Currently, the conservative approach remains the most common form of management in neurogenic bowel dysfunction and the number of individuals using any of the alternatives is small. More evidence is required to support conservative care and reduce the degree of trial and error required in developing effective individualized programmes. More work is needed to develop and validate new and innovative approaches, which can contribute significantly to the quality of life of these individuals.

References

1. Coggrave M, Norton C, Wilson-Barnett J. Management of neurogenic bowel dysfunction in the community after spinal cord injury: a postal survey in the United Kingdom. *Spinal Cord* 2009;**47**:323–30.

2. Bakke A, Myhr KM, Gronning M, Nyland H. Bladder, bowel and sexual dysfunction in patients with multiple sclerosis-a cohort study. *Scand J Urol Nephrol Suppl* 1996;**179**:61–6.

3. Chia YW, Fowler CJ, Kamm MA, et al. Prevalence of bowel dysfunction in patients with multiple sclerosis and bladder dysfunction. *J Neurol* 1995;**242**:105–8.

4. Hennessey A, Robertson NP, Swingler R, Compston DA. Urinary, faecal and sexual dysfunction in patients with multiple sclerosis. *J Neurol* 1999; **246**:1027–32.

5. Ponticelli A, Iacobelli BD, Silveri M, et al. Colorectal dysfunction and faecal incontinence in children with spina bifida. *Br J Urol* 1998;**81** (Suppl 3):117–9.

6. Edwards LL, Quigley EM, Pfeiffer RF. Gastrointestinal dysfunction in Parkinson's disease: frequency and pathophysiology. *Neurology* 1992;**42**:726–32.

7. Harari D, Coshall C, Rudd AG, Wolfe CD. New-onset fecal incontinence after stroke: prevalence, natural history, risk factors, and impact. *Stroke* 2003;**34**:144–50.

8. Del Giudice E, Staiano A, Capano G, et al. Gastrointestinal manifestations in children with cerebral palsy. *Brain Dev* 1999; **21**: 307–11.

9. Brittain KR, Peet SM, Castleden CM. Stroke and incontinence. *Stroke* 1998;**29**:524–8.

10. McDonnell GV, McCann JP. Issues of medical management in adults with spinal bifida. *Childs Nervous System* 2000;**16**:222–27.

11. Nakayama H, Jorgensen HS, Pedersen PM, Raaschou HO, Olsen TS. Prevalence and risk factors of incontinence after stroke: The Copenhagen Stroke Study. *Stroke* 1997;**28**:58–62.

12. Correa GI, Rotter KP. Clinical evaluation and management of neurogenic bowel after spinal cord injury. *Spinal Cord* 2000;**38**:301–8.

13. De Looze DA, Van Laere M, De Muynck MC, Beke R, Elewaut A. Constipation and other chronic gastrointestinal problems in spinal cord injury patients. *Spinal Cord* 1998;**36**:63–6.

14. Han RR, Kim JH, Kwon BS. Chronic gastrointestinal problems and bowel dysfunction in patients with spinal cord injury. *Spinal Cord* 1998;**36**:485–90.

15. Harari D, Sarkarati M, Gurwitz J, McGlinchey-Berroth G, Minaker K. Constipation-related symptoms and bowel program concerning individuals with spinal cord injury. *Spinal Cord* 1997;**35**:394–401.

16. Lynch AC, Antony A, Dobbs BR, Frizelle FA. Bowel dysfunction following spinal cord injury. *Spinal Cord* 2001;**39**:193–203.

17. Menter R, Weitzenkamp D, Cooper D, et al. Bowel management outcomes in individuals with long-term spinal cord injuries. *Spinal Cord* 1997;**35**:608–12.

18. Stone JM, Wolfe VA, Nino-Murcia M, Perkash I. Colostomy as treatment for complications of spinal cord injury. *Arch Phys Med Rehabil* 1990;**71**:514–18.

19. Showkathali R, Antonios T. Autonomic dysreflexia; a medical emergency. *J R Soc Med* 2007;**100**:382–3.

20. Kavchak-Keyes MA. Autonomic hyperreflexia. *Rehabil Nurs* 2000;**25**:31–5.

21. Colachis SC 3rd. Autonomic hyperreflexia with spinal cord injury. *J Am Paraplegia Soc* 1992;**15**:171–86.

22. Yoshimura M, Maejima H, Sasaki H. Bowel dysfunction and and disturbance of physical condition after evacuation in patients with chronic cervical spinal cord injury. *Journal of Physical Therapy Science* 2001;**13**:145–8.

23. De Lisa J, Kirshblum SA. Review: frustrations and needs in clinical care of spinal cord injury patients. *J Spinal Cord Med* 1997;**20**:384–90.

24. Ng C, Prott G, Rutkowski S, et al. Gastrointestinal symptoms in spinal cord injury: relationships with level of injury and psychologic factors. *Dis Colon Rectum* 2005;**48**:1562–8.

25. Glickman S, Kamm M. Bowel dysfunction in spinal-cord-injury patients. *Lancet* 1996;**347**:1651–3.

26. Coggrave M, Ingram R, Gardner B, Norton C. The impact of a stoma for bowel management after spinal cord injury. International Continence Society 2009. http://www.icsoffice.org/aspnet_membership/membership/Abstracts/AuthorIndex.aspx?EventID=47

27. Rogers, M. *Living with paraplegia*. London: Faber and Faber; 1991.

28. Anderson KD. Targeting recovery: priorities of the spinal cord injured population. *J Neurotrauma* 2004;**21**:1371–83.

29. Liu CW, Huang CC, Yang YH, et al. Relationship between neurogenic bowel dysfunction and health-related quality of life in persons with spinal cord injury. *J Rehabil Med* 2009;**41**:35–40.

30. Westgren N, Levi R. Quality of life and traumatic spinal cord injury. *Arch Phys Med Rehabil* 1998;**79**:1433–9.

31. Byrne CM, Pager CK, Rex J, Roberts R, Solomon MJ. Assessment of quality of life in the treatment of patients with neuropathic faecal incontinence. *Dis Colon Rectum* 1998;**45**:1431–6.

32. Stiens S, Bergman S, Goetz LL. Neurogenic bowel dysfunction after spinal cord injury: clinical evaluation and rehabilitative management. *Arch Phys Med Rehabil* 1997;**78**:S86–102.

33. Multidisciplinary Association of Spinal Cord Injury Professionals. *Guidelines for managing neurogenic bowel dysfunction after spinal cord injury 2009*. http://www.mascip.co.uk/pdfs/SIA-MASCIP_bowel_guidelines(1).pdf

34. Harari D, Norton C, Lockwood L, Swift C. Treatment of constipation and faecal incontinence in stroke patients: a randomised controlled trial. *Stroke* 2004;**35**:2549–55.

35. Krogh K, Christensen P, Sabroe S, Laurberg S. Neurogenic bowel dysfunction score. *Spinal Cord* 2005;**44**:625–31.

36. Heaton, KW, Radvan J, Cripps H, et al. Defecation frequency and timing, and stool form in the general population: a prospective study. *Gut* 1992;**33**:818–24.

37. Lewis SJ, Heaton KW. Stool form scale as a useful guide to intestinal transit time. *Scand J Gastroenterol* 1997;**32**:920–4.

38. Coggrave M. *Neurogenic bowel management in chronic spinal cord injury: evidence for nursing care*. King's College, London: unpublished PhD thesis, 2007.

39. Addison R, Smith M. *Digital rectal examination (DRE) – manual evacuation of faeces guidelines on the role of the nurse*. London: Royal College of Nursing UK; 1999.

40. Azpiroz F, Enck P, Whitehead E. Anorectal function testing: review of collective experience. *Am J Gastroenterol* 2002;**97**:232–40.

41. Kirk PM, King RB, Temple R, Bourjaily J, Thomas P. Long-term follow-up of bowel management after spinal cord injury. *SCI Nursing* 1997;**14**:56–63.

42. Creason N, Sparks D. Faecal impaction: a review. *Nursing Diagnosis* 2000;**11**:15–23.

43. Harari D. Bowel care in old age. In: Norton C, Chelvanayagam S, eds. *Bowel continence nursing*. Beaconsfield, UK: Beaconsfield Publishers; 2004:132–49.

44. Furasawa K, Sugiyama H, Tokuhiro A, et al. Topical anesthesia blunts the pressor response induced by bowel manipulation in subjects with cervical spinal cord injury. *Spinal Cord* 2008;**47**:144–8.

45. Cosman B, Vu T. Lidocaine anal block limits autonomic dysreflexia during anorectal procedures in spinal cord injury: a randomized, double-blind, placebo-controlled trial. *Dis Colon Rectum* 2005;**48**:1556–61.

46. Chen C; Su M; Tung S; Chang F; Wong J; Geraint M. Evaluation of polyethylene glycol plus electrolytes in the treatment of severe constipation and faecal

impaction in adults. *Current Medical Research Opinion* 2005;**21**:1595–602.

47. Coggrave M, Wiesel PH, Norton C. Management of faecal incontinence and constipation in adults with central neurological diseases. *Cochrane Database Syst Rev* 2006;(2):CD002115.

48. Kirshblum S, Gulati M, O'Connor K, Voorman S. Bowel care practices in chronic spinal cord injury patients. *Arch Phys Med Rehabil* 1998;**79**:20–3.

49. Department of Health. *Five a day – increasing fruit and vegetable consumption – a national priority*. London: Department of Health; 2003. http://www.doh.gov.uk/fiveaday/

50. British Dietetic Association. *Hydration*. British Dietetic Association; 2006. http://www.bda.uk.com/hot_topics_hydration.html

51. Norton C, Whitehead WE, Bliss DZ, Harari D, Lang J. Conservative and pharmacological management of faecal incontinence in adults. In: Abrams P, Cardozo L, Khoury S, Wein A, eds. *Incontinence*. Plymouth: Health Publications; 2009.

52. Aaronson MJ, Freed MM, Burakoff R. Colonic myoelectric activity in persons with spinal cord injury. *Dig Dis Sci* 1985;**30**:295–300.

53. Glick M, Meshkinpour H, Haldeman S, et al. Colonic dysfunction in patients with thoracic spinal cord injury. *Gastroenterology* 1984;**86**:287–94.

54. Menardo G, Bausano G, Corazziari E, et al. Large-bowel transit in paraplegic patients. *Dis Colon Rectum* 1987;**30**:294–8.

55. Walter SA, Morren GL, Ryn AK, Hallbook O. Rectal pressure responses to a meal in patients with high spinal cord injury. *Arch Phys Med Rehabil* 2003;**84**:108–11.

56. Albers B, Cramer H, Fischer A, et al. Abdominal massage as intervention for patients with paraplegia caused by spinal cord injury – a pilot study. *Pflege Z* 2006;**59**:2–8.

57. Emly M, Cooper S, Vail A. Colonic motility in profoundly disabled people: a comparison of massage and laxative therapy in the management of constipation. *Physiotherapy* 1998;**84**:178–83.

58. Klauser AG, Flaschentrager J, Gehrke A, Muller-Lissner SA. Abdominal wall massage: effect on colonic function in healthy volunteers and in patients with chronic constipation. *Z Gastroenterol* 1992;**30**:247–51.

59. Coggrave M, Norton C, Wilson-Barnett J. *Assessing interventions for bowel management using anorectal manometry*. International Continence Society; 2006. http://www.icsoffice.org/publications/2007/pdf/0031.pdf

60. Consortium for spinal cord medicine. Neurogenic bowel management in adults with spinal cord injury. Clinical practice guidelines. *Spinal Cord Medicine* 1998;**21**:248.

61. Fajardo NR, Pasiliao RV, Modeste-Duncan R, et al. Decreased colonic motility in persons with chronic spinal cord injury. *Am J Gastroenterol* 2003;**98**:128–34.

62. Wiesel P, Bell S. Bowel dysfunction: assessment and management in the neurological patient. In: Norton C, Chelvanayagam S, eds. *Bowel continence nursing*. Beaconsfield, UK: Beaconsfield Publishers; 2004:181–203.

63. Kyle G, Oliver H, Prynn P. *The procedure for the digital removal of faeces*. Norgine Ltd; 2005.

64. Haas U, Geng V, Evers G, Knecht H. Bowel management in patients with spinal cord injury – a multicentre study of the German speaking society of paraplegia. *Spinal Cord* 2005;**43**:724–30.

65. Grundy D, Swain I. *ABC of spinal cord injury*. Fourth edn. BMJ Books; 2002.

66. Frisbie JH. Improved bowel care with a polyethylene glycol based bisacodyl suppository. *J Spinal Cord Med* 1997;**20**:227–9.

67. House J, Stiens S. Pharmacologically initiated defecation for persons with spinal cord injury: effectiveness of three agents. *Arch Phys Med Rehabil* 1997;**78**:1062–5.

68. Paran H, Butnaru G, Neufeld D, Magen A, Freund U. Enema-induced perforation of the rectum in chronically constipated patients. *Dis Colon Rectum* 1999;**42**:1609–12.

69. Dunn K, Galka M. A comparison of the effectiveness of Therevac SB^{TM} and Bisacodyl suppositories in SCI patients bowel program. *Rehabil Nurs* 1994;**19**:334–8.

70. Amir IM, Sharma RM, Bauman WAM, Korsten MAM. Bowel care for individuals with spinal cord injury: comparison of four approaches. *J Spinal Cord Med* 1998;**21**:21–4.

71. Ehrenpreis E, Chang D, Eichenwald E. Pharmacotherapy for fecal incontinence: a review. *Dis Colon Rectum* 2007;**50**:641–9.

72. Wiesel PH, Norton C, Roy AJ, et al. Gut focused behavioural treatment (biofeedback) for constipation and faecal incontinence in multiple sclerosis. *J Neurol Neurosurg Psychiatry* 2000;**69**:240–3.

73. Norton C, Hosker G, Brazzelli M. Biofeedback and/or sphincter exercises for the treatment of faecal incontinence in adults. *Cochrane Database Syst Rev* 2000;(2):CD002111.

74. Shandling B, Gilmour RF. The enema continence catheter in spina bifida: successful bowel management. *J Pediatr Surg* 1987;**22**:271–3.

75. Christensen P, Krogh K, Buntzen S, Payandeh F, Laurberg S. Long-term outcome and safety of transanal irrigation for constipation and fecal incontinence. *Dis Colon Rectum* 2009;**52**:286–92.

76. Christensen P, Bazzocchi G, Coggrave M, et al. Treatment of fecal incontinence and constipation in patients with spinal cord injury – a prospective, randomized, controlled, multicentre trial of transanal irrigation vs. conservative bowel management. *Gastroenterology* 2006;**131**:738–47.

77. Del Popolo G, Mosiello G, Pilati C, et al. Treatment of neurogenic bowel dysfunction using transanal irrigation: a multicenter Italian study. *Spinal Cord* 2008;**46**:517–22.

78. Christensen P, Andreasen J, Ehlers L. Cost-effectiveness of transanal irrigation versus conservative bowel management for spinal cord injury patients. *Spinal Cord* 2009;**47**:138–43.

79. Christensen P, Bazzocchi G, Coggrave M, et al. Outcome of transanal irrigation for bowel dysfunction in patients with spinal cord injury. *J Spinal Cord Med* 2008;**31**:560–7.

80. Biering-Sørensen F, Bing J, Berggreen P, Olesen G. Rectum perforation during transanal irrigation: a case story. *Spinal Cord* 2009;**47**:266–7.

82. Teichman JM, Barber DB, Rogenes VJ, Harris JM. Malone antegrade continence enemas for autonomic dysreflexia secondary to neurogenic bowel. *J Spinal Cord Med* 1998;**21**:245–7.

83. Teichman JM, Zabihi N, Kraus SR, Harris JM, Barber DB. Long-term results for Malone antegrade continence enema for adults with neurogenic bowel disease. *Urology* 2003;**61**:502–6.

84. Gerharz EW, Vik V, Webb G, et al. The value of the MACE (Malone antegrade colonic enema) procedure in adult patients. *J Am Coll Surg* 1997;**185**:544–7.

85. Christensen, P, Kvitzau B, Krogh K, Buntzen S, Laurberg S. Neurogenic colorectal dysfunction – use of new antegrade and retrograde colonic wash-out methods. *Spinal Cord* 2000;**38**:255–61.

86. Bruce RG, el-Galley RE, Wells J, Galloway NT. Antegrade continence enema for the treatment of fecal incontinence in adults: use of gastric tube for catheterizable access to the descending colon. *J Urol* 1999;**161**:1813–6

87. National Institute for Health and Clinical Excellence. *Percutaneous endoscopic colostomy.* London: National Institute for Health and Clinical Excellence; 2006. http://guidance.nice.org.uk/IPG161

88. Cowlam S, Watson C, Elltringham M, et al. Percutaneous endoscopic colostomy of the left side of the colon. *Gastrointest Endosc* 2007;**65**:1007–14.

89. Stone J, Wolfe V, Nino-Murcia M, Perkash I. Colostomy as treatment for the complications of spinal cord injury. *Arch Phys Med Rehabil* 1990;**71**:514–18.

90. Kelly SR, Shashidharan M, Borwell B, et al. The role of intestinal stoma in patients with spinal cord injury. *Spinal Cord* 1999;**37**:211–14.

91. Branagan G, Tromans A, Finnis D. Effect of stoma formation on bowel care and quality of life in patients with spinal cord injury. *Spinal Cord* 2003;**41**:680–3.

92. Chia YW, Lee TK, Kour NW, Tung KH, Tan ES. Microchip implants on the anterior sacral roots in patients with spinal trauma: does it improve bowel function? *Dis Colon Rectum* 1996;**39**:690–4.

93. Creasey G, Grill J, Korsten M, et al. An implantable neuroprosthesis for restoring bladder and bowel control to patients with spinal cord injuries: a multicenter trial. *Arch Phys Med Rehabil* 2001;**82**:1512–19.

94. Binnie NR, Smith AN, Creasey GH, Edmond P. Constipation associated with chronic spinal cord injury: the effect of pelvic parasympathetic stimulation by the Brindley stimulator. *Paraplegia* 1991;**29**:463–9.

95. Valles M, Rodriguez A, Borau A, Mearin F. Effect of sacral anterior root stimulator on bowel dysfunction in patients with spinal cord injury. *Dis Colon Rectum* 2009;**52**:986–92.

96. Kenefick NJ, Christiansen J. A review of sacral nerve stimulation for the treatment of faecal incontinence. *Colorectal Dis* 2004; **6**:75–80.

97. Jarrett M, Mowatt G, Glazener C, et al. Systematic review of sacral nerve stimulation for faecal incontinence and constipation. *Br J Surg* 2004;**91**:1559–69.

Chapter 10

Evaluation and management of neurogenic sexual dysfunction

Charlotte Chaliha, Catherine M. Dalton, Sohier Elneil and Thomas M. Kessler

Introduction

Physiological sexual functioning is highly dependent on the integrity of the nervous system (Chapter 3) and is frequently affected by neurological disorders. Sexual function is recognized as an important factor determining quality of life and dysfunction in neurological patients may significantly add to the burden of their disease. The treatment of their sexual dysfunction (SD) should preferably involve a multidisciplinary, evidence-based approach and in addition to understanding medical therapies, healthcare professionals should appreciate the complex consequences of SD for a patient with neurological disease.

Classification of sexual dysfunction

Any disruption in the sexual response cycle (Chapter 3) results in SD. SD is therefore a general term that encompasses a broad group of categories, which although they have varied manifestations, can overlap with one another. Recently, attempts have been made to accurately define SD and its categories in the general population. These have provided a useful framework for clinically evaluating patients and planning a comprehensive therapeutic strategy [1, 2]. Accordingly, SD can be grouped into four broad categories (Table 10.1). It is likely that this system of analysis can be readily applied to patients with neurological disease as well.

Prevalence of sexual dysfunction

SD is highly prevalent in the general population with an incidence that increases with age, a fact that should be borne in mind when considering the problems of patients who develop neurological disease. A US National Health and Social Life Survey carried out in 1992 included data from a group of 1749 men and 1410

women aged 18–59 and found SD to be more prevalent in women (43%) than men (31%) [3]. SD was also more likely among women and men with poor physical and emotional health. A recent study performed between 2005 and 2006 in a group of older adults (1550 men and 1455 women) aged 57–85, living in the community [4], revealed a decline in sexual activity with age. Sexual activity, defined as sex within the previous 12 months, was 73% among those aged 57–64, 53% among those aged 65–74, and 26% among those aged 75–85. Women were significantly less likely than men at all ages to report sexual activity. Amongst the sexually active, about half of both men and women reported at least one bothersome sexual problem. The most prevalent sexual problems amongst women were low desire (43%) (although see Chapter 3 for background to this), difficulty with vaginal lubrication (39%) and inability to climax (34%). Amongst men, the most prevalent sexual problem was erectile dysfunction (ED) (37%). Fourteen percent of all men reported using medications or supplements to improve sexual function. Importantly, consistent with the study in the younger population, men and women who rated their health as being poor were less likely to be sexually active and among the respondents who were sexually active, more reported sexual problems. Despite the relatively high prevalence of SD, only 38% of men and 22% of women over the age of 50 had discussed their problem with a physician.

Sexual dysfunction in neurological disorders

From the foregoing it will be apparent that SD is a common problem in the general population such that it may sometimes be difficult to know if, in a patient

---

Pelvic Organ Dysfunction in Neurological Disease: Clinical Management and Rehabilitation, ed. Clare J. Fowler, Jalesh N. Panicker & Anton Emmanuel. Published by Cambridge University Press. © Cambridge University Press 2010.

Table 10.1. Overview of the categories of SD and potential therapeutic strategies. Adapted from [1, 2]

Dysfunction	Symptoms	Potential therapeutic strategies
Sexual interest/desire dysfunction (reduced libido)	Diminished or absent feelings of sexual interest or motivation	Relationship counselling, psychotherapy ?Hormonal replacement
Sexual arousal dysfunction	Poor/absent erections (males) (erectile dysfunction)	Treatment for erectile dysfunction
		PDE5 inhibitors
		Vacuum constriction devices
		Intracavernous/intraurethral prostaglandin therapy
	Diminished/absent feelings of sexual excitement and sexual pleasure (sexual arousal dysfunction) and/or vulval swelling or vaginal lubrication (genital arousal dysfunction) (females)	Vaginal lubricants ?Sildenafil
Orgasmic and ejaculatory dysfunctions	Delayed or absent ejaculation (males)	Yohimbine, midodrine
	Reduced or absent orgasms (males and females)	Psychosexual therapy, sensate focusing, cognitive behavior therapy
		Use of sex aids
		?Midodrine
Sexual pain disorder	Dyspareunia (females)	Anesthetic gels, pain modulation, specialist care

with neurological disease, it is or is not part of their neurological condition. In younger patients, such as a young man with MS, there is likely to be a close temporal relationship between the onset of ED and walking difficulties indicating relevant underlying spinal cord disease, whereas in an older man with Parkinson's disease ED could well be due to coincidental factors common in the aging male. There may be concomitant non-neurogenic factors contributing to SD as well, such as vascular disease or risk factors, endocrinopathies, genitourinary lesions, alcoholism or recreational drug use and polypharmacy.

Foley et al. studied sexual problems in patients with MS and proposed that they can stem from primary, secondary or tertiary sources. This model can be used to understand the complexity of SD in patients with other neurological diseases as well (Table 10.2) [5]. "Primary" SD results from the neurological lesions directly affecting the neural pathways subserving sexual functions, e.g. lesions in the spinal cord causing impairment of genital sensations. "Secondary" SD results from non-sexual physical changes due to the

neurological disease that have a bearing on sexual functions. "Tertiary" SD arises from the psychological, emotional or cultural impact of living with a neurological disease [6–10]. Organic and non-organic factors may co-exist, and a detailed evaluation is often required to uncover all the causes for SD.

Evaluation of sexual dysfunction

With increasing awareness of the impact of SD on quality of life, healthcare professionals have been encouraged to be proactive in this area. However, discussion about SD is often limited by lack of time during a consultation and feelings of embarrassment both on the part of the patient and the professional, the latter lacking confidence due to inadequate training in sexual medicine. One successful approach that can be taken in dealing with problems related to SD is the **PLISSIT** model [11] which focuses on four levels of intervention:

Permission (P): at this first level, patients are given the opportunity to open up about sexuality and relationship worries. The "permission-giving" should be

Table 10.2. Sexual dysfunction may be multifactorial. Adapted from [5]

Primary SD
Neurologic lesions in the nervous system impairing sexual response and/or sexual sensations

Secondary SD
Fatigue
Difficulties in attention and concentration
Bladder/bowel incontinence
Physical immobility: muscle weakness, leg spasms
Dysesthesia/allodynia
Other factors: incoordination, tremor, pain
Medications: antidepressants, baclofen, gabapentin
Presence of urethral indwelling catheter

Tertiary SD
Depression
Anxiety
Anger, guilt and fear
Altered self-image, low self-esteem
Relationship with the partner, change in family role

SD: sexual dysfunction

two-way and it may be helpful for the heathcare professional to indicate a willingness to talk about the topic by simply mentioning "sexual function can often be affected by neurological disorders which affect the bladder" when discussing urinary problems. The primary role of the healthcare professional at this stage is as a listener and this alone may be of immense therapeutic benefit for the patient.

Limited Information (LI): the healthcare professional can provide information to the patient and their partner about any areas of concern to help them address aspects of their disease that may affect sexual function and treatments. This can be done by the professional in whom the patient has confided or more formally by a professional attached to an SD clinic or counselling service.

Specific Suggestions (SS): suggestions about specific treatments appropriate for the patient can be offered. It would be useful to address the primary, secondary and tertiary factors predisposing to SD (Table 10.2).

Intensive Therapy (IT): the final step of the hierarchical model involves specialized psychosexual services and a formal treatment program for SD. This may not be suitable for all patients but can be considered once a formal evaluation has occurred and the patient is willing to engage in this process.

The PLISSIT model helps give a framework for counselling and treatment and has been successfully applied to patients with spinal cord disease [12, 13].

Factors that must be considered before addressing SD in a patient with neurological disease include the patient's attitude towards sex, sexual orientation and cultural influences. It is important to identify the component of SD that is most distressing for the patient. Involvement of the patient's partner is recommended if appropriate, when the quality of the relationship and the patient/partner needs and expectations of therapy have been assessed.

A detailed history, encompassing all components of SD that have been alluded to earlier (Table 10.2), and a focused clinical examination form the cornerstone of evaluation. Attention should be given to defining the problem and establishing the chronology and severity of symptoms. A typical history and onset of symptoms temporally related to neurological dysfunction would suggest that SD is likely to be due to the underlying neurological disorder. However, other factors contributing to SD may be uncovered as well such as cardiovascular disease or vascular risk factors (diabetes mellitus, systemic hypertension, hyperlipidemia or smoking), endocrinopathies, congenital or acquired genitourinary lesions or surgery, alcoholism, recreational drug use, psychiatric co-morbidities and medication history. In patients complaining of ED, it may be useful to enquire about the degree of the erectile response and the response at specific situations such as morning awakening, when presented with visual erotic stimuli, genital self-stimulation and during partner-related activity. This is because ED may be variable, with preserved nocturnal penile erections and erections on morning waking [14–16]. In the last 10–20 years the error of the neurological teaching that "if a man can get an erection at any time, impotence is likely to be psychogenic" has been recognized and nowadays ED is rarely attributed to emotional factors in the presence of neurological disease [8, 17]. With increasing neurological disability there may be a total failure of erectile function and also difficulty with ejaculation. Very few men with complete spinal cord injury can ejaculate (Chapter 15) [18, 19] and difficulty with ejaculation may become apparent when ED is successfully treated.

The use of validated questionnaires, e.g. the International Index for Erectile Function (IIEF) in men [20] and the Female Sexual Function Index (FSFI) in women [21], are helpful in assessing all sexual function domains and also in evaluating the impact of treatment. These have been used in research but may also be contributory in the clinical management of individual patients.

Most patients with neurological disease complain of reduced sexual functions, i.e. ED or reduced libido, but in some neurological conditions hypersexuality can be a problem. This can be the case in some patients with Parkinson's disease (in the context of dopamine dysregulation syndrome/hedonistic homeostatic dysregulation) (Chapter 12) or temporal lobe disease (Chapters 3 and 11). Hypersexuality may be assessed using the Sexual Compulsivity Scale developed by Kalichman and Rompa [22]. Although not validated in neurological patients, it has been used as a measure of the tendency of homosexual men to engage in sexual activity which may increase the risk of HIV infection. A higher score has been shown to be associated with lower self-esteem and resistance to adopting safer sexual practices. The scale is completed by the patient and may provide a means of obtaining information which might otherwise be embarrassing to elicit in a face-to-face consultation.

In general, as part of the workup of investigating SD in patients with a confirmed neurological deficit, physical examination evaluating the genitalia and secondary sexual characteristics may be performed if appropriate, but would be mandatory in a patient presenting with life-long complaints of SD. In patients with neurological disease with recent development of SD the focus may appropriately be on detecting relevant neurological disease, i.e. movement disorder, spinal cord or peripheral nerve disease.

Laboratory investigations
Blood tests

Laboratory testing should be tailored to the patient symptoms and risk factors. Fasting glucose and lipid profile may be measured to assess any atherosclerotic risk factors for ED. Hypothyroidism should be excluded. Total testosterone can be assayed if hypogonadism is suspected. Tests that measure the bioavailable or calculated free testosterone are, however, preferred as it is this fraction that is "bioavailable" to tissues and is better at establishing hypogonadism.

A morning sample should be sent in view of the circadian rhythm of testosterone levels. If low testosterone levels are detected, additional tests of pituitary function such as prolactin, follicle-stimulating hormone and luteinizing hormone may be ordered to distinguish hypogonadotrophic from hypergonadotrophic hypogonadism. There is no consensus recommended regarding routine laboratory tests in women. However, follicle-stimulating hormone and various androgen and estrogen values may be appropriate according to the clinical setting. Patients on neuroleptics should be aware of the possibility of hyperprolactinemia and should have prolactin levels measured if they report SD.

Uro-neurophysiological investigations

Although some years ago a number of papers were published reporting abnormalities of the bulbocavernosus reflex and pudendal evoked potentials in some men with ED, these tests proved to be of limited value and are not now routinely performed. Often the underlying neurological abnormality detected by these investigations was clinically readily apparent or could be demonstrated using testing outside the genital region such as nerve conduction studies and thermal thresholds to demonstrate peripheral neuropathy or lower limb evoked potentials to demonstrate spinal cord disease. However the fundamental flaw in the argument that these investigations tested relevant genital innervation was that the responses obtained were the result of conduction, albeit of the pudendal nerve, but in large myelinated nerve fibers responding to electrical stimulation [23]. Erectile responses, however, depend on the parasympathetic and sympathetic innervation which reaches the corpora through the cavernosal nerves (Chapter 3), fibers which cannot be depolarized by electrical stimuli of clinically acceptable intensity.

Activity purporting to be smooth muscle EMG recorded by a needle electrode from the corpus cavernosus and hence called "corpus cavernosum EMG" [24] had many biological features consistent with sympathetically derived electropotentials. However the exact nature was never fully resolved, the recordings did not prove to be of diagnostic value and its practical utility is limited [25].

Sensory testing

Complaints of impaired genital sensation may be a prominent feature of suspected neurogenic SD and a means of quantifying cutaneous sensations can be

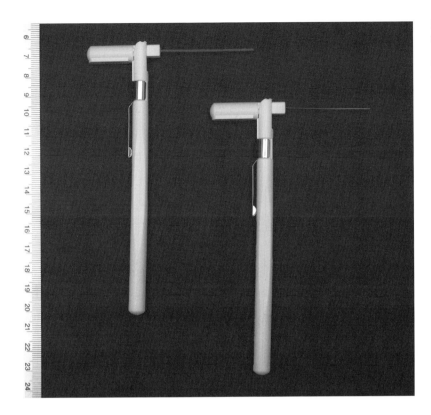

Fig. 10.1. Von Frey hairs consist of a series of calibrated filaments mounted on plexi-glass handles and can be used for quantitative mechanical stimulation of skin receptors. Reproduced with permission.

valuable in the investigation of such patients. Equipment offering a range of sensory tests which can be delivered according to semi-automated testing protocols, including light touch, vibration and thermal changes (Thermal Sensory Analyzer/Vibratory Sensory Analyzer system; TSA-3000 and VSA-3000; Medoc, Israel) has been used in research protocols to test both men and women with neurological disease.

More readily applicable, and a useful test in men complaining of loss of penile sensation, is sensory testing using von Frey hairs (Fig. 10.1). This is a type of esthesiometer and consists of a series of calibrated filaments to study single-point skin sensitivity to touch. This method is based on the principle that a fiber, pressed against the skin until it bends, produces a constant reproducible application of force. The bending force is proportional to the fiber diameter and inversely proportional to its length. We established in a small group of healthy, potent men, that the threshold for light touch on the glans penis should be comparable to that of the index finger in the same subject (unpublished data). Demonstration that such somatic sensation on the glans and shaft of the penis

is intact and there is not sensory impairment in a distribution indicating pudendal nerve damage (see Fig. 3.13B, p. 54) may be useful in the investigation of men who are complaining of "loss of sexual sensitivity." The underlying cause of that complaint is rarely established but analysis of symptoms frequently reveals the real problem is a change or loss of erotic sensations which are thought to be activated by hypothalamic-spinal pathways on sexual arousal (see Fig. 3.4, p. 43).

Therapeutic approaches

In neurological patients, multidimensional management of SD is often needed because of the heterogeneity of symptoms and the multiple contributory factors. Thus, a holistic approach, identifying all contributing factors for SD and planning a combination of therapeutic modalities, is optimal.

General measures

Alongside direct treatment for SD, associated co-morbidities should be identified and treated, and risk factors including obesity, smoking, alcoholism and

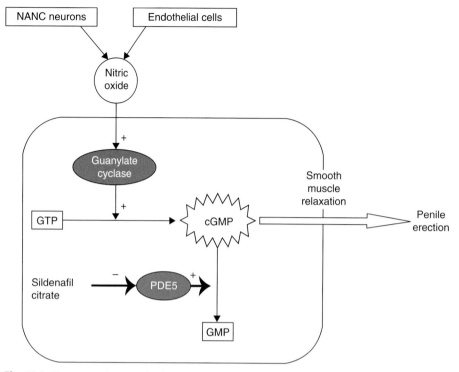

Fig. 10.2. Neurotransmitters involved in erection: sexual stimulation triggers the release of nitric oxide. Nitric oxide diffuses into cavernous smooth muscle cells and activates guanylate cyclase, which then catalyses the conversion of GTP to cGMP. This triggers a cascade of events that culminate in smooth muscle relaxation of the arteries and arterioles of the copora cavernosa and an erectile response. PDE5 inhibitors such as sildenafil prevent the degradation of cGMP and amplify the normal erectile physiology. Abbreviations: NANC = non-adrenergic non-cholinergic; GTP = guanosine-5'-triphosphate; cGMP = cyclic guanosine monophosphate; GMP = guanosine monophosphate; PDE5 = phosphodiesterase type 5 inhibitor.

substance abuse modified if possible. Depression and mood disorders need evaluation and treatment.

In chronic neurological disease, mobility, spasticity, trunk weakness and cognitive/behavioral disturbances may affect sexual activity. Antispasticity medications may be helpful in these situations as well as advice on sexual positioning. Fatigue is a feature in diseases such as MS and this can be addressed with drugs such as amantadine or modafinil that have been shown to improve sexual function [26].

Co-existent bowel and bladder dysfunction should be evaluated and treated by appropriate specialists. Fear of incontinence during sexual activity may have a negative impact not only on self-esteem but also personal relationships. For those with urinary incontinence, voiding before intercourse or drug therapy may promote continence. Intradetrusor botulinum A toxin injections have proven efficacy in promoting continence in people with neurogenic detrusor overactivity [27, 28]. For some patients with advanced disability, the use of an indwelling catheter, a

suprapubic in particular (Chapter 5), may be the preferred option. For those with anal incontinence, use of an enema before intercourse or the use of an anal plug may be helpful [26].

Concomitant medications should be reviewed, as drugs such as steroids, antidepressants, opiates and some diuretics and ß-blockers may impact sexual function. Serotonin reuptake inhibitors are associated with a reduction in sexual desire, arousal disorder and delayed or absent orgasm [29]. The resulting SD is a major contributor to non-compliance and discontinuation of treatment. Sustained-release bupropion has been shown to counter the effects of SSRIs [30]. In patients with concomitant depression and SD, it would be appropriate to use antidepressants having a different mechanism of action and less effect on sexual functions such as bupropion [31], a norepinephrine and dopamine reuptake inhibitor, or mirtazapine [32], a presynaptic alpha-2-adrenergic receptor blocker that inhibits the release of norepinephrine and serotonin.

Table 10.3. Phosphodiesterase type 5 (PDE5) inhibitors for the treatment of erectile dysfunction

Generic name	Sildenafil	Vardenafil	Tadalafil
Trade name	Viagra®	Levitra®	Cialis®
FDA approval	03/1998	08/2003	11/2003
Available doses	25, 50, 100 mg	5, 10, 20 mg	10, 20 mg
Starting dose	50 mg/d	10 mg/d	10 mg/d
Time to onset of action	30–60 minutes	30 minutes	30 minutes
Duration of effect	4 hours	4 hours	36 hours
Interaction with fatty meals	Yes	Yes	No
Trials in MS patients	Yes	No	No

FDA: Food and Drug Administration of the United States

Treatment options for men

Erectile dysfunction

First-line treatment

Oral drugs should be considered as first-line therapy for neurogenic ED. There are three phosphodiesterase type 5 (PDE5) inhibitors for oral use (Table 10.3), of which sildenafil (Viagra®) was the first available. The other drugs in this class are vardenafil (Levitra®) and tadalafil (Cialis®).

Phosphodiesterase catalyses the hydrolysis of cyclic adenosine monophosphate (cAMP) and cyclic guanosine monophosphate (cGMP), which are involved in the erectile function of the cavernous smooth muscle (Fig. 10.2). During sexual arousal, nitric oxide is released from the cavernous nerves and endothelium and activates guanylate cyclase that aids formation of cGMP. This triggers smooth muscle relaxation within the arterioles and arteries of the corpora cavernosa, resulting in increased blood flow and erection. PDE5 inhibitors slow the breakdown of cGMP and thereby amplify the normal erectile response. Therefore the PDE5 inhibitors do not cause spontaneous erections and sexual stimulation is necessary for their effect. There are several studies that demonstrate the efficacy of PDE5 inhibitors in men with neurological disease [33–35] and show that their response is often better than that in men with other medical conditions [36, 37] where vascular factors may predispose to ED (Fig. 10.3).

All three PDE5 inhibitors (Table 10.3) have similar efficacy and are well tolerated, though there are differences in onset of action, with sildenafil and vardenafil effective after 30–60 minutes and lasting for up to 4 hours, whereas tadalafil is effective after about 30 minutes, with peak effectiveness at 2 hours and lasting up to 36 hours [38]. A fatty meal may affect the absorption of sildenafil and vardenafil (but not tadalafil), with potential bearing on efficacy. Criteria to define "failure" of PDE5 inhibitors have recently been published, though not specifically for patients with neurological disease [39]. Use of PDE5 inhibitors may have an additional effect of improving lower urinary tract functions [40].

As PDE5 inhibitors increase the hypotensive effects of nitrates, they are contraindicated in patients who receive nitrates for angina [41]. Pre-existing hypotension and postural hypotension, as may occur in multiple system atrophy (MSA), are also relative contraindications [42]. Side-effects of PDE5 inhibitors are usually mild to moderate in nature and include headache, flushing, dyspepsia and nasal congestion. Of relevance to neurological patients, PDE5 inhibitors may rarely predispose to non-arteritic anterior ischemic optic neuritis [43].

Apomorphine (Uprima®, Ixense®), available as sublingual preparation, is a centrally acting dopamine agonist. It has modest efficacy and tolerability in mild ED [44, 45] although it was shown to be least preferred in a comparison trial with sildenafil [45]. It requires intact spinal pathways for action and its efficacy has not been established in neurological disease but it remains an option for patients who have contraindications for PDE5 use.

Vacuum constriction devices (VCDs) are an option for men who do not wish to consider, or have

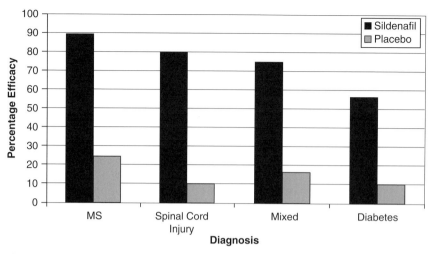

Fig. 10.3. Comparison of improvement in erections during individual trials of sildenafil patients with diabetes [37], mixed medical conditions [36], spinal cord injury [35] and multiple sclerosis [34] compared to placebo. The response is better in patients with neurological disorders compared to other medical conditions.

contraindications for, pharmacotherapy. These work by applying a negative pressure to the penis thereby drawing in blood and causing vasocongestion. A band is then applied to the base of the penis, constricting the outflow and maintaining tumescence. Patients are warned not to have the elastic bands in place continuously for more than 30 minutes because of the risk of venous anoxia. A certain amount of manual dexterity is required for use and side-effects include a sensation of trapped ejaculate, penile pain, numbness and bruising. Although they show good efficacy in spinal cord injured patients, satisfaction rates are low (Chapter 15) [46, 47] and they are generally more appropriate in older patients who are in a stable relationship.

Second-line treatment

Generally, if oral agents cannot be used or are not efficacious despite appropriate dosing and education, second-line treatments may be considered. However, the use of all second-line modalities is less suitable in neurological patients with advanced disability.

Intracavernous injections of prostaglandin E1, papaverine and phentolamine, are not licensed in the UK for ED but have good efficacy [48, 49]. However, a synthetic preparation of prostaglandin E1, alprostadil (Caverject®, Viridal®), is available. These vasoactive drugs, when injected into the corpora cavernosa of the penis, induce erection through smooth muscle relaxation, irrespective of sexual arousal. Adverse effects include penile pain, groin

pain, hypotension, prolonged erection (priapism) and in some instances, penile fibrosis when used over a long time. Intraurethral therapy of alprostadil (medicated urethral system for erection, MUSE®) is an alternative route of administration. Although efficacy rates over 60% have been reported in the general population [50], adverse effects including burning and irritation in the urethra make the therapy unpopular [51].

Surgical implantation of a penile prosthesis may be considered in men with ED refractory to other treatments. However, the procedure is invasive and irreversible and although there are high rates of patient and partner satisfaction, the infection rate is 1–5% and failure rates are 20% at five years and as high as 50% at 10 years [52, 53]. The potential for erosion and infection is higher in patients with neurological disease and a penile prosthesis should only be considered as a last resort. Lower urinary tract infections and spasticity mean the use of surgically implanted devices in progressive diseases are generally not advised. Anecdotally, a man with MS who had a device inserted when mildly disabled later regretted this when his condition deteriorated and he became dependent on others for toileting. Other surgical interventions for ED such as penile arterial revascularization or penile vein ligation have poor long-term success rates in general and are not used in patients with neurological disease.

Pelvic floor exercise may improve ED [54] and physiotherapy may be particularly effective in treating patients with veno-occlusive disease due to dysfunctional corporeal smooth muscle fibers, such as that due to sympathetic overactivity.

Ejaculation and orgasmic dysfunction

This often affects men with spinal cord lesions and the degree of dysfunction is dependent on the level and extent of injury. Yohimbine, derived from an alkaloid from the bark of the African tree *Pausinystalia yohimbe* and the South American herb quebracho *Aspidosperma quebracho-blanco*, is a monoamine oxidase inhibitor that has been shown to restore erotic sensitivity in a number of patients. Side-effects include an anxiogenic action, increased urinary frequency and elevation of blood pressure [55]. Sperling evaluated *Aspidosperma quebracho-blanco* binding to human penile alpha-adrenoceptors and concluded that the alpha-adrenoceptor mediated component of the pro-erectile effect was due to its yohimbine content [56]. The α-agonist midodrine given orally 30–120 minutes before stimulation has been shown to improve ejaculation and orgasm rates in spinal cord injured men [57].

When anejaculation is an issue in the setting of infertility treatment, two techniques may be used to aid semen collection. Vibratory stimulation employs a mechanical vibrator that is applied to the underside of the glans penis (Chapter 15) and set to vibrate at a designated frequency and wave amplitude. The technique only works in men with an intact ejaculatory reflex arc and the results are dependent on the level of neurological lesion. It does not require anesthesia or sedation.

The second technique, electroejaculation, is performed with a probe in the rectum which stimulates preganglionic efferent fibers with electric current (Chapter 3). The success rate is around 98% but it is an invasive method and there is a risk of rectal injury. Also, it is painful and has to be performed under general anesthesia or sedation for patients with incomplete spinal lesions.

Treatment options for women

There are fewer evidence-based therapeutic options for treatment of female SD. However it is an area of increasing interest and marketing of therapies by pharmaceutical companies. Therapies relate to treatment of sexual desire, arousal, orgasm and/or sexual pain. The term hypoactive sexual desire disorder (HSDD) is used to describe low sexual desire (Chapter 3) and distress, and many therapies aim to address this aspect of female sexual function.

There is no strong evidence to support hormone replacement therapy for HSDD, however local vaginal estrogen may be effective in SD related to vaginal atrophy. Vaginal atrophy may in itself cause dyspareunia and sexual pain and topical estrogen therapy is effective with a good safety profile [58]. Vaginal lubricants may also be of benefit in these cases.

Exogenous transdermal testosterone has been shown in small randomized trials to improve sexual desire, arousal and satisfaction. A large multicenter, phase III trial in 814 women with postmenopausal low libido called APHRODITE has shown testosterone patches to be effective, and testosterone gels are being evaluated in postmenopausal women. The side-effects include unwanted hair growth and there were four women on testosterone diagnosed with breast cancer during the study [59]. Tibolone has been shown to have a positive effect on climacteric symptoms and sexual function when compared with conventional hormone replacement therapy in postmenopausal women [60]. There are no data specifically for its use in neurological patients and the long-term effects of such a therapy are not known [61].

Sildenafil is not licensed for female SD but has been shown to have some beneficial effect in women with SD related to spinal cord injury [62]. In a placebo-controlled, cross-over trial, sildenafil resulted in significant increases of subjective arousal, especially when combined with manual and visual stimulation [62]. As in studies in men, the efficacy was best when stimulation was optimal and there were no significant side-effects. However, a double-blind cross-over study in female patients with MS did not reveal any clear benefit of sidenafil on sexual response [63].

Sex aids including vibrators and vacuum devices may be of some use in women with adequate dexterity or whose partners are willing to use them to aid stimulation and orgasm. The EROS-CTD system (Urometrics, St Paul, MN, USA) has been approved for orgasmic dysfunction in women (Fig. 10.4). This vacuum device is applied to the clitoris and works by increasing vaginal lubrication and enhancing orgasm ability. It can be used three or more times a week for up to five minutes and studies in non-neurogenical patients suggest an improvement in orgasm and sexual satisfaction [64]. It has, however, not been evaluated in women with an underlying neurological disease to date.

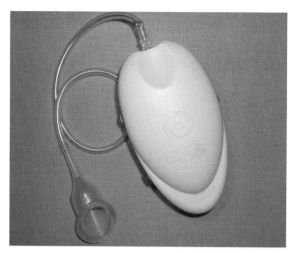

Fig. 10.4. The EROS-CTD system, which is FDA approved for orgasmic dysfunction in women. With kind permission from Beecourse Limited; www.beecourse.com

For some women, pelvic floor exercise may aid awareness of pelvic floor contractions and improve pelvic tone. The examiner can teach a patient to place a finger in the introitus and to contract her muscles. However, this requires some degree of dexterity and physical flexibility and may not be possible in those with minimal or no pelvic floor tone [65].

Genital prolapse is commonly seen in relation to parity and aging and in women with neurological disease, pelvic floor atrophy may further increase this risk. Both pelvic organ prolapse and urinary incontinence have a negative effect on sexual function. Severity of prolapse relates to symptoms of urinary incontinence, voiding dysfunction and SD but does not correlate to the location of the prolapse [66]. Correction of prolapse using either a ring pessary or surgery may improve sexual function though this may depend on the degree of prior SD, associated contributing factors and procedures performed.

Counselling and psychotherapy

In some patients, a formal treatment program for SD would also include specialized services involving psychotherapy, sensate focusing and behavioral counseling. Psychotherapy is time consuming and has been associated with variable results. Its value in patients with neurogenic SD is largely unknown but it may be reasonable to consider this option in some patients. Various strategies including individual, conjoint and group therapy approaches have been used. Psychotherapy

appears to be most effective when it is provided to the couple through a flexible and individualistic approach. In sensate focusing, couples are guided through a set of specific sexual exercises involving non-genital and genital touching. Cognitive-behavioral therapy emphasizes the role of thought patterns and beliefs in perpetuating maladaptive behavior and is useful when beliefs held by the patient or couple about norms or responses are contributing to the sexual problem [67]. In addition, treatments addressing interpersonal difficulties result in a better outcome than approaches focusing on problems in sexual functioning alone [68]. Psychosexual techniques that include setting of realistic couple goals, periodic psychosexual therapy follow-up, continual utilization of non-intercourse pleasuring sessions and initiating intimacy dates have been advocated as relapse prevention strategies [69].

Treatment outcomes

Many neurological diseases cause or contribute to SD so that neurogenic SD is not a homogenous but rather a widely heterogeneous entity. In addition, efficacy and safety data of the therapeutic modalities for treating SD are mainly based on studies enrolling non-neurological patients so that outcomes have often had to be extrapolated to the neurological population. Thus, although treatment outcome data for different therapeutic modalities are largely lacking in neurological patients, a similar treatment approach as in the non-neurological population is recommended.

Future perspectives

Sexual function is an important aspect of adult life and is impaired in many patients with neurological disorders, presenting various management challenges. Treatment should be tailored to the individual, with a holistic step-wise approach involving patient and partner education and counseling. Many men with an underlying neurological disorder fail to respond to PDE5 inhibitors and other lines of management and there is a need to study combination therapy. The role of newer therapies in neurological patients is yet to be established. In the general population, female SD is an area of considerable interest, especially for development of treatment options for arousal and orgasmic dysfunction. Sexual sensory dysfunction is a common problem in patients with neurological illnesses and there is a need for developing novel treatment options in this area. As awareness of the complexity of neurogenic SD grows, we can hope to understand how to target therapy better.

References

1. Lewis RW, Fugl-Meyer KS, Bosch R, et al. Epidemiology/risk factors of sexual dysfunction. *J Sex Med* 2004;**1**:35–9.

2. Hatzimouratidis K, Hatzichristou D. Sexual dysfunctions: classifications and definitions. *J Sex Med* 2007;**4**:241–50.

3. Laumann EO, Paik A, Rosen R. Sexual dysfunction in the United States: prevalence and predictors. *JAMA* 1999;**281**:537–44.

4. Lindau ST, Schumm LP, Laumann EO, et al. A study of sexuality and health among older adults in the United States. *N Engl J Med* 2007;**357**:762–74.

5. Foley F, Werner M. Sexuality and intimacy. In: Kalb R, ed. *Multiple sclerosis: the questions you ask, the answers you need.* New York: Demos Vermonde Press; 2000.

6. Hulter BM, Lundberg PO. Sexual function in women with advanced multiple sclerosis. *J Neurol Neurosurg Psychiatry* 1995;**59**:83–6.

7. Nortvedt MW, Riise T, Myhr KM, et al. Reduced quality of life among multiple sclerosis patients with sexual disturbance and bladder dysfunction. *Mult Scler* 2001;**7**:231–5.

8. Zivadinov R, Zorzon M, Bosco A, et al. Sexual dysfunction in multiple sclerosis: II. Correlation analysis. *Mult Scler* 1999;**5**:428–31.

9. Borello-France D, Leng W, O'Leary M, et al. Bladder and sexual function among women with multiple sclerosis. *Mult Scler* 2004;**10**:455–61.

10. Aisen M, Sanders A, eds. *Sexual dysfunction in neurologic disease: mechanisms of disease and counselling approaches.* AUA Update Series Lesson 35; 1998.

11. Annon JS. PLISSIT therapy. In: Corsini R, ed. *Handbook of Innovative Psychotherapies.* New York: Wiley & Sons; 1981:626–39.

12. Annon JS, Robinson CH. The use of various teaching models in treatment of sexual concerns. In: Piccolo JL, Piccolo LL, eds. *Handbook of sexual therapy.* New York: Plenum Press; 1978.

13. McBride KE, Rines B. Sexuality and spinal cord injury: a road map for nurses. *SCI Nurs* 2000;**17**:8–13.

14. Valleroy ML, Kraft GH. Sexual dysfunction in multiple sclerosis. *Arch Phys Med Rehabil* 1984;**65**:125–8.

15. Kirkeby HJ, Poulsen EU, Petersen T, Dorup J. Erectile dysfunction in multiple sclerosis. *Neurology* 1988;**38**:1366–71.

16. Staerman F, Guiraud P, Coeurdacier P, et al. Value of nocturnal penile tumescence and rigidity (NPTR) recording in impotent patients with multiple sclerosis. *Int J Impot Res* 1996;**8**:241–5.

17. Betts CD, Jones SJ, Fowler CG, Fowler CJ. Erectile dysfunction in multiple sclerosis. Associated neurological and neurophysiological deficits, and treatment of the condition. *Brain* 1994;**117**(Pt 6):1303–10.

18. Vas CJ. Sexual impotence and some autonomic disturbances in men with multiple sclerosis. *Acta Neurol Scand* 1969;**45**:166–82.

19. Witt MA, Grantmyre JE. Ejaculatory failure. *World J Urol* 1993;**11**:89–95.

20. Rosen RC, Riley A, Wagner G, et al. The international index of erectile function (IIEF): a multidimensional scale for assessment of erectile dysfunction. *Urology* 1997;**49**:822–30.

21. Rosen R, Brown C, Heiman J, et al. The Female Sexual Function Index (FSFI): a multidimensional self-report instrument for the assessment of female sexual function. *J Sex Marital Ther* 2000;**26**:191–208.

22. Kalichman SC, Rompa D. Sexual sensation seeking and sexual compulsivity scales: reliability, validity, and predicting HIV risk behavior. *J Pers Assess* 1995;**65**:586–601.

23. Fowler CJ. The neurology of male sexual dysfunction and its investigation by clinical neurophysiological methods. *Br J Urol* 1998;**81**:785–95.

24. Stief CG, Djamilian M, Anton P, et al. Single potential analysis of cavernous electrical activity in impotent patients: a possible diagnostic method for autonomic cavernous dysfunction and cavernous smooth muscle degeneration. *J Urol* 1991;**146**:771–6.

25. Jiang XG, Speel TG, Wagner G, Meuleman EJ, Wijkstra H. The value of corpus cavernosum electromyography in erectile dysfunction: current status and future prospect. *Eur Urol* 2003;**43**:211–8.

26. Ward-Abel N. *Sexuality & MS: a guide for women.* Letchworth Garden City, UK: Multiple Sclerosis Trust; 2007.

27. Kalsi V, Gonzales G, Popat R, et al. Botulinum injections for the treatment of bladder symptoms of multiple sclerosis. *Ann Neurol* 2007;**62**:452–7.

28. Karsenty G, Denys P, Amarenco G, et al. Botulinum toxin A (Botox) intradetrusor injections in adults with neurogenic detrusor overactivity/neurogenic overactive bladder: a systematic literature review. *Eur Urol* 2008;**53**:275–87.

29. Rosen RC, Lane RM, Menza M. Effects of SSRIs on sexual function: a critical review. *J Clin Psychopharmacol* 1999;**19**:67–85.

30. Clayton AH, Warnock JK, Kornstein SG, et al. A placebo-controlled trial of bupropion SR as an antidote for selective serotonin reuptake inhibitor-induced sexual dysfunction. *J Clin Psychiatry* 2004;**65**:62–7.

31. Clayton AH, Croft HA, Horrigan JP, et al. Bupropion extended release compared with escitalopram: effects on sexual functioning and antidepressant efficacy in 2 randomized, double-blind, placebo-controlled studies. *J Clin Psychiatry* 2006;**67**:736–46.

32. Saiz-Ruiz J, Montes JM, Ibanez A, et al. Assessment of sexual functioning in depressed patients treated with mirtazapine: a naturalistic 6-month study. *Hum Psychopharmacol* 2005;**20**:435–40.

33. Lombardi G, Macchiarella A, Cecconi F, Del Popolo G. Ten years of phosphodiesterase type 5 inhibitors in spinal cord injured patients. *J Sex Med* 2009; **6**:1248–58.

34. Fowler CJ, Miller JR, Sharief MK, et al. A double blind, randomised study of sildenafil citrate for erectile dysfunction in men with multiple sclerosis. *J Neurol Neurosurg Psychiatry* 2005;**76**:700–5.

35. Giuliano F, Hultling C, El Masry WS, et al. Randomized trial of sildenafil for the treatment of erectile dysfunction in spinal cord injury. Sildenafil Study Group. *Ann Neurol* 1999;**46**:15–21.

36. Padma-Nathan H, Steers WD, Wicker PA. Efficacy and safety of oral sildenafil in the treatment of erectile dysfunction: a double-blind, placebo-controlled study of 329 patients. Sildenafil Study Group. *Int J Clin Pract* 1998;**52**:375–9.

37. Rendell MS, Rajfer J, Wicker PA, Smith MD. Sildenafil for treatment of erectile dysfunction in men with diabetes: a randomized controlled trial. Sildenafil Diabetes Study Group. *JAMA* 1999;**281**:421–6.

38. Wespes E, Amar E, Hatzichristou D, et al. EAU guidelines on erectile dysfunction. http://www.uroweb. org/fileadmin/tx_eauguidelines/Erectile% 20Dysfunction.pdf. 2005:1–28.

39. Hackett G, Kell P, Ralph D, et al. British Society for Sexual Medicine guidelines on the management of erectile dysfunction. *J Sex Med* 2008;**5**:1841–65.

40. Gacci M, Del Popolo G, Macchiarella A, et al. Vardenafil improves urodynamic parameters in men with spinal cord injury: results from a single dose, pilot study. *J Urol* 2007;**178**:2040–3.

41. Brant WO, Bella AJ, Lue TF. Treatment options for erectile dysfunction. *Endocrinol Metab Clin North Am* 2007;**36**:465–79.

42. Hussain IF, Brady CM, Swinn MJ, Mathias CJ, Fowler CJ. Treatment of erectile dysfunction with sildenafil citrate (Viagra) in parkinsonism due to Parkinson's disease or multiple system atrophy with observations on orthostatic hypotension. *J Neurol Neurosurg Psychiatry* 2001;**71**:371–4.

43. Danesh-Meyer HV, Levin LA. Erectile dysfunction drugs and risk of anterior ischaemic optic neuropathy: casual or causal association? *Br J Ophthalmol* 2007;**91**:1551–5.

44. Pavone C, Curto F, Anello G, et al. Prospective, randomized, crossover comparison of sublingual apomorphine (3 mg) with oral sildenafil (50 mg) for male erectile dysfunction. *J Urol* 2004;**172**(6 Pt 1): 2347–9.

45. Eardley I, Wright P, MacDonagh R, Hole J, Edwards A. An open-label, randomized, flexible-dose, crossover study to assess the comparative efficacy and safety of sildenafil citrate and apomorphine hydrochloride in men with erectile dysfunction. *BJU Int* 2004; **93**:1271–5.

46. Levine LA, Dimitriou RJ. Vacuum constriction and external erection devices in erectile dysfunction. *Urol Clin North Am* 2001;**28**:335–41.

47. Jarow JP, Nana-Sinkam P, Sabbagh M, Eskew A. Outcome analysis of goal directed therapy for impotence. *J Urol* 1996;**155**:1609–12.

48. Hirsch IH, Smith RL, Chancellor MB, et al. Use of intracavernous injection of prostaglandin E1 for neuropathic erectile dysfunction. *Paraplegia* 1994;**32**:661–4.

49. Bella AJ, Brock GB. Intracavernous pharmacotherapy for erectile dysfunction. *Endocrine* 2004;**23**:149–55.

50. Padma-Nathan H, Hellstrom WJ, Kaiser FE, et al. Treatment of men with erectile dysfunction with transurethral alprostadil. Medicated Urethral System for Erection (MUSE) Study Group. *N Engl J Med* 1997;**336**:1–7.

51. Fulgham PF, Cochran JS, Denman JL, et al. Disappointing initial results with transurethral alprostadil for erectile dysfunction in a urology practice setting. *J Urol* 1998;**160**(6 Pt 1):2041–6.

52. Goldstein I, Newman L, Baum N, et al. Safety and efficacy outcome of mentor alpha-1 inflatable penile prosthesis implantation for impotence treatment. *J Urol* 1997;**157**:833–9.

53. Carson CC. Penile prostheses: are they still relevant? *BJU Int* 2003;**91**:176–7.

54. Claes H, van Hove J, van de Voorde W, et al. Pelvi-perineal rehabilitation for dysfunctioning erections. A clinical and anatomo-physiologic study. *Int J Impot Res* 1993;**5**:13–26.

55. Riley AJ. Yohimbine in the treatment of erectile disorder. *Br J Clin Pract* 1994;**48**:133–6.

56. Sperling H, Lorenz A, Krege S, Arndt R, Michel MC. An extract from the bark of Aspidosperma quebracho blanco binds to human penile alpha-adrenoceptors. *J Urol* 2002;**168**:160–3.

57. Soler JM, Previnaire JG, Plante P, Denys P, Chartier-Kastler E. Midodrine improves ejaculation in spinal cord injured men. *J Urol* 2007;**178**:2082–6.

58. Lara LA, Useche B, Ferriani RA, et al. The effects of hypoestrogenism on the vaginal wall: interference with the normal sexual response. *J Sex Med* 2009;**6**:30–9.

59. Davis SR, Moreau M, Kroll R, et al. Testosterone for low libido in postmenopausal women not taking estrogen. *N Engl J Med* 2008;**359**:2005–17.

60. Ziaei S, Moaya M, Faghihzadeh S. Comparative effects of continuous combined hormone therapy and tibolone on body composition in postmenopausal women. *Climacteric* 2010;**13**:249–53.

61. Bolour S, Braunstein G. Testosterone therapy in women: a review. *Int J Impot Res* 2005;**17**:399–408.

62. Sipski ML, Rosen RC, Alexander CJ, Hamer RM. Sildenafil effects on sexual and cardiovascular responses in women with spinal cord injury. *Urology* 2000;**55**:812–5.

63. Dasgupta R, Wiseman OJ, Kanabar G, Fowler CJ, Mikol DD. Efficacy of sildenafil in the treatment of female sexual dysfunction due to multiple sclerosis. *J Urol* 2004;**171**:1189–93.

64. Wilson SK, Delk JR, 2nd, Billups KL. Treating symptoms of female sexual arousal disorder with the Eros-Clitoral Therapy Device. *J Gend Specif Med* 2001;**4**:54–8.

65. Canavan TP, Heckman CD. Dyspareunia in women. Breaking the silence is the first step toward treatment. *Postgrad Med* 2000;**108**:149–52, 157–60, 164–6.

66. Ellerkmann RM, Cundiff GW, Melick CF, et al. Correlation of symptoms with location and severity of pelvic organ prolapse. *Am J Obstet Gynecol* 2001;**185**:1332–7.

67. Tiefer L, Schuetz-Mueller D. Psychological issues in diagnosis and treatment of erectile disorders. *Urol Clin North Am* 1995;**22**:767–73.

68. Stravynski A, Gaudette G, Lesage A, et al. The treatment of sexually dysfunctional men without partners: a controlled study of three behavioural group approaches. *Br J Psychiatry* 1997;**170**:338–44.

69. McCarthy BW. Relapse prevention strategies and techniques in sex therapy. *J Sex Marital Ther* 1993;**19**:142–6.

Cortical and subcortical disorders

Ryuji Sakakibara, Clare J. Fowler and Takamichi Hattori

Introduction

Description of the neural control of the individual pelvic organs can be found in Chapters 1–3. Much of that knowledge is based on recent data acquired by functional brain imaging but prior to the advent of those powerful techniques, what we knew about the role of the cortical and subcortical areas in the control of pelvic organs relied on a small number of carefully observed clinical cases: patients presenting with specific symptoms of bladder or bowel dysfunction or abnormalities of sexual behavior who had been found to have lesions at particular brain sites. Initially the lesion studies were based on observations made in life correlated with post-mortem or pathological specimens, but with increasingly better means of imaging it was possible to correlate symptoms with smaller, more discrete abnormalities. For various reasons, fewer case histories are now occupying space in journals and the majority of the case histories referred to in this chapter are more than 20 or 30 years old. The "lesion literature" is quite sparse for all three functional systems and is summarized in Tables 11.1–11.3 [1–45]. In this chapter, first the case histories and the "lesion literature" are discussed and the effects of injury or disease at focal sites described, and then the results of diffuse cortical and subcortical diseases, such as cerebrovascular disease, dementias and head injury, are considered.

Focal frontal lesions

Although the neural control for each pelvic organ function has been shown to differ considerably (Chapter 1–3), a general organizational principle is apparent. Each organ is innervated by its own set of peripheral nerves bringing it, through connections via sacral roots S_2–S_4, under the influence of the lowest sacral segments of the spinal cord. Although much reflex activity is organized at spinal levels, it is connections with subcortical centers, the hypothalamus in particular, which determine the coordinated control of each organ. However, the integration of bladder, bowel or sexual function into our human, social world requires the modulating influences of higher centers in the cortex. The concept of the "social brain," although introduced to account for "brain function which allows us to interact with other people" [46] proposes there are circumscribed regions of the brain which are dedicated to social interactions and these include the medial prefrontal and the orbital frontal cortex. The cortical control of the bladder is so far probably the best understood of the three functional systems and it appears that the medial prefrontal region maintains tonic inhibition of diencephalic centers, integrating bladder activity appropriately for our social behavior. It seems probable that a similar arrangement pertains for other pelvic organ functions and it is predominantly this aspect of control that is lost following frontal lobe damage or injury.

Bladder

Although Andrew and Nathan [2] were not the first to describe disturbances of micturition resulting from a variety of causes of frontal lobe pathology, their celebrated paper reporting the syndrome of frequency, urgency and in some patients fecal incontinence causing distress to the patient, is seminal. Their description of these patients cannot be improved upon:

"The patients described here were not demented, indifferent or lacking in social awareness; they were

Pelvic Organ Dysfunction in Neurological Disease: Clinical Management and Rehabilitation, ed. Clare J. Fowler,
Jalesh N. Panicker & Anton Emmanuel. Published by Cambridge University Press. © Cambridge University Press 2010.

Table 11.1. Lesion literature for bladder pathophysiology. Based on table in [1]

Key brain regions	Pathology	Number of cases	Effect on bladder behavior
Frontal			
	Various causes of frontal lobe pathology [2]	36	Altered bladder sensation and incontinence in absence of intellectual deterioration or retention 3 cases had retention
	Brain tumors [3]	50	Disturbances of micturition
	Frontal lobe tumors [4]	7	Frequency, urgency incontinence
	Frontal abscess [5]	1	Retention
	Frontal abscess/hematoma [6]	2	Retention
	Anterior cerebral vascular lesions [7]		Various bladder disorders and hemiparesis
ACG			
	Bilateral infarction of anterior cingulate gyri [8]	1	Complex behavioral changes and incontinence
	Glioma of ACG and supplementary motor cortex [9]	1	Urgency incontinence with loss of sensation
Insula			
	Glioma of insula and inferior frontal gyrus [9]	1	Incontinence without loss of bladder sensation
Hypothalamus			
	Ruptured anterior cerebral aneurysms [10]	6	Pre- or postoperative disturbances of micturition
	Pituitary tumors extending into the hypothalamus [11]	3	Urgency incontinence, weight loss, psychiatric symptoms
	Cystic lesion of hypothalamus [12]	1	Frequent incontinence
PAG			
	Presumed inflammatory lesion [13]	1	Urinary retention
Pons			
	Posterior fossa tumors [14]		Voiding difficulty
	Brain stem tumors [3]	46	Predominantly voiding difficulties
	Brainstem vascular lesions [15]	34	Predominantly voiding difficulties
	Brainstem gliomas in children [16]	24	Voiding difficulty
	Presumed dermoid [17]	1	Urinary retention and disordered eye movements
	Low grade glioma [18]	1	Paraparesis, urinary retention and disordered eye movements
	Herpes encephalitis [19]	1	Urinary retention and disordered eye movements
	Presumed rhombencephalitis [20]	1	Urinary retention and horizontal diplopia

Table 11.2. Lesion literature for bowel dysfunction

Key brain regions	Pathology	Number of cases	Effect on fecal continence
Frontal			
	Various causes of frontal lobe pathology [2]	36	"Defecation is involved less frequently and usually less severely than micturition"
	Frontal lobe disease [21]	7	Impaired sensation of bladder filling and rectal sensation and spontaneous rectal contractions
Pons			
	Pontine pathology [22]	3	Extreme constipation

Table 11.3. Lesion literature for sexual dysfunction. Adapted from [23]

Key brain regions	Pathology	Number of cases	Effect on sexual behavior
Frontal			
	Sexual behavior after lobotomy [24]	40	4 cases of increased sexual activity, 16 decreased
	Sexual automatisms [25]	10	Sexual automatisms and other complex motor behaviors
Parietal			
	Parasagittal pathology [26]	2	Genital sensations with sexual content
	Paracentral lobule [27]	10	Genital sensations without sexual resonance
Temporal			
	Sexuality in patients with psychomotor seizures [28]	36	26 had hyposexuality
	Effects on sexuality of temporal lobe surgery [29]	21	11 "grossly hyposexual" preoperatively
	Effects on sexuality of temporal lobe surgery [30, 31]	50	29 hyposexual and 7 hypersexual preoperatively.
	TLE and grand mal epilepsy compared [32]	140	Greater number TLE than grand mal were hyposexual
	Sexual behavior in women with epilepsy [33]		Lower marriage rate in women with TLE
	Reproductive endocrine disorders in women with TLE [34]	50	
	Reproductive endocrine disorders in men with TLE [35]	20	
	Hypersexuality after temporal lobe surgery [36]	7	Bilateral temporal lobe abnormalities in 5

Table 11.3. (cont.)

Key brain regions	Pathology	Number of cases	Effect on sexual behavior
	Kluver-Bucy due to various bi-temporal pathologies [37]		
	Hypersexuality and other behavioral symptoms [38]	8	4 hypersexuality, 4 altered sexual preference
	Sexual automatisms [39]	5	Grabbing or fondling genitals
	Postictal Kluver-Bucy [40]	1	Behavioral changes lasting 1–2 hours
	Orgasmic auras [41]	9	Ictal lateralizing sign to right hemisphere
	Fetishism [42]	1	Relieved by temporal lobectomy
Hypothalamic and septal region			
	Hypersexuality following septal injury [43]	2	VP shunt
	Hypersexuality [38]	1	VP shunt
	Hypersexuality and other behavioral symptoms [38]	1	Ruptured aneurysm with thalamic and hypothalamic infarct
	Cystic lesion of hypothalamus [12]	1	Incontinence and pathological libido preoperatively
Ansa lenticularis and pallidus			
	Myoclonus alleviated by bilateral ansotomy [44]	5	3 men and 1 women became alibidinous
	Pallidotomy for Parkinson's disease [45]	1	Immediate hypersexuality

much upset and embarrassed by these symptoms . . . The acts of micturition and defecation occur in a normal manner; what is disturbed by this frontal lesion is the higher control of these acts. The lesion causes frequency and extreme urgency of micturition when the patient is awake, incontinence when asleep. The sensation of gradual awareness of increasing fullness of the bladder and the sensation that micturition is imminent, are impaired. When the syndrome is less pronounced, the sensation underlying the desire to micturate is absent, whereas the sensation that micturition is imminent still occurs. Then the patient is waylaid by a sudden awareness that he is about to pass urine; when neither sensation is experienced, the patient is amazed to find that he has passed urine."

The infrequency with which such patients are encountered is illustrated by the fact that the authors tell us they had each been collecting cases separately over a period of 24 years and only just prior to writing did they learn of each other's interest and combined efforts to present a joint paper. In their paper the authors described 38 patients with disturbances of micturition as a result of lesions in the anterior frontal lobe (Fig. 1.14, p. 15) [47]. There were 10 patients with intracranial tumors, 2 with anterior frontal lobe damage following rupture of an aneurysm, 4 who had penetrating brain wounds and 22 patients who had undergone leucotomy. The authors explain that the leucotomy cases were the most useful in terms of localization of important brain structures and the significant plane of the lesion was that lying immediately anterior to the tips of the ventricles and the genu of the corpus callosum. Such lesions involved gray matter, in particular the superomedial part of the frontal lobe (see Fig. 1.14, p. 15) but they caused a permanent disorder of the control of micturition and of defecation only when they involved some of the white matter lateral to the anterior horns of the lateral ventricle, defecation being much less often affected than micturition. Lesions that did not affect this white

(a)

(b)

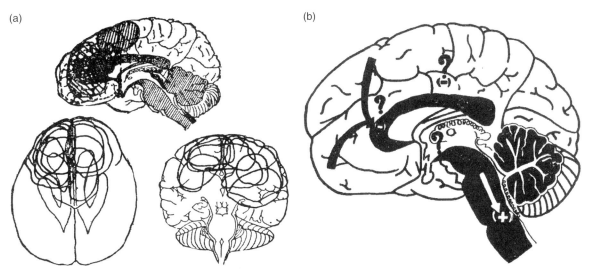

Fig. 11.1. A. Lesions by frontal lobe tumor that caused urinary incontinence. B. Schematic representation of cerebral control of micturition. From [48] with permission.

matter caused only transient disordered control of micturition. Correspondingly it was suggested that most of the critical lesion area was in this white matter (Fig. 1.14, p. 15) [2].

Subsequently the same features of bladder dysfunction were observed in 7 out of 50 consecutive patients with frontal tumors [4].

In three cases, Andrew and Nathan observed that lesions in similar areas to those discussed above led to urinary retention rather than incontinence (Table 11.1). Subsequently Yamamoto et al. [5] described a 70-year-old woman who was demonstrated to have urinary retention and detrusor hyporeflexia on cystometry. Her high fever and worsening cognitive state prompted brain imaging and she was found to have a right frontal lobe abscess. Both her general condition and her bladder function were improved by antibiotic administration which successfully treated the abscess. Lang et al. [6] reported two elderly female patients with frontal pathology and retention, one of whom recovered bladder function following a successful neurosurgical intervention.

Although the paper of Andrew and Nathan [2] has been the most influential in the study of frontal lobe control of the bladder, it was not in fact the first. In 1960 Ueki published a paper [3] of which Andrew and Nathan appear to have been unaware. A neurosurgeon in Japan, Ueki analysed the urinary symptoms of 462 patients who had come to surgery

for brain tumors. There were 34 cases of frontal lobectomy and 16 cases of bilateral anterior cingulectomy and he illustrated his conclusions with a diagram of the brain showing a strong positive influence on micturition of an area in the pons and an inhibitory input from the frontal lobe (Fig. 11.1) [48].

Urinary incontinence was a noted feature of the first patients described by Hakim and Adams [49] with normal pressure hydrocephalus, and Fisher found bladder symptoms were an early feature of 14 of the 30 patients in his series [50]. He speculates that fibers of tracts involved in the control of the urinary bladder must lie close to the dilated ventricles, as indeed is shown in Fig. 11.1. The stretching of tracts is thought to result in a physiological block which is reversible when the pressure is reduced.

Bowel

Andrew and Nathan wrote that in their series of patients defecation was affected much less often than micturition by cerebral diseases [2]. They found fecal frequency, incontinence and constipation in 3 of 10 patients with brain tumors, fecal incontinence in 1 of 2 patients after aneurysm surgery, and fecal incontinence in 2 of 4 patients with brain injury. Typically fecal incontinence could occur without warning in the daytime, or only when asleep. In a later study of 7 patients with frontal lobe injury, anorectal manometry was carried out and showed that in 2 patients there was an increased perception threshold for rectal distension, 5 had spontaneous rectal contractions, and 1 had lost the recto-anal inhibitory reflex [21].

Sexual behavior

In discussions about changes in sexual behavior due to neurological disease, Baird et al. [23] make the distinction between true hypersexuality and loss of social inhibition: it is the latter disorder that results from frontal lobe damage. Disinhibited sexual behavior has been reported following damage to the frontal lobes, particularly the orbitofrontal region of the limbic system [23].

At a time when prefrontal lobotomy was being performed for severe psychiatric disorders, a retrospective study of 40 cases examined the effect of surgery on sexual behavior [24]. Postoperatively 4 patients became a social problem on account of their sexual behavior, but in only 1 woman was this a completely new phenomenon. In 40% of all the cases (15 men and 25 women) there was considered to have been a decrease in sexual drive. The authors write "the expectation that loss of inhibitions was correlated with increased drive and vice versa was not borne out by the data. The only clear trend was that the apathetic patient with general loss of initiative and spontaneity usually has a decreased drive."

Sexual motor behaviors with pelvic and truncal movements are a form of "genital automatism" which appear to be peculiar to frontal lobe epilepsy [25] whereas complex partial seizures defined as repeated fondling or grabbing of the genitals occur possibly exclusively as a feature of temporal lobe epilepsy [39]. It is interesting to speculate that by analogy with the frontal control of micturition (an altogether less complex system), in health the frontal regions may exert a tonic inhibitory function over motor patterns with circuitry in mesencephalic structures such as the periaqueductal gray (PAG) and paroxysmal loss of this allows expression of primitive behaviors.

Parietal lobe

There are no reports of bladder or bowel dysfunction as a consequence of a focal parietal deficit.

Sexual behavior

The cortical representation of the genital region has been the subject of some debate over the years but

modern functional brain imaging techniques demonstrated light touch of the penis resulted in activation of the medial edge of the convexity of the contralateral postcentral gyrus, lateral to that of the toe representation and the lower abdominal wall, without any indication of representation in the mesial wall [51] (Figure 3.8, page 46). This evidence has only recently become available and until now Penfield was always cited that penile representation was on the mesial surface of the postcentral gyrus, i.e. the parietal "paracentral lobule." Bancaud et al. described 10 patients with seizures arising from paracentral lobule lesions which included lateralized genital sensations without sexual content, in contrast to patients experiencing temporal lobe sexual seizures [27]. In a review chapter, Toone cites case histories of parietal lesions in which abnormal genital sensation preceded orgasm in one woman with a right parasagital hemangioma originally described as having "nymphomania" [52] (Chapter 3) and another woman with a malignant glioma [26].

Temporal lesions

The temporal lobes have little or no apparent influence on bladder or bowel control but a major role in determining sexual behavior. Indeed the topic of human sexual activity and the appositely described "libidinous" temporal lobe [31] would alone justify a substantial tome. An attempt has been made to summarize what is known in Chapter 3 and here brief descriptions of the effect of various temporal lobe lesions is given.

In general terms the evidence is that the temporal lobes have a regulatory, largely inhibitory effect on the hypothalamus and septal regions, the neural centers for reproduction and sexual behavior (Chapter 3). Bilateral temporal lobectomy in rhesus monkeys results in profound behavioral abnormalities including hyperorality and hypersexuality, a condition known as the Kluver-Bucy syndrome. A comparable condition rarely has been seen in humans but as in animals it appears to follow bilateral temporal lobe damage [53]. The hypersexuality in animals consists of indiscriminate sexual responses to inappropriate objects and it is inappropriate sexual behavior which characterizes humans with this disorder. Less than full-blown expression of the syndrome has been described in patients with bilateral temporal lobe disease [37] following herpes encephalitis [38],

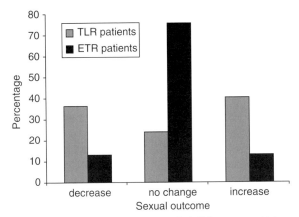

Fig. 11.2. Outcome following surgery [58]. TLR = temporal lobe resection; ETR = extra-temporal lobe resection.

adrenoleucodystrophy [54] or involvement in fronto-temporal dementia [55], a disease which leaves patients particularly prone to developing the syndrome [56].

Following temporal lobe resection for epilepsy, although abnormalities of the unoperated temporal lobe are present in the majority, the changes in behavior of patients that occur are unlike those of Kluver-Bucy syndrome: what is observed in some cases is a focused increased sexual drive rather than indiscriminate sexual behavior. This phenomenon was systematically analysed by Blumer and Walker in 26 patients who underwent unilateral temporal lobectomy for epilepsy [29]. Blumer [30] and Walker in his lecture five years later [31] described 47 patients with temporal lobe epilepsy (TLE) of whom 32 had had preoperative global hyposexuality (see below). Following temporal lobectomy, 15 patients had "greater sexuality." In a recent prospective study by Baird et al. of a series of patients undergoing surgery for TLE (58 patients) and extra-TLE (16 patients), sexual drive was estimated pre- and postsurgery by a self-administered questionnaire [57]. Temporal lobe resection was more commonly associated with postoperative change in sexual drive than extratemporal lobe resection, particularly right-sided temporal resections, and an increase in sexual drive was significantly more likely in women (Fig. 11.2). It was subsequently shown that those patients who reported an increase in sexual activity postoperatively had a significantly larger amygdala volume contralateral to the site of their resective surgery [58]. The authors hypothesize that the effect was due either to the control of the amygdala over endocrine substrates of sexual behavior or its role in processing potentially significant sexual stimuli.

Infrequently, hypersexuality occurs following temporal lobe resection: this was first reported by Blumer who noted that 7 out of 50 patients undergoing temporal lobe resection became hypersexual [30]. Some 30 years later Baird et al. described the self-reported hypersexuality [36] of 7 out of 60 cases who had had surgery.

Interictal hyposexuality in patients with temporal lobe epilepsy was a phenomenon first observed by Gastaut and Collomb in 1954 [28]. They noticed hyposexuality in several hundred patients with psychomotor seizures and on detailed examination confirmed its existence in 26 out of 36 patients. These patients had a "profound disinterest in all the usual libidinous aspects of life" with the onset of their global hyposexuality developing two to four years after the onset of seizures; a possible mechanism for this is discussed in Chapter 3. Although in more recent times the hyposexuality of patients with epilepsy was attributed to an effect of anticonvulsant medication [59, 60], some others have since confirmed the early observations and shown the problem to be greater in those with TLE than grand mal epilepsy [32]. Whereas a study from Egypt noted that women with early-onset TLE were more likely to be unmarried [33], a more recent UK study found no difference in desire and enjoyment of intercourse in women with treated TLE who had regular partners but did conclude that their study design might not have captured an abnormal group and that there could be a bimodal distribution of sexual interest in women with TLE. If temporal lobe damage occurs before the onset of puberty, "erotic apathy" [31] is characteristic, the subject showing no sexual interests and it was asserted "no concern about this." However, in the experience of one of the authors (CJF), this has not been the case – a young man who had had temporal lobe surgery for epilepsy in childhood has found his asexuality causes him great distress on account of his inability to form a dyadic relationship. The Asexual Visibility and Education Network (AVEN) may be a support to such patients in the future. Acquired temporal lobe damage in later life or sometimes following temporal lobe surgery for epilepsy can result in loss of sexual interests and appetites, with the expected consequences on interpersonal relationships.

Less commonly than hyposexuality, temporal lobe disease may be associated with hypersexuality or altered sexual preferences [38]. Some cases of

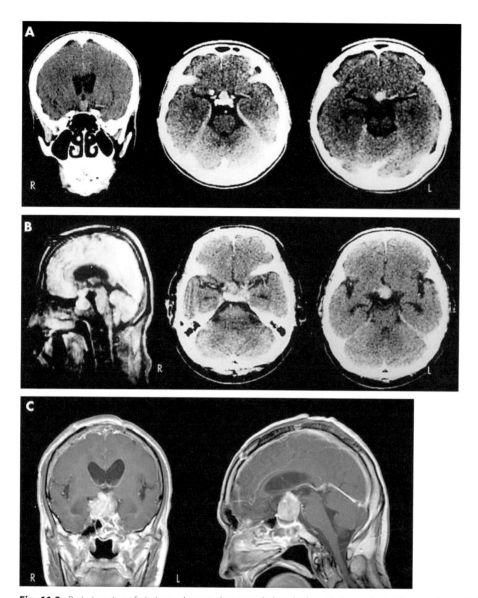

Fig. 11.3. Brain imaging of pituitary adenoma that extended to the hypothalamus. Brain CT scans of case 1. A. Coronal and axial planes with contrast enhancement showed a pituitary tumor extending upward to the hypothalamus and compressing the hypothalamus, optic chiasm, stria terminalis, septal area and supraoptic area. An MRI scan (sagittal plane, proton-weighted image) and CT scans (axial plane with contrast enhancement) of case 2 (B) showed a similar-sized pituitary tumor. MRI scans of case 3 (C) (coronal and sagital planes, Gadolinium-DTPA images) showed a pituitary tumor extending upward to the third ventricle and compressing the hypothalamus bilaterally. From [11] with permission.

paraphilias or sexual deviations have temporal lobe disease: in men it was thought that hypersexuality secondary to bilateral temporal lobe damage unmasked latent pedophilia [55]. That report also includes a helpful review of the relevant forensic psychiatric literature. Ictal phenomena with temporal lobe seizures include orgasmic auras [41], genital automatisms [39] and fetishisms [42].

Subcortical lesions
Hypothalamic and septal regions
The hypothalamus, part of the phylogenetically ancient diencephalon, is the major visceral control center of the brain. Many early animal experimental studies demonstrated that stimulation of anterior hypothalamus and septum pellucidum in an awake

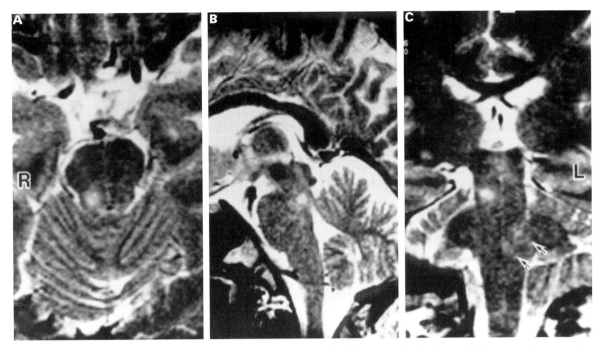

Fig. 11.4. Brain MRI of the patient. (A) Axial view, (B) sagittal view, (C) coronal MRI of patient with rhombencephalitis causing urinary retention and horizontal diplopia. T2-weighted images show a hyperintense focus in the right dorsolateral tegmentum of the rostral pon and arrows indicate amorphous lesions (C) [20]. Reproduced with permission.

cat resulted in the animal taking up its typical position for voiding or defecation [61]. Observations showing the importance of the hypothalamus in relation to phases of bladder activity have been repeatedly confirmed and refined by subsequent researchers [62, 63]. Functional brain imaging has shown activation of the hypothalamus during bladder filling [64] and the role of the hypothalamus in bladder control is centrally embedded in Griffith's "circuit 2" as described in Chapter 2.

Bladder and bowel

Much influenced by early experimental findings in animals and following their earlier work on the identification of regions of the frontal lobes important in the control of bladder and bowel function [2], Andrew and Nathan described six patients who had aneurysms affecting the region where the "rostral part of the diencephalon meets the telencephalon," i.e. septum and hypothalamus. Aneurysms of the anterior cerebral artery near the genu of the corpus callosum and the anterior communicating artery were thought to result in ischemic damage to the hypothalamus and septal regions and a disturbance of micturition was a

feature of all six cases either pre- or postoperatively [10]. In their discussion they observed that in the five boxers reported by Spillane (of what is now called "punch-drunk" syndrome) [65] urinary symptoms were a feature and postulated this was due to septal and hypothalamic damage. Based on these observations and their earlier findings the authors proposed that the acts of micturition and defecation were organized at the subcortical level but controlled by cortical input.

More recently, Yamamoto et al. [11] reported three cases of pituitary adenoma that extended to the hypothalamus (Fig. 11.3). None of these patients had diabetes inspidus with polyuria but instead, they complained of nocturnal frequency, urinary urgency, and either incontinence (case 1) or voiding difficulty and urinary retention (cases 2 and 3). Case 3 also had visual disturbance, anorexia, psychiatric symptoms, and syndrome of inappropriate secretion of antidiuretic hormone (SIADH). Cystometry showed DO in all three and in two, an underactive detrusor during the voiding phase.

Damage to the hypothalamus may lead to intestinal dysmotility; a woman reported by Krishna and Blenvis developed weight loss, nausea, vomiting and reversible gastroparesis due to a non-secreting pituitary tumor [66].

Sexual behavior

Comparable to the experimental data on the effect of hypothalamic stimulation and bladder activity, there is substantial literature on the role of the hypothalamus and septal areas in determining sexual behavior in animals (see Chapter 3). Stimulation of the preoptic nuclei in the monkey results in copulation behavior whereas ablation results in loss of sexual activity [67]. Hypothalamic activation is seen in functional imaging experiments when subjects view sexually arousing scenes (Chapter 3) and there are a number of clinical cases which indicate the strong influence of the hypothalamus and septal regions in human sexual behavior.

In the 1950s Heath and his colleagues at Tulane were pioneering neuropsychiatric interventions involving long-term placement of intracerebral electrodes and intraventicular canulae for drug delivery in patients with chronic psychiatric and epileptic disorders. In a report, many details of which now seem shocking, Heath described two patients in whom he was able to record from multiple in-depth electrodes whilst they experienced induced orgasm. The traces showed spike and large slow-wave activity superimposed on fast activity, restricted to and recorded from the septal electrodes. In other experiments, electrical self-stimulation of this region resulted in intensely pleasurable sensations, a compulsion to masturbate and sometimes orgasm [68]. These observations do not appear to have been further developed but more recently two male patients have been described who showed hypersexuality after the insertion of ventriculoperitoneal shunts for the treatment of hydrocephalus [43]. In both patients, CT scans revealed that the tip of the shunt catheter was lodged in the septum. Miller and colleagues reported a possible further case, although in that instance the patient had exhibited changes in sexual behavior prior to the shunt, attributed to an encephalitis [38]. One of the patients included in a series described by Andrew and Nathan with hypothalamic lesions [12] had a chiasmal cyst elevating the septal region and anterior hypothalamus, and had frequent urinary incontinence and pathologically excessive libido preoperatively, both problems being successfully resolved by surgery. Pathology in this area, which presumably had an overall "irritant" effect, has been reported in individuals causing hypersexuality [38, 69, 70].

Being the seat of integration of hormonal and autonomic aspects of sexual drive, damage to the hypothalamic region, as may occur with traumatic brain injury and middle fossa fracture [71], may result in central hypogonadism and loss of libido [72]. A decrease in sexual desire and erectile dysfunction was shown in men and women with hypothalamopituitary disorders, particularly those with hyperprolactinemia [73]. Intentional lesioning of the ventral medial hypothalamic nucleus resulted in a marked reduction or complete loss of libido in patients with troublesome sexual deviations [74].

Ansa lenticularis and globus pallidus

In their comprehensive review of the "neurological control of human sexual behavior," Baird et al. include the subcortical structures, the ansa lenticularis and pallidum as having a role in the mediation of sexual drive [23]. The ansa lenticularis is one of the pathways through which projections pass from the globus pallidus to the thalamus. In three men and one woman with movement disorders, a neurosurgical lesion to the ansa lenticularis resulted in loss of libido and erectile failure. The surgeon suggests the procedure probably produced incidental damage to the fornix, perifornical gray matter and posterior-inferior septal region (see Fig. 3.3, p. 42), regions presumed to be involved in central neural mechanisms essential to libido and erection [44].

There is an increasing awareness that hypersexuality may occur in patients with Parkinson's disease being treated with dopamine and dompamine agonists who then undergo deep brain stimulation. Among 30 Parkinson's disease patients who received high-frequency stimulation of the subthalamic nucleus, 2 men developed mania and hypersexuality which came on a few days after the implant was switched on and lasted for some months before gradually resolving [75]. A similar case history was reported from another center following a deep-brain stimulator electrode in the left globus pallidus [76]. How this relates to the dopamine dysregulation syndrome [77] is as yet unknown.

Immediately after a pallidotomy a man who had had Parkinson's disease for 16 years became disruptively and grossly hypersexual. His antiparkinsonism treatment had not been reduced postoperatively but when it was, and with the addition of valproate, his behavior improved somewhat [45]. The site of the pallidotomy was considered "atypical," being somewhat more anteriolateral than usual.

Cerebellum

Although the cerebellum has not been included in the circuits outlined in Chapter 2, it is certainly thought to have some influence on the micturition reflex and appears in Fig. 1.11 (p. 12) as well as Ueki's summary figure (Fig. 11.1), in addition to the pictorial meta-analysis of functional brain imaging experiments during bladder filling [78]. In experimental animals, stimulation of the cerebellum and fastigial nucleus can either inhibit or facilitate the micturition reflex [79–83]. Neural connections between the bladder preganglionic neurons and the cerebellar vermis have been demonstrated both morphologically and electrophysiologically [84], [85].

Clinically, patients with advanced cerebellar atrophy or those with cerebellar stroke [86, 87] have been found to have detrusor overactivity. Also an MRI study of lesion sites in multiple sclerosis revealed a correlation between urinary dysfunction and the cerebellum [88] although spinal cord involvement must have been an additional significant factor. In patients with MSA, activation seen on SPECT imaging in the cerebellar vermis was reduced in the bladder full and voiding phase [89]. Following posterior fossa surgery for malignant childhood tumors, a disturbance of bladder control may be part of the syndrome of persisting neurological deficit [90].

Taken together, the clinical and experimental data suggest that the cerebellum has mainly an inhibitory influence on the micturition reflex and that either difficulty with emptying or detrusor overactivity may ensue in patients with disease involving the cerebellum.

Brainstem lesions

Bladder

In 1926 Holman [14] noted that voiding difficulty could be a sign of posterior fossa tumors and in the series of patients with brain tumors reported by Ueki (1960), voiding difficulty occurred in 46 (30%) of 152 patients with posterior fossa tumors and urinary incontinence in 3 (2%). Looked at in greater detail, voiding difficulty occurred in 77% with lesions of pons, 67% with fourth ventricle, 41% with midline

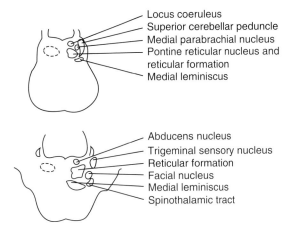

Fig. 11.5. Responsible sites of brainstem lesions for voiding disturbance within the dashed circle outline on the left and the organization of neural structures at this level shown on the right. Redrawn from [15], with permission.

of cerebellum, 24% with cerebellar hemisphere and 9% with cerebellopontine angle in posterior fossa tumors [3].

Urinary retention was described in children with pontine tumors [16]. Betts et al. [17] reported, in brief, voiding dysfunction and diplopia as the presenting symptoms in a young man with a probable dermoid involving the upper pons. Other case histories have been described of patients with retention and focal pontine lesions [13, 18, 20, 91] (Fig. 11.5). The proximity of the medial longitudinal fasciculus in the dorsal pons to the presumed pontine micturition center means that a disorder of eye movements such as an internuclear opthalmoplegia is highly likely in patients with pontine pathology causing a voiding disorder.

An analysis of urinary symptoms of 39 patients who had had brainstem strokes showed that it was dorsally situated lesions (Fig. 11.5) that resulted in disturbance of micturition [15]. Forty-nine percent of all the patients had urinary symptoms, with nocturnal urinary frequency and voiding difficulty in 28%, urinary retention in 21% and urinary incontinence in 8%. The problems were more common in those following hemorrhage, possibly because the damage was usually bilateral. MR scanning showed that the responsible lesions were in the pontine reticular nucleus and the reticular formation, adjacent to the medial parabrachial nucleus and the locus ceruleus. A correlation was found between urinary symptoms and sensory disturbance, abnormal eye movement and incoordination. Urodynamics in 11 symptomatic patients showed detrusor hyperreflexia in 8 (73%),

(a)

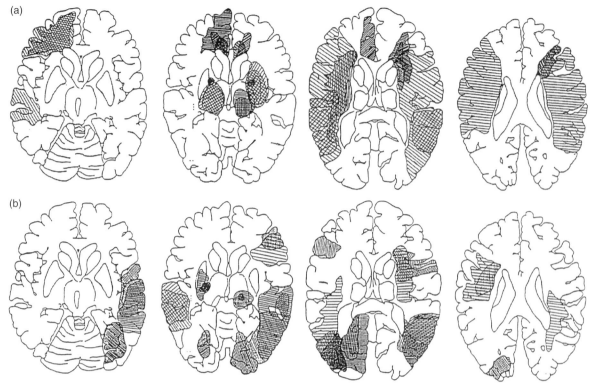

(b)

Fig. 11.6. A. Lesions on brain CT or MRI in patients with micturitonal disturbance. Most of the patients had lesions of anterior and medial surface of the frontal lobe, anterior edge of the paraventricular white matter, genu of the internal capsule, large lesion of the putamen and large lesion of the thalamus adjacent to or including the genu of the internal capsule. B. Lesions on brain CT or MRI in patients without disturbance of micturiton. Most of the patients had lesions of the occipital, temporal or parietal lobe, posterior lateral surface of the frontal lobe, crus posterius of the internal capsule and small lesion of the putamen or the thalamus. Reproduced from [7], with permission.

low compliance bladder in 1 (9%), detrusor areflexia in 3 (27%), non-relaxing sphincter on voiding in 5 (45%) and uninhibited sphincter relaxation in 3 (27%). Three asymptomatic patients had normal findings.

Brainstem stroke cases suggested the region is located in the dorsolateral pons including the pontine reticular nucleus and the reticular formation, adjacent to the medial parabrachial nucleus and the locus ceruleus [15].

Bowel

A "pontine defecation center" is thought to have been demonstrated in experimental animals, located adjacent to the pontine micturition center and the locus celureus [92, 93]. Weber et al. [22] reported three patients with pontine lesions in whom there was prolonged right CTT and absence of rectoanal inhibitor reflex in the first case; and poor esophageal coordination and prolonged left CTT in cases 2 and 3,

resulting in extreme constipation. It is perhaps surprising that there are no other reports of disturbed bowel function due to focal pontine pathology if centers in the pons are critical for supraspinal control of colonic and anorectal motility.

Cerebrovascular disease
Bladder

Cerebrovascular disease is often accompanied by bladder dysfunction. Khan et al. followed up their first report of 1981 [94] on bladder dysfunction following stroke with a further study of a similar design [95]. In that later study there were 33 patients with voiding problems and the predominant finding was of involuntary contractions of the bladder. This was present in 26, all of whom had normal coordinated voiding. The majority of patients with cerebral cortex and/or internal capsular lesions had uninhibited relaxation of the sphincter during

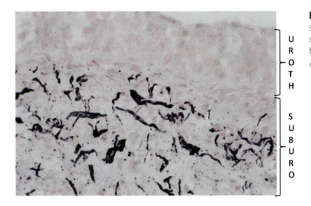

Fig. 1.1. Immunohistochemical staining of a human bladder specimen obtained via flexible cystoscopy with the pan-neuronal marker PGP9.5 depicts the dense network of suburothelial nerve fibers laying immediately below the basal lamina of the urothelium. Abbreviations: UROTH = urothelium, SUBURO = suburothelium.

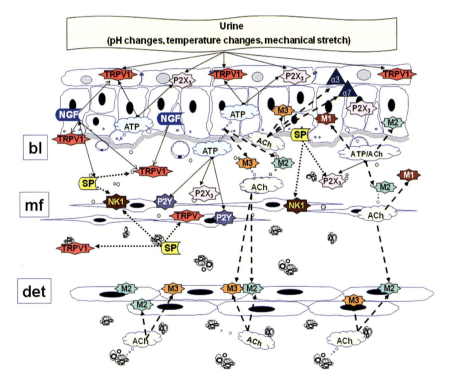

Fig. 1.6. In this cartoon representation of the ultrastructural components of the human bladder wall, the known or proposed location of receptors and sites of release of neuropeptides, neurotransmitters and growth factors thought to be involved in bladder mechanosensation are shown (updated from figure in [117]). A complex system of interactions has been proposed between the neurotransmitters and neuropeptides released and their respective receptors, which are thought to be up-regulated in DO. Fine-line arrows refer to the proposed activation of urothelial and suburothelial purinergic receptors and potentiation of the response of TRPV1 to irritative stimuli by urothelially released ATP. Dotted arrows refer to the proposed activation of suburothelial and detrusor muscarinic receptors by ACh released from the urothelium and suburothelial nerves. Dashed arrows refer to proposed activation of NK1 receptors on myofibroblasts and potentiation of suburothelial TRPV1 and P2X$_3$ receptors by SP. A reciprocal relationship appears to exist between SP and NGF, also identified by such arrows. Finally, thick-line arrows refer to the known effect of NGF on the expression of TRPV1. Abbreviations: bl = basal lamina of urothelium; mf = myofibroblast layer; det = detrusor muscle; TRPV1 = transient receptor potential vanilloid 1; P2X$_3$ = ionotropic purinergic receptor type 3; P2Y = metabotropic purinergic receptors types 2, 4 and 6; M2/M3 = muscarinic acetylcholine receptors types 2 and 3; α$_3$/α$_7$ = nicotinic acetylcholine receptors types 3 and 7; NK1 = neurokinin receptor type 1 (SP receptor); SP = substance P; NGF = nerve growth factor; ACh = acetylcholine; ATP = adenosine triphosphate.

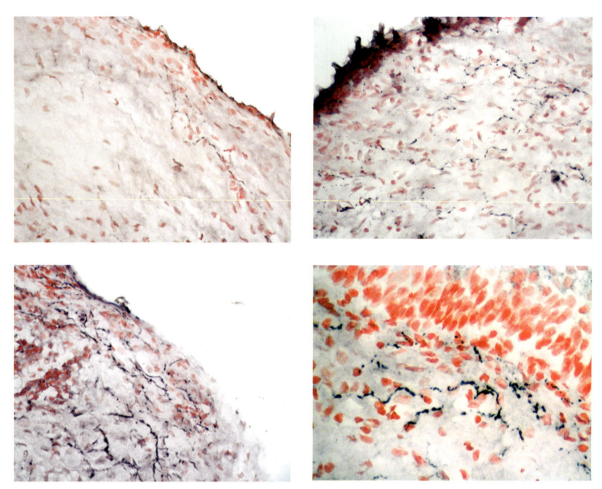

Fig. 1.7. Immunohistochemical staining of human bladder specimens obtained via flexible cystoscopy with specific antibodies to the vanilloid receptor TRPV1 (top left – suburothelial fiber-like staining, magnification x20), substance P (top right – urothelial cell and suburothelial fiber-like staining, magnification x20), vesicular acetylcholine transporter VAChT (bottom left – suburothelial fiber-like staining, magnification x20) and CGRP (bottom right – suburothelial fiber-like staining, magnification x40).

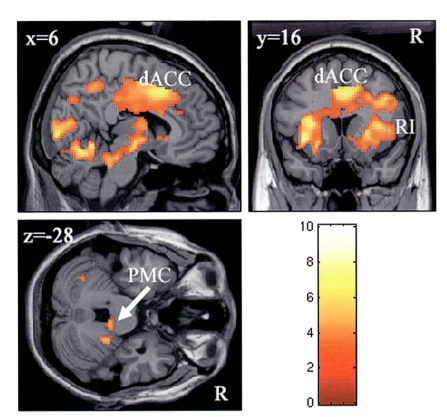

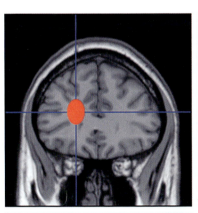

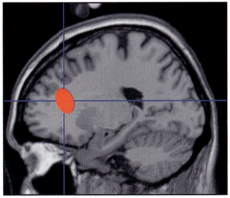

Fig. 1.13. Activation in response to bladder filling in subjects with urge incontinence (P < 0.01 uncorrected). Abbreviations: dACC = dorsal anterior cingulate cortex; RI = right insula; x, y and z are Montreal Neurological Institute (MNI) coordinates for the three sections shown. Adapted from reference [118] with permission.

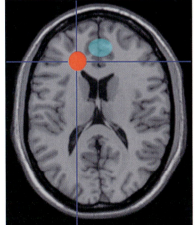

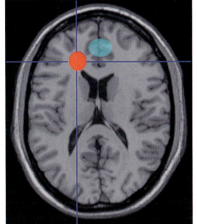

Fig. 1.14. Location of lesions causing incontinence (or occasionally retention) in the group of patients studied by Andrew and Nathan [103]. The red ellipse shows where white-matter lesions caused lasting urinary tract dysfunction. The cyan ellipse shows the location of gray-matter lesions that caused transient dysfunction. (Nathan, personal communication.)

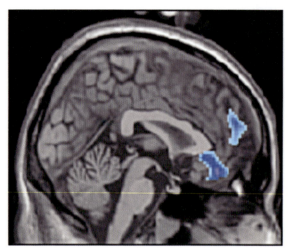

Fig. 1.15. Medial PFC deactivation in response to bladder filling in patients with urge incontinence (P < 0.05 uncorrected). Two regions appear to be involved: the medial prefrontal cortex (BA 9) and the orbitofrontal cortex (BA 11/32 plus pregenual ACC). The medial prefrontal cortex is near the cyan ellipse shown in Fig. 1.14.

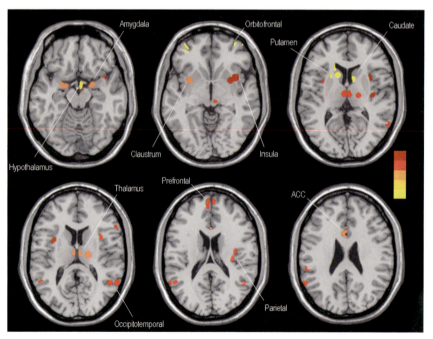

Fig. 3.9. Summary of patterns of brain activity with sexual stimulation (visual, olfactory, auditory or tactile). Dark red seen in 8, light red in 7, orange in 5, dark yellow in 4 and light yellow in 3 out of 13 published reports (listed in Table 3.2).

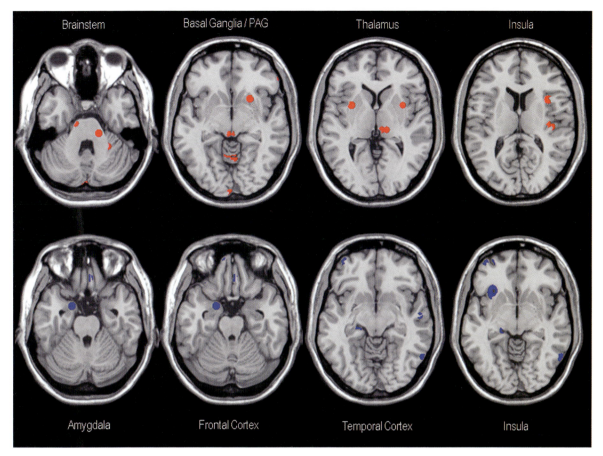

Fig. 3.10. Brain activations (red) and deactivations (blue) seen with orgasm in 16 males and females. Summary figures created using MNI coordinates from three datasets [68, 70, 75]. Figure created using MRIcro.

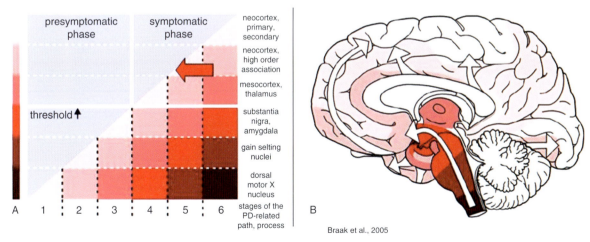

Braak et al., 2005

Fig. 12.2. The presymptomatic phase is marked by the appearance of Lewy neurites/bodies in the brains of asymptomatic persons. A. In the symptomatic phase, the individual neuropathological threshold is exceeded (black arrow). The increasing slope and intensity of the colored areas below the diagonal indicate the growing severity of the pathology in vulnerable brain regions (right). The severity of the pathology is indicated by darker degrees of shading in the colored upright arrow (left). B. Diagram showing the ascending pathological process (white arrows). The shading intensity of the colored areas corresponds to that in A. (From [5] with permission.) The large arrow pointing just above stage 4 indicates the stage at which bladder symptoms become common.

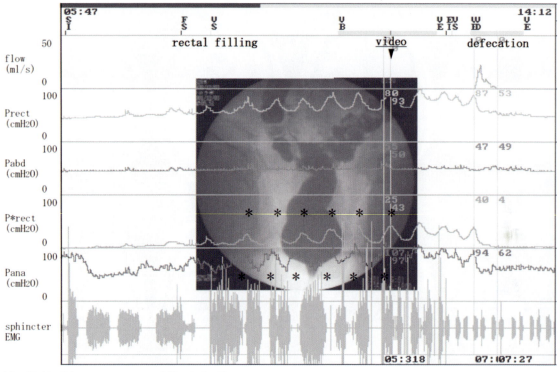

Fig. 13.10. Videomanometry – rectal filling in health.

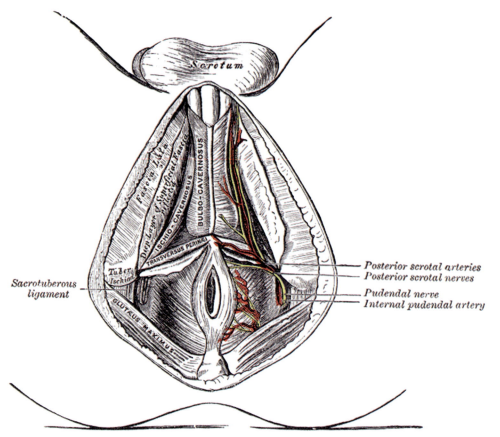

Fig. 18.3. Course of the pudendal nerve in the perineum. Reproduced from *Gray's Anatomy*, with permission.

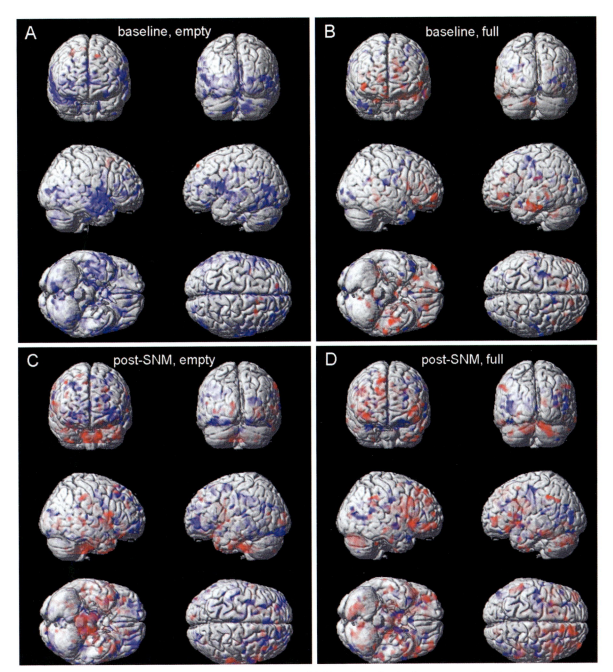

Fig. 19.4. Functional MRI study in Fowler's syndrome. Responses to bladder infusion for the six women, rendered (projected) on the brain surface. Red = activation; blue = negative response. A. Session at baseline with a near-empty bladder. B. at baseline with a full bladder. C. After SNM and a near-empty bladder. D. After SNM and a full bladder. Positive responses (red) indicate activation by bladder infusion. Negative responses (blue) indicate that the fMRI signal is smaller during infusion than during withdrawal. For the session at baseline with an empty bladder (Fig. 19.2A), the brain responses to bladder infusion (relative to withdrawal) were almost exclusively negative.

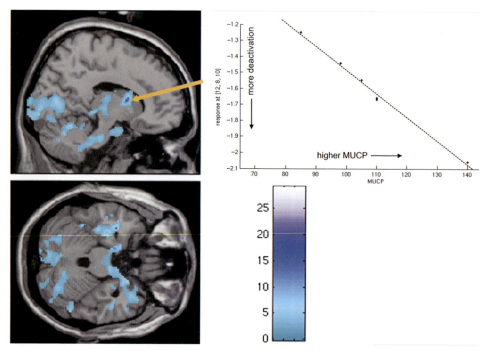

Fig. 19.5. Correlation between the defect in the interoception of filling, i.e. an abnormal negative response, and the maximum urethral closure pressure (MUCP), a proxy measure of the abnormality of sphincter activity, in the individual subjects.

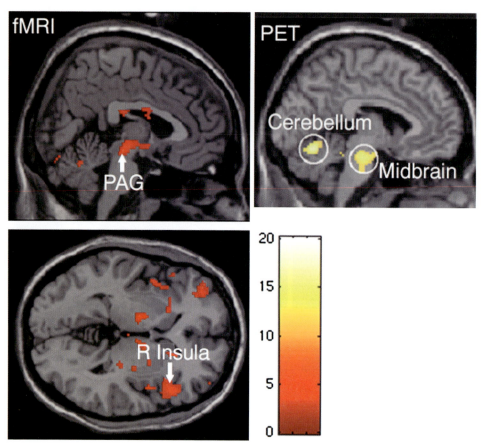

Fig. 19.7. PET imaging showed that with SNM afferent activity reached the midbrain [34] and more recently with functional magnetic resonance imaging (fMRI) [31] the PAG and right insula showed activation. Reproduced with permission.

involuntary bladder contractions while all of the patients with lesions only in the basal ganglia or thalamus had normal sphincter function.

Subsequently Sakakibara et al. [7] reported on the bladder symptoms of 72 patients who had been admitted with an acute hemispheric stroke. When assessed at three months, 53% were found to have significant urinary complaints. The most common problem was of nocturnal urinary frequency which affected 36%, while urge incontinence affected 29% and a difficulty in voiding 25%. Urinary retention was seen in the acute phase of illness in 6%. A significant correlation was found between the occurrence of a urinary disturbance and hemiparesis ($p<0.05$) and a negative correlation with hemianopia ($p<0.05$), brain imaging techniques confirming a more anterior location of brain lesions in the former group (Fig. 11.6). Urodynamic studies of 22 symptomatic patients showed detrusor hyperreflexia in 68%, detrusor-sphincter dyssynergia in 14% and uninhibited sphincter relaxation in 36%. Patients with urinary retention had detrusor areflexia and an unrelaxing sphincter. No statistically significant correlation could be demonstrated between any particular lesion site and urodynamic findings. In this study no preponderance of right-sided lesions in the group of patients with urinary symptoms was found. There was some indication that lesion size was related to the occurrence of urinary symptoms. These findings further supported the idea that lesions of the anteromedial frontal lobe and its descending pathway and the basal ganglia are mainly responsible for bladder dysfunction in stroke patients.

That urinary incontinence within seven days of acute stroke has a highly predictive prognostic value for long-term outcome was observed by Wade and Hewer in 1985 [96]. It proved more accurate than the level of consciousness at the time of admission for predicting recovery and of more than 500 patients, when assessed at six months 53% of those who had had incontinence in the first week were dead whereas only 19% of the continent group had died. The level of disability in the two groups was similarly different: 57% were moderately or severely disabled in the incontinent group compared to 20% in the continent group. This important observation was subsequently confirmed by other research groups and recovery from urinary incontinence following stroke has been found to be associated with better stroke outcome at three months [97]. The underlying mechanism for this is as yet unknown.

Bowel

The prevalence of bowel dysfunction after stroke varies from 23% to 60%. Rovain et al. studied 152 post-stroke patients, and found a positive correlation between constipation and Barthel index ($p<0.003$) [98], suggesting that either brain disease or immobility is a contributing factor to the bowel dysfunction.

Bracci et al. studied 90 post-stroke patients and found they had a significantly higher incidence of constipation than a group of orthopedic patients who experienced the same degree of immobility (Table 11.4). It seems likely therefore that constipation after stroke does not result from impaired mobility alone, but from the brain's modulatory effect on the gut [99]. Whole gut transit studies in stroke patients stratified for immobility would be the way to address this research question. Otegbayo et al. showed that the most common bowel dysfunction after stroke was constipation 14 (25.9%), followed by incomplete bowel evacuation and fecal incontinence [100]. Constipation and incomplete evacuation were more common in ischemic stroke than in hemorrhagic stroke. Since gut function tests have rarely been performed in patients with stroke, the mechanism underlying the bowel dysfunction remains unclear but may well include prolonged colonic transit, decreased phasic rectal contraction and decreased straining as occurs in Parkinson's disease [101, 102].

Fecal incontinence after stroke was shown to be related to immobility and the size of the cerebral lesion [103], and was also more common in diabetics [104], suggesting that fecal incontinence in stroke cases might be a result of immobility or cognitive problems, or co-morbid diabetic neuropathy. However, anal sphincter function in post-stroke patients needs further investigation.

Sexual behavior

Marked changes in sexual activity have been shown to occur following a stroke. Some specific changes of sexual function such as erectile dysfunction have been noted using Rigiscan under audiovisual sexual stimulation (AVSS). Jeong and colleagues reported that 47% of 44 stroke survivors who complained of erectile dysfunction (ED) (International Index of Erectile Function Questionnaire [IIEF] < 22) had objective

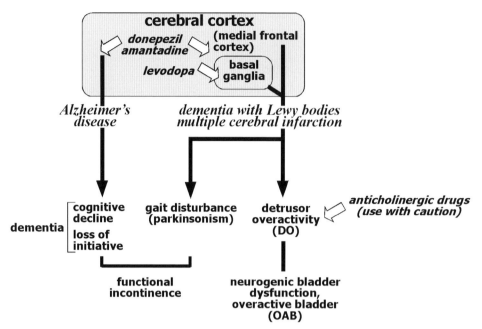

Fig. 11.7. Relationship between functional incontinence and neurogenic incontinence. From [112] with permission.

Table 11.4. Constipation and effect of cerebral or orthopedic disease. Comparing two groups with the same motor deficits, those with hemiplegics had more severe constipation. Modified from [99].

	Constipation			
	+	–	Odds ratio	p-value
	n=33 (19.3%)	n=138 (80.7%)		
mean age (years)	68.4	71.4	0.94	0.64
male	13	48	0.82	0.62
female	20	90	1	
hemiplegics	27	63	5.36	0.01
orthopedics (fracture)	6	75	1	

ED [105]. In their study, organic ED was more common in the thalamic stroke than any other brain areas. Severe ED was more common in patients with diabetes as a vascular risk factor [106].

However, the major effect of stroke on sexual activity is a reduction in libido and coital frequency. This appears to be primarily the result of a change in attitude towards sexuality with an unwillingness for sex by the patient and their partner [107]. In a study by Korpelainen and colleagues, 14 (28%) patients at 2 months post-stroke and 6 (14%) patients at 6 months had ceased having sexual intercourse [108]. There was a fear that having sex might adversely affect blood pressure and cause another stroke [109]. Depression has also been identified as a possible contributing factor.

Rarely, hypersexuality has been described as part of marked behavioral changes resulting from bilateral thalamic infarction [110].

Dementia

The role of diffuse brain disease, such as dementia, in causing incontinence is not entirely clear, although this is a problem of immense socio-economic importance because of the cost of caring for demented incontinent patients. Urinary incontinence is common in patients with dementia, and is more prevalent in demented than in non-demented older individuals [111].

Neurogenic incontinence is a common feature of patients with multiple cerebral infarction or dementia with Lewy bodies, and in both diseases walking difficulty and falls are common. In contrast, functional or secondary incontinence is common in Alzheimer's disease due to cognitive disability and decreased motivation (Fig. 11.7) [112].

Bowel dysfunction in demented elderly people is a concern. It includes constipation and fecal incontinence. Patients with dementia with Lewy bodies (DLB) often have constipation. In our 32 patients with DLB (all of whom had low cardiac MIBG uptake), constipation (less than three times a week) was noted in 56%, difficult expulsion in 44%, and fecal incontinence in 16%. This may reflect peripheral Lewy body pathology in the gut, which is thought to predate motor disorder in DLB/Parkinson's disease patients [113]. Constipation is reported to be more common in DLB than in Alzheimer's disease [114]. Fecal incontinence is a social as well as hygienic problem, and is more problematic than urinary incontinence for patients and their caregivers.

Toileting difficulties are early occurrences in the sequence of disturbed behaviors in dementia [115]. This results from a mixture of neurological and recurring behavioral characteristics. Aphasia impairs the patient's capacity to communicate their need to void, whilst agnosia and apraxia cause an inability to recognize and use the normal toilet facilities. The range of behavioral disturbances is equally wide. Initially some patients become apathetic about the effort required to maintain continence; alternatively there may be fear of failing to be continent with the implications of incompetence that go with that. The fear of humiliating dependence on others for bowel care may result in incontinence, which unfortunately worsens the embarrassment. In advanced dementia there may be aspects of curiosity and manipulation that result in fecal smearing behaviors [115]. In summary, toileting behaviors relate to neurological and biographic factors which may vary with time.

The use of central cholinergic stimulation in the treatment of cognitive decline (Fig. 11.7) would be expected, on theoretical grounds, to exacerbate urinary dysfunction and increase the risk of DO [112]. However, in a study of elderly individuals with both dementia and urinary dysfunction, the combined use of donepezil, a central AChE inhibitor, and propiverine, a peripheral muscarine receptor antagonist, ameliorated overactive bladder in elderly individuals with dementia without any changes in cognitive scales [116].

Sexual behavior

In long-term care settings, staff members might tend to view a resident's attempts at sexual expression as "problem" behavior. However, there is also recognition of interest in, and the right to, sexual expression among older adults. Sexuality and intimacy exist throughout the life-span and are important for quality of life. From an autonomic point of view, erectile dysfunction was reported in 53% of 55 patients with Alzheimer's disease (mean age 70.2 years old) [117], which might reflect central hypothalamic dysfunction, peripheral vascular pathology or both.

Head injury

The severity, extent and site of brain damage following brain injury is so variable that generalizations about the effect of traumatic brain injury on pelvic organ dysfunction are impossible.

Sexual behavior

A review of the literature on head injury and sexual dysfunction written in 1996 summarizes the situation, saying "there is controversy as to whether desire increases, decreases or stays the same" [118] and there is the added difficulty that it may be difficult to differentiate between primary and secondary sexual problems [119].

As might be expected, those who had had frontal damage, a common site for brain injury, may be disinhibited, sexually demanding [120] or less insightful, or more willing to report sexual arousal and experiences [121]. Other studies have shown hyposexuality associated with apathy to be the commoner problem [122]. A major factor determining frequency of intercourse following a head injury is the impact of the damage on the behavior and personality of the injured: approximately one-quarter of men and women discontinue sex with their partners after severe brain injury [123]. A comparison of partners of Israeli soldiers who had fought and either not been injured or who had had spinal cord or head injury found that sexual desire and enjoyment for the head-injured patients' wife was "drastically reduced" and significantly worse than for the control groups [124]. In recent years there has been the realization that traumatic brain injury may cause damage to the hypothalamus or pituitary and a consensus view is that following a moderate-to-severe brain injury, screening pituitary function tests should be performed if there is reason to suspect hormonal deficiency [125]. Recommendations have been made to treat specific aspects of sexual dysfunction following traumatic brain injury [72].

Bladder

An expected, correlation is seen between the occurrence of a neurogenic bladder and the severity and extent of brain damage so that urodynamic abnormalities have been associated with motor deficits [126].

There has been little written about bladder behavior in patients in a coma or in a vegetative state but Wyndaele studied the ability to void spontaneously in 135 comatose patients of various etiologies [127]. Of these, 76% emptied their bladder as soon as the indwelling catheter was removed although elderly men had more difficulties in becoming independent of an indwelling catheter. Krimchansky performed urodynamics in 17 patients in a vegetative state, 1–6 months after brain injury. Cystometry results indicated that 100% of the patients had a neurogenic DO bladder but none showed detrusor-sphincter dyssynergia [128].

References

1. Birder L, Drake M. Neural control. In: Abrams P, Cardozo L, Khoury S, Wein A, eds. *Incontinence*. Paris: Health Publications Ltd; 2009:167–254.

2. Andrew J, Nathan PW. Lesions on the anterior frontal lobes and disturbances of micturition and defaecation. *Brain* 1964;**87**:233–62.

3. Ueki K. Disturbances of micturition observed in some patients with brain tumour. *Neurologica Medica Chirugia* 1960;**2**:25–33.

4. Maurice-Williams RS. Micturition symptoms in frontal tumours. *J Neurol Neurosurg Psychiatry* 1974;**37**:431–6.

5. Yamamoto S, Soma T, Hatayama T, Mori H, Yoshimura N. Neurogenic bladder induced by brain abscess. *Br J Urol* 1995;**76**:272.

6. Lang EW, Chesnut RM, Hennerici M. Urinary retention and space-occupying lesions of the frontal cortex. *Eur Neurol* 1996;**36**:43–7.

7. Sakakibara R, Hattori T, Yasuda K, Yamanishi T. Micturitional disturbance after acute hemispheric stroke: analysis of the lesion site by CT and MRI. *J Neurol Sci* 1996;**137**:47–56.

8. Laplane D, Degos JD, Baulac M, Gray F. Bilateral infarction of the anterior cingulate gyri and of the fornices. Report of a case. *J Neurol Sci* 1981; **51**:289–300.

9. Duffau H, Capelle L. Incontinence after brain glioma surgery: new insights into the cortical control of micturition and continence. Case report. *J Neurosurg* 2005;**102**:148–51.

10. Andrew J, Nathan PW, Spanos NC. Disturbances of micturition and defaecation due to aneurysms of anterior communicating or anterior cerebral arteries. *J Neurosurg* 1966;**24**:1–10.

11. Yamamoto T, Sakakibara R, Uchiyama T, et al. Lower urinary tract function in patients with pituitary adenoma compressing hypothalamus. *J Neurol Neurosurg Psychiatry* 2005;**76**:390–4.

12. Andrew J, Nathan PW. The cerebral control of micturition. *Proc RSM* 1965;**58**:553–5.

13. Yaguchi H, Soma H, Miyazaki Y, et al. A case of acute urinary retention caused by periaqueductal grey lesion. *J Neurol Neurosurg Psychiatry* 2004;**75**:1202–3.

14. Holman E. Difficult urination associated with intracranial tumours of the posterior fossa. A physiologic and clinical study. *Arch Neurol Psychiat* 1926;**15**:371–80.

15. Sakakibara R, Hattori T, Yasuda K, Yamanishi T. Micturitional disturbance and the pontine tegmental lesion: urodynamic and MRI analyses of vascular cases. *J Neurol Sci* 1996;**141**:105–10.

16. Renier WO, Gabreels FJ. Evaluation of diagnosis and non-surgical therapy in 24 children with a pontine tumour. *Neuropediatrics* 1980;**11**:262–73.

17. Betts CD, Kapoor R, Fowler CJ. Pontine pathology and voiding dysfunction. *Br J Urol* 1992;**70**:100–2.

18. Manente G, Melchionda D, Uncini A. Urinary retention in bilateral pontine tumour: evidence for a pontine micturition centre in humans. *J Neurol Neurosurg Psychiatry* 1996;**61**:528–36.

19. Sakakibara R, Hattori T, Fukutake T, et al. Micturitional disturbance in herpetic brainstem encephalitis; contribution of the pontine micturition centre. *J Neurol Neurosurg Psychiatry* 1998;**64**:269–72.

20. Komiyama A, Kubota A, Hidai H. Urinary retention associated with a unilateral lesion in the dorsolateral tegmentum of the rostral pons. *J Neurol Neurosurg Psychiatry* 1998;**65**:953–4.

21. Weber J, Delangre T, Hannequin D, Beuret-Blanquart F, Denis P. Anorectal manometric anomalies in seven patients with frontal lobe brain damage. *Dig Dis Sci* 1990;**35**:225–30.

22. Weber J, Denis P, Mihout B, et al. Effect of brain-stem lesion on colonic and anorectal motility. Study of three patients. *Dig Dis Sci* 1985;**30**:419–25.

23. Baird AD, Wilson SJ, Bladin PF, Saling MM, Reutens DC. Neurological control of human sexual behaviour: insights from lesion studies. *J Neurol Neurosurg Psychiatry* 2007;**78**:1042–9.

24. Levine J, Albert H. Sexual behavior after lobotomy. *J Nerv Ment Dis* 1951;**113**:332–41.

25. Williamson PD, Spencer DD, Spencer SS, Novelly RA, Mattson RH. Complex partial seizures of frontal lobe origin. *Ann Neurol* 1985;**18**:497–504.

26. Toone BK. Sex, sexual seizure and the female with epilepsy. In: Trimble MR, ed. *Women and epilepsy*. Chichester: Wiley; 1991:201–6.

27. Bancaud J, Favel P, Bonis A, et al. Paroxysmal sexual manifestations and temporal lobe epilepsy. Clinical, EEG and SEEG study of a case of epilepsy of tumoral origin. *Rev Neurol (Paris)* 1970;**123**:217–30.

28. Gastaut H, Collomb H. Sexual behavior in psychomotor epileptics. *Ann Med Psychol (Paris)* 1954;**112**(2 Pt 5):657–96.

29. Blumer D, Walker AE. Sexual behavior in temporal lobe epilepsy. A study of the effects of temporal lobectomy on sexual behavior. *Arch Neurol* 1967;**16**:37–43.

30. Blumer D. Hypersexual episodes in temporal lobe epilepsy. *Am J Psychiatry* 1970;**126**:1099–106.

31. Walker AE. The libidinous temporal lobe. *Schweiz Arch Neurol Neurochir Psychiatr* 1972;**111**:473–84.

32. Shukla GD, Srivastava ON, Katiyar BC. Sexual disturbances in temporal lobe epilepsy: a controlled study. *Br J Psychiatry* 1979;**134**:288–92.

33. Demerdash A, Shaalan M, Midani A, Kamel F, Bahri M. Sexual behavior of a sample of females with epilepsy. *Epilepsia* 1991;**32**:82–5.

34. Herzog AG, Seibel MM, Schomer DL, Vaitukaitis JL, Geschwind N. Reproductive endocrine disorders in men with partial seizures of temporal lobe origin. *Arch Neurol* 1986;**43**:347–50.

35. Herzog AG, Seibel MM, Schomer DL, Vaitukaitis JL, Geschwind N. Reproductive endocrine disorders in women with partial seizures of temporal lobe origin. *Arch Neurol* 1986;**43**:341–6.

36. Baird AD, Wilson SJ, Bladin PF, Saling MM, Reutens DC. Hypersexuality after temporal lobe resection. *Epilepsy Behav* 2002; **3**:173–81.

37. Lilly R, Cummings JL, Benson DF, Frankel M. The human Kluver-Bucy syndrome. *Neurology* 1983;**33**:1141–5.

38. Miller BL, Cummings JL, McIntyre H, Ebers G, Grode M. Hypersexuality or altered sexual preference following brain injury. *J Neurol Neurosurg Psychiatry* 1986;**49**:867–73.

39. Leutmezer F, Serles W, Bacher J, et al. Genital automatisms in complex partial seizures. *Neurology* 1999;**52**:1188–91.

40. Anson JA, Kuhlman DT. Postictal Kluver-Bucy syndrome after temporal lobectomy. *J Neurol Neurosurg Psychiatry* 1993;**56**:311–3.

41. Janszky J, Szucs A, Halasz P, et al. Orgasmic aura originates from the right hemisphere. *Neurology* 2002;**58**:302–4.

42. Mitchell W, Falconer MA, Hill D. Epilepsy with fetishism relieved by temporal lobectomy. *Lancet* 1954;**267**:626–30.

43. Gorman DG, Cummings JL. Hypersexuality following septal injury. *Arch Neurol* 1992;**49**:308–10.

44. Meyers R. Three cases of myoclonus alleviated by bilateral ansotomy, with a note on postoperative alibido and impotence. *J Neurosurg* 1962;**19**:71–81.

45. Mendez MF, O'Connor SM, Lim GT. Hypersexuality after right pallidotomy for Parkinson's disease. *J Neuropsychiatry Clin Neurosci* 2004;**16**:37–40.

46. Frith CD. The social brain? *Philos Trans R Soc Lond B Biol Sci* 2007;**362**:671–8.

47. Fowler CJ, Griffiths DJ. A decade of functional brain imaging applied to bladder control. *Neurourol Urodyn* 2010;**29**:49–55.

48. Ueki Y. Micturitional disturbance in patients with brain tumour. *Sogo Rinsho* 1960;**9**:1361–70.

49. Hakim S, Adams RD. The special clinical problem of symptomatic hydrocephalus with normal cerebrospinal fluid pressure. Observations on cerebrospinal fluid hydrodynamics. *J Neurol Sci* 1965;**2**:307–27.

50. Fisher CM. Hydrocephalus as a cause of disturbances of gait in the elderly. *Neurology* 1982;**32**:1358–63.

51. Kell CA, von Kriegstein K, Rosler A, Kleinschmidt A, Laufs H. The sensory cortical representation of the human penis: revisiting somatotopy in the male homunculus. *J Neurosci* 2005;**25**:5984–7.

52. Erickson TC. Erotomania (nymphomania) as an expression of cortical epileptiform discharge. *Arch Neurol Psych* 1945;**53**:226–31.

53. Terzian H, Ore GD. Syndrome of Kluver and Bucy; reproduced in man by bilateral removal of the temporal lobes. *Neurology* 1955;**5**:373–80.

54. Powers JM, Schaumburg HH, Gaffney CL. Kluver-Bucy syndrome caused by adreno-leukodystrophy. *Neurology* 1980;**30**:1231–2.

55. Mendez MF, Chow T, Ringman J, Twitchell G, Hinkin CH. Pedophilia and temporal lobe disturbances. *J Neuropsychiatry Clin Neurosci* 2000;**12**:71–6.

56. Edwards-Lee T, Miller BL, Benson DF, et al. The temporal variant of frontotemporal dementia. *Brain* 1997;**120**(Pt 6):1027–40.

57. Baird AD, Wilson SJ, Bladin PF, Saling MM, Reutens DC. Sexual outcome after epilepsy surgery. *Epilepsy Behav* 2003;**4**:268–78.

58. Baird AD, Wilson SJ, Bladin PF, Saling MM, Reutens DC. The amygdala and sexual drive: insights from temporal lobe epilepsy surgery. *Ann Neurol* 2004;**55**:87–96.

59. Toone BK, Wheeler M, Nanjee M, Fenwick P, Grant R. Sex hormones, sexual activity and plasma anticonvulsant levels in male epileptics. *J Neurol Neurosurg Psychiatry* 1983;**46**:824–6.

60. Rattya J, Turkka J, Pakarinen AJ, et al. Reproductive effects of valproate, carbamazepine, and oxcarbazepine in men with epilepsy. *Neurology* 2001;**56**:31–6.

61. Ranson SW. Some functions of the hypothalamus: Harvey lecture, December 17, 1936. *Bull N Y Acad Med* 1937;**13**:241–71.

62. Stuart DG, Portner RW, Adey WR, Kamikawa Y. Hypothalamic unit activity: visceral and somatic influences. *Electroencephalogr Clin Neurophysiol* 1964;**16**:237–41.

63. Enoch DM, Kerr FW. Hypothalamic vasopressor and vesicopressor pathways. II. Anatomic study of their course and connections. *Arch Neurol* 1967;**16**:307–20.

64. Blok B, Willemsen T, Holstege G. A PET study of brain control of micturition in humans. *Brain* 1997;**120**:111–21.

65. Spillane JD. Five boxers. *Br Med J* 1962;**2**:1205–10.

66. Krishna AY, Blevins LS, Jr. Case report: reversible gastroparesis in patients with hypopituitary disease. *Am J Med Sci* 1996;**312**:43–5.

67. MacLean PD, Ploog DW. Cerebral representation of penile erection. *J Neurophysiol* 1962;**25**:29–55.

68. Heath RG. Pleasure and brain activity in man. Deep and surface electroencephalograms during orgasm. *J Nerv Ment Dis* 1972;**154**:3–18.

69. Poeck K, Pilleri G. Release of hypersexual behaviour due to lesion in the limbic system. *Acta Neurol Scand* 1965;**41**:233–44.

70. Frohman EM, Frohman TC, Moreault AM. Acquired sexual paraphilia in patients with multiple sclerosis. *Arch Neurol* 2002;**59**:1006–10.

71. Crompton MR. Hypothalamic lesions following closed head injury. *Brain* 1971;**94**:165–72.

72. Rees PM, Fowler CJ, Maas CP. Sexual function in men and women with neurological disorders. *Lancet* 2007;**369**:512–25.

73. Casanueva FF, Molitch ME, Schlechte JA, et al. Guidelines of the Pituitary Society for the diagnosis and management of prolactinomas. *Clin Endocrinol (Oxf)* 2006;**65**:265–73.

74. Muller D, Roeder F, Orthner H. Further results of stereotaxis in the human hypothalamus in sexual deviations. First use of this operation in addiction to drugs. *Neurochirurgia (Stuttg)* 1973;**16**:113–26.

75. Romito LM, Raja M, Daniele A, et al. Transient mania with hypersexuality after surgery for high frequency stimulation of the subthalamic nucleus in Parkinson's disease. *Mov Disord* 2002;**17**:1371–4.

76. Roane DM, Yu M, Feinberg TE, Rogers JD. Hypersexuality after pallidal surgery in Parkinson disease. *Neuropsychiatry Neuropsychol Behav Neurol* 2002;**15**:247–51.

77. Giovannoni G, O'sullivan JD, Turner K, Manson AJ, Lees AJ. Hedonistic homeostatic dysregulation in patients with Parkinson's disease on dopamine replacement therapies. *J Neurol Neurosurg Psychiatry* 2000;**68**:423–8.

78. DasGupta R, Kavia RB, Fowler CJ. Cerebral mechanisms and voiding function. *BJU Int* 2007;**99**:731–4.

79. Bradley WE, Teague CT. Cerebellar regulation of the micturition reflex. *J Urol* 1969;**101**:396–9.

80. Rasheed BM, Manchanda SK, Anand BK. Effects of the stimulation of paleocerebellum on certain vegetative functions in the cat. *Brain Res* 1970;**20**:293–308.

81. Martner J. Influences on the defaecation and micturition reflexes by the cerebellar fastigial nucleus. *Acta Physiol Scan* 1975;**94**:95–104.

82. Huang TF, Yang CP, Yang SL. The role of the fastigial nucleus in bladder control. *Exp Neurol* 1979;**66**:674–81.

83. Nishizawa O, Ebina K, Sugaya K, et al. Effect of cerebellectomy on reflex micturition in the decerebrate dog as determined by urodynamic evaluation. *Urol Int* 1989;**44**:152–6.

84. Dietrichs E, Haines DE. Possible pathways for cerebellar modulation of autonomic responses: micturition. *Scand J Urol Nephrol Suppl* 2002;**210**:16–20.

85. Zhu JN, Yung WH, Kwok-Chong Chow B, Chan YS, Wang JJ. The cerebellar-hypothalamic circuits: potential pathways underlying cerebellar involvement in somatic-visceral integration. *Brain Res Rev* 2006;**52**:93–106.

86. Nardulli R, Monitillo V, Losavio E, et al. Urodynamic evaluation of 12 ataxic subjects: neurophysiopathologic considerations. *Funct Neurol* 1992;**7**:223–5.

87. Leach G, Farsaii A, Kark P, Raz S. Urodynamic manifestations of cerebellar ataxia. *J Urol* 1982;**128**:348–50.

88. Charil A, Zijdenbos AP, Taylor J, et al. Statistical mapping analysis of lesion location and neurological disability in multiple sclerosis: application to 452 patient data sets. *Neuroimage* 2003;**19**:532–44.

89. Sakakibara R, Uchida Y, Uchiyama T, Yamanishi T, Hattori T. Reduced cerebellar vermis activation during urinary storage and micturition in multiple system atrophy: 99mTc-labelled ECD SPECT study. *Eur J Neurol* 2004;**11**:705–8.

90. Pollack IF, Polinko P, Albright AL, Towbin R, Fitz C. Mutism and pseudobulbar symptoms after resection of posterior fossa tumors in children: incidence and pathophysiology. *Neurosurgery* 1995;**37**:885–93.

91. Sakakibara R, Hattori T, Fukutake T, et al. Micturitional disturbance in herpetic brainstem encephalitis; contribution of the pontine micturition center (PMC). *J Neurol Neurosurg Psychiatry* 1998;**64**:269–72.

92. Nagano M, Ishimizu Y, Saitoh S, Okada H, Fukuda H. The defecation reflex in rats: fundamental properties and the reflex center. *Auton Neurosci* 2004;**111**:48–56.

93. Valentino RJ, Miselis RR, Pavcovich LA. Pontine regulation of pelvic viscera: pharmacological target for pelvic visceral dysfunctions. *Trends Pharmacol Sci* 1999;**20**:253–60.

94. Khan Z, Hertanu J, Yang W, Melman A, Leiter E. Predictive correlation of urodynamic dysfunction and brain injury after cerebrovascular accident. *J Urol* 1981;**126**:86–8.

95. Khan Z, Starer P, Yang WC, Bhola A. Analysis of voiding disorders in patients with cerebrovascular accidents. *Urology* 1990;**35**:265–70.

96. Wade DT, Hewer RL. Outlook after an acute stroke: urinary incontinence and loss of consciousness compared in 532 patients. *Q J Med* 1985;**56**:601–8.

97. Patel M, Coshall C, Lawrence E, Rudd AG, Wolfe CD. Recovery from poststroke urinary incontinence: associated factors and impact on outcome. *J Am Geriatr Soc* 2001;**49**:1229–33.

98. Robain G, Chennevelle JM, Petit F, Piera JB. Incidence of constipation after recent vascular hemiplegia: a prospective cohort of 152 patients. *Rev Neurol (Paris)* 2002;**158**(5 Pt 1):589–92.

99. Bracci F, Badiali D, Pezzotti P, et al. Chronic constipation in hemiplegic patients. *World J Gastroenterol* 2007;**13**:3967–72.

100. Otegbayo JA, Talabi OA, Akere A, et al. Gastrointestinal complications in stroke survivors. *Trop Gastroenterol* 2006;**27**:127–30.

101. Harari D, Coshall C, Rudd AG, Wolfe CD. New-onset fecal incontinence after stroke: prevalence, natural history, risk factors, and impact. *Stroke* 2003;**34**:144–50.

102. Shamliyan T, Wyman J, Bliss DZ, Kane RL, Wilt TJ. Prevention of urinary and fecal incontinence in adults. *Evid Rep Technol Assess (Full Rep)* 2007;**161**:1–379.

103. Brittain K, Perry S, Shaw C, et al. Isolated urinary, fecal, and double incontinence: prevalence and degree of soiling in stroke survivors. *J Am Geriatr Soc* 2006;**54**:1915–9.

104. Nakayama H, Jorgensen HS, Pedersen PM, Raaschou HO, Olsen TS. Prevalence and risk factors of incontinence after stroke. The Copenhagen Stroke Study. *Stroke* 1997;**28**:58–62.

105. Jeon SW, Yoo KH, Kim TH, Kim JI, Lee CH. Correlation of the erectile dysfunction with lesions of cerebrovascular accidents. *J Sex Med* 2009;**6**:251–6.

106. Tang B, Zhou GQ, Zhao WX, et al. Characteristics of erectile dysfunction in old males with lacunar infarction. *Zhonghua Nan Ke Xue* 2006;**12**:798–9, 802.

107. Giaquinto S, Buzzelli S, Di Francesco L, Nolfe G. Evaluation of sexual changes after stroke. *J Clin Psychiatry* 2003;**64**:302–7.

108. Korpelainen JT, Kauhanen ML, Kemola H, Malinen U, Myllyla VV. Sexual dysfunction in stroke patients. *Acta Neurol Scand* 1998;**98**:400–5.

109. Monga TN, Lawson JS, Inglis J. Sexual dysfunction in stroke patients. *Arch Phys Med Rehabil* 1986;**67**:19–22.

110. Mutarelli EG, Omuro AM, Adoni T. Hypersexuality following bilateral thalamic infarction: case report. *Arq Neuropsiquiatr* 2006;**64**:146–8.

111. Resnick NM. Urinary incontinence. *Lancet* 1995;**346**:94–9.

112. Sakakibara R, Uchiyama T, Yamanishi T, Kishi M. Dementia and lower urinary dysfunction: with a reference to anticholinergic use in elderly population. *Int J Urol* 2008;**15**:778–88.

113. Abbott RD, Ross GW, Petrovitch H, et al. Bowel movement frequency in late-life and incidental Lewy bodies. *Mov Disord* 2007;**22**:1581–6.

114. Allan L, McKeith I, Ballard C, Kenny RA. The prevalence of autonomic symptoms in dementia and their association with physical activity, activities of daily living and quality of life. *Dement Geriatr Cogn Disord* 2006;**22**:230–7.

115. Stokes G. Psychological approaches to bowel care in older people with dementia. In: Potter J, Norton C, Cottenden A, eds. *Bowel care in older people*. London: Royal College of Physicians; 2002.

116. Sakakibara R, Ogata T, Uchiyama T, et al. How to manage overactive bladder in elderly individuals with dementia? A combined use of donepezil, a central acetylcholinesterase inhibitor, and propiverine,

a peripheral muscarine receptor antagonist. *J Am Geriatr Soc* 2009;**57**:1515–7.

117. Zeiss AM, Davies HD, Wood M, Tinklenberg JR. The incidence and correlates of erectile problems in patients with Alzheimer's disease. *Arch Sex Behav* 1990;**19**:325–31.

118. Elliott ML, Biever LS. Head injury and sexual dysfunction. *Brain Inj* 1996;**10**:703–17.

119. Aloni R, Katz S. A review of the effect of traumatic brain injury on the human sexual response. *Brain Inj* 1999;**13**:269–80.

120. Bruckner FE, Randle AP. Return to work after severe head injuries. *Rheumatol Phys Med* 1972;**11**:344–8.

121. Sandel ME, Williams KS, Dellapietra L, Derogatis LR. Sexual functioning following traumatic brain injury. *Brain Inj* 1996;**10**:719–28.

122. Hibbard MR, Gordon WA, Flanagan S, Haddad L, Labinsky E. Sexual dysfunction after traumatic brain injury. *NeuroRehabilitation* 2000;**15**:107–20.

123. Kreuter M, Dahllof AG, Gudjonsson G, Sullivan M, Siosteen A. Sexual adjustment and its predictors after traumatic brain injury. *Brain Inj* 1998;**12**:349–68.

124. Rosenbaum M, Najenson T. Changes in life patterns and symptoms of low mood as reported by wives of severly brain-injured soldiers. *J Consult Clin Psychol* 1976;**44**:881–8.

125. Ghigo E, Masel B, Aimaretti G, et al. Consensus guidelines on screening for hypopituitarism following traumatic brain injury. *Brain Inj* 2005;**19**:711–24.

126. Moiyadi AV, Devi BI, Nair KP. Urinary disturbances following traumatic brain injury: clinical and urodynamic evaluation. *NeuroRehabilitation* 2007;**22**:93–8.

127. Wyndaele JJ. Micturition in comatose patients. *J Urol* 1986;**135**:1209–11.

128. Krimchansky BZ, Sazbon L, Heller L, Kosteff H, Luttwak Z. Bladder tone in patients in post-traumatic vegetative state. *Brain Inj* 1999;**13**:899–903.

Parkinson's disease

Ryuji Sakakibara, Clare J. Fowler and Takamichi Hattori

Introduction

Although the major therapeutic target of Parkinson's disease (PD) has so far been the motor symptoms, there is increasing recognition that the disease involves many brain regions other than the substantia nigra. These include brainstem structures such as the locus ceruleus, raphe and vagal nuclei with consequent loss of neurotransmitters other than dopamine, namely noradrenaline, serotonin and acetylcholine, and it has been suggested that the non-motor symptoms of the condition may reflect this multisystem involvement [1]. Whilst motor symptoms can to a large extent be managed so that patients live longer, non-motor neurological deficits accumulate as the disease advances with consequent adverse effects on quality of life. Prominent amongst the non-motor symptoms are those relating to pelvic organ function (Fig. 12.1) [2]. Unlike the motor symptoms, pelvic organ dysfunctions are generally not responsive to levodopa and require other therapeutic approaches.

Bowel dysfunction

Bowel dysfunction is a common and troublesome problem in patients with PD and constipation may even be a premonitory symptom. This information first became apparent from the Honolulu Heart Program when, between 1971 and 1974, information was collected from 6790 men aged 51 to 75 years. Amongst the data was information about their frequency of bowel movements and at follow-up some 24 years later, 96 men had developed PD. The risk of PD in men with bowel frequency of less than one bowel movement per day increased 4.5-fold compared to men with bowel movements more than twice

a day [3], leading the authors to speculate whether constipation is part of early PD processes or is a marker of susceptibility or may be due to environmental factors that may cause PD. The observation that bowel infrequency might be a predictor for the risk of developing PD was further supported by a retrospective study of lifestyle risk factors in a group of Japanese patients with PD. Constipation was defined as less than one bowel movement in three days and in 71% of 94 patients this was a complaint. In 33 patients out of 74 (44.6%), the onset of constipation had preceded motor disturbance by an average time of 18.1 ± 18.8 years. A correlation with lifelong reduced water intake, possibly predating the onset of constipation, was also demonstrated [4].

Based on neuropathological studies, Braak and colleagues have identified that the disease process may start in the dorsal motor nucleus of the vagus in the brainstem and in the olfactory bulb and tract. They have staged the disease according to the ascending progression of Lewy bodies, only involving the substantia nigra at stage 3 of a total of six stages (Fig. 12.2) [5]. Phases 1–3 may predate the onset of motor symptoms by many years and, according to this system, constipation is a feature of the "presymptomatic phase." However, the connection may be even more significant and Braak et al. have hypothesized that an unidentified toxin passes through the mucosal barrier of the intestine and is transported in a retrograde manner by the vagus nerve axon, leading to vagus nerve neuron damage [6]. Why the olfactory bulb should also be involved so early in the course of the disease with the established premonitory feature of anosmia leads to the proposal that there is pathogenic access to the brain through the stomach and nose – the "dual-hit" theory [7].

Pelvic Organ Dysfunction in Neurological Disease: Clinical Management and Rehabilitation, ed. Clare J. Fowler, Jalesh N. Panicker & Anton Emmanuel. Published by Cambridge University Press. © Cambridge University Press 2010.

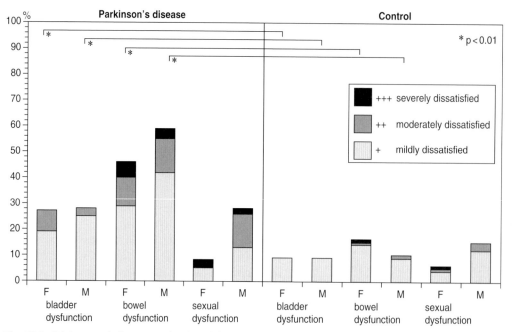

Fig. 12.1. Pelvic organ dysfunction and quality of life (dissatisfaction) in PD compared with age-matched controls. From [2] with permission.

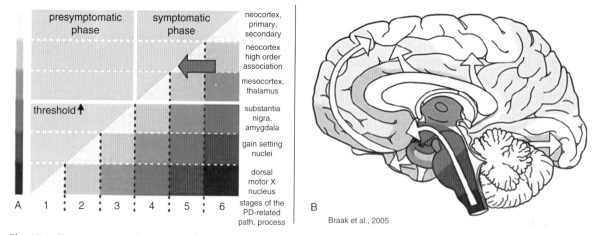

Fig. 12.2. The presymptomatic phase is marked by the appearance of Lewy neurites/bodies in the brains of asymptomatic persons. A. In the symptomatic phase, the individual neuropathological threshold is exceeded (black arrow). The increasing slope and intensity of the colored areas below the diagonal indicate the growing severity of the pathology in vulnerable brain regions (right). The severity of the pathology is indicated by darker degrees of shading in the colored upright arrow (left). B. Diagram showing the ascending pathological process (white arrows). The shading intensity of the colored areas corresponds to that in A. (From [5] with permission.) The large arrow pointing just above stage 4 indicates the stage at which bladder symptoms become common. See plate section for color version.

The neural regulation of bowel function is described in Chapter 2 and will only be briefly summarized here with a particular emphasis on the role of dopamine. The enteric nervous system plays the most important role in regulating the peristaltic reflex of the lower gastrointestinal tract [8] and the strength of cholinergic transmission in the enteric nervous system is thought to be regulated by opposing receptors; serotonin 5-HT4 receptor mediating excitation [9, 10] and dopamine D2 receptor mediating inhibition [11, 12]. However, the situation is not straightforward and in some studies dopamine has been demonstrated to increase motility of the colon (which has a low density of dopamine receptors), whilst having less effect on the stomach (which has a high density of dopamine receptors) [13], presumably due to effects mediated by other receptor populations, such as adrenergic or serotonergic receptors, or other central mechanisms [13]. It has been shown in a knockout model that the function of this small proportion of enteric dopaminergic nerves is to inhibit gut motility through a presynaptic D2 receptor mechanism upon cholinegic nerves. However, MPTP/salsolinol-induced parkinsonian animals showed decreased gastrointestinal motility [14] and decreased c-Kit expression in interstitial cells of Cajal [15]. These cells are primarily located in the right colon, and are regarded as the enteric pacemakers [16]. Wakabayashi et al. have shown that in addition to enteric dopaminergic neurons, VIP-containing enteric neurones are susceptible to Lewy body formation. One could speculate that there is some enteric neurotoxin that is transported across the synapse, supported by Braak's classic finding that IPANs are uninvolved in PD (hence the unmyelinated axons may be the vector for central transmission).

Pathological studies have demonstrated that PD affects the enteric nervous system showing a decrease in dopaminergic myenteric neurons and the appearance of Lewy bodies along the proximal-distal axis, being most frequent in the lower esophagus and scarce in the rectum [17, 18]. Presumably, degeneration of not only the inhibitory (dopaminergic) fibers, but also of facilitatory fibers, may also contribute to the slow colonic transit in PD. The extra-enteric nervous system relevant to PD pathology may include the spinal parasympathetic preganglionic neurons [19], although to a lesser degree than can be shown in MSA, and no Lewy bodies have been found in the Onuf's nucleus innervating the anal sphincter in PD. Constipation in PD occurs commonly with a low coefficient of variation in electrocardiographic R to R intervals [20] suggesting that a parasympathetic deficit may underlie these abnormalities.

In PD, neuronal cell loss and the appearance of Lewy bodies in the vagus nuclei [19, 21] and the Barrington's nucleus [21] (both facilitatory) have been documented. The basal ganglia modulate the bowel motility, with mainly an inhibitory effect [22, 23]. However, in rats under stressful conditions, administration of dopamine may facilitate colonic spike activity, presumably via the hypothalamus [24]. Furthermore bowel function seems to be modulated by the higher brain structures (Chapter 2). However, the contribution of higher neural structures and their failing output in PD causing bowel dysfunction awaits further clarification.

Lower gastrointestinal tract symptoms

The reported prevalence of bowel symptoms in PD is more than 50% [25]. In controlled studies [2, 25–27] the incidence rate of a stool frequency of less than three times a week ranged from 20% to 81% in PD patients, difficulty in stool expulsion in 57–67% and diarrhea in 21% (Fig. 12.3). All of these figures are significantly different from those in control populations where a decreased stool frequency occurred in 0–33%, difficulty in stool expulsion 26–28% and diarrhea 10%. Fecal incontinence has been reported to be 10–24% in PD [25, 2]. Therefore, constipation is the most prominent bowel symptom in patients with PD.

Indeed, PD is a risk factor for elderly nursing home residents to have constipation [28]. Of particular importance is that bowel dysfunction affects the quality of life in patients with PD [2]. Among three pelvic organ dysfunctions in PD, the rate of dissatisfaction for bowel dysfunction (59%) was significantly higher than that for urinary (28%) or sexual dysfunction (29%) and is significantly higher than in healthy controls (16%) (Fig. 12.1).

Difficulty in stool evacuation and diarrhea are more common in the higher grades of Hoehn and Yahr staging [2, 25, 29], suggesting a relationship between dopaminergic degeneration and lower gastrointestinal tract symptoms. However, there are also studies in which no such relationship was found [29]. Fecal incontinence in PD occurs commonly together with urinary incontinence, whereas no significant relation has been seen between bowel and sexual dysfunction [2].

Paralytic ileus or so-called "intestinal pseudo-obstruction" [30] was reported with a frequency of 7.1% in 112 patients with PD [31]. The clinical features of this extreme bowel condition include abdominal bloating, pain, nausea and/or vomiting. On clinical examination, the abdomen is found to be tympanic and on plain abdominal x-ray dilated loops of colon and small intestine are seen [32]. This condition demands prompt medical intervention.

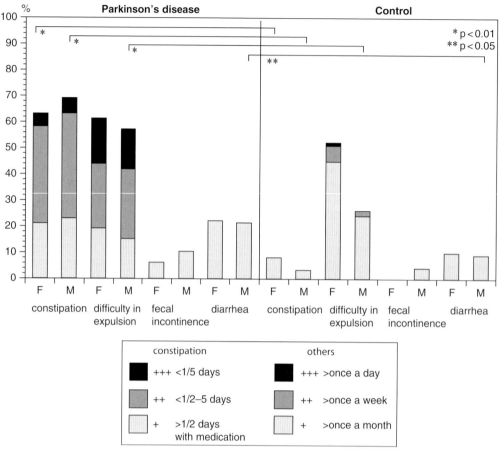

Fig. 12.3. Bowel dysfunction in Parkinson's disease. From [2] with permission.

Lower gastrointestinal tract function tests

Lower gastrointestinal tract function primarily consists of (1) colonic transport of the bowel content to the anorectum, (2) transient rectal reservoir function and (3) defecation with the aid of voluntary strain (Chapter 2). In PD, constipation results primarily from decreased transport and/or disturbed anorectal evacuation. Fecal incontinence may result from disturbed rectal reservoir capacity, or overflow secondary to constipation.

Transit time study

Studies have shown that total colonic transit time is increased in 80% of PD patients, which translates into an increased average colonic transit time ranging from 44 to 130 hours in PD and 89 hours in de novo PD patients [33, 34], all of which are significantly longer than those of controls (range 20–39 hours). Slow colonic transit is the major cause of decreased stool

frequency. Among right, left and rectosigmoid segments of the colonic transit time, the rectosigmoid transit time is significantly prolonged in PD patients [33–35]. Several explanations for this finding have been put forward: that the enteric nervous system innervated by the sacral cord is more severely affected than that innervated by the dorsal motor nucleus of the vagus or that this is simply a reflection of normal colonic transit time distribution which is slowest in the rectosigmoid segment [34]. Alternatively, it could be an artefact of measurement technique, such that problems with rectal voiding are reflected as delayed distal colonic transit.

Recto-anal videomanometry and sphincter electromyography

In PD, resting and squeezing anal pressure and motor unit potential analysis of the external sphincter muscles are mostly normal except in patients with

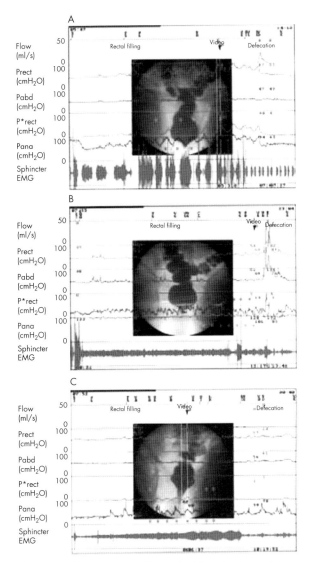

Fig. 12.4. Videomanometry. Flow = fecal flow; Prect = rectal pressure, Pabd = abdominal (bladder) pressure; P*rect = differential rectal pressure = Prect – Pabd; Pana = anal pressure. (A) and (B) During filling, the control subject had spontaneous phasic rectal contractions (P*rect). The Parkinson's disease patient had smaller phasic rectal contractions. During defecation, the control subject showed as rectal contraction type defecation (P*rect). In this subject, anal pressure increased mildly. (C) However, the Parkinson's disease patient showed paradoxical sphincter contraction on defecation (Pana) with minimum strain (Pabd), and this patient was almost unable to defecate with large post-defecation residuals. From [34, 39] with permission.

longstanding disease [36]. During slow rectal filling, PD patients have mostly normal rectal volume at first sensation and a maximum desire to defecate, and normal rectal compliance compared with control subjects [34, 37]. However, the amplitude of the

spontaneous phasic rectal contraction in PD patients is significantly less than that in control subjects [34]. The decreased spontaneous phasic rectal contractions may share the same enteric nervous system pathology with the decrease in colonic transit time.

In addition to slow transit constipation, anorectal (outlet type) constipation is a common feature in PD. A videomanometry study showed that most PD patients could not defecate completely and had post-defecation residuals [34]. Whereas healthy subjects utilized the final wave of spontaneous phasic rectal contractions for defecation [38], rectal contraction on defecation in PD patients is smaller than that in controls (Fig. 12.4) [34, 39].

Straining plays a physiological role in defecation and is achieved by co-contraction of the glottis, diaphragm and abdominal wall [40]. However, PD patients show a less pronounced increase in abdominal pressure on coughing, [34, 41], during the Valsalva maneuver and in the defecation phase [34, 42] than do controls. The mechanism of the impaired straining in PD may include rigidity and reduced contractility of the axial muscles, and a failure of coordinated glottis closure. Patients with PD may show paradoxical sphincter contraction on defecation, so called "anismus" [34, 37, 42]. Mathers and colleagues considered this to be a form of focal dystonia. Apomorphine was shown to lessen this disorder [42, 43]. Whether such drug approaches also improve other pathophysiological aspects of parkinsonian constipation remains to be explored. Both weak abdominal strain and anismus seem to be the major causes of difficulty in stool expulsion in PD patients.

Medication for bowel symptoms

The management of neurogenic bowel disorders is discussed in Chapter 3 but data specific to PD are presented here. An increase in dietary fiber has been shown to improve stool consistency and increase stool frequency in PD [44]. In addition, insoluble fiber treatment appears to improve levodopa absorption [44]. Dietary fibers such as psyllium [44, 45] and polyethylene glycol 3350 [46], or the highly hydrophilic agent polycarbophil [47], improve constipation in various neurodegenerative disorders, including PD. Polycarbophil shortens the total colonic transit time, particularly in the proximal bowel segments [47].

Endogenous dopamine, which does not penetrate the blood–brain barrier, is thought to inhibit intestinal motility. However, it is not well known whether levo-dopa alters gut function in treatment-naive PD patients. As for somatic sphincter function, levodopa improves voluntary anal squeezing in PD patients, which parallels an improvement in gait difficulty [45]. The effect of apomorphine on lessening anismus [42, 43] is not antagonized by domperidone, which does not cross the blood-brain barrier, suggesting that apomorphine may be acting centrally. Domperidone is widely used as a gastrointestinal prokinetic, antagonizing dopamine's inhibitory effects on motility, particularly through the effect of D2 receptor blockade. Domperidone pretreatment caused a mean 12% increase in peak plasma levodopa concentrations compared to the effect of levodopa when given alone [48, 49]. Dopaminergic blockers that do penetrate the blood–brain barrier, such as metoclopramide or levosulpiride, are not recommended because of their potential to worsen the extrapyramidal motor disorder of PD.

The selective 5-HT4 receptor agonist cisapride [50], when still licensed, and newer agents, such as mosapride [51] and tegaserod [52], have been shown to significantly reduce colonic transit time and ameliorate constipation in PD. However, safety concerns mean that none of these are currently available for prescription.

Individual series have shown a role for botulinum toxin A injections into the puborectalis muscle [53] and biofeedback to be of some benefit [54] in lessening anismus in PD. It is certainly fair to say that much work remains to be done in both the understanding of pathophysiology and the treatment of bowel dysfunction in PD. This is ironic given the emerging evidence that the gut may be etiologically important in the development of the a-synuclein changes that are central to the development of the condition.

Bladder dysfunction

In contrast to constipation and disorders of the bowel, bladder dysfunction as part of PD occurs relatively late and is thought to result from central rather than peripheral nervous system abnormalities. Not all patients with PD develop bladder symptoms, although as the disease advances bladder symptoms are more predictably troublesome. A lack of correlation between the severity of neurological deficit in the early stages and onset of bladder symptoms in PD means that there may be considerable diagnostic difficulties, particularly in men with mild PD and lower urinary tract symptoms (LUTS), and coincidental urological conditions, such as prostate disease, must be considered.

Prostate disease in aging men

Prostatic cancer is the second most common cause of death from malignancy in men. A recent large European study showed a reduction in mortality following large-scale screening by PSA blood measurements [55] and as a result, it seems likely that screening of men over the age of 50 may be introduced in a number of European countries in the near future. Prostate cancer can be either a silent condition until the patient presents with metastatic disease, or can, in a proportion of patients, present with LUTS. Thus in a man in whom bladder dysfunction cannot be certainly attributed to a neurological condition, screening for prostate cancer with the measurement of blood PSA would seem a sensible recommendation.

Benign prostatic outflow obstruction typically affects men over the age of 60 and there is an obvious overlap in the populations of those with PD and those with benign prostatic hypertrophy. The symptoms of benign prostatic outflow include voiding difficulty, i.e. a weak or interrupted stream and post-micturition dribble, but also symptoms which reflect the compensatory reaction and hypertrophy of the detrusor muscle to obstruction, which include frequency and urgency. Night-time frequency is a particularly common and troublesome symptom. Thus these symptoms are very similar to those that can be attributed to PD in its later stages.

Surgery for prostate disease in men with PD

A highly influential paper which described the onset of urinary incontinence following prostatic surgery in patients with parkinsonism and poor voluntary sphincter contractions has deterred urologists from operating on men with PD for many years [56]. However, a re-examination of the patients included in that study shows that a number of them, particularly those who subsequently developed incontinence, probably had multiple system atrophy (MSA) rather than PD. This is known because the authors divided the patients into those who could and those who could not voluntarily contract their sphincters prior to surgery, as measured by sphincter EMG and it was commented that many of those who could not had changes of denervation and chronic reinnervation, as is known to occur in MSA. Since the publication of that important paper, the features of MSA have become more commonly recognized and that these patients do not do well following transurethral resection is generally agreed. However, men with PD and coincidental benign prostatic outflow obstruction should be investigated appropriately.

A study which looked at the incidence of incontinence in men undergoing radical prostatectomy for prostate cancer found no difference between men with PD and those without [57]. A retrospective study of 23 men with benign prostatic outflow obstruction who underwent a TURP showed a 70% response rate. The authors concluded "in case of refractory voiding symptoms, the risk of de-novo urinary incontinence seems minimal. Thus, TURP should not be considered contraindicated in patients with PD provided that preoperative investigations including urodynamic assessment indicate prostatic bladder outlet obstruction" [58].

Differential diagnosis of MSA and PD

The uro-genital symptoms of MSA are detailed in the following chapter but when reading literature about bladder dysfunction in PD dating back more than a decade, it should be borne in mind that it was only relatively recently that the importance of this differential diagnosis was recognized. Since almost 50% of patients with MSA-parkinsonism are initially misdiagnosed as having PD, any such misclassifications are likely to have confounded early studies.

Prevalence of bladder symptoms in PD

There was almost certainly an element of preselection in the prevalence studies lead by urologists who looked at lower urinary tract symptoms in PD and found a very high incidence of neurogenic detrusor overactivity (DO) [59–61]. A study in 2000 found that 27% of those attending a neurology clinic had LUTS [62]. Most recently, an international survey used the recently devised questionnaire to assess non-motor symptoms of PD (NMSQuest) in 545 patients with a mean Hoehn and Yahr stage of 2.5 [63]. This survey found that 56% answered positively to the question "have you experienced a sense of urgency to pass urine which makes you rush to the toilet?" and the most common

complaint of all was of nocturia, with 62% answering in the affirmative to the question "have you experienced getting up regularly at night to pass urine?" From that study it emerged that the "urinary domain" had the highest percentage positive answers of all nine [64]. An earlier questionnaire study from Japan [2] focusing only on pelvic organ symptoms, when given to 115 patients with PD and a mean Hoehn and Yahr stage of 3, found that 42% of women and 54% of men complained of urinary urgency, which was significantly higher than an age-matched control group (Fig. 12.5).

Correlation with severity of neurological disease

Several studies have demonstrated a correlation between increasing severity of neurological disease and increasing bladder problems: both the NMSQuest survey and the Japanese pelvic organ questionnaire provided data which supported this [2, 64]. In a study which used the international prostate symptom score (IPSS) (and found it to be equally effective tool in men and women), an almost linear relationship was found between the Hoehn and Yahr stage (with the introduction of a classification grade 3.5 for patients requiring assistance to walk outside) and IPSS score [62] (Fig. 12.6).

Detailed studies in individual patients using SPECT imaging of dopamine transporters have shown a correlation between urinary dysfunction and the extent of degeneration of the nigro-striated dopaminergic cells. Loss was pronounced in the striatum in patients with bladder symptoms compared to those without [65], whilst a recent Danish study showed that the severity of bladder dysfunction correlated with the relative degeneration of the caudate nucleus compared with the putamen [66].

Braak's hypothesis [5] and the staging of the neuropathology of PD (Fig. 12.2) serves as a valuable framework for understanding how it is that the bladder symptoms occur in the context of a patient with more severe disability than simply motor symptoms. In the authors' opinion and based on the demonstrated correlation of severity of neurological deficit and the occurrence of bladder symptoms, it is reasonable to put the clinical threshold for bladder symptomatology above Braak stage 4, i.e. when the neuropathology is starting to affect the neocortex (see large arrow, Fig. 12.2).

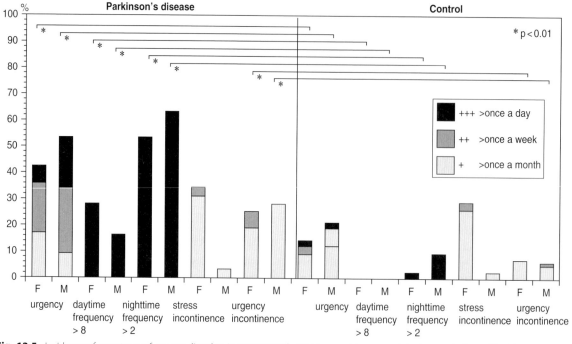

Fig. 12.5. Incidence of symptoms of storage disorders in patients with PD compared to age-matched controls. From [2] with permission.

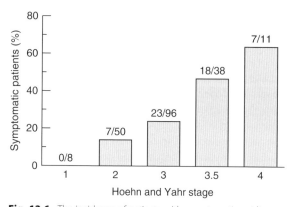

Fig. 12.6. The incidence of patients with symptomatic voiding dysfunction with IPSS score >12 at different Hoehn and Yahr stages of disability. The incidence is given as a percentage relative to the total number of patients at each stage. From [39] with permission.

Underlying pathophysiology of symptoms

Animal experimental data has shown that D1 receptors in the striatum have an inhibitory effect of on the pontine micturition center, whereas D2 receptor activation facilitates the micturition reflex [67, 68]. Recent studies in cats have shown a relationship between striatal neuronal activity and bladder function: electrical stimulation of the striatum inhibited spontaneous bladder contractions [69]. Thus it has

been proposed that the overactive bladder which underlies many of the symptoms that affect patients with PD is due to a failure of D1 activation, with the addition of possible exacerbation by the D2 content of many medications (Fig. 12.7).

The pathophysiology, however, is probably more complicated than that as the results of deep brain stimulation have largely shown an improvement in bladder function with the stimulator on [70–74]. A PET study that looked at this effect in some detail proposed that the amelioration may result from facilitated processing of afferent activity by the basal ganglia [74] (Fig. 12.8). It has been shown that subthalamic nucleus deep brain stimulation leads to improved sensory motor integration [75] and there is evidence that it is a higher-order processing of afferent activity that is improved in patients with PD whose bladder symptoms are ameliorated by medication [76]. Thus the notion that DO is the main underlying problem resulting from loss of dopamine-mediated inhibition may be an oversimplification.

It is widely accepted that the complaint of urinary urgency reflects underlying DO. Repeatedly DO has been shown to be the commonest urodynamic abnormality in patients with PD and symptoms of an overactive bladder, but symptoms of voiding difficulty are

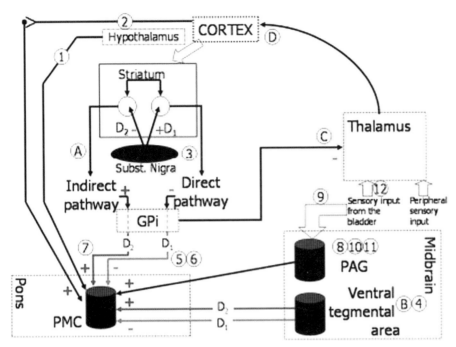

Fig. 12.7. Diagram showing model of cortical, basal ganglia and brainstem structures in bladder control in health and PD. See Chapter 1 for the proposed roles of the named structures. From [70] with permission.

also known to occur: Fig. 12.5 shows the occurrence of symptoms related to bladder filling whereas Fig. 12.9 shows that hesitancy, abnormal stream, difficulty voiding and a sensation of incomplete emptying are also common [2]. The explanation for difficulty with voiding is not altogether clear, although a disorder of bladder contractility has been suggested as the underlying pathophysiology [77] in addition to an abnormality of sphincter relaxation, or "bradykinesia" of the sphincter. This was shown to be reversible by apomorphine [78].

Nocturia appears to be a particular problem for patients with PD. As already mentioned, the NMSQuest study showed this to be the most common of all non-motor symptoms, reported by 62% of patients. Likewise the Japanese pelvic organ questionnaire showed that this affected 63% of men and 58% of women where night-time frequency was defined as having to get up more than twice. The reason for the frequency of this complaint has not been properly elucidated and possible explanations lie with an increased urine output at night, reduced bladder capacity or impairment of sleep. Although the DO which commonly affected patients with PD would be expected to result in a reduced bladder capacity and thus frequency, in the view of the authors, the night-

time frequency of patients with PD appears to be disproportionate compared to their daytime frequency. Night-time urine output has yet to be fully investigated as a contributing factor, but impairment of sleep, a common and pronounced problem for patients with PD, may well be a significant additional factor.

Bladder symptoms and PD therapies

The effect of antiparkinsonian medication on the bladder is unpredictable. The only agreed finding from various studies is that voiding difficulty is less in all subjects when "on."

Several studies have shown that l-dopa can in individual patients either worsen or ameliorate (less common) urgency and other symptoms of DO [78–80]. In the most recent study, 18 PD patients with a median Hoehn and Yahr score of 5 during the off phase and 3 during the on phase had urodynamic studies before and about one hour after the patients had taken 100 mg of l-dopa with dopa-decarboxylase inhibitor (DCI). After taking the l-dopa/DCI, urinary urgency and urge incontinence aggravated, whereas voiding difficulty was alleviated in all 12 patients [77].

A study which observed that l-dopa alone worsened DO but that l-sulpride (a central and peripheral

STN-DBS and control of urinary bladder

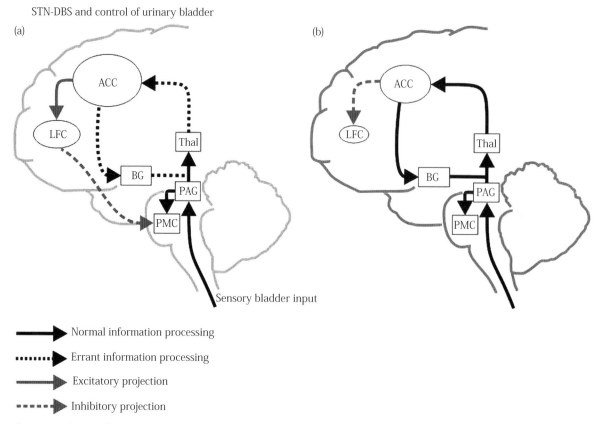

Fig. 12.8. Influence of STN-DBS on cortical centers of urinary bladder control in stimulation OFF condition (A) and stimulation ON condition (B). In STN-DBS OFF, errant processing of urinary bladder input, which is relayed to the higher centers by the PAG, in the basal ganglia (BG) loop may lead to an increase in activation of the ACC. As a compensatory mechanism, the LFC is activated and exerts its inhibitory influence on the PMC. This allows maintenance of continence. In STN-DBS ON, sensory information processing in the BG loop may be restored, which consecutively results in normalization (i.e. a relative decrease) of ACC activity. As a consequence, inhibitory influence of the LFC on the PMC is no longer necessary for maintenance of continence. Thal = thalamus. From [74] with permission.

D2 antagonist) counteracted the worsening in a dose-dependent manner found that domperidone (a peripheral D2 antagonist) failed to show the same counteraction, and so concluded that central acute D2 stimulation appears to reduce bladder capacity and worsen DO in patients with mild PD [81]. Because of the differential effect of D1 and D2 agonists on bladder control, attempts in an animal model were made to see if pergolide (D1 agonist) has a more beneficial effect on bladder control than D1 and D2 acting agonists [82]. An ambitious study aimed at examining the effect on nocturia of changing from bromocriptine to pergolide failed to recruit more than three women, but in all nocturia became less frequent [83].

Management of bladder symptoms in PD

Investigations

A good history, often from the patient's carer, is an essential starting point. If appropriate, the patient and their carer should be asked to keep a 3-day, 24-hour bladder diary. On this is recorded the time and volume of each void together with sensation preceding the void (i.e. strong desire or urgency). Additional useful information is fluid intake and the time the patient went to bed and got up in the morning. From this it may be possible to establish the possible role of excessive fluid intake, probable DO, nocturnal

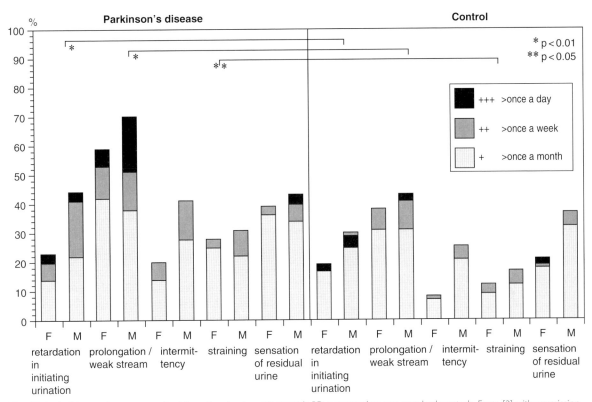

Fig. 12.9. Incidence of symptoms of voiding disorders in patients with PD compared to age-matched controls. From [2] with permission.

polyuria and sleep disorder as etiological factors in a patient's symptoms.

Medication for bladder symptoms

If symptoms of urgency and frequency suggest DO and a voiding diary confirms frequent, small-volume voids both day and night, a trial of an antimuscarinic is appropriate. However, it is important to balance the possible therapeutic benefits with the potential adverse effects of such drugs. These are discussed in Chapter 6 but particularly relevant in PD is the potential effect of these medications on cognition. Anticholinergics should be used with caution, particularly in elderly patients who have hallucination or cognitive decline (i.e. PD with dementia, also called "Lewy body dementia") [84, 85], and an antimuscarinic which does not cross the blood–brain barrier or that does not act on central nervous system M1 receptors (these include trospium, tolterodine and darifenacin) is recommended [86]. Oxybutynin has been shown to have a detrimental effect on cognitive function, memory in particular in elderly patients [87]. Somewhat worryingly, a recent study has shown that cognitive decline in patients with PD over an

eight-year period was higher in those taking drugs with anticholinergic activity (this included a variety of types of medication and rarely those for bladder symptoms), and recommended that such drugs be avoided [88].

Whereas night-time polyuria is a common consequence of postural hypotension in multiple system atrophy, it is not thought to be a major factor in the nocturia that affects so many patients with PD. The use of DDAVP is generally not advised in patients over 60 to treat night-time frequency in the absence of nocturnal polyuria and if inappropriately given may result in hyponatremia with an exacerbation of confusion.

If a voiding diary chart shows night-time frequency disproportionate to the number of voids during the day, further investigation of sleep disturbance and appropriate treatment would be indicated.

Flow rate, residual volume and cystometry

As a general rule it would seem reasonable to restrict the level of investigation to that which would have a determining role in any considered future management. A simple flow rate and measurement of the residual volume can exclude major outflow obstruction and show that incomplete bladder emptying is not a contributing factor to urinary frequency and urgency. If these initial investigations do suggest an element of prostatic outflow obstruction, cystometry with insertion of urethral and rectal catheters may be appropriate so that pressure/flow studies can be made. The question of prostatic surgery in elderly men with bladder symptoms is particularly difficult and a man with advanced PD may not wish to have a TURP even if pressure flow studies show obstructed outflow.

Possible future treatments

As mentioned in the opening paragraph, in idiopathic PD, in addition to the loss of dopaminergic pathways, there is also neuronal cell loss in the serotonergic raphe nucleus [89]. The main action of serotonergic pathways on the lower urinary tract is facilitation of urine storage [90]. Up to now there has been little published on the use of serotonergic drugs for overactive bladder [91]. However, this might be a rational approach if patients with PD also have co-morbid depression. When prescribing these drugs, their gastrointestinal and sedative actions should be considered.

Detrusor injection of botulinum toxin has proved to be of immense benefit in patients with neurogenic DO due to spinal cord disease [92] or MS [93] but little is known about its value in patients with PD. A small study from Italy reported that four women with PD and intractable DO treated with detrusor injections of botulinum toxin A had good symptomatic improvement without the need for intermittent self-catheterization [94]. Patients with advanced PD troubled by symptoms of DO may not be capable of clean intermittent self-catheterization nor their carers willing to do this for them.

There have not as yet been published studies looking at the effect of sacral neuromodulation in patients with PD but whilst the current techniques for this intervention require not inconsiderable surgical procedures, careful patient selection will be necessary if this treatment is to be considered.

Sexual behavior

Whether or not specific genital dysfunction is a feature of PD is not resolved although sexual dysfunction in patients with PD is common [2]. In animal studies the medial preoptic area (MPO) of the hypothalamus has been shown to regulate sexual drive, and selective stimulation of D2 dopaminergic receptors in this region increases sexual activity in rats [95, 96]. The MPO receives projections from the nigral dopaminergic neurons and changes in the hypothalamus can be seen in patients with PD [97]. Some untreated patients with PD have been found to have hyperprolactinemia [98], which may also contribute to erectile dysfunction (ED). A role for testosterone deficiency as a contributing cause of apathy and sexual dysfunction in elderly men has been suggested [99].

Sexual dysfunction in PD

Although ED, premature ejaculation in men and difficulty in arousal and reaching orgasm in women with PD may be complaints [2, 100, 101], unless age- and disability-matched groups are compared it is difficult to know how specific these complaints are. ED is known to have a major increase in incidence with increasing age [102] and early studies that found a high incidence of ED in men with PD may not have excluded men with MSA. A study that compared a group of married men with PD to a group with arthritis found a similar pattern of sexual functioning in the two groups but suggested that although sexual dysfunction was common in PD, it was not more so than in men with a chronic illness that does not involve the nervous system [103]. Age, severity of disease and depression seem to be major determinants of sexual dysfunction, as they are in other neurological diseases [104].

The reported prevalence of sexual symptoms in patients with PD ranges from 37% to 65% [2, 101, 105, 106]. Jacobs et al. studied 121 men with PD (mean age 45 years) and 126 age- and sex-matched, community derived controls [106]. Using questionnaire surveys, several studies have shown that dissatisfaction with the quality of sexual experiences in men [106] and women [106–108] with PD is more likely than in control subjects. A survey of young patients with PD and their partners revealed a high level of dissatisfaction, with the most severely affected couples being those in which the patient was male and who complained of ED and premature ejaculation [100]. Patients were more dissatisfied with their present sexual functioning and relationship, whereas no differences were found for the frequency of sexual intercourse itself. A study which divided PD patients and

(a)

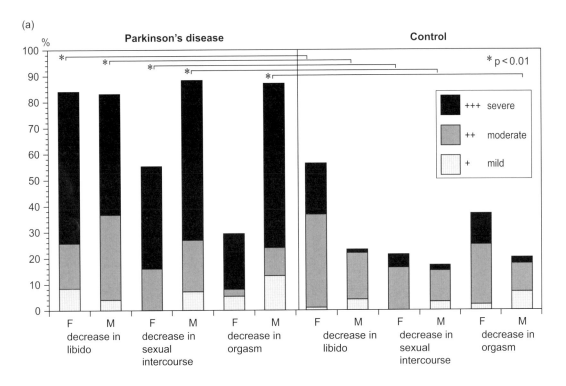

(b)

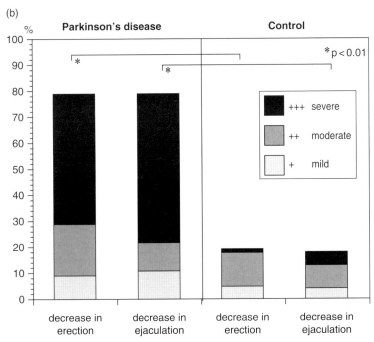

Fig. 12.10. Sexual function in the patients with Parkinson's disease and control subjects: (a) libido, intercourse, orgasm; (b) erection, ejaculation.

controls into four age subgroups (subjects in their 30s, 40s, 50s and 60s) found the frequency of sexual intercourse and of orgasm was significantly lower in older individuals [2]. In the PD group, only the frequency of orgasm was lower in older men (p<0.05). Comparing the results between both sexes in the control group, decrease of libido and orgasm were more common in women (p<0.01). In the PD group, there was no significant difference in sexual function items. Bronner et al. reported that use of medications (selective serotonin reuptake inhibitors used for co-morbid depression) and advanced PD stage contributed to the development of ED [101].

In their study on the effect of pelvic organ dysfunction on quality of life, Sakakibara and colleagues compared 84 PD patients (46 men, 38 women, age 35–70 years) with 356 healthy control subjects (258 men, 98 women, age 30–70 years) and found that in the patients there was a significant reduction in libido (84% men, 83% women), decrease in sexual intercourse (55% men, 88% women), decrease of orgasm (87% men) and decrease of erection (79%) and ejaculation (79%) in men [2] (Fig. 12.10). Increase in sexual dysfunction increased with age but not with disability as measured by Hoehn and Yahr stage. Interestingly, the prevalence of dissatisfaction with sexual conditions did not differ between the controls and patients with PD despite there being greater sexual dysfunction in the patients with PD (Fig. 12.1).

Treatment

It is not entirely clear to what extent levodopa ameliorates sexual dysfunction in PD. Apomorphine is thought to stimulate dopamine D2 receptors and activate oxytocinergic neurons in the paraventricular nucleus of the anterior hypothalamus. The pro-erectile effect of sublingual apomorphine was exploited as a licensed worldwide treatment of erectile dysfunction in 2001 [109] although a head-to-head comparison with sildenafil since showed this latter medication to be more effective [110]. Nausea was a common side-effect of apomorphine. Some men with PD being treated with apomorphine took advantage of its pro-erectile effect [111]. Cabergoline [112] and pergolide [113] have also been reported to improve sexual dysfunction in PD. Men with PD and erectile dysfunction respond satisfactorily to treatment with sildenafil citrate [114, 115].

A small but positive response in sexual well-being was reported in men, but not women, after deep brain stimulation of the subthalamic nucleus [116]. The effect was greatest in younger men.

Impulse control disorders and dopamine dysregulation syndrome

The role of dopamine in reward-seeking behavior, gambling addiction and hypersexuality is complex. An increase in libido in some patients with PD treated with l-dopa is a well-observed problem although the extent to which this occurs is not known. Some years following the introduction of l-dopa as a treatment for PD, a troublesome increase in libido was reported as an adverse effect [117–119]. Since then, features of the disorder have been characterized, showing an element of dose dependency between antiparkinsonian drugs, dopamine agonists in particular, and hypersexual behavior [120–122]. The behavior may be an isolated aberration and not be part of hypomania or a more diffuse psychiatric disturbance [123] although other features of compulsive-like behaviors such as gambling may also co-exist. It has been estimated that almost 3% of patients treated for PD develop hypersexuality with the incidence rising in those treated with dopamine agonists [124].

It was suggested that hypersexuality following antiparkinsonian drugs was a consequence of inhibition of prolactin secretion [123], but most recently excessive stimulation of D3 receptors has been implicated [125]. Change of therapy or dose adjustment appears to offer the best chance of controlling the behavior [120] but improvements with neuroleptics [126] or carbamazepine [127] have been reported.

Hypersexuality has also been described after deep brain stimulation: among 30 PD patients who received high-frequency stimulation of the subthalamic nucleus, two men developed mania and hypersexuality which came on a few days after the implant was switched on and lasted for some months before gradually resolving [128], and a similar case history was described from a second center [129].

References

1.   Lang AE, Obeso JA. Challenges in Parkinson's disease: restoration of the nigrostriatal dopamine system is not enough. *Lancet Neurol* 2004;**3**:309–16.

2.   Sakakibara R, Shinotoh H, Uchiyama T, et al. Questionnaire-based assessment of pelvic organ dysfunction in Parkinson's disease. *Auton Neurosci* 2001;**92**:76–85.

3. Abbott RD, Petrovitch H, White LR, et al. Frequency of bowel movements and the future risk of Parkinson's disease. *Neurology* 2001;**57**:456–62.

4. Ueki A, Otsuka M. Life style risks of Parkinson's disease: association between decreased water intake and constipation. *J Neurol* 2004;**251**(Suppl 7):18–23.

5. Braak H, Ghebremedhin E, Rub U, Bratzke H, Del Tredici K. Stages in the development of Parkinson's disease-related pathology. *Cell Tissue Res* 2004;**318**:121–34.

6. Braak H, Rub U, Gai WP, Del Tredici K. Idiopathic Parkinson's disease: possible routes by which vulnerable neuronal types may be subject to neuroinvasion by an unknown pathogen. *J Neural Transm* 2003;**110**:517–36.

7. Hawkes CH, Del Tredici K, Braak H. Parkinson's disease: a dual-hit hypothesis. *Neuropathol Appl Neurobiol* 2007;**33**:599–614.

8. Hansen MB. Neurohumoral control of gastrointestinal motility. *Physiol Res* 2003;**52**:1–30.

9. Liu MT, Rayport S, Jiang Y, Murphy DL, Gershon MD. Expression and function of 5-HT3 receptors in the enteric neurons of mice lacking the serotonin transporter. *Am J Physiol Gastrointest Liver Physiol* 2002;**283**:G1398–411.

10. Tonini M. 5-Hydroxytryptamine effects in the gut: the 3, 4, and 7 receptors. *Neurogastroenterol Motil* 2005;**17**:637–42.

11. Walker JK, Gainetdinov RR, Mangel AW, Caron MG, Shetzline MA. Mice lacking the dopamine transporter display altered regulation of distal colonic motility. *Am J Physiol Gastrointest Liver Physiol* 2000;**279**:G311–8.

12. Anlauf M, Schafer MK, Eiden L, Weihe E. Chemical coding of the human gastrointestinal nervous system: cholinergic, VIPergic, and catecholaminergic phenotypes. *J Comp Neurol* 2003;**459**:90–111.

13. Vaughan CJ, Aherne AM, Lane E, et al. Identification and regional distribution of the dopamine D(1A) receptor in the gastrointestinal tract. *Am J Physiol Regul Integr Comp Physiol* 2000;**279**:R599–609.

14. Haskel Y, Hanani M. Inhibition of gastrointestinal motility by MPTP via adrenergic and dopaminergic mechanisms. *Dig Dis Sci* 1994;**39**:2364–7.

15. Banach T, Zurowski D, Gil K, et al. Peripheral mechanisms of intestinal dysmotility in rats with salsolinol induced experimental Parkinson's disease. *J Physiol Pharmacol* 2006;**57**:291–300.

16. Miyamoto-Kikuta S, Ezaki T, Komuro T. Distribution and morphological characteristics of the interstitial cells of Cajal in the ileocaecal junction of the guinea-pig. *Cell Tissue Res* 2009;**338**:29–35.

17. Braak H, de Vos RA, Bohl J, Del Tredici K. Gastric alpha-synuclein immunoreactive inclusions in Meissner's and Auerbach's plexuses in cases staged for Parkinson's disease-related brain pathology. *Neurosci Lett* 2006;**396**:67–72.

18. Qualman SJ, Haupt HM, Yang P, Hamilton SR. Esophageal Lewy bodies associated with ganglion cell loss in achalasia. Similarity to Parkinson's disease. *Gastroenterology* 1984;**87**:848–56.

19. Wakabayashi K, Takahashi H. Neuropathology of autonomic nervous system in Parkinson's disease. *Eur Neurol* 1997;**38**(Suppl 2):2–7.

20. Wang SJ, Fuh JL, Shan DE, et al. Sympathetic skin response and R-R interval variation in Parkinson's disease. *Mov Disord* 1993;**8**:151–7.

21. Gai WP, Blessing WW, Blumbergs PC. Ubiquitin-positive degenerating neurites in the brainstem in Parkinson's disease. *Brain* 1995;**118**(Pt 6):1447–59.

22. Gravante G, Sabatino M, Sorbera F, Ferraro G, La Grutta V. Effects of substantia nigra stimulation on electrical and mechanical activities of the duodeno-jejunal loop, in the cat. *Arch Int Physiol Biochim* 1985;**93**:93–100.

23. Jing H, Lin KW, Mei MH. Participation of dopamine on the muscarinic inhibitory effect of substance P on gastric myoelectric activity and motility. *Sheng Li Xue Bao* 1995;**47**:245–52.

24. Bueno L, Gue M, Fabre C, Junien JL. Involvement of central dopamine and D1 receptors in stress-induced colonic motor alterations in rats. *Brain Res Bull* 1992;**29**:135–40.

25. Edwards LL, Pfeiffer RF, Quigley EM, Hofman R, Balluff M. Gastrointestinal symptoms in Parkinson's disease. *Mov Disord* 1991;**6**:151–6.

26. Singer C, Weiner W, Sanchez-Ramos JR. Autonomic dysfunction in men with Parkinson's disease. *European Neurology* 1992;**32**:134–40.

27. Siddiqui MF, Rast S, Lynn MJ, Auchus AP, Pfeiffer RF. Autonomic dysfunction in Parkinson's disease: a comprehensive symptom survey. *Parkinsonism Relat Disord* 2002;**8**:277–84.

28. Robson KM, Kiely DK, Lembo T. Development of constipation in nursing home residents. *Dis Colon Rectum* 2000;**43**:940–3.

29. Jost WH. Gastrointestinal motility problems in patients with Parkinson's disease. Effects of antiparkinsonian treatment and guidelines for management. *Drugs Aging* 1997;**10**:249–58.

30. Shimada J, Sakakibara R, Uchiyama T, et al. Intestinal pseudo-obstruction and neuroleptic malignant syndrome in a chronically constipated parkinsonian patient. *Eur J Neurol* 2006;**13**:306–7.

31. Yokoyama T, Hasegawa I. Ileus in Parkinson's disease. *Neurological Medicine* 2007;**66**:6–11.

32. Rosenthal MJ, Marshall CE. Sigmoid volvulus in association with parkinsonism. Report of four cases. *J Am Geriatr Soc* 1987;**35**:683–4.

33. Jost WH, Schrank B. Defecatory disorders in de novo Parkinsonians – colonic transit and electromyogram of the external anal sphincter. *Wien Klin Wochenschr* 1998;**110**:535–7.

34. Sakakibara R, Odaka T, Uchiyama T, et al. Colonic transit time and rectoanal videomanometry in Parkinson's disease. *J Neurol Neurosurg Psychiatry* 2003;**74**:268–72.

35. Ashraf W, Pfeiffer RF, Park F, Lof J, Quigley EM. Constipation in Parkinson's disease: objective assessment and response to psyllium. *Mov Disord* 1997;**12**:946–51.

36. Libelius R, Johanson JF. Quantitative electromyography of the external anal sphincter in Parkinson's disease and multiple system atrophy. *Muscle & Nerve* 2000;**23**:1250–6.

37. Stocchi F, Badiali D, Vacca L, et al. Anorectal function in multiple system atrophy and Parkinson's disease. *Mov Disord* 2000;**15**:71–6.

38. Ito T, Sakakibara R, Uchiyama T, et al. Videomanometry of the pelvic organs: a comparison of the normal lower urinary and gastrointestinal tracts. *Int J Urol* 2006;**13**:29–35.

39. Araki I, Kitahara M, Oida T, Kuno S. Voiding dysfunction and Parkinson's disease: urodynamic abnormalities and urinary symptoms. *J Urol* 2000;**164**:1640–3.

40. Iscoe S. Control of abdominal muscles. *Prog Neurobiol* 1998;**56**:433–506.

41. Fontana GA, Pantaleo T, Lavorini F, Benvenuti F, Gangemi S. Defective motor control of coughing in Parkinson's disease. *Am J Respir Crit Care Med* 1998;**158**:458–64.

42. Mathers SE, Kempster PA, Law PJ, et al. Anal sphincter dysfunction in Parkinson's disease. *Arch Neurol* 1989;**46**:1061–4.

43. Edwards LL, Quigley EM, Harned RK, Hofman R, Pfeiffer RF. Defecatory function in Parkinson's disease: response to apomorphine. *Ann Neurol* 1993;**33**:490–3.

44. Astarloa R, Mena MA, Sanchez V, de la Vega L, de Yebenes JG. Clinical and pharmacokinetic effects of a diet rich in insoluble fiber on Parkinson disease. *Clin Neuropharmacol* 1992;**15**:375–80.

45. Ashraf W, Wszolek ZK, Pfeiffer RF, et al. Anorectal function in fluctuating (on-off) Parkinson's disease: evaluation by combined anorectal manometry and electromyography. *Mov Disord* 1995;**10**:650–7.

46. Eichhorn TE, Oertel WH. Macrogol 3350/electrolyte improves constipation in Parkinson's disease and multiple system atrophy. *Mov Disord* 2001;**16**:1176–7.

47. Sakakibara R, Yamaguchi T, Uchiyama T, et al. Calcium polycarbophil improves constipation in primary autonomic failure and multiple system atrophy subjects. *Mov Disord* 2007;**22**:1672–3.

48. Soykan I, Sarosiek I, Shifflett J, Wooten GF, McCallum RW. Effect of chronic oral domperidone therapy on gastrointestinal symptoms and gastric emptying in patients with Parkinson's disease. 1997;**12**:952–7.

49. Shindler JS, Finnerty GT, Towlson K, et al. Domperidone and levodopa in Parkinson's disease. *Br J Clin Pharmacol* 1984;**18**:959–62.

50. Djaldetti R, Koren M, Ziv I, Achiron A, Melamed E. Effect of cisapride on response fluctuations in Parkinson's disease. *Mov Disord* 1995;**10**:81–4.

51. Liu Z, Sakakibara R, Odaka T, et al. Mosapride citrate, a novel 5-HT4 agonist and partial 5-HT3 antagonist, ameliorates constipation in parkinsonian patients. *Mov Disord* 2005;**20**:680–6.

52. Sullivan KL, Staffetti JF, Hauser RA, Dunne PB, Zesiewicz TA. Tegaserod (Zelnorm) for the treatment of constipation in Parkinson's disease. *Mov Disord* 2006;**21**:115–6.

53. Cadeddu F, Bentivoglio AR, Brandara F, et al. Outlet type constipation in Parkinson's disease: results of botulinum toxin treatment. *Aliment Pharmacol Ther* 2005;**22**:997–1003.

54. Chiarioni G, Heymen S, Whitehead WE. Biofeedback therapy for dyssynergic defecation. *World J Gastroenterol* 2006;**12**:7069–74.

55. Schroder FH, Hugosson J, Roobol MJ, et al. Screening and prostate-cancer mortality in a randomized European study. *N Engl J Med* 2009;**360**:1320–8.

56. Staskin DS, Vardi Y, Siroky MA. Post-prostatectomy incontinence in the parkinsonian patient: the significance of poor voluntary sphincter control. *J Urol* 1988;**140**:117–8.

57. Routh JC, Crimmins CR, Leibovich BC, Elliott DS. Impact of Parkinson's disease on continence after radical prostatectomy. *Urology* 2006;**68**:575–7.

58. Roth B, Studer UE, Fowler CJ, Kessler TM. Benign prostatic obstruction and parkinson's disease – should transurethral resection of the prostate be avoided? *J Urol* 2009;**181**:2209–13.

59. Andersen JT, Bradley WE. Cystometric, sphincter and electromyelographic abnormalities in Parkinson's disease. *J Urol* 1976;**116**:75–8.

60. Berger Y, Blaivas JG, DeLaRocha ER, Salinas JM. Urodynamic findings in Parkinson's disease. *J Urol* 1987;**138**:836–8.

61. Pavlakis AJ, Siroky MB, Goldstein I, Krane RJ. Neurourologic findings in Parkinson's disease. *J Urol* 1983;**129**:80–3.

62. Araki I, Kuno S. Assessment of voiding dysfunction in Parkinson's disease by the international prostate symptom score. *J Neurol Neurosurg Psychiatry* 2000;**68**:429–33.

63. Chaudhuri KR, Martinez-Martin P, Schapira AH, et al. International multicenter pilot study of the first comprehensive self-completed nonmotor symptoms questionnaire for Parkinson's disease: the NMSQuest study. *Mov Disord* 2006;**21**:916–23.

64. Martinez-Martin P, Schapira AH, Stocchi F, et al. Prevalence of nonmotor symptoms in Parkinson's disease in an international setting; study using nonmotor symptoms questionnaire in 545 patients. *Mov Disord* 2007;**22**:1623–9.

65. Sakakibara R, Shinotoh H, Uchiyama T, et al. SPECT imaging of the dopamine transporter with [(123)I]-beta-CIT reveals marked decline of nigrostriatal dopaminergic function in Parkinson's disease with urinary dysfunction. *J Neurol Sci* 2001;**187**:55–9.

66. Winge K, Friberg L, Werdelin L, Nielsen KK, Stimpel H. Relationship between nigrostriatal dopaminergic degeneration, urinary symptoms, and bladder control in Parkinson's disease. *Eur J Neurol* 2005;**12**:842–50.

67. Yoshimura N, Sasa M, Yoshida O, Takaori S. Mediation of micturition reflex by central norepinephrine from the locus coeruleus in the cat. *J Urol* 1990;**143**:840–3.

68. Seki S, Igawa Y, Kaidoh K, et al. Role of dopamine D1 and D1 receptors in the micturition reflex in conscious rats. *Neurourol Urodyn* 2001;**20**:105–13.

69. Yamamoto T, Sakakibara R, Nakazawa K, et al. Effects of electrical stimulation of the striatum on bladder activity in cats. *Neurourol Urodyn* 2009;**28**:549–54.

70. Winge K, Fowler CJ. Bladder dysfunction in Parkinsonism: mechanisms, prevalence, symptoms, and management. *Mov Disord* 2006;**21**:737–45.

71. Finazzi-Agro E, Peppe A, D'Amico A, et al. Effects of subthalamic nucleus stimulation on urodynamic findings in patients with Parkinson's disease. *J Urol* 2003;**169**:1388–91.

72. Sakakibara R, Nakazawa K, Uchiyama T, et al. Effects of subthalamic nucleus stimulation on the micturation reflex in cats. *Neuroscience* 2003;**120**:871–5.

73. Seif C, Herzog J, van der Horst C, et al. Effect of subthalamic deep brain stimulation on the function of the urinary bladder. *Ann Neurol* 2004;**55**:118–20.

74. Herzog J, Weiss PH, Assmus A, et al. Subthalamic stimulation modulates cortical control of urinary bladder in Parkinson's disease. *Brain* 2006;**129**:3366–75.

75. Gerschlager W, Alesch F, Cunnington R, et al. Bilateral subthalamic nucleus stimulation improves frontal cortex function in Parkinson's disease. An electrophysiological study of the contingent negative variation. *Brain* 1999;**122**(Pt 12):2365–73.

76. Winge K, Werdelin LM, Nielsen KK, Stimpel H. Effects of dopaminergic treatment on bladder function in Parkinson's disease. *Neurourol Urodyn* 2004;**23**:689–96.

77. Uchiyama T, Sakakibara R, Hattori T, Yamanishi T. Short-term effect of a single levodopa dose on micturition disturbance in Parkinson's disease patients with the wearing-off phenomenon. *Mov Disord* 2003;**18**:573–8.

78. Christmas T, Kempster P, Chapple C, et al. Role of subcutaneous apomorphine in parkinsonian voiding dysfunction. *Lancet* 1988;**2**:1451–3.

79. Fitzmaurice H, Fowler CJ, Rickards D, et al. Micturition disturbance in Parkinson's disease. *Br J Urol* 1985;**57**:652–6.

80. Aranda B, Cramer P. Effects of apomorphine and L-dopa on the parkinsonian bladder. *Neurourol Urodyn* 1993;**12**:203–9.

81. Brusa L, Petta F, Pisani A, et al. Central acute D2 stimulation worsens bladder function in patients with mild Parkinson's disease. *J Urol* 2006;**175**:202–6.

82. Yoshimura N, Mizuta E, Yoshida O, Kuno S. Therapeutic effects of dopamine D1/D2 receptor agonists on detrusor hyperreflexia in 1-methyl-4-phenyl-1,2,3,6-tetrahydropyridine-lesioned parkinsonian cynomolgus monkeys. *J Pharmacol Exp Ther* 1998;**286**:228–33.

83. Kuno S, Mizuta E, Yamasaki S, Araki I. Effects of pergolide on nocturia in Parkinson's disease: three female cases selected from over 400 patients. *Parkinsonism Relat Disord* 2004;**10**:181–7.

84. McKeith IG, Dickson DW, Lowe J, et al. Diagnosis and management of dementia with Lewy bodies: third report of the DLB Consortium. *Neurology* 2005;**65**:1863–72.

85. Sakakibara R, Ito T, Uchiyama T, et al. Lower urinary tract function in dementia of Lewy body type. *J Neurol Neurosurg Psychiatry* 2005;**76**:729–32.

86. Kay GG, Abou-Donia MB, Messer WS, Jr., et al. Antimuscarinic drugs for overactive bladder and their potential effects on cognitive function in older patients. *J Am Geriatr Soc* 2005;**53**:2195–201.

87. Kay GG, Granville LJ. Antimuscarinic agents: implications and concerns in the management of overactive bladder in the elderly. *Clin Ther* 2005;**27**:127–38.

88. Ehrt U, Broich K, Larsen JP, Ballard C, Aarsland D. Use of drugs with anticholinergic effect and impact on cognition in Parkinson's disease: a cohort study. *J Neurol Neurosurg Psychiatry* 2010;**81**:160–5.

89. Halliday GM, Blumbergs PC, Cotton RG, Blessing WW, Geffen LB. Loss of brainstem serotonin- and substance P-containing neurons in Parkinson's disease. *Brain Res* 1990;**510**:104–7.

90. Ito T, Sakakibara R, Nakazawa K, et al. Effects of electrical stimulation of the raphe area on the micturition reflex in cats. *Neuroscience* 2006; **142**:1273–80.

91. Andersson KE. Treatment of overactive bladder: other drug mechanisms. *Urology* 2000;**55**:51–7.

92. Schurch B, Hauri D, Rodic B, et al. Botulinum-A toxin as a treatment of detrusor-sphincter dyssynergia: a prospective study in 24 spinal cord injury patients. *J Urol* 1996;**155**:1023–9.

93. Kalsi V, Gonzales G, Popat R, et al. Botulinum injections for the treatment of bladder symptoms of multiple sclerosis. *Ann Neurol* 2007;**62**:452–7.

94. Giannantoni A, Rossi A, Mearini E, et al. Botulinum toxin A for overactive bladder and detrusor muscle overactivity in patients with Parkinson's disease and multiple system atrophy. *J Urol* 2009;**182**:1453–7.

95. Andersson KE. Pharmacology of penile erection. *Pharmacol Rev* 2001;**53**:417–50.

96. Montorsi F, Perani D, Anchisi D, et al. Apomorphine-induced brain modulation during sexual stimulation: a new look at central phenomena related to erectile dysfunction. *Int J Impot Res* 2003; **15**:203–9.

97. Langston JW, Forno LS. The hypothalamus in Parkinson disease. *Ann Neurol* 1978;**3**:129–33.

98. Bellomo G, Santambrogio L, Fiacconi M, Scarponi AM, Ciuffetti G. Plasma profiles of adrenocorticotropic hormone, cortisol, growth hormone and prolactin in patients with untreated Parkinson's disease. *J Neurol* 1991; **238**:19–22.

99. Ready RE, Friedman J, Grace J, Fernandez H. Testosterone deficiency and apathy in Parkinson's disease: a pilot study. *J Neurol Neurosurg Psychiatry* 2004;**75**:1323–6.

100. Brown RG, Jahanshahi M, Quinn N, Marsden CD. Sexual function in patients with Parkinson's disease and their partners. *J Neurol Neurosurg Psychiatry* 1990;**53**:480–6.

101. Bronner G, Royter V, Korczyn AD, Giladi N. Sexual dysfunction in Parkinson's disease. *J Sex Marital Ther* 2004;**30**:95–105.

102. Feldman H, Goldstein I, Hatzichristou D, Krane R, McKinlay J. Impotence and its medical and psychosocial correlates: results of the Massachusetts Male Aging Study. *J Urol* 1994;**151**:54–61.

103. Lipe H, Longstreth WT, Jr., Bird TD, Linde M. Sexual function in married men with Parkinson's disease compared to married men with arthritis. *Neurology* 1990;**40**:1347–9.

104. Chandler BJ, Brown S. Sex and relationship dysfunction in neurological disability. *J Neurol Neurosurg Psychiatry* 1998;**65**:877–80.

105. Papatsoris AG, Deliveliotis C, Singer C, Papapetropoulos S. Erectile dysfunction in Parkinson's disease. *Urology* 2006;**67**:447–51.

106. Jacobs H, Vieregge A, Vieregge P. Sexuality in young patients with Parkinson's disease: a population based comparison with healthy controls. *J Neurol Neurosurg Psychiatry* 2000;**69**:550–2.

107. Welsh M, Hung L, Waters CH. Sexuality in women with Parkinson's disease. *Mov Disord* 1997;**12**:923–7.

108. Wermuth L, Stenager E. Sexual problems in young patients with Parkinson's disease. *Acta Neurol Scand* 1995;**91**:453–5.

109. Heaton J. Central neuropharmacological agents and mechanisms in erectile dysfunction: the role of dopamine. *Neuroscience and Behavioral Reviews* 2000;**24**:561–9.

110. Eardley I, Wright P, MacDonagh R, Hole J, Edwards A. An open-label, randomized, flexible-dose, crossover study to assess the comparative efficacy and safety of sildenafil citrate and apomorphine hydrochloride in men with erectile dysfunction. *BJU Int* 2004;**93**:1271–5.

111. O'Sullivan J, Hughes A. Apomorphine-induced penile erections in Parkinson's disease. *Mov Disord* 1998;**13**:536–9.

112. Safarinejad MR. Salvage of sildenafil failures with cabergoline: a randomized, double-blind, placebo-controlled study. *Int J Impot Res* 2006; **18**:550–8.

113. Pohanka M, Kanovsky P, Bares M, Pulkrabek J, Rektor I. The long-lasting improvement of sexual dysfunction in patients with advanced, fluctuating Parkinson's disease induced by pergolide: evidence from the results of an open, prospective, one-year trial. *Parkinsonism Relat Disord* 2005;**11**:509–12.

114. Zesiewicz TA, Helal M, Hauser RA. Sildenafil citrate (Viagra) for the treatment of erectile dysfunction in men with Parkinson's disease. *Mov Disord* 2000;**15**:305–8.

115. Hussain IF, Brady CM, Swinn MJ, Mathias CJ, Fowler CJ. Treatment of erectile dysfunction with sildenafil citrate (Viagra) in parkinsonism due to Parkinson's disease or multiple system atrophy with observations on orthostatic hypotension. *J Neurol Neurosurg Psychiatry* 2001;**71**:371–4.

116. Castelli L, Perozzo P, Genesia ML, et al. Sexual well being in parkinsonian patients after deep brain stimulation of the subthalamic nucleus. *J Neurol Neurosurg Psychiatry* 2004;**75**:1260–4.

117. Ballivet J, Marin A, Gisselmann A. Aspects of hypersexuality observed in parkinsonian patients treated by L-dopa. *Ann Med Psychol (Paris)* 1973;**2**:515–22.

118. Gisselmann A. Hypersexuality and L dopa. *Nouv Presse Med* 1973;**2**:1616.

119. Brown E, Brown GM, Kofman O, Quarrington B. Sexual function and affect in parkinsonian men treated with L-dopa. *Am J Psychiatry* 1978;**135**:1552.

120. Klos KJ, Bower JH, Josephs KA, Matsumoto JY, Ahlskog JE. Pathological hypersexuality predominantly linked to adjuvant dopamine agonist therapy in Parkinson's disease and multiple system atrophy. *Parkinsonism Relat Disord* 2005;**11**:381–6.

121. Kanovsky P, Bares M, Pohanka M, Rektor I. Penile erections and hypersexuality induced by pergolide treatment in advanced, fluctuating Parkinson's disease. *J Neurol* 2002;**249**:112–4.

122. Shapiro MA, Chang YL, Munson SK, Okun MS, Fernandez HH. Hypersexuality and paraphilia induced by selegiline in Parkinson's disease: report of 2 cases. *Parkinsonism Relat Disord* 2006;**12**:392–5.

123. Uitti RJ, Tanner CM, Rajput AH, et al. Hypersexuality with antiparkinsonian therapy. *Clin Neuropharmacol* 1989;**12**:375–83.

124. Voon V, Hassan K, Zurowski M, et al. Prevalence of repetitive and reward-seeking behaviors in Parkinson disease. *Neurology* 2006;**67**:1254–7.

125. Fenu S, Wardas J, Morelli M. Impulse control disorders and dopamine dysregulation syndrome associated with dopamine agonist therapy in Parkinson's disease. *Behav Pharmacol* 2009;**20**:363–79.

126. O'Sullivan SS, Evans AH, Lees AJ. Dopamine dysregulation syndrome: an overview of its epidemiology, mechanisms and management. *CNS Drugs* 2009;**23**:157–70.

127. Bach JP, Oertel WH, Dodel R, Jessen F. Treatment of hypersexuality in Parkinson's disease with carbamazepine – a case report. *Mov Disord* 2009;**24**:1241–2.

128. Romito LM, Raja M, Daniele A, et al. Transient mania with hypersexuality after surgery for high frequency stimulation of the subthalamic nucleus in Parkinson's disease. *Mov Disord* 2002;**17**:1371–4.

129. Roane DM, Yu M, Feinberg TE, Rogers JD. Hypersexuality after pallidal surgery in Parkinson disease. *Neuropsychiatry Neuropsychol Behav Neurol* 2002;**15**:247–51.

Multiple system atrophy

Ryuji Sakakibara, Clare J. Fowler and Takamichi Hattori

Introduction

Despite its many various modes of presentation, multiple system atrophy (MSA) is now a recognized single disease entity. The condition can present either as a poorly levodopa-responsive parkinsonism (MSA-P) or cerebellar dysfunction (MSA-C), the criteria for diagnosis requiring additionally bladder dysfunction or postural hypotension [1]. The discovery in 1989 that glial cytoplasmic inclusions (GCIs) [2] are the pathological hallmark of the disease led to an improved understanding of the condition, its presentation and evolution. Immunocytochemistry has shown that the GCIs of MSA are comprised of ubiquitin-, tau- and alpha-synuclein-positive material, possibly representing a cytoskeletal alteration in glial cells. The severity of neuronal cell loss and gliosis have been shown to be correlated and the clinical phenotype depends on the distribution of pathology within the basal ganglia or cerebellum [3].

The differential diagnosis between MSA-P, the most common clinical form, and PD is difficult even for movement disorder specialists but a symmetric akinetic rigid syndrome, poor response to levodopa and rapid progression are all red flags indicating MSA [4]. Genetic testing is helpful in distinguishing hereditary spinocerebellar ataxias from MSA-C. Pelvic organ dysfunction, e.g. bladder, bowel and sexual symptoms, are prominent in MSA and affect patients with both MSA-P or MSA-C. This involvement is important diagnostically and also because such symptoms affect the quality of life (QOL) of the patient and their carer (Fig. 13.1).

Bladder dysfunction

The second consensus statement on the diagnosis of MSA recognizes that the disease frequently begins with bladder dysfunction [1] (although erectile dysfunction (ED) usually precedes that complaint). Patients may present with urinary incontinence, urinary retention or a combination of incontinence and incomplete bladder emptying. It is important that other common causes of poor bladder control are excluded by a urologist or uro-gynecologist before the disorder is attributed to the neurological condition [5].

Figs. 13.2 and 13.3 show the frequency of troublesome urinary symptoms in 256 patients with MSA compared with 158 age-matched control subjects [6].

Patients with MSA had significantly higher prevalence of daytime frequency (45% of women, 43% of men), night-time frequency (65%, 69%), urinary urgency (64% of men) and urgency incontinence (75%, 66%) than did the controls (Fig. 13.2). They also had more hesitancy of micturition (62%, 73%), prolonged, poor (71%, 81%) or intermittent stream (61%, 47%), or the need to strain to void (48%, 55%) (Fig. 13.3). Of particular importance is that the QoL index in the MSA group was significantly higher (i.e. worse) in MSA patients for bladder dysfunction (70%, 76%) than that in controls.

Detrusor overactivity

Urodynamic investigations in patients with MSA commonly show detrusor overactivity (DO) [7–10] as the underlying cause of decreased bladder volumes at first sensation, reduced bladder capacity and urgency incontinence. Uninhibited sphincter relaxation has also been observed in patients with MSA and when this occurs in combination with DO, severe incontinence results. It seems likely that DO results from the central pathology of MSA, which includes neuronal loss of neuromelanin-containing cells in the locus ceruleus as well as in the nigrostriatal dopaminergic system ("putaminal slit sign") and cerebellum,

---

Pelvic Organ Dysfunction in Neurological Disease: Clinical Management and Rehabilitation, ed. Clare J. Fowler, Jalesh N. Panicker & Anton Emmanuel. Published by Cambridge University Press. © Cambridge University Press 2010.

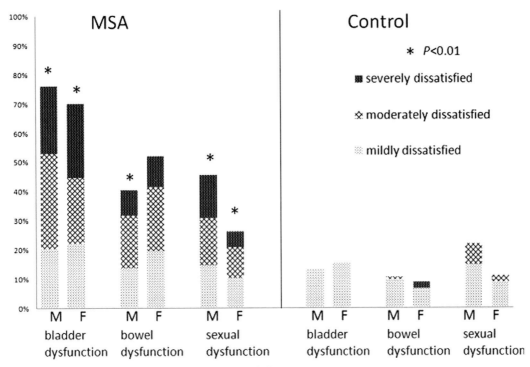

Fig. 13.1. Pelvic organ dysfunction affecting the quality of life.

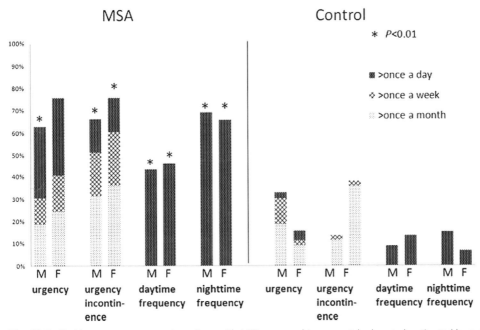

Fig. 13.2. Bladder storage symptoms in patients with MSA compared to age-matched controls estimated by questionnaire.

and to a lesser extent in the ponto-medullary raphe ("pontine cross sign") and the frontal cortex. [11, 12]. Many of these regions have been shown to be involved in the central neural control of the bladder (Chapter 1). A single photon emission computed tomography (SPECT) study showed that in the bladder full and

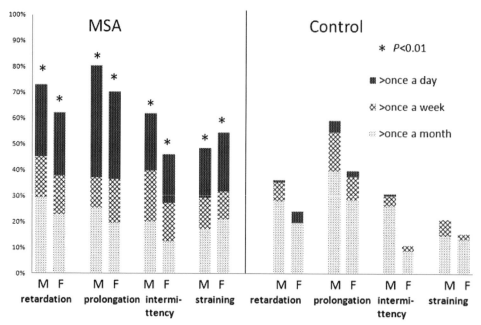

Fig. 13.3. Voiding symptoms in patients with MSA were significantly worse than age-matched controls. They had a significantly higher prevalence of voiding symptoms, particularly retardation in initiating urination (hesitancy) than the controls.

micturition phases, but not bladder empty, activation of the cerebellar vermis was significantly lower in MSA patients than in control subjects [13].

Bladder underactivity and detrusor-sphincter dyssynergia causing incomplete bladder emptying

Incomplete bladder emptying is a significant feature of MSA and worsens with progression of the illness. A study which measured the post-void residual (PVR) volume in a large number of patients with MSA found that the mean value was 71 ml in the first year after the onset of illness, 129 ml in the second year (which exceeded the threshold volume for the start of clean intermittent catheterization), and 170 ml in the fifth year (Fig. 13.4) [14]. It has been suggested that the finding of a raised PVR volume is a useful discriminator in the differential diagnosis of MSA and PD [15].

The underlying mechanisms for incomplete bladder emptying include impaired detrusor contraction and urethral obstruction due to detrusor-sphincter dyssynergia. Poor detrusor contraction has been found to be more common in MSA (71% in women and 63% in men) than in PD (66% in women and 40% in men) [10], but outflow obstruction as indicated by an Abrams-Griffiths (AG) number >40 was less

common in patients with MSA (12 in women and 28 in men) than in those with PD (40 in women and 43 in men) [10]. However, there is a subset of patients with MSA who have an obstructive pattern presumably due to detrusor-sphincter dyssynergia. There is also a group of patients with MSA who have detrusor overactivity during storage but underactivity during voiding [16]. The exact mechanisms underlying this phenomenon have yet to be ascertained but it may reflect the fact that the central mechanisms for bladder filling and voiding are distinct from each other (Chapter 1) and both systems may be involved in the pathology of MSA.

Open bladder neck

The bladder neck, also known as the internal (smooth) urethral sphincter, is an important component in the maintenance of continence and receives sympathetic innervation from the hypogastric nerve. In MSA the intermediolateral (IML) cell columns in the thoracic cord which convey the descending sympathetic innervation are frequently involved by the pathology of MSA and it is the resulting deficit which is thought to underlie the postural hypotension, as well as the open bladder neck, which are features of this condition [7]. In another early study an open

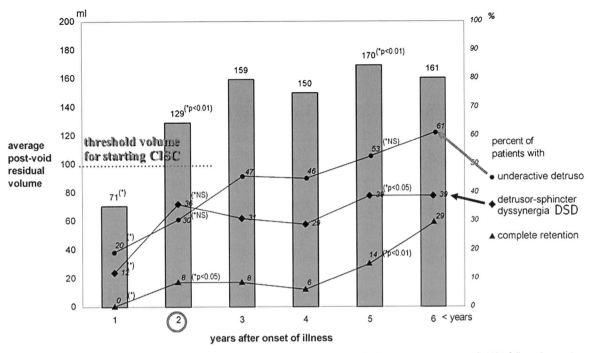

Fig. 13.4. Incomplete bladder emptying as shown by the average post-void residual volume in 245 patients with MSA followed over six years. The post-void residual volume in MSA patients exceeded 100 ml (the threshold volume for the start of clean intermittent self-catheterization (CISC)) in the second year. It appears that an underactive detrusor is the major factor contributing to a large residual volume.

bladder neck was found in all five patients who had cystometry [8]. Most recently, an open bladder neck at the start of bladder filling without the accompanying bladder overactivity was not found in any patients with PD but was found in 53% of those with MSA ($p<0.01$) [10]. An open bladder neck may be asymptomatic in women, but, in combination with the other disorders of bladder function seen in MSA, may contribute to incontinence.

Neurogenic changes in sphincter electromyography (EMG)

The group of anterior horn cells in the sacral spinal cord, which project fibers to the external sphincters, were first described by Onufrowicz in 1900 and hence became known as "Onuf's nuclei." Postmortem studies in patients dying with MSA demonstrated a selective loss of anterior horn cells in Onuf's nuclei whereas this was spared in those with amyotrophic lateral sclerosis [17]. Since in PD the anterior horn cells of Onuf's nuclei are spared [18], sphincter EMG was proposed as a valuable means of distinguishing between MSA-P and PD [19, 20], although others

have not found the technique valuable [21]. It appears that the sensitivity of the test is highly dependent on the exact method that is used and that automated methods for capturing individual motor units tend to "truncate" the satellites of the long-duration, reinnervated motor units that are so characteristic of this condition. An abnormal result with prolonged mean duration is only found if the "total MUP duration" is included [22].

A study which examined the neurogenic changes in the anal sphincter motor units in patients with MSA found abnormalities in 52% in the first year, which increased to 83% in the fifth year from the onset of illness [23]. This confirmed the earlier observation that the test was increasingly likely to become abnormal as the disease progresses [9]. Although denervation can be found in the other skeletal muscles in MSA, it occurs much earlier in the external sphincter muscles [24]. The test may be abnormal in other forms of parkinsonism [23] but in a patient with the onset of a cerebellar or akinetic rigid syndrome within five years and with significant urinary symptoms, a normal result makes a diagnosis of MSA unlikely [25].

The external (striated) urethral sphincter is a critical component in the maintenance of continence and up to 40% of patients with MSA have a low resting urethral pressure [10] reflecting the sphincter weakness and further contributing to the urgency incontinence. Sphincter weakness in MSA may also result in continuous urinary incontinence, which occurs particularly in female patients [26].

Changing bladder patterns

The bethanechol test may be used to demonstrate denervation supersensitivity of the bladder. When the bladder loses its parasympathetic innervation, the postjunctional cholinergic receptor density increases so that a small dose (2.5 mg subcutaneous injection) of bethanechol results in a rise in detrusor pressure of 15 cmH$_2$O for 30 minutes' observation [27]. Repeated measurements in patients with MSA have shown that cystometric changes occur with progression of the disease and that the bethanechol test changes from negative to positive [28]. Clinically this is reflected in a change of symptoms from urinary urgency and frequency to symptoms due to worsening of incomplete bladder emptying [14]. Together these findings suggest that the responsible neuropathology underlying bladder dysfunction changes from being "central" to "peripheral" during the course of the illness. Since MSA primarily affects the preganglionic neurons in the autonomic nervous system, these bladder findings suggest that postganglionic lesions may reflect transsynaptic degeneration of the cholinergic fibers.

With the evolution of the pathological changes in the course of MSA, bladder emptying becomes most dominant, so that if patients are performing clean intermittent self-catheterization they may become increasingly reliant on that technique but their tendency to incontinence diminishes. Thus the patient may find that their bladder symptomatically improves at a time when they are neurologically deteriorating; indeed bladder control is the only aspect of this condition that may "get better" with progression.

Autonomic and motor disorders in MSA

It is important to avoid inappropriate urological surgery in patients with MSA and the neurological basis for bladder symptoms may be missed in the early stages of the disease. Approximately 60% of patients with MSA develop urinary symptoms either prior to or at the time of presentation with a motor disorder [28, 29] (Fig. 13.5) so that many of the patients seek urological advice early in the course of their disease. Since incontinence can be severe, surgical intervention may be considered and male patients with MSA undergo urological surgery for prostatic outflow obstruction with an almost inevitable poor outcome. Urologists have been cautioned to consider carefully the advisability of surgical intervention in patients with early parkinsonism or ataxic features and incontinence [5]. Furthermore these patients generally respond well to medical management [29]. Neurologists encountering a patient with marked urinary symptoms and an early movement disorder might consider future investigation by brain MRI and sphincter EMG.

Differential diagnosis of PD and MSA-P

A careful analysis of bladder abnormalities can be helpful in distinguishing between MSA-P and PD, because although DO causing urgency and frequency occurs in both conditions, patients with MSA are more likely to have a high (>100 ml) PVR [14, 15], detrusor-sphincter dyssynergia and an open bladder neck at the start of bladder filling on videocystometrogram [10] and a neurogenic EMG of the anal sphincter [7, 19, 20]. Urinary dysfunction is almost never the initial presentation in PD and in general bladder symptoms should usually only be attributed to PD in the later stages of that condition, after treatment of more than 10 years (see Chapter 12).

Although there has been a tendency to group bladder dysfunction and postural hypotension together as symptoms of "autonomic failure," retrospective studies have shown that urinary symptoms (96%) are more common than symptoms of orthostatic hypotension (43%) (p<0.01) [28] (Fig. 13.6) and occur earlier [30]. Furthermore, in 53 patients with MSA, bladder symptoms were the initial symptoms in 48% whereas orthostatic symptoms occurred first in 29%. In 23% the onset of both symptoms was considered to be simultaneous [28]. In no patient were there symptoms of orthostatic hypotension without bladder symptoms. In another retrospective study, bladder symptoms preceded symptoms of orthostatic hypotension in 76% of male patients [31]. Since a *single* feature of "autonomic failure" is a requirement for the diagnosis of probable MSA [1], postural hypotension

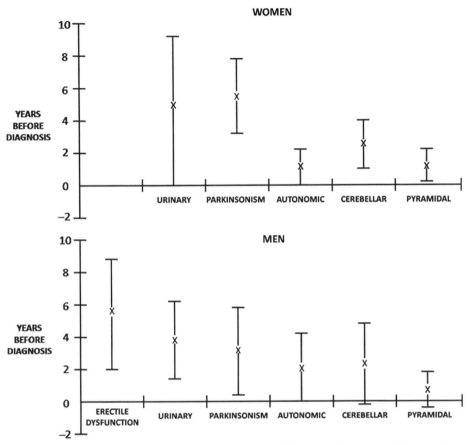

Fig. 13.5. Retrospective analysis of duration (average + 2 standard deviations) of symptoms before the diagnosis of multiple system atrophy. Based on [29], with permission.

becomes less critical for the diagnosis of the disease in its early stages.

Management

Treatment of DO

In the early stages of their disease patients should be offered oral antimuscarinics (Chapter 6) to control DO after measurement of the PVR (Chapter 4). There is very little published data to date on the use of detrusor injection of Botox in patients with MSA but in cases where oral antimuscarinic medication proves insufficiently effective, this would seem to be a reasonable option. As the disease progresses, clean intermittent self-catheterization may become increasingly important but those unable to manage the technique are helped by an indwelling catheter [32]. Recurrent urinary tract infections are a major cause of morbidity in patients with MSA and about 25% die of complications related to them [33].

Other medications

Since incomplete bladder emptying in patients with MSA is due mostly to bladder underactivity, drugs acting on outflow obstruction are unlikely to benefit all patients. However, occasionally α-adrenergic blockers may be effective in lessening PVR volumes [34]. It is, however, important to use "uro-selective" blockers such as tamsulosin and naftopidil to reduce the risk of developing or exacerbating existing postural hypotension.

Some recent research has suggested that pyridostigmine may be effective in lessening PVR volumes and postural hypotension, presumably by enhancing nicotinic acetylcholine receptor transmission in the sympathetic ganglia [35].

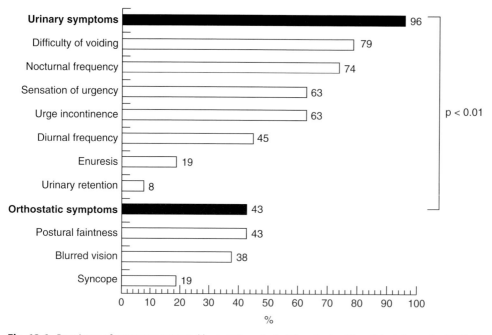

Fig. 13.6. Prevalence of symptoms estimated by questionnaire in 121 patients with a clinical diagnosis of MSA. From [28], with permission.

Desmopressin may be particularly effective in treating night-time frequency in patients with MSA because these patients develop a vasopressin deficiency, secondary to degeneration of arginine vasopressin-secreting neurones in the suprachiasmatic nucleus [36–38]. Obstructive sleep apnea may also exacerbate nocturnal polyuria. Desmopressin has been found to be effective in treating postural hypotension [39] as well as reducing nocturnal polyuria. In the elderly this should be used with caution because of their risk of hyponatremia or cardiac failure.

Many patients with postural hypotension are treated with α-agonists such as midodrine or amezinium, medications which theoretically increase bladder neck outflow and thus impair emptying.

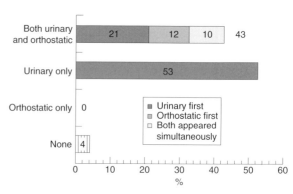

Fig. 13.7. A retrospective questionnaire survey of urinary and orthostatic symptoms in patients with MSA at the time of presentation, i.e. 0.5–2 years after the onset of their disease in most cases.

Bowel dysfunction

Mechanisms underlying the bowel dysfunction of MSA include prolonged colonic transit, weak spontaneous phasic rectal contraction (rectal propulsive activity), weak strain and paradoxical sphincter contraction on defecation (PSCD or anismus), abnormalities which are also seen in PD. The anorectal dysfunction that affects disproportionately more patients with MSA is fecal incontinence, possibly reflecting degeneration in the sacral Onuf's nucleus.

Bowel symptoms

A recent questionnaire survey by Yamamoto and colleagues of 256 patients with MSA compared with 158 age-matched controls [6] found that the MSA patients had significantly higher prevalence of difficulty in expulsion of feces (66% in men, 59% in women) (Fig. 13.8). Constipation was an equal problem for both groups but fecal incontinence was significantly more common in the female MSA group. Constipation and fecal incontinence were found to

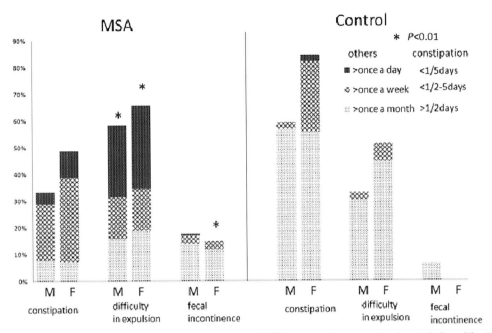

Fig. 13.8. Prevalence of bowel symptoms in patients with MSA compared to age-matched controls. From [6], with permission.

worsen the QOL in patients with MSA, as well as that of their caregivers.

Bowel dysfunction in MSA

Prolonged colonic transit

In a colonic transit time (CTT) study of 15 patients with MSA (10 men and 5 women; mean age 63.5 years; mean duration of disease 3 years) and 10 age-matched control subjects, those with MSA had more prolonged right and left CTT than control subjects, though these differences did not reach the statistical significance [40] (Table 13.1 and Fig. 13.9). However, the rectosigmoid CTT of 38.2 hours and total CTT of 71.8 hours in the patients with MSA were significantly prolonged compared to control subjects (18.0 hours and 39.0 hours, respectively). In the control subjects transit time was also longest in the rectosigmoid segment so the extreme prolongation in this segment in MSA may simply reflect proportionate slowing or there may be additional pathology affecting motility in this segment. A similar prolonged CTT has also been seen in PD [18] which may represent an artefact of the measurement technique in that rectal evacuatory function is reflected as delayed distal colonic transit. Alternatively, it may reflect a real reduction in contraction of colonic smooth muscle, and in both MSA and PD this is likely to reflect both central

Table 13.1. Colonic transit time study and the times taken in each segment

	MSA	control	p-value	PD*
Total	71.8	39.0	<0.05	82.4
Right	11.2	6.9	NS	28.8
Left	22.2	14.1	NS	20.5
Rectosigmoid	38.2	18.0	<0.05	34.0

and peripheral pathology. Sites of relevant central nervous system pathology include centers in the pons [41] and pre- and postganglionic autonomic fibers in the intrinsic myenteric nerve plexus (Auerbach's plexus) [40].

Weak sphincter

Anal sphincter EMG has been found to show changes of denervation and reinnervation causing prolongation of the mean duration of individual motor units in 75–100% of patients with MSA [23, 25], reflecting the loss of anterior horn cells that occurs in Onuf's nucleus in MSA [17]. Patients with MSA had a significantly lower anal squeeze pressure than control subjects (p<0.01) (Table 13.1) [40, 42], in contrast to patients with PD in whom such changes were rarely observed except during "off" periods in patients

213

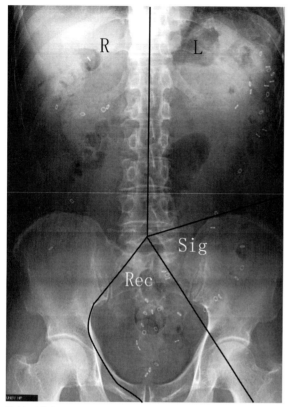

Table 13.1

	MSA	control	p-value	PD*
total	71.8	39	<0.05	82.4
right	11.2	6.9	NS	28.8
left	22.2	14.1	NS	20.5
rectosigmoid	38.2	18	<0.05	34

Fig. 13.9. Colonic transit time study and the times taken in each segment shown in Table 13.1 for patients with MSA, controls

with a long disease duration [43]. Thus, external sphincter denervation and weakness appears to be a significant factor for fecal incontinence in MSA.

Weak spontaneous phasic rectal contraction

During rectal filling, the amplitude of the phasic rectal contraction in MSA patients was small (p<0.01) (Fig. 13.10 and Table 13.2) [40]. The reduced phasic rectal contractions may share the same pathogenesis as the slowed CTT.

Whereas in controls there is a close correlation between an increase in rectal pressure and decrease in anal pressure, resembling the recto-anal inhibitory

reflex (Chapter 2), in patients with MSA both rectal and anal pressures tended to increase together. This resembles PSCD or anismus, already discussed in Chapter 12. However it seems more likely that the fecal incontinence which occurs is patients with advanced MSA is due to sphincter denervation.

Impaired defecation

Both rectal contraction and abdominal strain on attempts at defecation in patients with MSA were abnormally reduced and the patients had a less pronounced increase in abdominal pressure on coughing than that in control subjects (p<0.01) (Table 13.2). This impairment may be due to general axial rigidity as well as a failure of coordinated glottis closure in MSA.

Management

Polyethylene glycol 3350, an osmotic agent with high water-binding capacity, was shown to improve stool frequency and reduce difficulty with defecation in two patients with MSA [44], while calcium polycarbophil, an osmotic and bulking agent, was found to reduce total and right segment CTT significantly in four patients with MSA [45]. Mosapride citrate, a novel selective 5-HT4 receptor agonist, reduced total and rectosigmoid segment CTT, as well as reducing first sensation and augmenting the amplitude of phasic rectal contractions in seven patients with MSA [46]. Similar results were obtained in a study in which a Japanese dietary herb extract, Dai-Kenchu-To, an active component of which is 5-HT3 receptor agonist, was prescribed [47]. Other general measures for managing neurogenic bowel disorders are described in Chapter 8.

Sexual dysfunction

Sexual dysfunction may be a premonitory symptom in MSA, often preceding urinary symptoms and sometimes occurring several years before any motor symptoms (Fig. 13.5) [29].

Sexual symptoms

In the questionnaire survey by Yamamoto and colleagues, already referred to in the earlier sections of this chapter [6], the differences between the patient and control group for aspects of sexual function (Fig. 13.11A) were significant (p<0.01), although this did not impact on QOL as greatly as bladder

Table 13.2. Results of anorectal videomanometry in patients with MSA and PD compared to age-matched controls [40]

		MSA	control	p-value	PD*
resting phase					
anal pressure (cmH$_2$O)	rest	51.1	63.8	NS	48.4
	squeeze	38.8	96.1	<0.01	88.3
abdominal pressure (cmH$_2$O)	strain	42.2	71.0	NS	29.2
	cough	41.5	98.4	<0.01	62.9
storage phase					
first sensation (ml)		125.4	127.8	NS	131.1
maximum capacity (ml)		337.4	302.2	NS	345.6
rectal compliance (ml/cmH$_2$O)		84.2	69.3	NS	73.1
phasic rectal contraction (cmH$_2$O)		10.2	22.2	<0.01	12.2
anal contraction (cmH$_2$O)		11.7	−11.2	NS	14.4
defecation phase					
rectal contraction (cmH$_2$O)		2.9	11.1	NS	4.4
anal contraction (cmH$_2$O)		29.5	19.6	NS	49.6
abdominal pressure (cmH$_2$O)		49.8	67.3	NS	53.9
residual feces (ml)		92	15	<0.05	133

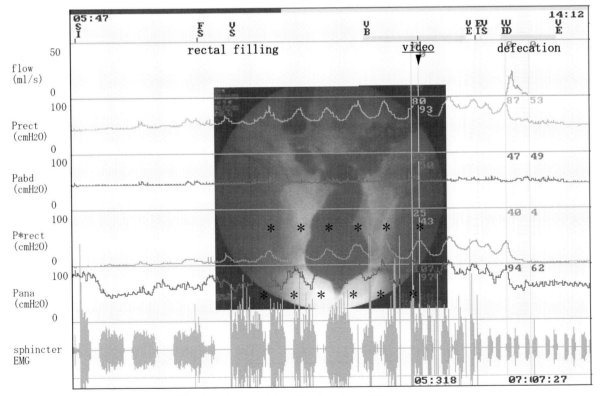

Fig. 13.10. Videomanometry – rectal filling in health. See plate section for color version.

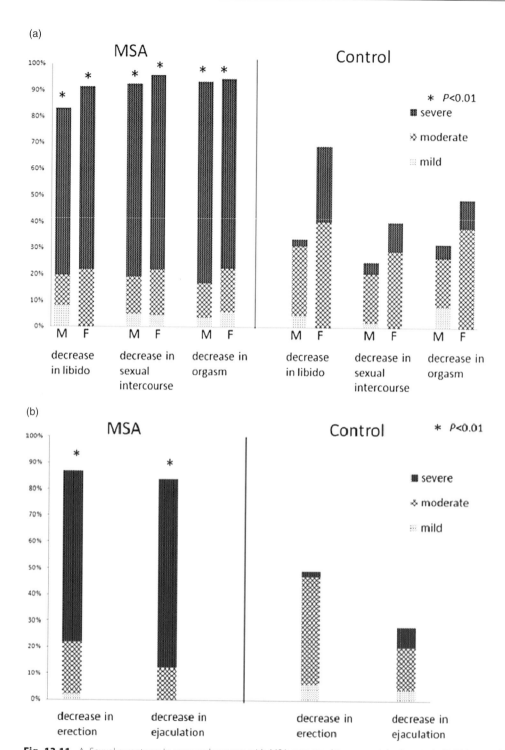

Fig. 13.11. A. Sexual symptoms in men and women with MSA compared to age-matched controls. B. Male sexual symptoms.

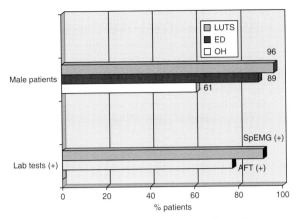

Fig. 13.12. Lower urinary tract symptoms (LUTS), erectile dysfunction (ED) and orthostatic hypotension (OH) in MSA. SpEMG: sphincter EMG; AFT: autonomic function test.

dysfunction (see Fig. 13.1). The patients with MSA had a marked decrease in libido (92% of men, 84% of women), reduction in frequency of sexual intercourse (95%, 92%), decrease in orgasm (93%, 94%) (Fig. 13.11A) and in men, problems with erection (88%) and ejaculation (84%) (Fig. 13.11B). The findings of this survey were in keeping with the results of earlier studies of sexual dysfunction in MSA [29, 31].

It was previously thought that the ED that is such a common problem in men with MSA was associated with hypotension but a retrospective study showed this was not the case: in 71 men with MSA the onset of ED had preceded the onset of bladder symptoms in 58% and the onset of symptoms of orthostatic hypotension in 91% (Fig. 13.12) [31]. By contrast, urogenital symptoms are almost never the initial presentation in PD.

Female sexual dysfunction with MSA has been little scrutinized but in a study of women with MSA-P, PD and healthy controls, 47% of the MSA patients admitted to "reduced genital sensitivity" but only 4% of the PD patients and 4% of the control group did so. Furthermore, the appearance of reduced genital sensitivity in female MSA patients showed a close temporal relation to the onset of the disease [48].

Sexual dysfunction in MSA

The pathophysiology underlying the early occurrence of sexual dysfunction in MSA is not yet known but loss of dopaminergic neurons in the paraventricular hypothalamic region or the intermediolateral cell columns is a potential cause [49].

That erectile responses can be restored in men with MSA through treatment with sildenafil citrate, a peripheral phosphodiesterase-5 inhibitor [50], suggests a central etiology. Some men with MSA have mild hyperprolactinemia [51], which may be a contributing factor. Since ED occurs so early in the course of this disease it will be important to understand its neurological basis better, both because the explanations might give clues as to the cause of this progressive degenerative disease and because if a neuroprotective treatment is discovered it will be most effective if given early.

Management

A study of six men with MSA showed that in those with pre-existing postural hypotension, sildenafil citrate exacerbated this disorder to a potentially dangerous degree, whereas those without postural hypotension did not show the same changes [50]. From this, the recommendation arose that lying and standing blood pressure should be checked in men with parkinsonism before prescribing oral phosphodiesterase-5 inhibitors. Furthermore it would seem preferable to use the shorter-acting phosphodiesterase-5 inhibitors sildenafil or vardenafil in MSA rather than tadalafil, which has a half-life of 18 hours (see Chapter 10).

Two patients with MSA, amongst a larger group of 13 men with PD, have been described who developed hypersexuality within 8 months of starting a dopamine agonist, together with additional compulsive or addictive behaviors in 9 [52].

References

1. Gilman S, Wenning GK, Low PA, et al. Second consensus statement on the diagnosis of multiple system atrophy. *Neurology* 2008;**71**:670–6.

2. Papp MI, Kahn JE, Lantos PL. Glial cytoplasmic inclusions in the CNS of patients with multiple system atrophy (striatonigral degeneration, olivopontocerebellar atrophy and Shy-Drager syndrome). *J Neurol Sci* 1989;**94**:79–100.

3. Ozawa T, Paviour D, Quinn NP, et al. The spectrum of pathological involvement of the striatonigral and olivopontocerebellar systems in multiple system atrophy: clinicopathological correlations. *Brain* 2004;**127**(Pt 12):2657–71.

4. Quinn N. Parkinsonism – recognition and differential diagnosis. *BMJ* 1995;**310**:447–52.

5. Chandiramani VA, Palace J, Fowler CJ. How to recognize patients with parkinsonism who should not have urological surgery. *Br J Urol* 1997;**80**:100–4.

6. Yamamoto T, Sakakibara R, Uchiyama T, et al. Questionnaire-based assessment of pelvic organ dysfunction in multiple system atrophy. *Mov Disord* 2009;**24**:972–8.

7. Kirby R, Fowler C, Gosling J, Bannister R. Urethro-vesical dysfunction in progressive autonomic failure with multiple system atrophy. *J Neurol Neurosurg Psychiatry* 1986;**49**:554–562.

8. Salinas JM, Berger Y, De La Rocha RE, Blaivas JG. Urological evaluation in the Shy Drager syndrome. *J Urol* 1986;**135**:741–3.

9. Stocchi F, Carbone A, Inghilleri M, et al. Urodynamic and neurophysiological evaluation in Parkinson's disease and multiple system atrophy. *J Neurol Neurosurg Psychiatry* 1997;**62**:507–11.

10. Sakakibara R, Hattori T, Uchiyama T, Yamanishi T. Videourodynamic and sphincter motor unit potential analyses in Parkinson's disease and multiple system atrophy. *J Neurol Neurosurg Psychiatry* 2001;**71**:600–6.

11. Yoshida M. Multiple system atrophy: alpha-synuclein and neuronal degeneration. *Neuropathology* 2007;**27**:484–93.

12. Benarroch EE, Schmeichel AM, Low PA, Parisi JE. Involvement of medullary serotonergic groups in multiple system atrophy. *Ann Neurol* 2004;**55**:418–22.

13. Sakakibara R, Uchida Y, Uchiyama T, Yamanishi T, Hattori T. Reduced cerebellar vermis activation during urinary storage and micturition in multiple system atrophy: 99mTc-labelled ECD SPECT study. *Eur J Neurol* 2004;**11**:705–8.

14. Ito T, Sakakibara R, Yasuda K, et al. Incomplete emptying and urinary retention in multiple-system atrophy: when does it occur and how do we manage it? *Mov Disord* 2006;**21**:816–23.

15. Hahn K, Ebersbach G. Sonographic assessment of urinary retention in multiple system atrophy and idiopathic Parkinson's disease. *Mov Disord* 2005;**20**:1499–502.

16. Yamamoto T, Sakakibara R, Uchiyama T, et al. Neurological diseases that cause detrusor hyperactivity with impaired contractile function. *Neurourol Urodyn* 2006;**25**:356–60.

17. Mannen T, Iwata M, Toyokura Y, Nagashima K. The Onuf's nucleus and the external anal sphincter muscle in ALS and Shy-Drager syndrome. *Acta Neuropathol* 1982;**58**:255–60.

18. Sakakibara R, Uchiyama T, Yamanishi T, Shirai K, Hattori T. Bladder and bowel dysfunction in Parkinson's disease. *J Neural Transm* 2008;**115**:443–60.

19. Palace J, Chandiramani VA, Fowler CJ. Value of sphincter electromyography in the diagnosis of multiple system atrophy. *Muscle Nerve* 1997;**20**:1396–403.

20. Tison F, Arne P, Sourgen C, Chrysostome V, Yeklef F. The value of external anal sphincter electromyography for the diagnsosis of multiple system atrophy. *Mov Disord* 2000;**15**:1148–57.

21. Giladi N, Simon ES, Korczyn AD, et al. Anal sphincter EMG does not distinguish between multiple system atrophy and parkinson's disease. *Muscle Nerve* 2000;**23**:731–4.

22. Podnar S, Fowler CJ. Sphincter electromyography in diagnosis of multiple system atrophy: technical issues. *Muscle Nerve* 2004;**29**:151–6.

23. Sakakibara R, Uchiyama T, Yamanishi T, Kishi M. Sphincter EMG as a diagnostic tool in autonomic disorders. *Clin Auton Res* 2009;**19**:20–31.

24. Pramstaller PP, Wenning GK, Smith SJ, et al. Nerve conduction studies, skeletal muscle EMG, and sphincter EMG in multiple system atrophy. *J Neurol Neurosurg Psychiatry* 1995;**58**:618–21.

25. Paviour DC, Williams D, Fowler CJ, Quinn NP, Lees AJ. Is sphincter electromyography a helpful investigation in the diagnosis of multiple system atrophy? A retrospective study with pathological diagnosis. *Mov Disord* 2005;**20**:1425–30.

26. Mashidori T, Yamanishi T, Yoshida K, et al. Continuous urinary incontinence presenting as the initial symptoms demonstrating acontractile detrusor and intrinsic sphincter deficiency in multiple system atrophy. *Int J Urol* 2007;**14**:972–4.

27. Lapides J, Friend CR, Ajemian EP, Reus WF. A new method for diagnosing the neurogenic bladder. *Med Bull (Ann Arbor)* 1962;**28**:166–80.

28. Sakakibara R, Hattori T, Uchiyama T, et al. Urinary dysfunction and orthostatic hypotension in multiple system atrophy: which is the more common and earlier manifestation? *J Neurol Neurosurg Psychiatry* 2000;**68**:65–9.

29. Beck RO, Betts CD, Fowler CJ. Genitourinary dysfunction in multiple system atrophy: clinical features and treatment in 62 cases. *J Urol* 1994;**151**:1336–41.

30. Wenning GK, Scherfler C, Granata R, et al. Time course of symptomatic orthostatic hypotension and urinary incontinence in patients with postmortem confirmed parkinsonian syndromes: a clinicopathological study. *J Neurol Neurosurg Psychiatry* 1999;**67**:620–3.

31. Kirchhof K, Apostolidis AN, Mathias CJ, Fowler CJ. Erectile and urinary dysfunction may be the presenting

features in patients with multiple system atrophy: a retrospective study. *Int J Impot Res* 2003;**15**:293–8.

32. Papatsoris AG, Papapetropoulos S, Singer C, Deliveliotis C. Urinary and erectile dysfunction in multiple system atrophy (MSA). *Neurourol Urodyn* 2008;**27**:22–7.

33. Papapetropoulos S, Tuchman A, Laufer D, et al. Causes of death in multiple system atrophy. *J Neurol Neurosurg Psychiatry* 2007;**78**:327–9.

34. Sakakibara R, Hattori T, Uchiyama T, et al. Are alpha-blockers involved in lower urinary tract dysfunction in multiple system atrophy? A comparison of prazosin and moxisylyte. *J Auton Nerv Syst* 2000;**79**:191–5.

35. Yamamoto T, Sakakibara R, Yamanaka Y, et al. Pyridostigmine in autonomic failure: can we treat postural hypotension and bladder dysfunction with one drug? *Clin Auton Res* 2006;**16**:296–8.

36. Ozawa T, Tanaka H, Nakano R, et al. Nocturnal decrease in vasopressin secretion into plasma in patients with multiple system atrophy. *J Neurol Neurosurg Psychiatry* 1999;**67**:542–5.

37. Sakakibara R, Matsuda S, Uchiyama T, et al. The effect of intranasal desmopressin on nocturnal waking in urination in multiple system atrophy patients with nocturnal polyuria. *Clin Auton Res* 2003;**13**:106–8.

38. Benarroch EE, Schmeichel AM, Sandroni P, Low PA, Parisi JE. Differential involvement of hypothalamic vasopressin neurons in multiple system atrophy. *Brain* 2006;**129**(Pt 10):2688–96.

39. Mathias CJ, Fosbraey P, da Costa DF, Thornley A, Bannister R. The effect of desmopressin on nocturnal polyuria, overnight weight loss, and morning postural hypotension in patients with autonomic failure. *Br Med J (Clin Res Ed)* 1986;**293**:353–4.

40. Sakakibara R, Odaka T, Uchiyama T, et al. Colonic transit time, sphincter EMG, and rectoanal videomanometry in multiple system atrophy. *Mov Disord* 2004;**19**:924–9.

41. Valentino RJ, Miselis RR, Pavcovich LA. Pontine regulation of pelvic viscera: pharmacological target for pelvic visceral dysfunctions. *Trends Pharmacol Sci* 1999;**20**:253–60.

42. Stocchi F, Badiali D, Vacca L, et al. Anorectal function in multiple system atrophy and Parkinson's disease. *Mov Disord* 2000;**15**:71–6.

43. Ashraf W, Wszolek ZK, Pfeiffer RF, et al. Anorectal function in fluctuating (on-off) Parkinson's disease: evaluation by combined anorectal manometry and electromyography. *Mov Disord* 1995;**10**:650–7.

44. Eichhorn TE, Oertel WH. Macrogol 3350/electrolyte improves constipation in Parkinson's disease and multiple system atrophy. *Mov Disord* 2001;**16**:1176–7.

45. Sakakibara R, Yamaguchi T, Uchiyama T, et al. Calcium polycarbophil improves constipation in primary autonomic failure and multiple system atrophy subjects. *Mov Disord* 2007;**22**:1672–3.

46. Liu Z, Sakakibara R, Odaka T, et al. Mosapride citrate, a novel 5-HT4 agonist and partial 5-HT3 antagonist, ameliorates constipation in parkinsonian patients. *Mov Disord* 2005;**20**:680–6.

47. Sakakibara R, Odaka T, Lui Z, et al. Dietary herb extract dai-kenchu-to ameliorates constipation in parkinsonian patients (Parkinson's disease and multiple system atrophy). *Mov Disord* 2005;**20**:261–2.

48. Oertel WH, Wachter T, Quinn NP, Ulm G, Brandstadter D. Reduced genital sensitivity in female patients with multiple system atrophy of parkinsonian type. *Mov Disord* 2003;**18**:430–2.

49. Dominguez JM, Hull EM. Dopamine, the medial preoptic area, and male sexual behavior. *Physiol Behav* 2005;**86**:356–68.

50. Hussain IF, Brady CM, Swinn MJ, Mathias CJ, Fowler CJ. Treatment of erectile dysfunction with sildenafil citrate (Viagra) in parkinsonism due to Parkinson's disease or multiple system atrophy with observations on orthostatic hypotension. *J Neurol Neurosurg Psychiatry* 2001;**71**:371–4.

51. Winkler AS, Landau S, Chaudhuri KR. Serum prolactin levels in Parkinson's disease and multiple system atrophy. *Clin Auton Res* 2002;**12**:393–8.

52. Klos KJ, Bower JH, Josephs KA, Matsumoto JY, Ahlskog JE. Pathological hypersexuality predominantly linked to adjuvant dopamine agonist therapy in Parkinson's disease and multiple system atrophy. *Parkinsonism Relat Disord* 2005;**11**:381–6.

Multiple sclerosis and other non-compressive myelopathies

Catherine M. Dalton, Giuseppi Preziosi, Shahid Khan and Marianne de Sèze

Introduction

Multiple sclerosis (MS) is the most common progressive neurological disorder of young people, affecting around 100,000 people in the United Kingdom [1], with a prevalence of 163.7 per 100,000. However the highest prevalence is in Scotland, where in the Orkney Islands it reaches 220 per 100,000 [2].

MS is a chronic inflammatory demyelinating disease of the central nervous system, characterized by the sustained autoimmune response of aggressive T-cells which disrupt the myelin sheaths in the central nervous system, causing focal demyelinating plaques in the white matter and finally gliosis. According to the clinical course, four subtypes have been identified. Relapsing remitting MS (RRMS) is the most common type (85% of patients) but nearly half of these patients convert to secondary progressive MS (SPMS) over a median time period of 11 years [3]. About 10% of patients may have progressive symptoms from the onset (primary progressive MS; PPMS) and a minority have progressive relapsing MS (PRMS) [4]. Pathologically, RRMS is characterized by new and active focal inflammatory demyelinating lesions in the white matter while diffuse injury of the normal appearing white matter, cortical demyelination and axonal loss are characteristic of PPMS and SPMS [5, 6]. Recent studies have suggested that inflammation is also the driving force in progressive MS although anti-inflammatory and immunomodulatory therapies do not appear to have a significant effect on this [7].

The accumulation and progression of disability is often measured using the Kurtzke expanded disability status scale (EDSS) which ranges from 0–10, the score being largely determined after EDSS Level 4 by loss of mobility [8]. The rating for bladder dysfunction in this scale is not satisfactory since it is considered together with bowel symptoms and does not recognize the effect of incomplete bladder emptying and its management as a discrete step in progression. Nevertheless the scale reflecting increasing spinal cord dysfunction is highly relevant to pelvic organ symptoms as there is, not unsurprisingly, a general correlation between worsening mobility and increasing difficulties with bladder and bowel control and sexual function. Although patients may present with bladder dysfunction early in the disease if the initial clinically isolated syndrome is due to a spinal cord lesion [9], in general bladder dysfunction is related to the duration of MS [10] and degree of pyramidal symptoms in the lower limbs [11, 12], bladder symptoms becoming more difficult to manage with increasing disability.

The sustained disability of EDSS Level 4 (at which patients can walk some 500 m without aid or rest) is thought to the herald the onset of SPMS and reflects the burden of axonal injury [13]. The mean time from disability level EDSS 4 to 6 (when there is intermittent or constant assistance required to walk 100 metres) has been estimated to be 6–8.4 years [3, 13, 14] irrespective of any factors which at the onset may have been regarded as indicative of a good prognosis. It is during this period of inexorable progression that bladder management may become particularly difficult but the surgical solutions successfully applied to patients following traumatic spinal cord injury (Chapter 15) are not suitable for those with deteriorating neurological function. Sexual dysfunction also correlates with the severity of spinal cord disease although the problems of bowel control in MS are not so clearly linked.

This chapter describes first the bladder problems which occurs in MS, then the bowel and finally sexual dysfunction, which characterize the disease, and

Pelvic Organ Dysfunction in Neurological Disease: Clinical Management and Rehabilitation, ed. Clare J. Fowler, Jalesh N. Panicker & Anton Emmanuel. Published by Cambridge University Press. © Cambridge University Press 2010.

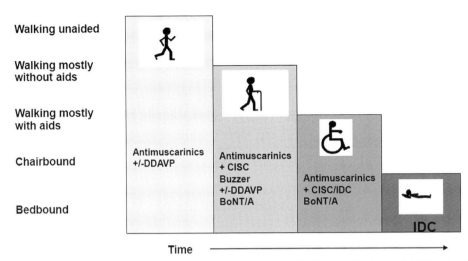

Fig. 14.1. Bladder management options with progression of disability (see text for details). BoNT/A = botulinum toxin A; "buzzer" = suprapubic vibration device; CISC = clean intermittent self-catherterization; DDAVP = desmopressin; IDC = indwelling catheter. From [12] with permission.

concludes with brief mention of the various other non-compressive diseases which may affect the spinal cord and cause pelvic organ dysfunction.

Bladder dysfunction in MS

Introduction

Estimates of the proportion of patients with MS who have lower urinary tract symptoms (LUTS) vary according to the severity of the neurological disability in the group under study, but a figure of about 75% is frequently cited [15]. The importance of this topic is demonstrated by the effect incontinence has on quality of life. Several studies have shown that urinary incontinence is considered to be one of the worst aspects of the disease, with 70% of a self-selected group of patients with MS responding to a questionnaire as classifying the impact bladder symptoms had on their life as "high" or "moderate" [16]. Urinary incontinence represents a considerable psychosocial burden to patients and their carers, while urinary tract infections (UTIs) and their complications may result in multiple hospital admissions.

Pathophysiology

The weight of clinical evidence points to the occurrence of bladder dysfunction becoming increasingly likely as the duration of the neurological illness gets longer and the level of disability increases [11, 17–19]. In most instances the severity of bladder dysfunction

is in keeping with the patient's impairment of mobility, both features reflecting the extent of spinal cord involvement. This is illustrated in Fig. 14.1.

The consequences of spinal cord disease on bladder control are outlined in Chapter 1 but essentially the problems are those of detrusor overactivity (DO) with or without detrusor sphincter dyssynergia (DSD) and incomplete bladder emptying. Cystometric studies in groups of patients with MS have found that the most frequent abnormality on filling cystometry is DO (mean occurrence 65%) followed by detrusor underactivity (mean occurrence 25%) and poor bladder compliance (2–10%). The prevalence of DSD in studies is very varied, probably due to technical difficulties in detecting abnormal sphincter contraction, but with a median prevalence of 35%, becoming more common if patients are followed up over time [20].

Symptoms

The most common bladder complaints of patients with MS are urgency, urinary frequency and urgency incontinence reflecting the underlying DO. Less commonly mentioned by patients initially at least, but often also present, are symptoms which reflect loss of voiding ability, such as hesitancy, poor stream and a feeling of incomplete bladder emptying. In fact the self-observation that the short intervals between voids ("I can pass urine and go back again five minutes later and pass the same amount") is probably more often

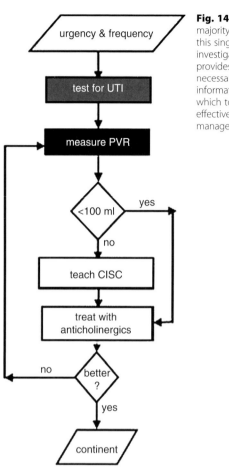

Fig. 14.2. In the majority of cases, this single investigation provides the necessary information on which to base effective management.

published in France by GENULF (Groupe d'Etudes de Neuro-Urologie de Langue Française; http://www.genulf.com/) [18] and more recently in the UK [12]. Both sets of guidelines underline the need for multidisciplinary uro-neurological long-term follow-up in MS. Ideally this should involve a urologist, neurologist, rehabilitation physician, continence advisor and the patient's carer, to define the best therapeutic options, taking both the neurological disability and patient's environment into consideration.

General measures

Inevitably, patients with overactive bladder symptoms tend to cut down on what they drink and 1.5 to 2.5 litres a day is the generally recommended intake. The amount should be individualized but an assessment of fluid balance using a voiding diary is often helpful (Chapter 4). Caffeine reduction below 100 mg/day has been shown to reduce symptoms of urgency and frequency, though not specifically in patients with MS [21].

Physical treatments

There are a number of therapeutic interventions which can be of benefit to patients with overactive bladder symptoms (Chapter 5). These are physically based and the same treatments are often offered as alternatives to oral medication in patients with symptoms of bladder overactivity of non-neurological origin. Pelvic floor exercises can enhance the inhibitory effect of pelvic floor contraction on the detrusor. Bladder retraining involves the patient voluntarily "holding on" for increasingly longer periods, often an incremental program supervised by specialist continence advisors or physiotherapists. Of course these interventions can only be expected to be effective in patients with intact neural pathways to pelvic floor muscles and an assessment of pelvic floor contractions should be made prior to initiating treatment. "Neuromuscular stimulation" has also been used in patients with MS, which involves electrically stimulating pudendal afferents with an appropriately designed stimulator, and it is thought that the resulting reflex pelvic floor contraction has the same inhibitory effect on detrusor activity as does a voluntary contraction of pelvic floor muscles. Both these procedures may be effective and there is certainly no evidence that they are harmful [22, 23].

given as evidence of voiding dysfunction than an actual sensation of persisting post-void residual urine.

Often incomplete bladder emptying and an overactive bladder co-exist, the residual urine exacerbating symptoms due to the already impaired bladder capacity. However, whereas the symptoms of an overactive bladder were found to be a reliable indicator of underlying DO, patient reports of incomplete bladder emptying are not: those patients who thought they did not empty their bladders were usually correct, but half of those who thought they did, were wrong [11]. It is for this reason that measurement of the post-void residual volume (PVR) is such a critical investigation in the management of bladder symptoms in patients with MS (Fig. 14.2).

Management

Consensus guidelines for MS bladder management and long-term urological follow-up have been

Investigations for planning management

Urine testing

Combined rapid tests of urine, "dipstick" tests, using reagent strips for urinalysis, are advisable for all patients with MS presenting with new bladder symptoms (Fig. 14.2). Their negative predictive value for excluding UTI is excellent (>98%) but their positive predictive value for confirming UTI is only 50% [24]. Hematuria should always be fully investigated (Chapter 4).

Measurement of the post-micturition residual volume

The post-micturition residual urine should be measured as part of the initial assessment and preferably before antimuscarinic treatment is started (see Fig. 14.2). Furthermore, if there is any reason to suspect a patient already established on treatment has developed incomplete emptying (either from history or from their failure to respond to antimuscarinics) or has had more than one confirmed or two suspected episodes of UTI in a period of one year, the post-micturition residual volume should be measured by ultrasound, or alternatively in-out catheterization if ultrasound is not available.

In the majority of cases, this single investigation provides the necessary information on which to base effective management.

Urodynamics

The UK consensus paper recommended that urodynamics should be carried out only in those who are refractory to conservative treatment or bothered by their symptoms and wish to undergo further interventions. This is somewhat different to the French approach in which these tests are more central in management planning [18].

"Urodynamics" (referring here to multichannel cystometry and pressure/flow studies of voiding), with or without additional synchronous fluoroscopic screening (video-urodynamics), are essential in the management of patients following spinal cord injury to ensure bladder pressures are "safe" and silent upper tract damage is not a risk (Chapter 15). Risk factors predisposing to upper tract damage in MS were identified in an evidence-based review of literature (Table 14.1) [18] but for some unknown reason,

Table 14.1. Risk factors of upper urinary tract complications in MS [18]

Definite risk factors[*]	Probable risk factors[*]
Duration of disease >15 years	Detrusor sphincter dyssynergia
Indwelling urinary catheter	Age over 50 years
High-amplitude uninhibited detrusor contractions	Male
High detrusor pressure	

Note: *Patients at risk of upper tract damage have either ≥1 definite risk factor or ≥2 probable risk factors

upper tract complications are much less common in patients with MS than in those following spinal cord injury. Although urinary sepsis, stone formation and upper tract dilatation may occur in patients with MS, this is usually in the context of advanced disease (Fig. 14.1) and rarely as a clinically silent, isolated problem. Reassuringly, there is no increase in the risk of renal failure in patients with MS compared to the general UK population [25].

Upper tract problems include infections or upper tract dilatation (8%), vesicoureteral reflux (5%) and urinary lithiasis (2% to 11%) [11, 18–20, 26–29]. Morphologic changes to the bladder wall, including diverticula, trabeculations or wall thickening are observed in 30% of patients with longstanding disease. Any patient with such complications is likely to already be under urological supervision and may well have a long-term indwelling catheter.

However, a variety of other symptoms may need to be investigated using urodynamics. For example, some women with MS will complain of stress urinary incontinence in addition to urgency incontinence and if surgical treatment is being considered, full urodynamic evaluation, ideally by videourodynamics, is necessary.

Management of impaired voiding

Clean intermittent self-catheterization (CISC)

The expert panel of the UK consensus report considered CISC to be of the greatest importance in the management of patients with neurogenic bladder dysfunction due to MS [12], although there is no formal evidence base for this. In patients with impaired voiding, a PVR more than 100 ml or more than one-third of bladder capacity is thought likely to contribute to bladder dysfunction and be the indication to learn CISC. It is recognized that a single measurement of the PVR is not representative and when possible, a series of measurements should be made over the course of one or two weeks. Moreover the figure of 100 ml is not universally agreed for the PVR at which to initiate CISC but notwithstanding it is often helpful to be able to start management based on a single figure.

The UK recommendation is that any patient with a persistent PVR in excess of 100 ml should be offered the opportunity to learn CISC. This should be taught by a urology specialist nurse or continence advisor, either in an outpatient setting or in the patient's home (see Chapter 5). Frequency of catheterization depends upon the PVR but 2–6 catheterizations per day are usually recommended, so that the maximum volume obtained is 400–500 ml.

CISC is rarely necessary in the early stages of MS but becomes increasingly likely to be needed as mobility deteriorates (Fig. 14.1). Factors that can impede a patient's ability to perform CISC include impaired manual dexterity and motivation. The ability of patients with MS to learn CISC may be influenced by the EDSS but cognitive decline seems not be a limitation [30].

Long-term indwelling catheter

If CISC is no longer possible (Fig. 14.1), a long-term indwelling catheter should be offered, preferably a suprapubic rather than urethral one (Chapters 7); progressive urethral damage is a condition too often seen in MS patients managed by indwelling urethral catheters. However, the possible hazard of bowel perforation with suprapubic catheter insertion in a patient with a small, contracted bladder should not be overlooked (Chapter 7). Choice of the type of catheter may determine the incidence of UTIs and consideration should be given to the individual's propensity for catheter blockage and encrustation (Chapter 5). Use of a catheter valve may enable intermittent bladder drainage rather than continuous drainage into a leg bag, although often DO may be so severe as to preclude this.

Other measures

Although a small study of patients with MS showed α-blocker medication reduced PVR [31], experience in clinical practice does not often show a consistent benefit with this medication. However, "diagnostic shadowing" should not be allowed to obscure the fact that men with symptoms of poor voiding may have outflow obstruction of prostatic origin. If so, they may benefit from a combination of α-blockers and 5-α-reductase inhibitors (Chapter 6) [32].

Suprapubic vibration ("buzzer") (Fig. 14.1) can help initiate detrusor contractions and improve bladder emptying in some patients with incomplete bladder emptying and DO [33], but its effect is limited.

Use of the Credé's maneuver is not recommended in patients following spinal cord injury (Chapter 15) [34]. Nothing is known about the possible long-term risks of using this in patients with MS.

Treatment of impaired storage
Antimuscarinics

There is a clinical impression that antimuscarinics (Chapter 6) are particularly effective in neurogenic DO but the data do not exist to allow a comparison of effectiveness in patients with MS to be made against those with idiopathic DO.

Often it is a combination of CISC and oral antimuscarinics that is most effective. In the presence of raised PVR, detrusor contractions will continue despite the use of antimuscarinics. Consequently, antimuscarinics may exacerbate the situation by further impairing the efficiency of bladder emptying; it is for this reason that the algorithm shown in Fig. 14.2 is recommended. The PVR should be re-checked in patients who have not responded to antimuscarinics.

There are a small number of studies which provide evidence for the efficacy of antimuscarinics in reducing incontinence, frequency and urgency, specifically in MS [35, 36]. Not all the antimuscarinics currently available (Chapter 6) have been systematically investigated and their use is often by inference of efficacy. Dual therapy (combinations of oxybutynin, tolterodine and trospium) has been shown to be effective and well tolerated in a few patients [37].

In the cognitively impaired, antimuscarinics should be prescribed with a warning for carers to be vigilant about possible deterioration in cognitive function [38] or the onset of confusion. In the absence of positive evidence, it seems sensible at this time to recommend the use of antimuscarinics which do not cross the blood–brain barrier, i.e. trospium chloride, or darifenacin, a selective blocker of the M3 receptor which is not known to be involved in cognition (Chapter 6).

Other measures

Other measures that can be used to treat the neurogenic DO of MS are discussed in Chapter 6.

Desmopressin or DDAVP (100–400 µg orally or 10–40 µg intranasally) has been shown to be of benefit in the treatment of daytime frequency or nocturia in MS [39]. However, it should be prescribed with caution and not be used more than once in 24 hours (Chapter 6).

No specific data for patients with MS exist but patients with nocturnal polyuria (i.e. more than one-third of the 24-hour urine output overnight) have been shown to have a reduction in night-time frequency if given an afternoon diuretic in a standard dosage [40]. This is particularly effective in those with dependent edema.

In patients with advanced MS and LUTS refractory to first-line treatment, sublingual spray containing delta-9-tetrahydrocannabinol (THC) and/or cannabidiol (CBD) significantly reduced urinary urgency, the number and volume of incontinence episodes, daytime frequency and nocturia [41]. In a large placebo-controlled study of 647 patients with MS, an oral cannabis extract of delta-9-THC reduced urge incontinence episodes and pad weight significantly more than the placebo drug [42]. A multicenter, double-blind, placebo-controlled trial specifically studying LUTS in patients with advanced MS used sublingual Sativex, a medicinal plant extract of cannabis. Daytime frequency, nocturia and the Patient's Global Impression of Change improved significantly in the active treatment arm and reductions were also noted in urgency and urge incontinence episodes, but not significantly better than the placebo [43].

Intravesical capsaicin significantly improved clinical and urodynamic parameters of DO in patients with spinal cord damage, including MS [44], but is unlicensed. Resiniferatoxin, a capsaicin analogue, has also been shown to improve urodynamic parameters and incontinence and appeared promising [45], but like capsaicin it is currently not licensed (Chapter 6).

Detrusor injection of botulinum toxin A

The demonstrated efficacy of detrusor injections of BoNT/A in the treatment of neurogenic DO (Chapter 6) has transformed the management of

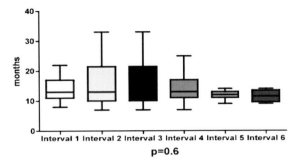

Fig. 14.3. Mean intervals between successive detrusor injections of Botox in a series of 112 patients with MS and neurogenic DO. The numbers in the later groups are relatively small but this shows that the treatment is not losing its duration of efficacy with repeated treatments.

urgency incontinence for patients with MS who have not responded adequately to antimuscarinics and CISC. Two placebo-controlled trials included a small number of patients with MS [46, 47] and an open-label study showed it was highly efficacious in improving symptoms, urodynamic parameters and quality of life [48]. That study also demonstrated almost all patients (42 out of 43) receiving this treatment needed to do CISC afterwards [48], in contrast to patients with non-neurogenic DO. However, the need for CISC did not affect the patients' estimates of improvement in quality of life.

All patients with MS should have been taught or agreed to learn to do CISC before being treated with detrusor BoNT/A. However, because this is usually only recommended for patients who have failed to respond to two or more oral antimuscarinics, many of them have already reached the stage when CISC has also become necessary (Fig. 14.1).

In our department, 112 patients with MS and intractable incontinence have so far been treated and re-treated as necessary with detrusor injections of 300 U of Botox®. Re-injections were arranged when patients reported a return of symptoms and the median duration of effect was found to be 13 months (Fig. 14.3) [49].

Importantly, patients' quality of life improved dramatically after each repeat treatment session [49] (Fig. 14.4).

Encouraging evidence is emerging that detrusor BoNT-A treatment may benefit patients with an indwelling urethral catheter and catheter bypassing [50], and may also reduce the frequency of UTIs [51]. However, at the time of writing, BoNT-A for treatment of DO is still unlicensed and it is unlikely to

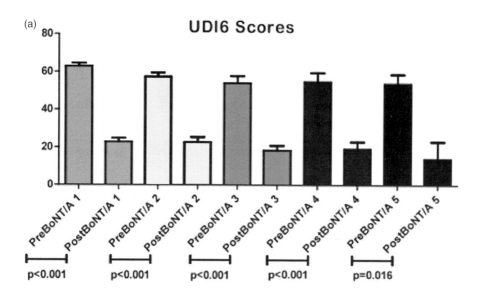

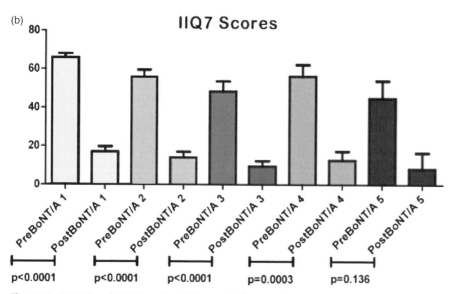

Fig. 14.4. UDI6 (A) and IIQ7 (B) quality of life scores before and after detrusor injections of BoNT-A, repeated five times.

receive regulatory approval in Europe before 2011–2012. This means that its use should only be undertaken provided national and local regulations are complied with.

Details of the method of administration are given in Chapter 6.

Surgical treatments

Sacral nerve neuromodulation has been tried in a very small number of patients with MS (13 in Europe and 13 in the United States) with limited success [52, 53] (Chapter 7). The problem has been loss of efficacy if the patient experiences a relapse of their disease. It is possible that, with the introduction of disease-modifying treatments for MS reducing the relapse rate, this intervention may become a more suitable treatment in the future.

There is no evidence that patients with MS will suffer neurological deterioration following bladder surgery. Where surgery is offered, it should be carried out in centers that regularly undertake anesthesia and surgery on MS patients.

Women with MS who suffer from stress urinary incontinence should be offered surgical treatment for this problem.

The need for surgical intervention for intractable urge incontinence appears to have diminished since the advent of botulinum toxin treatment. However, a proportion of patients will still have intractable urgency incontinence and may benefit from surgery. The use of surgical interventions is higher in France than the UK (Chapter 7). Although there is a good deal of literature relating to these techniques, it is unusual for MS patients to be singled out for separate analysis in the reporting of results.

Surgical options such as urinary diversion are guided by discussions in the setting of a multidisciplinary approach [34, 54]. Occasional patients who have been managed with long-term catheters become catheter-intolerant with frequent catheter blockages, recurrent UTIs, systemic sepsis or frequent pericatheter leakage, and some of these may benefit from urinary diversion. An ileal conduit allows for ease of practical management of urinary incontinence because bags are easily changed by the patient or carer. The procedure may be complicated by recurrent pyocystis and consideration should be given to simultaneous removal of the bladder, a simple cystectomy (Chapter 7).

Containment

A range of penile sheaths and disposable body-worn pads may be helpful for containing incontinence when other measures are unsatisfactory (see Chapter 5). Men should be assessed by an appropriately trained practitioner, be fitted with external drainage systems if needed and be reviewed on an annual basis, or sooner if clinically indicated.

Infections

Lower urinary infections are reported in 30% of patients, but true prevalence is difficult to define, owing to variability in diagnostic criteria. A high PVR and female gender are both factors which predispose to infections [29]. It is worthwhile to "dipstick" test the urine if there are unexplained changes in bladder symptoms [12]. Asymptomatic bacteriuria alone in a patient performing CISC is not an indication for antibiotic treatment, as bacteriuria is not correlated with symptomatic UTIs [55]. Antibiotic treatment should be limited to symptomatic UTIs since unrestricted use of prophylactic antibiotics can lead to antibiotic resistance.

In patients with proven recurrent UTIs, in whom no anatomical or urological abnormality has been identified and in whom the catheterization technique cannot be improved, it is reasonable to start prophylactic low-dose antibiotics [12]. Otherwise, antibiotic prophylaxis is limited only to situations where there is increased chance for complications, such as urinary tract instrumentation. Although the value of cranberry preparations in preventing UTIs is beneficial in spinal cord injury [56], its role in MS has not been fully evaluated.

Infections have been associated with MS relapses and disability measured by EDSS has been more sustained compared to exacerbations in the absence of infection [57]. During a relapse, all patients should have a urine "dipstick" test to ensure no UTI is present. Prior to steroid use for managing relapse, all treatment centers (primary care practices and hospitals) should have an internal protocol for treatment of possible infections (often using trimethoprim) until the formal culture and sensitivity is available.

Bladder cancer

The incidence of bladder cancer in MS patients is poorly documented, but may be greater than in the general population due to chronic indwelling suprapubic catheter and chemotherapeutic agents such as cyclophosphamide [58].

Follow-up review

An annual evaluation should include a bladder diary, uroflowmetry (measurement of urinary flow rate) and bladder scan. Patients doing CISC should be under the regular care of a nurse who can advise regarding the type of catheter and its use (see Chapter 5).

Increased vigilance is required to monitor risk factors for urinary tract damage (Table 14.1) and follow up patients with known upper urinary tract problems [59]. In this group, multidisciplinary urological involvement with cystoscopy is necessary with imaging including cystourethrography and functional evaluations such as urinary creatinine clearance and renal scintigraphy. Lastly, in patients with a risk for bladder cancer, regular cytology and cystoscopy are recommended.

Bowel dysfunction

Introduction

Bowel dysfunction, comprising constipation and/or fecal incontinence, affects between 39% and 73% of patients with MS [60–65]. The mechanisms are often multiple and complex. The neurological contributions are thought to include dysfunction of descending cortical modulation, and disturbed extrinsic afferent and efferent autonomic pathways [66]. Impaired mobility, altered behavioral patterns, pelvic floor dysfunction and polypharmacy may all contribute to symptom generation [67].

Bowel pathophysiology

Defecation, essentially a reflex act controlled and modulated by cortical efferents (Chapter 2), may be impaired in MS since there is disruption in neural control of the gut at both brain and spinal cord levels. At cortical level, voluntary control of bowel function may be impaired, and psychosocial behavioral disturbances occur [66, 68]. Abnormalities in the spinal cord are a common feature of progressive MS [69–72], resulting in disturbed control of colonic motility.

Motility may be altered to cause either constipation or loose stools. Interruption of the normal cortical inhibition of colonic motor activity generates high intracolonic pressures and uncontrolled peristalsis. The resulting loose or liquid stool can cause incontinence. Rectal impaction of feces and overflow may also cause incontinence in some cases. At the other extreme, disturbed colonic motility results in prolonged colonic transit time, particularly in the left colon [73–77]. The etiology of the altered colonic motility is frequently related to attenuated parasympathetic outflow. Loss of parasympathetic tone results in the twin effects of impairment of the gastrocolic reflex and interruption of normal cortical inhibition of colonic motor activity [73–75, 78]. Slowing of left colonic transit, along with reduced anorectal sensation [63, 76, 78], results in difficulty with rectal evacuation [78, 79]. A similar physiological pattern is seen in cauda equina syndrome, and hence demyelination of the conus medullaris may result in rectal evacuatory dysfunction [80].

In addition to these colonic transit changes, MS patients may have anorectal disturbances contributing to their symptoms. Weakness of the external sphincter [63, 73, 74, 81–84] is common and may contribute to fecal incontinence. It is important to remember that such disturbance may result from unrelated co-morbidity – obstetric perineal trauma, diabetes and lumbar disc prolapse [82].

Another consequence of MS-related autonomic dysfunction is reduced rectal compliance [63, 75, 76, 79] with increased basal tone [74, 78, 79]. Taken together these changes result in reduced rectal capacity, and a tendency to fecal incontinence owing to failure of reservoir function. At the other end of the spectrum, involvement of the pudendal nerve and other pelvic floor innervations may result in pelvic floor incoordination [73], paradoxical contraction of puborectalis on straining [83] and attenuation of the recto-anal inhibitory reflex [74]. These result in failure of external anal sphincter relaxation and disturbed defecation.

Finally, reduced rectal sensation reduces the urge to defecate and contributes to failure of relaxation of the pelvic floor on straining [86]. Failure of puborectalis and external anal sphincter relaxation, allied to inability to generate adequate expulsive forces, limit the ability to overcome anal resisting pressure despite a full rectum [85], and hence cause evacuatory dysfunction.

Constipation

Constipation affects up to two-thirds of patients with MS [63]. It is often accompanied by the symptom of fecal incontinence, and a typical presentation is of reduced stool frequency with varying degrees of fecal urgency. Attempts to relieve the constipation frequently precipitate incontinence. In addition to the neurological changes detailed above, other contributory factors towards constipation include immobility (associated with disease duration), presence of pelvic floor incoordination (signaled as co-morbid bladder dysfunction) and the use of medications [61, 85].

Urinary urgency and incontinence induces patients to reduce fluid intake, which dehydrates the stools, making expulsion difficult. Sometimes the quality of diet (high calorie, low fiber) may be poor. Medication for spasticity (baclofen), pain (opiates, gabapentin) and depression (tricyclic antidepressants), as well as anticholinergic drugs used for bladder dysfunction, all can lead to worsening constipation.

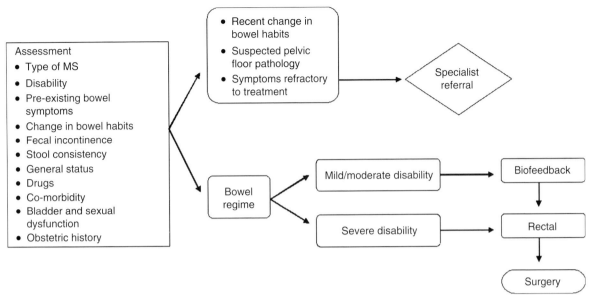

Fig. 14.5. Bowel management algorithm.

Incontinence

Fecal incontinence occurs regularly in about 25% of MS patients and occasionally in 50% [61, 62]. The involuntary loss of stools is related to lack of anorectal sensation and anal sphincter weakness [87], to which previous childbirth or age-related sphincter atrophy may be contributing factors. Dietary contributions from caffeine, sweeteners, alcohol and medications that reduce spasticity in striated muscle may be etiologically important.

Assessment

Bowel symptoms in neurological diseases should be fully evaluated to exclude co-morbidity such as ulcerative colitis, colorectal cancer, thyroid dysfunction, diabetes and anal sphincter disruption. Sudden changes in bowel habits should prompt a specialist referral to rule out primary gut pathology. Diet, degree of disability and presence of other pelvic floor symptoms should be detailed.

Anorectal physiology has a role in establishing the extent of hind-gut denervation, sphincter function and rectal compliance. Endo-anal ultrasound detects sphincter injuries, and MR or barium defecating proctography helps identify significant structural deficits of the pelvic organs and pelvic floor: rectoceles, enteroceles, rectal prolapse, pelvic floor descent and incoordination may all be detected on imaging.

Treatment

A bowel regimen should be drawn up following a simple algorithm (Fig. 14.5), escalating in a stepwise fashion and adjusted according to symptom severity [68]. This is similar to the approach described in neurogenic bowel dysfunction of any cause, discussed in detail in Chapter 8. The aim of treatment, whether the prevalent symptom is constipation or incontinence, is to achieve regular and predictable bowel motion. Input from a continence nurse has been shown to be especially effective in instigating a bowel regimen and providing support to the patient and carer [88].

Biofeedback has a specific role in managing bowel dysfunction in MS in patients with mild to moderate disability and mild alteration of anorectal function [88–90]. If biofeedback fails, or the patient is severely disabled, rectal irrigation using the Peristeen enema system (Chapter 8) can offer symptom relief. Surgical options such as sacral nerve stimulation should be contemplated if all else fails and the patient is otherwise suitable (Chapter 7). In view of the paucity of specific evidence in MS, most of the current recommendations are based on spinal cord injuries.

Conclusions

Bowel dysfunction is highly prevalent in MS and other demyelinating diseases. The neurological control of bowel function can be affected at a variety of

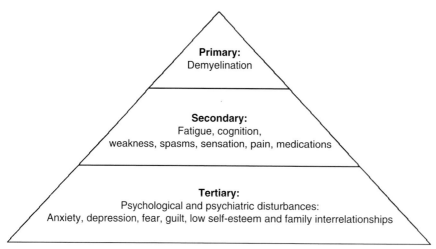

Fig. 14.6. Multifactorial causes for sexual dysfunction in MS.

different levels of the neuraxis. Reduced anorectal sensation, pelvic floor incoordination and alteration in motility secondary to the loss of autonomic (parasympathetic) outflow to the colon may all have a role in constipation and incontinence.

Full evaluation should exclude organic bowel pathology and quantify hind-gut involvement. Bowel management strategies should be simple and clear with realistic goals, involving the patient and carer to actively titrate laxatives and constipating agents. Where lifestyle modification, drugs, biofeedback and rectal irrigation have failed, surgical options should be contemplated.

Sexual dysfunction in MS
Introduction

Sexual dysfunction (SD) is a common, underestimated problem in MS [91] which seriously reduces quality of life. It is often associated with the bladder and bowel complaints which have been discussed earlier in this chapter. SD may occur early at the time of diagnosis of MS or later associated with increasing disability.

Understanding and treating SD in MS requires knowledge of the normal sexual response cycle in both males and females (Chapter 3) and an understanding of the neurological determinants of each phase of the cycle. Most commonly the problems arise secondary to spinal cord disease but brain lesions can contribute. General physical disability (secondary indirect physical dysfunction) and psychological and emotional issues including fatigue and depression (tertiary psychosocial dysfunction) can also be factors (Fig. 14.6).

A multidisciplinary holistic approach is required to address the pathophysiological causative factors, and appropriate pharmacological and non-pharmacological treatments can do much to improve this aspect of life for patients with MS.

Prevalence

Studies specifically focusing on patients with MS and SD reveal 50–90% of men and 40–80% of women are affected by SD, depending on disease duration and disability [92–94].

Pathophysiology of SD in men

In men, erectile dysfunction (ED) is the most common manifestation of sexual dysfunction and the evidence generally points to spinal cord involvement [95, 96]. Cord involvement in MS may initially result in a partial deficit so that ED is variable, with preserved nocturnal penile erections and erections on morning waking [97–99]. In the last 10–20 years the error of the neurological teaching that "if a man can get an erection at anytime, impotence is likely to be psychogenic" has been recognized. In contrast to earlier times, nowadays ED, the preferred term being less pejorative and diagnostically more informative, is rarely attributed to emotional factors in the presence of neurological disease [96, 100]. With increasing neurological disability there may be a total failure of erectile function and also difficulty with ejaculation.

Very few men with complete spinal cord injury can ejaculate (Chapter 15) [101, 102] and a study of ED in men with MS in which pudendal evoked potentials were measured showed greater difficulty with ejaculation in men with more delayed potentials [96]. Difficulty with ejaculation may become apparent when ED is successfully treated.

Pathophysiology of SD in women

The most common symptoms include impaired or absent genital sensations, vaginal dryness, orgasmic dysfunction, loss of libido and dysperunia.

There is a complex relationship between SD and disability in MS. Nortvedt's Norwegian study looking at disability and SD in 194 patients with MS (duration 9 ± 19 years) found that 53% of patients with an EDSS less than or equal to 4 reported disease-related SD, compared to 86% of patients with an EDSS greater than 4 [103]. A significant positive relationship has been shown between SD and all other MS disability scales [104]. However, SD may occur early in patients newly diagnosed with MS (34.9%) with very little disability (mean EDSS 2.5), although that same study estimated a prevalence of 21% in healthy female controls [105]. Case reports of hypersexuality and paraphilias in women with MS are extremely rare and occur in the context of widespread cortical and subcortical disease [106–108] (Chapter 3).

Diagnosis of SD and appropriate investigations

A history including all aspects of the sexual cycle is required. This includes questions about sexual desire (libido), arousal (erectile function), orgasmic ejaculatory function and sexual pain. The use of validated questionnaires such as the International Index of Erectile Function (IIEF) in men and the Female Sexual Function Index (FSFI) (Appendix 1) [109–111] may be helpful to open discussion but have mostly been used for research purposes.

General physical examination, as well as a neurological examination, should be performed with particular attention to eliciting long tract signs. Referral to an endocrinology clinic may be appropriate if hypogonadism is suspected.

Gruenwald performed quantitative sensory testing (QST) of the female genitalia in 41 MS patients and found sensory deficits were common. Using responses to a questionnaire, it was established that 25 (61%) of the patients had SD, most commonly decreased libido (61%) and orgasmic disturbances (54%). There were correlations between high sensory thresholds and SD parameters; the most significant correlation was between clitoral vibratory sensation and orgasmic dysfunction [112].

Treatments of SD

Treatment should involve a comprehensive approach identifying the area of the sexual response cycle involved and contributing factors. As well as focusing on medications for treatment of primary SD, treatments of secondary and tertiary problems (Fig. 14.6) should not be overlooked.

Treatments for men

Patients with MS responded better to sildenafil than most other patient groups in the early clinical trials (Chapter 10). Sildenafil in men with MS resulted in significant improvements in both general and disease-specific quality of life variables [113] although a more recent study cast doubt on those findings. Safarinejad reported little effect of sildenafil in men with MS and recommended against its use in the routine treatment of ED in this disease [114]. The explanation for this discrepancy is unclear but a difference in patient selection may have contributed. There is no data regarding the efficacy of vardenafil (Levitra®) and tadalafil (Cialis®) (see Chapter 10) specifically in patients with MS but in clinical practice in the UK many men report considerable benefit in erectile function from these medications.

Effective second-line therapeutic agents include the intracavernous injection of prostaglandin E1 or, less often, paparervine and phentolamine (Chapter 10). However, administration may be difficult in patients with increasing disability and reduced hand function.

The dopamine agonist apomorphine is also available as a pro-erectile agent, but has been shown in two studies to have a lower efficacy than sildenafil [115, 116] (Chapter 10), and since its mode of action is thought to depend on spinal cord integrity, it is unlikely to prove effective in men with MS.

Vacuum constriction devices (VCDs) with constriction tension bands to maintain tumescence are the simplest non-medicinal treatment for ED (Chapter 10). Success with this technique depends upon a local champion who is able to demonstrate how the device should be used and some men do use it in combination with oral treatments.

Surgical implantation of a penile prosthesis is not recommended in men with MS (see Chapter 10).

As yet there are no medications to restore ejaculatory function. Yohimbine (from the bark of the *Pausinystalia yohimbe* tree) has been associated with improvement in erotic sensitivity in some non-neurological patients [117], at 5–10 mg taken 1–2 hours before intercourse. Side-effects due to monoamine oxidase inhibition stimulating release of norepinephrine include elevated blood pressure, anxiety and increased frequency of micturition. The α-1-agonist midrodine enhances orgasm and improves ejaculatory function in patients with spinal cord injury but its effect has not been investigated in MS [118, 119].

Treatments for women

In contrast to the many therapeutic options available for men, treatment for female sexual dysfunction (FSD) is limited (Fig. 14.7). Sildenafil was assessed in a small, double-blinded trial involving 19 women with MS and resulted in only a modest increase in vaginal lubrication [120].

Education can be important in helping women explore other means of achieving orgasm and additional erogenous zones. Poor vaginal lubrication can be managed by liberal application of water-based lubricants such as KY jelly. Anesthetic agents are useful for treatment of dyspareunia. Altered sensations and neuropathic pain in the genital area may respond to treatment such as carbamazepine or amitriptyline.

Some women find that the use of vibrators and other sexual aids increases the intensity of stimulation. In particular, the EROS CTD system has been approved by the FDA (Chapter 10). Partners are advised to experiment and find new ways to approach altered sexual functioning whilst retaining a sense of fun!

Female SD is an area of interest for a number of pharmaceutical companies, in particular addressing options for arousal and orgasmic dysfunction.

Addressing secondary and tertiary sources of SD in men and women

Addressing secondary and tertiary causes of SD involves treatment of fatigue, depression and spasticity (Fig. 14.6). Lower limb spasticity with adductor spasms impacting on sexual function can be ameliorated by physical therapy, suggestions about alternative positions and medication, although baclofen used for treatment of spasticity can cause sexual dysfunction [121, 122]. Antidepressant medication including all SSRIs can also significantly contribute to sexual dysfunction (see Chapter 10).

Practical suggestions include bladder emptying, possibly by catheterization prior to intercourse, or using a micro-enema to alleviate bowel symptoms.

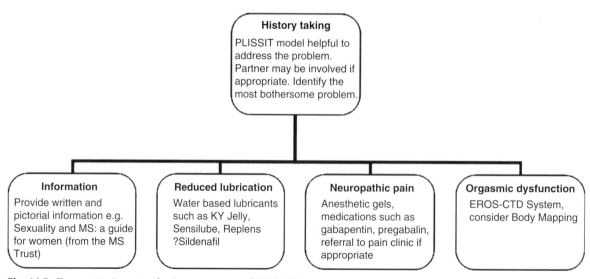

Fig. 14.7. Therapeutic alternatives for the management of FSD in MS.

Table 14.2. Summary of urodynamic findings in a variety of inflammatory and demyelinating disorders of the brain and spinal cord

Neurological Diagnosis	Author	Year	Patients	Urodynamic findings	Follow-up	Results and recovery
ADEM	Sakakibara [126]	1996	11	DH (6/10), low compliance (2/10), DU (1/10) and DSD (2/10). External sphincter polyphasic neurogenic changes (1/4)	3–38 months	7/9 with retention became able to urinate (5/9 had voiding difficulty and 4/9 frequency or urge incontinence). Two remained in retention
ADEM	Panicker [127]	2009	20/61	DO (4), DU (4)	3 months	5/20 hesitancy, 5/20 urgency
Meningitis retention syndrome	Sakakibara [128]	2006	3	Voiding DU and unrelaxed sphincter (1)	3 weeks	Complete
Adenomyeloneuropathy	Sakakibara [129]	1998	1	Age 31, PVR = 50ml, DO	26 years	Age 38, PVR = 200 ml, bladder capacity down with marked DO
Central pontine myelinolysis	Alberca [130]	1985	1	NA		Mental confusion and urinary incontinence at 12 months
Central pontine myelinolysis	Ito [125]	2005	1	DO during storage and a DU during voiding		Continent
Systemic lupus erythematosis	Sakakibara [131]	2003	8	Decreased urinary flow (5), PVR (3) (mean 97 ml), DO (5), impaired detrusor contractility (5), DSD (4) and neurogenic motor unit potentials of the external sphincter in 2/4 patients studied	2–8 years	Loss of bladder sensation (1), low compliance bladder (1), DO and decreased bladder capacity from 470 to 40 ml
Subacute myelo-optico-neuropathy (SMON)	Sakakibara [132]	2001	6	Increased maximum urethral closure pressure (2/4), decreased bladder volume at first sensation (2), DO (3), absent bulbocavernosus reflex (1). No DSD or PVR	Up to 10 years	Repeated in one patient with DO, showed the same findings
Neuromyelitis optica	Graber [133]	2009	1	Urinary retention (no results)	8 months	Patient death
Neurosarcoidosis	Sakakibara [134]	2000	1	Marked DO. Exaggerated bulbocavernosus reflex	6 months	Relapse with urgency, frequency and incontinence
Transverse myelitis	Hiraga [135]	2006	24/32	Two patients with retention: DO during bladder filling, impaired contractility during voiding and spared bladder sensation	9 months (not specified for all patients)	2/3 with retention became able to urinate. One needed CIC during a 9-month follow-up, despite neurological improvement

Table 14.2. (cont.)

Neurological Diagnosis	Author	Year	Patients	Urodynamic findings	Follow-up	Results and recovery
Transverse myelitis	Kalita [9]	2002	18	Areflexic bladder (10), DO with poor compliance (2) and DSD (3). Persistent abnormalities at 12 months: DO, DSD and DU	12 months	Bladder function restored: 2/18. Retention (6), storage symptoms (10), emptying difficulties (5)
Transverse myelitis	DaJusta [124]	2008	14 children	Acute phase (3): DU. Recovery phase (in patients with no or partial recovery): DU (7) or DO ± DSD (3)	9 years	Full recovery 4, partial recovery 2 and no recovery 8. No bladder recovery seen beyond 4 months
Transverse myelitis	Pidcock [136]	2007	47 children	Not given	Not given	Dependent for spincter control: 24% (8/33). Normal sphincter control 46% (15/33)
Parainfectious conus myelitis	Pradhan [137]	1998	12	Normal bladder compliance, normal/reduced bladder sensations and no involuntary contraction during filling in 8 patients. Voiding DU and high PVR	24 months follow-up	Good outcome = 6, fair=4 (passing urine independently), poor=2
Schistosomiasis (conus lesion)	Olsen [138]	2001	1 case report	Catheter drained 1400 ml (no urodynamics)	6 months	Resolved at 6 months
Schistosomiasis	Gomes [139]	2005	26	DO with DSD in 14, DO (6), DO with no DSD (4) and DU (2)	36 months	18 performed CIC. 7 voided spontaneously. 5 developed bladder stones. Failed conservative DO treatment (3): botulinum-A toxin (2) and one had an ileocystoplasty
Brown–Séquard syndrome	Sakakibara [140]	2001		Urodynamic abnormalities (5) with urological symptoms: PVR (4) average 149 ml, high urethral closure pressure (2), increased bladder volume at first sensation (1), DO (4), voiding DU (3) and DSD (4). Asymptomatic (3)	Disease course 2 days to 12 years	Combination treatment for the neurological disorder with alpha-blockers and CIC
Subacute combined degeneration of the cord	Misra [141]	2008	8	DU (2), DO with high pressure voiding in 3 and normal in 2 patients. A repeat study (2) showed DU improvement	6 months	Urinary symptoms improved: complete recovery (3), partial (4) and poor (1)

DH = detrusor hyperactivity; Do = detrusor overactivity; DSD = detrusor sphincter dyssynergia; DU = detrusor underactivity; PVR = post-void residual; CIC = clean intermittent catheterization

Role for healthcare professionals

With increasing awareness of SD and its impact on quality of life, there is a move for healthcare professionals to be proactive in this area. However, this attempt is often limited by lack of time during the consultation and feelings of embarrassment, compounded by a lack of confidence due to inadequate training in sexual medicine.

One of the approaches used in handling problems related to sexuality is the PLISSIT model, which is described in Chapter 10 [123]. Further details about it are available from the MS Trust website at http://www.mstrust.org.uk/professionals/information/msinfo/sexuality.jsp.

Other non-compressive myelopathies

Pelvic organ dysfunction may occur in several other inflammatory and/or demyelinating neurological conditions, such as acute demyelinating encephalomyelitis (ADEM), central pontine myelinolysis, leucodystrophies, Devic's disease, transverse myelitis and B12 deficiency. Bladder dysfunction has been evaluated in many of these conditions and the results of urodynamic studies are summarized in Table 14.2.

Studies in adults with transverse myelitis highlight that whereas there may be good recovery of motor functions over time and indeed patients may become fully ambulant, bladder dysfunction may persist [9]. However, in children, it appears that improvement in bladder function does parallel neurological recovery if recovery occurs in the first four months [124].

From studies in central pontine myelinolysis, anatomical-pathological correlates are possible where brain MRI has confirmed basis pontis lesions that extend to the tegmentum and middle cerebellar peduncle and involve the pontine micturition center [125] (Chapter 11). Lesions in the pontine micturition center can result in severe bladder dysfunction, such as urinary retention (detrusor areflexia) or urinary incontinence (DO) (Chapter 11).

References

1. World Health Organization, Multiple Sclerosis International Federation. *Atlas: multiple sclerosis resources in the world.* Geneva: World Health Organization; 2008.

2. Pugliatti M, Sotgiu S, Rosati G. The worldwide prevalence of multiple sclerosis. *Clin Neurol Neurosurg* 2002;**104**:182–91.

3. Confavreux C, Aimard G, Devic M. Course and prognosis of multiple sclerosis assessed by the computerized data processing of 349 patients. *Brain* 1980;**103**:281–300.

4. Compston A, Confavreux C, Lassmann H, et al., eds. *McAlpine's multiple sclerosis.* London: Churchill Livingstone; 2006.

5. Kutzelnigg A, Lucchinetti CF, Stadelmann C, et al. Cortical demyelination and diffuse white matter injury in multiple sclerosis. *Brain* 2005;**128**(Pt 11):2705–12.

6. Furby J, Hayton T, Anderson V, et al. Magnetic resonance imaging measures of brain and spinal cord atrophy correlate with clinical impairment in secondary progressive multiple sclerosis. *Mult Scler* 2008;**14**:1068–75.

7. Bradl M, Lassmann H. Progressive multiple sclerosis. *Semin Immunopathol* 2009;**31**:455–65.

8. Kurtzke JF. Rating neurological impairment in multiple sclerosis: an expanded disability status scale (EDSS). *Neurology* 1983;**33**:1444–52.

9. Kalita J, Shah S, Kapoor R, Misra UK. Bladder dysfunction in acute transverse myelitis: magnetic resonance imaging and neurophysiological and urodynamic correlations. *J Neurol Neurosurg Psychiatry* 2002;**73**:154–9.

10. Awad SA, Gajewski JB, Sogbein SK, Murray TJ, Field CA. Relationship between neurological and urological status in patients with multiple sclerosis. *J Urol* 1984;**132**:499–502.

11. Betts CD, D'Mellow MT, Fowler CJ. Urinary symptoms and the neurological features of bladder dysfunction in multiple sclerosis. *J Neurol Neurosurg Psychiatry* 1993;**56**:245–50.

12. Fowler CJ, Panicker JN, Drake M, et al. A UK consensus on the management of the bladder in multiple sclerosis. *J Neurol Neurosurg Psychiatry* 2009;**80**:470–7.

13. Confavreux C, Vukusic S, Moreau T, Adeleine P. Relapses and progression of disability in multiple sclerosis. *N Engl J Med* 2000;**343**:1430–8.

14. Confavreux C, Vukusic S, Adeleine P. Early clinical predictors and progression of irreversible disability in multiple sclerosis: an amnesic process. *Brain* 2003;**126** (Pt 4):770–82.

15. Marrie RA, Cutter G, Tyry T, Vollmer T, Campagnolo D. Disparities in the management of multiple sclerosis-related bladder symptoms. *Neurology* 2007;**68**:1971–8.

16. Hemmett L, Holmes J, Barnes M, Russell N. What drives quality of life in multiple sclerosis? *QJM* 2004;**97**:671–6.

17. Giannantoni A, Scivoletto G, Di Stasi SM, et al. Lower urinary tract dysfunction and disability status in patients with multiple sclerosis. *Arch Phys Med Rehabil* 1999;**80**(4):437–41.

18. de Sèze M, Ruffion A, Denys P, Joseph PA, Perrouin-Verbe B. The neurogenic bladder in multiple sclerosis: review of the literature and proposal of management guidelines. *Mult Scler* 2007;**13**:915–28.

19. Koldewijn E, Hommes O, Lemmens W, Debruyne F, van Kerrebroeck P. Relationship between lower urinary tract abnormalities and disease-related parameters in multiple sclerosis. *J Urol* 1995;**154**:169–73.

20. Porru D, Campus G, Garau A, et al. Urinary tract dysfunction in multiple sclerosis: is there a relation with disease-related parameters? *Spinal Cord* 1997;**35**:33–6.

21. Bryant CM, Dowell CJ, Fairbrother G. Caffeine reduction education to improve urinary symptoms. *Br J Nurs* 2002;**11**:560–5.

22. McClurg D, Ashe RG, Marshall K, Lowe-Strong AS. Comparison of pelvic floor muscle training, electromyography biofeedback, and neuromuscular electrical stimulation for bladder dysfunction in people with multiple sclerosis: a randomized pilot study. *Neurourol Urodyn* 2006;**25**:337–48.

23. Vahtera T, Haaranen M, Viramo-Koskela AL, Ruutiainen J. Pelvic floor rehabilitation is effective in patients with multiple sclerosis. *Clin Rehabil* 1997;**11**:211–9.

24. Fowlis GA, Waters J, Williams G. The cost effectiveness of combined rapid tests (Multistix) in screening for urinary tract infections. *J R Soc Med* 1994;**87**:681–2.

25. Lawrenson R, Wyndaele JJ, Vlachonikolis I, Farmer C, Glickman S. Renal failure in patients with neurogenic lower urinary tract dysfunction. *Neuroepidemiology* 2001;**20**:138–43.

26. Bemelmans BL, Hommes OR, Van Kerrebroeck PE, et al. Evidence for early lower urinary tract dysfunction in clinically silent multiple sclerosis. *J Urol* 1991;**145**:1219–24.

27. Sirls LT, Zimmern PE, Leach GE. Role of limited evaluation and aggressive medical management in multiple sclerosis: a review of 113 patients. *J Urol* 1994;**151**:946–50.

28. Kasabian N, Krause I, Brown W, Khan Z, Nagler H. Fate of the upper urinary tract in multiple sclerosis. *Neurourol Urodyn* 1995;**14**:81–5.

29. Gallien P, Robineau S, Nicolas B, et al. Vesicourethral dysfunction and urodynamic findings in multiple sclerosis: a study of 149 cases. *Arch Phys Med Rehabil* 1998;**79**:255–7.

30. Vahter L, Zopp I, Kreegipuu M, et al. Clean intermittent self-catheterization in persons with multiple sclerosis: the influence of cognitive dysfunction. *Mult Scler* 2009;**15**:379–84.

31. O'Riordan JI, Doherty C, Javed M, et al. Do alpha-blockers have a role in lower urinary tract dysfunction in multiple sclerosis? *J Urol* 1995;**153**:1114–6.

32. McConnell JD, Roehrborn CG, Bautista OM, et al. The long-term effect of doxazosin, finasteride, and combination therapy on the clinical progression of benign prostatic hyperplasia. *N Engl J Med* 2003;**349**:2387–98.

33. Prasad RS, Smith SJ, Wright H. Lower abdominal pressure versus external bladder stimulation to aid bladder emptying in multiple sclerosis: a randomized controlled study. *Clin Rehabil* 2003;**17**:42–7.

34. Abrams P, Agarwal M, Drake M, et al. A proposed guideline for the urological management of patients with spinal cord injury. *BJU Int* 2008;**101**:989–94.

35. Gajewski JB, Awad SA. Oxybutynin versus propantheline in patients with multiple sclerosis and detrusor hyperreflexia. *J Urol* 1986;**135**:966–8.

36. Ethans KD, Nance PW, Bard RJ, Casey AR, Schryvers OI. Efficacy and safety of tolterodine in people with neurogenic detrusor overactivity. *J Spinal Cord Med* 2004;**27**:214–8.

37. Amend B, Hennenlotter J, Schafer T, et al. Effective treatment of neurogenic detrusor dysfunction by combined high-dosed antimuscarinics without increased side-effects. *Eur Urol* 2008;**53**:1021–8.

38. Kay G, Crook T, Rekeda L, et al. Differential effects of the antimuscarinic agents darifenacin and oxybutynin ER on memory in older subjects. *Eur Urol* 2006;**50**:317–26.

39. Bosma R, Wynia K, Havlikova E, De Keyser J, Middel B. Efficacy of desmopressin in patients with multiple sclerosis suffering from bladder dysfunction: a meta-analysis. *Acta Neurol Scand* 2005;**112**:1–5.

40. Reynard JM, Cannon A, Yang Q, Abrams P. A novel therapy for nocturnal polyuria: a double-blind randomized trial of frusemide against placebo. *Br J Urol* 1998;**81**:215–8.

41. Brady CM, DasGupta R, Dalton C, et al. An open-label pilot study of cannabis-based extracts for bladder dysfunction in advanced multiple sclerosis. *Mult Scler* 2004;**10**:425–33.

42. Freeman RM, Adekanmi O, Waterfield MR, et al. The effect of cannabis on urge incontinence in patients with multiple sclerosis: a multicentre, randomised placebo-controlled trial (CAMS-LUTS). *Int Urogynecol J Pelvic Floor Dysfunct* 2006;**17**:636–41.

43. Kavia R, De Ridder D, Constantinescu S, Fowler C. Randomised controlled trial of Sativex to treat detrusor over activity in multiple sclerosis. *Multiple Sclerosis* 2010;submitted.

44. de Sèze M, Wiart L, Joseph PA, et al. Capsaicin and neurogenic detrusor hyperreflexia: a double-blind placebo-controlled study in 20 patients with spinal cord lesions. *Neurourol Urodyn* 1998;**17**:513–23.

45. Kim JH, Rivas DA, Shenot PJ, et al. Intravesical resiniferatoxin for refractory detrusor hyperreflexia: a multicenter, blinded, randomized, placebo-controlled trial. *J Spinal Cord Med* 2003;**26**:358–63.

46. Schurch B, de Sèze M, Denys P, et al. Botulinum toxin type A is a safe and effective treatment for neurogenic urinary incontinence: results of a single treatment, randomized, placebo controlled 6-month study. *J Urol* 2005;**174**:196–200.

47. Ehren I, Volz D, Farrelly E, et al. Efficacy and impact of botulinum toxin A on quality of life in patients with neurogenic detrusor overactivity: a randomised, placebo-controlled, double-blind study. *Scand J Urol Nephrol* 2007;**41**:335–40.

48. Kalsi V, Gonzales G, Popat R, et al. Botulinum injections for the treatment of bladder symptoms of multiple sclerosis. *Ann Neurol* 2007;**62**:452–7.

49. Khan S, Kessler TM, Panicker J, et al. Sustained and significant quality of life improvement after intra-detrusor botulinum toxin type A injections for neurogenic detrusor overactivity secondary to multiple sclerosis. *Br J Urol [Presentation]*2009;**103**:37.

50. Lekka E, Lee LK. Successful treatment with intradetrusor botulinum-A toxin for urethral urinary leakage (catheter bypassing) in patients with end-staged multiple sclerosis and indwelling suprapubic catheters. *Eur Urol* 2006;**50**:806–9.

51. Game X, Castel-Lacanal E, Bentaleb Y, et al. Botulinum toxin A detrusor injections in patients with neurogenic detrusor overactivity significantly decrease the incidence of symptomatic urinary tract infections. *Eur Urol* 2008;**53**:613–8.

52. Wallace PA, Lane FL, Noblett KL. Sacral nerve neuromodulation in patients with underlying neurologic disease.*Am J Obstet Gynecol* 2007;**197**:96.e1–5.

53. Cappellano F, Bertapelle P, Spinelli M, et al. Quality of life assessment in patients who undergo sacral neuromodulation implantation for urge incontinence: an additional tool for evaluating outcome. *J Urol* 2001;**166**:2277–80.

54. Ruffion A, de Sèze M, Denys P, Perrouin-Verbe B, Chartier-Kastler E. Groupe d'Etudes de Neuro-Urologie de Langue Francaise (GENULF) guidelines

for the management of spinal cord injury and spina bifida patients. *Prog Urol* 2007;**17**:631–3.

55. Stohrer M, Castro-Diaz D, Chartier-Kastler E, et al. Guidelines on neurogenic lower urinary tract dysfunction. *Prog Urol* 2007;**17**:687–99.

56. Hess MJ, Hess PE, Sullivan MR, Nee M, Yalla SV. Evaluation of cranberry tablets for the prevention of urinary tract infections in spinal cord injured patients with neurogenic bladder. *Spinal Cord* 2008;**46**:622–6.

57. Buljevac D, Flach HZ, Hop WC, et al. Prospective study on the relationship between infections and multiple sclerosis exacerbations. *Brain* 2002;**125**(Pt 5):952–60.

58. De Ridder D, van Poppel H, Demonty L, et al. Bladder cancer in patients with multiple sclerosis treated with cyclophosphamide. *J Urol* 1998;**159**:1881–4.

59. Bonniaud V, Bryant D, Parratte B, Guyatt G. Development and validation of the short form of a urinary quality of life questionnaire: SF-Qualiveen. *J Urol* 2008;**180**:2592–8.

60. Hinds J, Wald A. Colonic and anorectal dysfunction associated with multiple sclerosis. *Am J Gastroenterol* 1989;**84**:587–95.

61. Hinds J, Eidelman B, Wald A. Prevalence of bowel dysfunction in multiple sclerosis. A population survey. *Gastroenterology* 1990;**98**:1538–42.

62. Chia Y-W, Fowler C, Kamm M, et al. Prevalence of bowel dysfunction in patients with multiple sclerosis and bladder dysfunction. *J Neurol* 1995;**242**:105–8.

63. Nordenbo A, Andersen J, Andersen J. Disturbances of ano-rectal function in multiple sclerosis. *J Neurol* 1996;**243**:445–51.

64. Bakke A, Myhr K, Gronning M, Nyland H. Bladder, bowel and sexual dysfunction in patients with multiple sclerosis – a cohort study. *Scand J Urol Nephrol* 1996;**179**(Suppl):61–6.

65. Munteis E, Andreu M, Tellez MJ, et al. Anorectal dysfunction in multiple sclerosis. *Mult Scler* 2006;**12**:215–8.

66. Wiesel PH, Norton C, Glickman S, Kamm MA. Pathophysiology and management of bowel dysfunction in multiple sclerosis. *Eur J Gastroenterol Hepatol* 2001;**13**:441–8.

67. National Institute for Clinical Excellence. *Management of multiple sclerosis in primary and secondary care.* London: NICE, 2003.

68. Preziosi G, Emmanuel A. Neurogenic bowel dysfunction: pathophysiology, clinical manifestations and treatment. *Expert Rev Gastroenterol Hepatol* 2009;**3**:417–23.

69. Gore RM, Mintzer RA, Calenoff L. Gastrointestinal complications of spinal cord injury. *Spine (Phila Pa 1976)* 1981;**6**:538–44.

70. Glick ME, Meshkinpour H, Haldeman S, et al. Colonic dysfunction in patients with thoracic spinal cord injury. *Gastroenterology* 1984;**86**:287–94.

71. Aaronson MJ, Freed MM, Burakoff R. Colonic myoelectric activity in persons with spinal cord injury. *Dig Dis Sci* 1985;**30**:295–300.

72. Sun WM, Read NW, Donnelly TC. Anorectal function in incontinent patients with cerebrospinal disease. *Gastroenterology* 1990;**99**:1372–9.

73. Chia Y, Gill K, Jameson J, et al. Paradoxical puborectalis contraction is a feature of constipation in patients with multiple sclerosis. *J Neurol Neurosurg Psychiatry* 1996;**60**:31–5.

74. Weber J, Grise P, Roquebert M, et al. Radiopaque markers transit and anorectal manometry in 16 patients with multiple sclerosis and urinary bladder dysfunction. *Dis Colon Rectum* 1987;**30**:95–100.

75. Waldron D, Horgan P, Patel F, Maguire R, Given H. Multiple sclerosis assessment of colonic and anorectal function in the presence of faecal incontinence. *Int J Colorectal Dis* 1993;**8**:220–4.

76. Preziosi G, Emmanuel A. Evidence of reduced rectal compliance in constipated patients with multiple sclerosis. In: Emmanuel A, ed. *Association of Coloproctology of Great Britain and Ireland*, Harrogate 8–11/06/2009 (Poster).

77. Nicoletti R, Mina A, Balzaretti G, Tessera G, Ghezzi A. Intestinal transit studied with radiopaque markers in patients with multiple sclerosis. *Radiol Med* 1992;**83**:428–30.

78. Glick E, Meshkinpour H, Haldeman S, Bhatia N, Bradley W. Colonic dysfunction in multiple sclerosis. *Gastroenterology* 1982;**83**:1002–7.

79. Haldeman S, Glick M, Bhatia NN, Bradley WE, Johnson B. Colonometry, cystometry, and evoked potentials in multiple sclerosis. *Arch Neurol* 1982;**39**:698–701.

80. Taylor MC, Bradley WE, Bhatia N, Glick M, Haldeman S. The conus demyelination syndrome in multiple sclerosis. *Acta Neurol Scand* 1984;**69**:80–9.

81. Jameson JS, Rogers J, Chia YW, et al. Pelvic floor function in multiple sclerosis. *Gut* 1994;**35**:388–90.

82. Swash M, Snooks SJ, Chalmers DHK. Parity as a factor in incontinence in multiple sclerosis. *Arch Neurol* 1987;**44**:504–8.

83. Mathers SE, Ingram DA, Swash M. Electrophysiology of motor pathways for sphincter control in multiple sclerosis. *J Neurol Neurosurg Psychiatry* 1990;**53**:955–60.

84. Snooks SJ, Swash M. Motor conduction velocity in the human spinal cord: slowed conduction in multiple sclerosis and radiation myelopathy. *J Neurol Neurosurg Psychiatry* 1985;**48**:1135–9.

85. Halligan S, Bartram CI, Park HJ, Kamm MA. Proctographic features of anismus. *Radiology* 1995;**197**:679–82.

86. Read NW, Timms JM, Barfield LJ, Donnelly TC, Bannister JJ. Impairment of defecation in young women with severe constipation. *Gastroenterology* 1986;**90**:53–60.

87. Speakman CT, Kamm MA. Abnormal visceral autonomic innervation in neurogenic faecal incontinence. *Gut* 1993;**34**:215–21.

88. Wiesel PH, Norton C, Roy AJ, et al. Gut focused behavioural treatment (biofeedback) for constipation and faecal incontinence in multiple sclerosis. *J Neurol Neurosurg Psychiatry* 2000;**69**:240–3.

89. Preziosi G, Thirupathy K, Boulos P, Emmanuel A. Successful biofeedback in patients with multiple sclerosis is related to disability and mood factors more than anorectal physiology variables. *Gastroenterology* 2009;**136**(5 Suppl 1):A380.

90. Munteis E, Andreu M, Martinez-Rodriguez J, et al. Manometric correlations of anorectal dysfunction and biofeedback outcome in patients with multiple sclerosis. *Mult Scler* 2008;**14**:237–42.

91. DasGupta R, Fowler CJ. Sexual and urological dysfunction in multiple sclerosis: better understanding and improved therapies. *Curr Opin Neurol* 2002;**15**:271–8.

92. Tepavcevic DK, Kostic J, Basuroski ID, et al. The impact of sexual dysfunction on the quality of life measured by MSQoL-54 in patients with multiple sclerosis. *Mult Scler* 2008;**14**:1131–6.

93. Foley FW, LaRocca NG, Sanders AS, Zemon V. Rehabilitation of intimacy and sexual dysfunction in couples with multiple sclerosis. *Mult Scler* 2001;**7**:417–21.

94. Zorzon M, Zivadinov R, Monti Bragadin L, et al. Sexual dysfunction in multiple sclerosis: a 2 year follow-up study. *J Neurol Sci* 2001;**187**:1–5.

95. Zivadinov R, Zorzon M, Bosco A, et al. Sexual dysfunction in multiple sclerosis: II. Correlation analysis. *Mult Scler* 1999;**5**:428–31.

96. Betts CD, Jones SJ, Fowler CG, Fowler CJ. Erectile dysfunction in multiple sclerosis. Associated neurological and neurophysiological deficits, and treatment of the condition. *Brain* 1994;**117** (Pt 6):1303–10.

97. Valleroy ML, Kraft GH. Sexual dysfunction in multiple sclerosis. *Arch Phys Med Rehab* 1984;**65**:125–8.

98. Kirkeby HJ, Poulsen EU, Petersen T, Dorup J. Erectile dysfunction in multiple sclerosis. *Neurol* 1988;**38**:1366–71.

99. Staerman F, Guiraud P, Coeurdacier P, et al. Value of nocturnal penile tumescence and rigidity (NPTR) recording in impotent patients with multiple sclerosis. *Int J Impot Res* 1996;**8**:241–5.

100. Zivadinov R, Zorzon M, Bosco A, et al. Sexual dysfunction in multiple sclerosis: II. Correlation analysis. *Mult Scler* 1999;**5**:428–31.

101. Vas CJ. Sexual impotence and some autonomic disturbances in men with multiple sclerosis. *Acta Neurol Scand* 1969;**45**:166–82.

102. Witt MA, Grantmyre JE. Ejaculatory failure. *World J Urol* 1993;**11**:89–95.

103. Nortvedt MW, Riise T, Myhr KM, et al. Reduced quality of life among multiple sclerosis patients with sexual disturbance and bladder dysfunction. *Mult Scler* 2001;**7**(4):231–5.

104. Fraser C, Mahoney J, McGurl J. Correlates of sexual dysfunction in men and women with multiple sclerosis. *J Neurosci Nurs* 2008;**40**:312–7.

105. Tzortzis V, Skriapas K, Hadjigeorgiou G, et al. Sexual dysfunction in newly diagnosed multiple sclerosis women. *Mult Scler* 2008;**14**:561–3.

106. Gondim FA, Thomas FP. Episodic hyperlibidinism in multiple sclerosis. *Mult Scler* 2001;**7**:67–70.

107. Huws R, Shubsachs AP, Taylor PJ. Hypersexuality, fetishism and multiple sclerosis. *Br J Psychiatry* 1991;**158**:280–1.

108. Frohman EM, Frohman TC, Moreault AM. Acquired sexual paraphilia in patients with multiple sclerosis. *Arch Neurol* 2002;**59**:1006–10.

109. Rosen RC, Riley A, Wagner G, et al. The international index of erectile function (IIEF): a multidimensional scale for assessment of erectile dysfunction. *Urol* 1997;**49**:822–30.

110. Rosen R, Brown C, Heiman J, et al. The Female Sexual Function Index (FSFI): a multidimensional self-report instrument for the assessment of female sexual function. *J Sex Marital Ther* 2000;**26**:191–208.

111. Wiegel M, Meston C, Rosen R. The female sexual function index (FSFI): cross-validation and development of clinical cutoff scores. *J Sex Marital Ther* 2005;**31**:1–20.

112. Gruenwald I, Vardi Y, Gartman I, et al. Sexual dysfunction in females with multiple sclerosis: quantitative sensory testing. *Mult Scler* 2007;**13**:95–105.

113. Fowler CJ, Miller JR, Sharief MK, et al. A double blind, randomised study of sildenafil citrate for erectile dysfunction in men with multiple sclerosis. *J Neurol Neurosurg Psychiatry* 2005 May;**76**(5):700–5.

114. Safarinejad MR. Evaluation of the safety and efficacy of sildenafil citrate for erectile dysfunction in men with multiple sclerosis: a double-blind, placebo controlled, randomized study. *J Urol* 2009;**181**:252–8.

115. Pavone C, Curto F, Anello G, et al. Prospective, randomized, crossover comparison of sublingual apomorphine (3 mg) with oral sildenafil (50 mg) for male erectile dysfunction. *J Urol* 2008;**179**(5 Suppl): S92–4.

116. Eardley I, Wright P, MacDonagh R, Hole J, Edwards A. An open-label, randomized, flexible-dose, crossover study to assess the comparative efficacy and safety of sildenafil citrate and apomorphine hydrochloride in men with erectile dysfunction. *BJU Int* 2004;**93**:1271–5.

117. Riley AJ. Yohimbine in the treatment of erectile disorder. *Br J Clin Pract* 1994;**48**:133–6.

118. Tam SW, Worcel M, Wyllie M. Yohimbine: a clinical review. *Pharmacol Ther* 2001;**91**:215–43.

119. Soler JM, Previnaire JG, Plante P, Denys P, Chartier-Kastler E. Midodrine improves orgasm in spinal cord-injured men: the effects of autonomic stimulation. *J Sex Med* 2008;**5**:2935–41.

120. Dasgupta R, Wiseman OJ, Kanabar G, Fowler CJ, Mikol DD. Efficacy of sildenafil in the treatment of female sexual dysfunction due to multiple sclerosis. *J Urol* 2004;**171**:1189–93.

121. Saval A, Chiodo AE. Sexual dysfunction associated with intrathecal baclofen use: a report of two cases. *J Spinal Cord Med* 2008;**31**:103–5.

122. McGehee M, Hornyak JE, Lin C, Kelly BM. Baclofen-induced sexual dysfunction. *Neurology* 2006;**67**:1097–8.

123. Annon J. PLISSIT Therapy. In: Corsini R, ed. *Handbook of innovative psychotherapies*. New York: Wiley and Sons; 1981:626–39.

124. DaJusta DG, Wosnitzer MS, Barone JG. Persistent motor deficits predict long-term bladder dysfunction in children following acute transverse myelitis. *J Urol* 2008;**180**(4 Suppl):1774–7.

125. Ito T, Sakakibara R, Uchiyama T, et al. Lower urinary tract dysfunction in central pontine myelinolysis: possible contribution of the pontine micturition centre. *Eur J Neurol* 2005;**12**:812–3.

126. Sakakibara R, Hattori T, Yasuda K, Yamanishi T. Micturitional disturbance in acute disseminated encephalomyelitis (ADEM). *J Auton Nerv Syst* 1996;**60**:200–5.

127. Panicker J, Nagaraja D, Kovoor J, Nair K, Subbakrishna D. Lower urinary tract dysfunction in

acute disseminated encephalomyelitis. *Mult Scler* 2009;**15**:1118–22.

128. Sakakibara R, Uchiyama T, Liu Z, et al. Meningitis-retention syndrome. An unrecognized clinical condition. *J Neurol* 2005;**252**:1495–9.

129. Sakakibara R, Hattori T, Fukutake T, et al. Micturitional disturbance in a patient with adrenomyeloneuropathy (AMN). *Neurourol Urodyn* 1998;**17**:207–12.

130. Alberca R, Iriarte LM, Rasero P, Villalobos F. Brachial diplegia in central pontine myelinolysis. *J Neurol* 1985;**231**:345–6.

131. Sakakibara R, Uchiyama T, Yoshiyama M, Yamanishi T, Hattori T. Urinary dysfunction in patients with systemic lupus erythematosis. *Neurourol Urodyn* 2003;**22**:593–6.

132. Sakakibara R, Hattori T, Uchiyama T, Yamanishi T. Micturitional disturbance in subacute myelo-optico-neuropathy (SMON). *Auton Neurosci* 2001;**87**:282–5.

133. Graber JJ, Kister I, Geyer H, Khaund M, Herbert J. Neuromyelitis optica and concentric rings of Balo in the brainstem. *Arch Neurol* 2009;**66**:274–5.

134. Sakakibara R, Hattori T, Uchiyama T, Yamanishi T. Micturitional disturbance in a patient with neurosarcoidosis. *Neurourol Urodyn* 2000;**19**:273–7.

135. Hiraga A, Sakakibara R, Mori M, et al. Urinary retention can be the sole initial manifestation of acute myelitis. *J Neurol Sci* 2006;**251**:110–2.

136. Pidcock FS, Krishnan C, Crawford TO, et al. Acute transverse myelitis in childhood: center-based analysis of 47 cases. *Neurology* 2007;**68**:1474–80.

137. Pradhan S, Gupta RK, Kapoor R, Shashank S, Kathuria MK. Parainfectious conus myelitis. *J Neurol Sci* 1998;**161**:156–62.

138. Olson S, Rossato R, Guazzo E. Spinal schistosomiasis. *J Clin Neurosci* 2002;**9**:317–20.

139. Gomes CM, Trigo-Rocha F, Arap MA, et al. Schistosomal myelopathy: urologic manifestations and urodynamic findings. *Urology* 2002;**59**:195–200.

140. Sakakibara R, Hattori T, Uchiyama T, Yamanishi T. Urinary dysfunction in Brown-Sequard syndrome. *Neurourol Urodyn* 2001;**20**:661–7.

141. Misra UK, Kalita J, Kumar G, Kapoor R. Bladder dysfunction in subacute combined degeneration: a clinical, MRI and urodynamic study. *J Neurol* 2008;**255**:1881–8.

Spinal cord injury

Xavier Gamé and Rizwan Hamid

Epidemiology

Spinal cord injury (SCI) can be a devastating consequence of motor vehicle accidents, sports injury, violence, spinal vascular events, infections, disc prolapse or spinal surgery. Because of road safety improvements and the new participation of women in dangerous sports, the epidemiology of SCI patients has changed over the last 30 years. The incidence in women has increased over that period and the male-to-female ratio is now 4:1. In 2000–2003, the mean age at time of injury was 37.7 ± 17.5 years [1]. The largest group is comprised of incomplete quadriplegics (28%), followed by complete paraplegics (26%), complete quadriplegics (24%) and then incomplete paraplegics (18%) [2].

The life expectancy and quality of life have improved in SCI patients especially from the 1970s onwards and now the life expectancy of paraplegic patients is similar to that of the general population. This improvement is a consequence of the development of multidisciplinary teams, the introduction of clean intermittent self-catheterization (CISC) and better follow-up.

SCI is classified by the neurological level of motor and sensory function on the American Spinal Injury Association (ASIA) impairment scale [3]. Recent proposals have been to add an additional scale to assess autonomic function [4] as this was not previously taken into account, although autonomic function is almost always impaired in SCI. This new scale item involves a clinical assessment of general autonomic function, lower urinary tract, bowel, sexual function and a urodynamic evaluation. The impact of the SCI on pelvic organ function constitutes a major part of the classification. It is well known that pelvic organ dysfunction has a significant effect on quality of life

and furthermore neurogenic bladder dysfunction, if untreated, can lead to upper urinary tract damage. Unlike the situation with most neurological diseases where progressive disability is expected, after the acute phase, the neurological condition of patients who have had an SCI is usually stable.

Bladder dysfunction

Bladder dysfunction after SCI can be divided into two phases; a period of spinal shock and a chronic phase. The injury can also be classified according to the level, i.e. suprasacral or sacral and degree of completeness.

"Spinal shock"

The consequences of "spinal shock" immediately follow the injury and last, on an average, three months. It is characterized by the loss of muscle tone and segmental spinal reflexes caudal to the level of the SCI. The detrusor is areflexic.

During the acute phase, an indwelling urethral catheter is usually required since fluid resuscitation and volume management contribute to a high urinary output. Once the patient no longer requires supplemental fluids or nutrition, and the 24-hour urinary output is approximately 2000 ml, the recommendation is to change to an alternative form of bladder management as soon as is practical, such as CISC or intermittent catheterization by nurses or carers. CISC decreases the incidence of genitourinary tract infections and bladder stones. Catheterization is recommended every 4–5 hours by the clock because the patient may have lost bladder sensation and the desire to void, and the bladder should not be distended to a capacity of more than 500 ml.

Pelvic Organ Dysfunction in Neurological Disease: Clinical Management and Rehabilitation, ed. Clare J. Fowler, Jalesh N. Panicker & Anton Emmanuel. Published by Cambridge University Press. © Cambridge University Press 2010.

Chronic neurogenic bladder dysfunction

Recovery of bladder function usually follows that of skeletal muscle reflexes. It is sometimes said "the bladder is the last thing to come back."

Suprasacral lesions

In patients with suprasacral lesions the acute period is followed by the chronic phase, when there may be both storage and voiding dysfunction [5]. The major abnormality causing a storage dysfunction is detrusor overactivity (DO) which is due to the emergence of a segmental spinal reflex subserved by unmyelinated C-fiber afferents (Chapter 1). The result is neurogenic detrusor overactivity (NDO) and in addition to this there is a loss of the detrusor-sphincter coordination which in spinal health emanates from the pontine micturition centre (Chapter 1). Instead of the reciprocal relaxation of the sphincter which occurs with detrusor contraction, there is dyssynergic sphincter contraction. Detrusor sphincter dyssynergia (DSD) is defined as intermittent or complete failure of relaxation of the striated urinary sphincter during a bladder contraction and voiding, and has been reported in 96% of individuals with suprasacral lesions. DSD can occur with both complete and incomplete lesions, but it is much more common with complete injuries [6]. Smooth muscle sphincter dyssynergia may also occur at the same time as the striated muscle dyssynergia, becoming apparent when the striated muscle component is successfully managed, for example by stenting.

Ambulatory patients with incomplete spinal cord damage may have significantly fewer urinary tract symptoms [7], but the urodynamic parameters may be as abnormal as in patients with complete injury [8].

Infrasacral lesions

In patients with infrasacral lesions, there may be damage to the conus together with root injury. Following cauda equina injury (Chapter 17) bladder dysfunction can be unpredictable but is not inevitably hypotonic. This is thought to be because the bladder has been decentralized rather than denervated, the postganglionic parasympathetic fibers originating in the pelvic plexus being intact (Chapter 1). Although patients may present with hesitancy, a poor, slow and interrupted stream and a feeling of incomplete emptying, symptoms of overactivity can also be present. Furthermore, because of loss of compliance of the bladder wall, the bladder may develop high intravesical pressures during filling, especially in individuals with conus medullaris lesions or with partial injuries. Following a cauda equina injury, sphincter electromyography commonly shows denervation and changes of chronic reinnervation as well as a reduced number of spontaneously firing motor units, changes characteristic of a lower motor neuron affecting the sacral roots (Chapter 4). Following a conus lesion, denervation of the sphincter and pelvic floor is not expected and the guarding reflex may be intact.

Symptoms

Urinary incontinence

Urinary incontinence is a frequent problem in SCI patients, the mechanism varying according to the level of injury. In patients with suprasacral lesions, incontinence is secondary to NDO. In patients with infrasacral lesions, it can be secondary to overflow incontinence and sphincter weakness, but sometimes also due to DO.

Frequency/urgency

Frequency and urgency can be complaints of patients with incomplete suprasacral or infrasacral lesions. In suprasacral patients, they are related to NDO and incomplete emptying whereas in infrasacral patients, they are often related to incomplete emptying and overflow incontinence.

Incomplete bladder emptying

Patients present with hesitancy, a poor, slow and interrupted stream and incomplete emptying, and often retain high residual volumes. Patients with both suprasacral and infrasacral lesions may have incomplete bladder emptying. In suprasacral patients, this can be secondary to outlet obstruction caused by DSD and poorly sustained detrusor contractions. In patients with infrasacral damage, the cause is often poor voluntary bladder contraction.

Autonomic dysreflexia

In patients who have an SCI at level T6 or above, autonomic dysreflexia may be a recurrent problem presenting as a clinical emergency. It is caused by a massive sympathetic discharge triggered by either a noxious or non-noxious stimulus originating below the level of the injury, commonly irritation of the bladder or colon. However, many other stimuli can trigger episodes of autonomic dysreflexia including pressure sores, infected ingrowing toenails or skin irritation.

Several mechanisms have been proposed for the development of autonomic dysreflexia: it may result from changes occurring within the spinal and peripheral autonomic circuits or the destruction of the descending vasomotor pathways resulting in the loss of inhibitory and excitatory supraspinal input to the sympathetic preganglionic neurons. Altered sensitivity of peripheral α-adrenergic receptors is currently considered to be a predominant factor resulting in unstable blood pressure [9].

Autonomic dysreflexia is characterized by acute hypertension with systolic increase of more than 20–30 mmHg and commonly bradycardia. This is associated with a constellation of symptoms including severe headache, blurred vision, nasal congestion, cardiac arrhythmias, atrial fibrillation, feeling of anxiety, profuse sweating, flushing and piloerection above the injury and dry, pale skin below the level of injury. It can vary in intensity from being asymptomatic, to mild discomfort and headache, to a life-threatening emergency, such as when systolic blood pressure reaches 300 mmHg. Untreated episodes may result in intracranial hemorrhage, retinal detachment, seizures and death.

The higher the level of injury, the greater the likelihood of autonomic dysfunction. Another important factor relating to the severity of autonomic dysreflexia is the completeness of the spinal injury: it affects 27% of patients with incomplete tetraplegia but 91% of patients with complete tetraplegia [10].

The first line of treatment of autonomic dysreflexia, if triggered by the bladder, is to ensure complete emptying. Then, according to the Guidelines of the Consortium for Spinal Cord Medicine, non-pharmacologic measures should be performed, such as placing the patient in an upright position to take advantage of orthostatic reduction in blood pressure, and then loosening any tight clothing or constrictive devices. If these measures fail and systolic blood pressure continues at or above 150 mmHg in an adult, 140 mmHg in an adolescent, 130 mmHg in a child 6–12 years old, or 120 mmHg in a child under 5 years old, a pharmacologic agent, such as sublingual nifedipine 10 mg in adults and 250–500 mg/kg in children, should be given [11].

Assessment and investigations in "chronic phase"

Practical guidelines for management of the bladder following SCI [12–15] emphasize the need for a complete assessment of patients for upper urinary tract damage and evaluation of the risk factors for urinary tract complications. The first detailed assessment should be performed between the third and the sixth month after the injury and is usually performed once the patient has recovered from spinal shock.

Assessment includes a complete clinical history including date of SCI and medical history since, medications, prior surgery and other past medical events. The neurological status, spasticity, mental status and comprehension, mobility and hand function are assessed, with a special focus on urinary symptoms, bowel and sexual functions, and tendency to develop autonomic dysreflexia.

A two- or three-day bladder diary should be recorded, although the Spinal Cord Outcomes Partnership Endeavor considers that diary-based measures of continence and voiding are not well standardized and have limited sensitivity, accuracy and reliability [16].

Laboratory investigations will include kidney and bladder ultrasonography, creatinine clearance, video-urodynamics or urodynamics and urethrocystogram. If indicated, other investigations such as dimethylmercaptosuccinic acid (DMSA) renography or mercaptoacetly-triglycine (MAG3) renography, cystoscopy and abdominal CT scan should be performed. A renal ultrasound can be undertaken to look for upper urinary tract dilation, stones, pyelonephritic scars and parenchymal atrophy. The bladder ultrasound scan detects stones, bladder wall thickness and any large mucosal lesions. A post-void residual volume assessment is performed if the patient can pass urine spontaneously. Renal function should also be assessed and it is currently recommended to measure creatinine clearance rather than simply creatinine since there may have been significant loss of muscle mass. In the future, cystatine C may be recommended for assessing renal function in neurological patients [17].

A video-cystometrogram (VCMG) is regarded as the gold standard of investigation (see Chapter 4) for understanding bladder and urethral sphincter functioning and for assessing the risks of upper urinary tract damage of SCI patients. The filling phase allows assessment of bladder and urethral behavior during the storage phase, cystometric capacity, compliance and external urethral sphincter activity. The voiding phase assesses bladder and urethral behavior, pressure-flow, and will identify an underactive detrusor, DSD and any unsuspected abnormalities in the urethra. In patients passing urine spontaneously, a uroflowmetry study can be obtained. A classical VCMG tracing demonstrating NDO with DSD is shown in Fig. 15.1.

If VCMG facilities are not available, an x-ray cystogram with voiding phase can be done (Fig. 15.2). This will reveal vesico-ureteral reflux and indicate the level of bladder outlet obstruction (bladder neck obstruction, external urethral sphincter) and the appearance of the bladder wall.

Urinary tract complications in patients with spinal cord injury

Prior to the 1950s, upper urinary tract damage (urinary sepsis and renal failure) was the primary cause of death following SCI. Nowadays, urinary complications constitute the fifth most common cause of mortality in these patients.

Urinary tract complications include urinary tract infections (UTIs), stones, renal failure, morphological damage to the lower urinary tract and bladder cancer.

Stones

The incidence of renal stones is higher in the spinal cord injured than in the general population, especially during the first two years after injury, but it may also occur 10 or 20 years later [18]. The reported prevalence of kidney stones varies between 1.2% and 35.1% depending on the time since injury and on bladder management [18, 19]. The major risk factors for the development of urolithiasis amongst the spinal cord injured are immobilization hypercalcuria, recurrent UTIs, indwelling catheters, vesico-ureteral reflux, and ileal conduit urinary diversion.

Bladder stones are also frequent after SCI with an estimated prevalence of 9% to 29% [20, 21]. This is related to bladder management, the prevalence increasing with indwelling catheters, suprapubic catheters and augmentation cystoplasty.

The principles of stone management are same in SCI patients as for the general population, i.e. extracorporeal shockwave lithotripsy, percutaneous nephrolithotomy and endoscopic surgery.

Renal failure

Before 1950, the prevalence of renal failure in SCI was 50%, but since the 1970s and the introduction of CISC, this has decreased significantly. However, the age-standardized ratio of renal failure in patients with paraplegia or quadriplegia is still five times greater than in the general population [22]. Risk factors include an indwelling catheter, suprapubic catheter, Credé maneuver, vesico-ureteric reflux, quadriplegia and age at the time of injury [18, 19, 23].

Urinary tract infections

Because of a lack of consensus on the bacteriological definition of a UTI [24–26] and the absence of specific symptoms, the prevalence of UTIs in SCI is not known. Around 50–80% of those who use CISC have bacteriuria [27] but such colonizations do not threaten the urinary apparatus in the long term, are not a risk factor of symptomatic UTI and do not require treatment. However, genuine infections are a major cause of morbidity and are one of the main reasons for hospitalization in patients with SCI [28, 29].

Symptomatic urinary infections (prostatitis, pyelonephritis, epididimo-orchitis) threaten the urinary tract and require treatment. In case of symptomatic recurrent UTI, possible risk factors should be investigated and treated accordingly. These include high bladder pressure, which promotes vesico-ureteral reflux and ischemic injury to the bladder wall, creating favorable conditions for infection, stones and bladder cancer. The use of non-hydrophilic-coated catheters and trauma whilst performing CISC may also be risk factors. If no risk factors are found and treated and UTIs recur, prophylactic treatment with an oral antibiotic has been proposed [30, 31]. Ingestion with cranberry extract rather than juice has been shown to result in a 60% reduction both in the number of UTIs and the number of subjects who experience UTIs, but this should not be taken patients being treated with warfarin [30].

Ureteric reflux

Reflux is mostly caused by high bladder pressure secondary to low bladder compliance or to NDO and less commonly by an abnormality of the urethro-vesical junction. McGuire observed that reflux was likely when bladder pressure was over 40 cmH$_2$O [32]. Reflux can induce reflux nephropathy, hydronephrosis, upper UTIs and stones. A classical VCMG of reflux in a neuropathic patient is shown in Fig. 15.3.

(a)

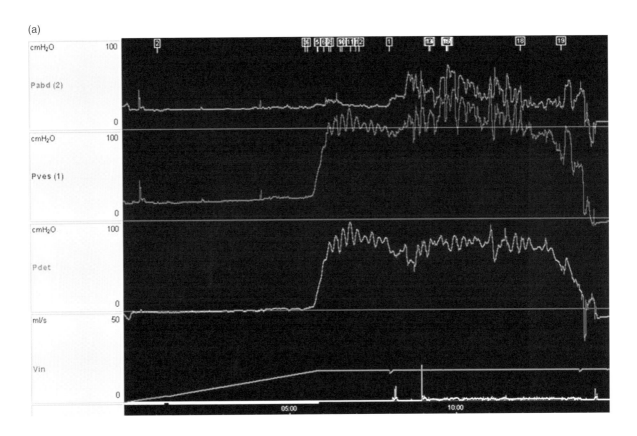

(b)

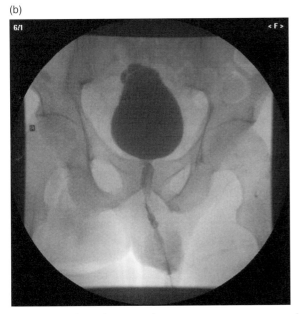

Fig. 15.1. A. This is classic trace for an upper motor neuron type of spinal cord injury resulting in high-pressure neurogenic detrusor overactivity, known as saw-toothed appearance. There is high-pressure, sustained detrusor overactivity with a pressure of around 80 cmH$_2$O which lasts for more than five minutes, during which urine flow is weak due to detrusor sphincter dyssynergia. B. This shows hold-up of urine at the level of the external sphincter, confirming the presence of DSD.

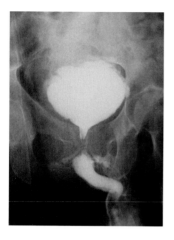

Fig. 15.2. Voiding phase of cystogram in a T5 ASIA A patient showing detrusor sphincter dyssynergia, irregular bladder wall with diverticulae and ejaculatory duct reflux.

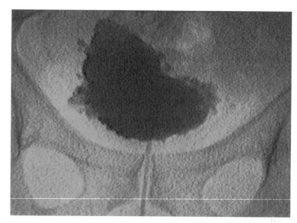

Fig. 15.4. This is a classical neuropathic bladder sometimes referred to as a "fir tree" because of its shape and multiple diverticulae.

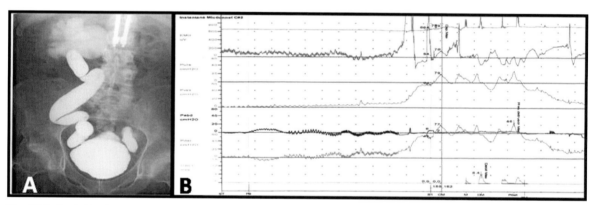

Fig. 15.3. Grade IV right vesico-ureteric reflux and grade I left vesico-ureteric reflux in a T6 ASIA A male quadriplegic patient (A) with high bladder pressure over 40 cmH_2O secondary to detrusor overactivity and detrusor sphincter dyssynergia.

Morphological damage to lower urinary tract

Morphological damage to the lower urinary tract is common, including bladder diverticula, trabeculae and parietal thickening (Fig. 15.4). It is caused by high bladder pressure, multiple phasic contractions and bladder outlet obstruction and may lead to decreased bladder compliance and ureteric stenosis.

Bladder cancer

The reported prevalence of bladder cancer in SCI patients is between 0.1% and 10% (mean prevalence in the general population: 17 per 100,000) [33, 34]. The histological subtype is a squamous cell carcinoma in up to 80% of the cases, a tumor type with a poor prognosis. Symptoms are often non-specific and may include recurrent UTIs or worsening incontinence. The diagnosis is often delayed. Risk factors include

an indwelling catheter, stones and recurrent UTIs, so that it is recommended that in patients with long-term catheters a surveillance cystoscopy and biopsies should be performed [35]. However, a contrary view is that surveillance cystoscopies are not helpful, failing to detect any cancers. Cytology is often abnormal due to chronic inflammation [36, 37].

Prolapse

In the general population, it is well known that straining to void or to pass stool, common activities for SCI patients, are associated with pelvic organ prolapse. The Credé maneuver may also be a risk factor for prolapse in SCI patients. The prevalence of pelvic organ prolapse in SCI patients is unknown but does not appear to be much higher than in the general population.

Treatment of neurogenic bladder dysfunction

As with other causes of NDO, the goal of bladder management in SCI patients is to preserve the upper urinary tract and renal function, to avoid urological complications and to improve patients' quality of life by restoring independence and continence. Continence can be achieved by creating a low-pressure reservoir and accomplishing complete bladder emptying with or without the use of a urinary drainage device. Management must be adapted to suit the patient's disability, cognitive functions and hand functions and is based on a multidisciplinary approach by a team (Chapter 4) which includes a urologist, rehabilitation physician, physiotherapists, specialist nurses and a sometimes a neurosurgeon and gastroenterologist. Several practical guidelines for management of SCI related neurogenic bladder have been proposed [13–15, 38].

Quality of life should be assessed and a validated questionnaire, such as "Qualiveen," which has been specifically developed for assessing quality of life in relation to bladder function after SCI [39], may be helpful.

Since the management aims and treatment options are common to those of other causes of NDO, each aspect is covered systematically in the relevant chapters as shown in Table 15.1. Only treatment or management specific to SCI is detailed here. Differences between management of the bladder of patients who have had SCI and those with progressive neurological disease relate to the much greater risk of upper tract complications in the SCI group and consequently surgery is more frequently performed in them as an effective definitive procedure. The treatment of bladder dysfunction following an SCI can be divided according to the level of injury (Table 15.1).

Bladder dysfunction in suprasacral injuries

Treatments to manage neurogenic detrusor overactivity

Medications

The first-line treatment of NDO in SCI patients is based on antimuscarinics which, together with other pharmacological agents, are discussed in Chapter 6. SCI patients, especially those with cervical level

Table 15.1. Treatment of bladder dysfunction in spinal cord injured patients showing which chapters in this book cover the specific topic

Bladder dysfunction in suprasacral injuries	See Chapter
To decrease neurogenic detrusor overactivity	
Pharmacotherapy	6
Clean intermittent self-catheterization	5
Neurotoxins (vanilloids)	6
Botulinum toxin A	6
Sacral neuromodulation	7
Sacral anterior root stimulator	7
Clam cystoplasty	7
Continent urinary diversion	7
Ileal conduit	7
Reduction of external sphincter dyssynergia	
Pharmacotherapy	6
Botulinum toxin A	6
Sphincterotomy	7
Urethral stents	7
Bladder dysfunction in sacral or subsacral injuries (conus or cauda equina syndrome)	See also 17
To improve bladder emptying	
Pharmacotherapy	6
Clean intermittent self-catheterization	5
Valsalva or Credé maneuver	5
To improve sphincter function	
Pharmacotherapy	6
Bulking agents	7
Slings	7
Artificial urinary sphincter	7
Bladder neck closure (females)	7
Catheters and sheaths	5

injury or with associated brain trauma, often have an increase in urine production during the night which can cause nocturnal enuresis. Desmopressin has been shown to be useful for the treatment of polyuria in SCI [40].

Intravesical agents

At a time when intravesical vanilloids (Chapter 6) were available, they were used in patients with SCI but with apparently lesser effect than in patients with MS. However, the original description of detrusor injections of botulinum toxin to treat DO was in spinal cord injured patients [41] and the treatment has since transformed the lives of numerous patients with neurogenic DO, many with SCI (Chapter 6). Many studies have shown this treatment to be highly effective, resulting in a significant improvement in urinary continence (40–80% of patients became completely dry), a decrease in mean maximum detrusor pressure to less than 40 cmH$_2$O in most studies, an increase in maximum bladder capacity and an improvement of patients' quality of life [42]. A recent study of the repeated effectiveness in patients with SCI showed that in 17 patients, followed over 6 years with repeated clinical, urodynamic and upper tract investigations and assessments of quality of life, botulinum toxin detrusor injections remained constantly effective and that the mean interval between 2 consecutive injections did not shorten but remained at 11.0 months [43].

Clean intermittent self-catheterization

A combination of antimuscarinics and CISC is the mainstay of management of bladder dysfunction in suprasacral SCI. This maintains a low pressure bladder, prevents NDO-related incontinence and facilitates complete bladder emptying (Chapter 5).

CISC should be started during the spinal shock phase once the fracture site is stable. Four to six catheterizations per day are usually recommended, so that the maximal volumes are between 300 and 500 ml.

Several factors can impede an SCI patient's ability to perform CISC, including impaired manual dexterity if quadriplegic or persistent cognitive dysfunction due to concomitant brain injury. In quadriplegics, a tendon transfer surgery, such as extensor carpi radialis longus to flexor digitorum profundus tendon, may be needed before a patient can perform CISC. Alternatively the patient may be unable to master the technique due to body habitus.

Neuromodulation

Sacral neuromodulation can be used as a second-line treatment in the care of neurological urinary incontinence related to NDO in incomplete SCI [44]. The effectiveness of neuromodulation on DSD is not yet defined and currently neuromodulation is only recommended in patients without DSD and with incomplete SCI (see Chapter 7).

Very recently, sacral neuromodulation has been used in the acute SCI setting, i.e. in the state of spinal shock, and been found to prevent DO emerging. Continence is maintained with CISC reducing urinary infections as well as improving bowel function. So far the benefit has been sustained for more than two years [45]. If this striking effect can be confirmed in a larger study following SCI, it could transform the management of NDO in SCI patients.

Sacral anterior root stimulation

Sacral anterior root stimulation with sacral deafferentation for patients with SCI was introduced by Brindley in the 1970s [46]. During a neurosurgical procedure, sacral deafferentation was achieved by posterior sacral root section, which was necessary to abolish DO. Electrodes were then placed on the sacral anterior roots S$_2$, S$_3$ and S$_4$ [47] (see Chapter 17 for discussion as to the function of each root). The electrodes were tunnelled to a radio receiver positioned subcutaneously over the lower anterior chest wall and when micturition was desired, the patient placed a radio transmitter over the receiver and activated the device with settings for micturition, defecation and even erection. Bladder emptying was accomplished usually by stimulation of S$_3$ with a bladder emptying success rate of 70% (see Chapter 7 for further details).

This device could only be used in individuals with complete suprasacral SCI because those with incomplete lesions found even anterior root stimulation painful. However, because of the posterior rhizotomy which was required to abolish DO, men lost reflex erections and it is probably because of this destructive component of the intervention that it is now little used. It was not used in patients with progressive neurological disease.

Bladder augmentation (clam cystoplasty)

Following the introduction of detrusor injection of botulinum toxin to treat DO, clam cystoplasty is rarely performed in the UK for patients with progressive neurological disease such as MS [48] but it remains the preferred treatment option for many patients following SCI. Augmentation cystoplasty can provide a long-term definitive solution for the management of severe DO, which is important for a young person who is not expected to undergo further neurological deterioration and with an otherwise almost normal life expectancy. Furthermore patients with cervical level injury may not want to come back for repeated botulinum toxin injections, even if the treatment had been previously efficacious, since returning to hospital every six to nine months can be very disruptive for them.

The various surgical techniques that have been proposed to increase bladder capacity and decrease overactivity [49] are described in Chapter 7. Cutaneous continent diversion and ileal conduits are also described in Chapter 7.

Treatments to overcome external sphincter dyssynergia

Medications

Although external sphincter dyssynergia is more likely to be troublesome in patients following SCI than those with other causes of spinal cord disease, the pharmacological and surgical treatment for this problem, including stenting, are covered in Chapters 6 and 7 respectively.

Treatments to improve bladder emptying

The medical treatment of the poorly contractile bladder is not as impressive as the drugs used to treat overactivity but the agents that can be tried are discussed in Chapter 6.

The Valsalva or Credé maneuvers are not generally recommended but for some SCI patients these work well if they do not have outflow obstruction. In the absence of recurrent UTI, raising intra-abdominal pressure to empty can be an acceptable solution although CISC remains the mainstay of management, as described in Chapter 5. However, in the long term, many patients with SCI abandon CISC [50].

Treatments to improve sphincter function

A variety of drugs have been used with very limited benefit, and are discussed in Chapter 6. Bulking agents, slings, the use of the artificial urinary sphincter and bladder neck closure are described in Chapter 7.

Catheters and sheaths

If the bladder does not empty, the ideal technique is CISC but in some patients this is simply not possible.

This is generally the case in quadriplegics but also some patients find it difficult and if this interferes with rehabilitation then a permanent catheter drainage system has to be employed. This can be either a urethral or a suprapubic (SPC). The SPC is preferred over urethral as the latter can cause pressure necrosis with cleavage of urethra in males and that of bladder neck in females. The SPC is also hygienically superior. The SPC is easier to change although it can have all the other problems of a urethral catheter, like blockages, recurrent infections and falling out. The specific problems of a long-term catheter are discussed in Chapter 7.

Follow-up

SCI patients need urological follow-up for the rest of their lives. No studies have been done on the optimum frequency of follow-up evaluations but most of guidelines propose an assessment of the upper urinary tract function using creatinine clearance or serum creatinine and kidney and bladder ultrasound every year [13–15, 38]. Other evaluations should be performed according to the kidney damage risks, symptoms and complications such as UTIs, urinary incontinence and hematuria.

Bowel

Fecal incontinence and constipation are common following SCI. The prevalence of fecal incontinence is up to 75% and constipation up to 80%, and these problems frequently co-exist. Not only are gut symptoms highly prevalent, but they also have a major negative effect on quality of life, the ability to socially integrate and the ability to live independently. People with SCI rated loss of bowel control as among the most restrictive consequences of their injury [51].

The frequency and length of time spent on bowel management have major service implications for carers and community nursing teams. Bowel symptoms arise due to a mixture of sensory and motor neurological injury, compromised mobility, polypharmacy, lifestyle and behavioral factors.

Assessment and management of the bowel has to be started immediately after the injury, and this is discussed in detail in Chapter 8. In brief, this begins with optimizing the scheduled bowel regimen, using laxatives and/or suppositories as dictated by symptoms. Bowel irrigation approaches (whether antegrade or retrograde) are of proven value, at least in the short term. Options for electrical stimulation may represent the future for carefully selected patients.

Sexual dysfunction

The vast majority experience alterations in sexual function following SCI. The degree of sexual dysfunction depends on the level and completeness of injury.

Male sexual dysfunction

Erectile dysfunction

Patients with complete lesions above T_{10} have preserved reflex erections and stimulation of the penis will result in an erection in about 80% although this is not usually adequate for penetration (Chapter 3). In men who have sustained injury to the lower lumbar spine without extensive damage to the sacral roots, psychogenic erections may be more readily induced than erection following genital stimulation, mediated by sympathetic innervation (Chapter 3). Men with a complete lesion below S_2 have psychogenic erections but have no reflex erections, but damage to the cauda equina results in almost complete loss of erectile responses (Chapter 17).

Nowadays, erectile dysfunction management is based on sexual rehabilitation including management of sexuality-impairing factors such as urinary incontinence, penile retraction associated with spasticity and drugs. Courtois has also reported improvement in penile rigidity in 10 SCI males after biofeedback followed by home perineal muscle training exercises. However, this treatment can be used only in men with incomplete lesions [52].

The three PDE5 inhibitors currently available (Chapter 10) are moderately effective in treating erectile dysfunction in this patient group. Most of the studies reporting the impact of PDE5 inhibitors in SCI used sildenafil and showed a functional improvement of more than 90% [53]. However, the effectiveness of the medication is related to the completeness of the lesion, higher doses frequently being necessary for men with complete lesions. The efficacy of the other PDE5 inhibitors is thought to be similar but trials in SCI have not been done. In general these medications are well tolerated and adverse events are mild to moderate and transient, commonly consisting of headache and facial flushing. A notable clinical improvement of ejaculation rates and orgasmic function in men with partial SCI compared with baseline has also been reported [54].

In case of failure of PDE5 inhibitors, the majority of SCI patients are dissatisfied with using the vacuum erection device (Chapter 10). They find it difficult to use, especially men with poor dexterity and the ring used on the base of the penis can cause excoriation in those who lack penile sensitivity. Intracavernous injections of vasoactive substances are effective with a reported intercourse rate of up to 90% and are well tolerated [55]. The injections require manual dexterity but can be performed by the patient's partner. However, priapisms are frequent and patients must be aware of this complication and how to manage it.

When all conservative treatments fail, a penile prosthesis can be implanted. However, this is associated with high morbidity such as infections, mechanical failures and late erosion.

Ejaculation

Preservation of ejaculation following SCI at any level is exceptional (Chapter 3). The most commonly employed technique to obtain semen is vibro-ejaculation which may be achieved using a specially designed vibrator, the "Ferticare" (Fig. 15.5).

The plate is placed underneath the glans penis and the vibrations are performed for 1–3 minutes. It is only effective in upper motor neuron lesions as it relies on an intact spinal reflex arc to facilitate ejaculation but even then has a success rate of 60–80%. It can cause retrograde ejaculation as can be confirmed by performing catheterization

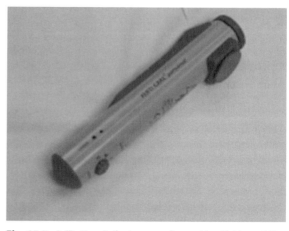

Fig. 15.5. A "Ferticare" vibrator, manufactured by Multicept A/S, Denmark.

after stimulation if there has not been any ante-grade ejaculation. Midodrine, an orally selective α-adrenoreceptor agonist, may prevent retrograde ejaculation by closing the bladder neck, and has been shown to improve ejaculation and orgasm in SCI patients [56]. However, it should be used with caution because it can induce hypertension and increase autonomic dysreflexia.

The complications include bruising and autonomic dysreflexia.

In unsuccessful cases, and for all patients with a sacral root lesion, the ejaculate can be obtained by electroejaculation. This is performed with a probe in the rectum and stimulating preganglionic efferent fibers with electric current [57] (Chapter 3). The success rate is around 98% but this is an invasive method and there is a risk of rectal injury. Also, it is painful and has to be performed under general anesthesia or sedation for patients with incomplete spinal lesions.

Fertility

SCI is associated with impaired fertility due most obviously to erectile dysfunction and ejaculatory failure but also abnormal semen characteristics. These are the results of urinary tract and genital infections, hormonal and hypothalamic-pituitary testicular axis abnormality, local temperature change and sympathetic nerve alteration [58]. The main semen abnormality is asthenozoospermia.

Currently, practice is to retrieve sperm early after SCI for cryopreservation, using vibro- or electroejaculation as described above. In the majority of cases assisted conception techniques are required to achieve conception.

Female sexual dysfunction
Vaginal lubrication

Reports on the effects of SCI on sexual function in women are limited. The pathophysiological principles are similar to those in men in that the level and completeness of the injury determine preservation of psychogenic and reflex lubrication, the process analogous to erectile function (Chapter 3). Following damage above the lower thoracic region reflex responses to genital stimulation are preserved and women with incomplete SCI who are able to perceive pinprick in the T_{12}–L_2 segment may retain the ability for

psychogenic genital vasocongestion. Women with sacral root damage have little in the way of arousal responses.

Orgasmic capacity

By comparison with healthy women, about 50% of women following SCI are able to achieve orgasm. Only 17% of women with complete lower motor neuron dysfunction and 59% of women with other levels can achieve orgasm [59]. In a study which used physiological measurements and written accounts of sensations to record orgasm, 44% of women with SCI were able to achieve orgasm in the laboratory setting although the time to do so was much longer than in control, able-bodied women [59]. It has been suggested that the preserved vaginal-cervical "awareness" is provided by vagal innervation which provides a "spinal cord bypass" [60] (Chapter 3).

A pilot study found a positive effect of sildenafil on sexual dysfunction in SCI women but these results have to be confirmed [61].

Sexual rehabilitation

In an excellent review of sexual rehabilitation following SCI in women it was pointed out that urinary and bowel incontinence, spasticity, vaginal lubrication and autonomic dysreflexia are the physical consequences of SCI that appear to have most impact on sexual activity. However psychosocial factors, such as age and partnership status, may also affect sexual rehabilitation [62].

Discussions with women with SCI in Denmark and Sweden on their reactions to information and counselling offered during rehabilitation revealed an overwhelming need for the exchange of information and experience with other women with SCI, and a desire for opportunities for counselling after initial rehabilitation [62].

Pregnancy

The first months after injury are associated with amenorrhea but menstruation soon resumes and the fertility in SCI women is not compromised. There are no medical restrictions on the contraceptive methods that can be used.

When planning pregnancy, ongoing treatment of bladder dysfunction can present a problem. Pregnancy is not recommended within six months of detrusor botulinum toxin A injections and none of the manufacturers of antimuscarinics state that their medication is safe during pregnancy.

The usual problems in pregnancy are UTIs, management of DO, anemia, pedal edema, weight-transfer problems and thrombophlebitis. It is recommended to check the urine for infection every month and treat all infections or bacteriuria. CISC should be maintained and often an increased number of daily catheterizations.

Pregnant SCI women require frequent check-ups and early hospitalization is often necessary. Pregnancy in SCI is more frequently associated with premature cervical dilatation and labour and "small-for-dates" infants. Management of labor, especially if the woman cannot perceive labor pains, may present special difficulties and such patients should be managed by an experienced multidisciplinary team. Women with an injury at level T_6 and above are at an increased risk of developing autonomic dysreflexia. Autonomic dysreflexia can be stimulated by induction, labor, delivery or even breast-feeding. During labor, autonomic dysreflexia can be prevented by early epidural anesthesia and most women will have successful vaginal deliveries: SCI does not constitute an indication for Cesarean section.

The lactation may cease after three months, for reasons not yet understood.

References

1. Jackson AB, Dijkers M, Devivo MJ, Poczatek RB. A demographic profile of new traumatic spinal cord injuries: change and stability over 30 years. *Arch Phys Med Rehabil* 2004;**85**:1740–8.

2. Stover SL, Fine PR. The epidemiology and economics of spinal cord injury. *Paraplegia* 1987;**25**:225–8.

3. Ditunno JF, Jr., Young W, Donovan WH, Creasey G. The international standards booklet for neurological and functional classification of spinal cord injury. American Spinal Injury Association. *Paraplegia* 1994;**32**:70–80.

4. Alexander MS, Biering-Sorensen F, Bodner D, et al. International standards to document remaining autonomic function after spinal cord injury. *Spinal Cord* 2009;**47**:36–43.

5. Norris JP, Staskin DR. History, physical examination, and classification of neurogenic voiding dysfunction. *Urol Clin North Am* 1996;**23**:337–43.

6. Weld KJ, Graney MJ, Dmochowski RR. Clinical significance of detrusor sphincter dyssynergia type in patients with post-traumatic spinal cord injury. *Urology* 2000;**56**:565–8.

7. Patki P, Woodhouse J, Hamid R, Shah J, Craggs M. Lower urinary tract dysfunction in ambulatory patients with incomplete spinal cord injury. *J Urol* 2006;**175**:1784–7.

8. Moslavac S, Dzidic I, Kejla Z. Neurogenic detrusor overactivity: comparison between complete and incomplete spinal cord injury patients. *Neurourol Urodyn* 2008;**27**:504–6.

9. Krassioukov A, Warburton DE, Teasell R, Eng JJ. A systematic review of the management of autonomic dysreflexia after spinal cord injury. *Arch Phys Med Rehabil* 2009;**90**:682–95.

10. Curt A, Nitsche B, Rodic B, Schurch B, Dietz V. Assessment of autonomic dysreflexia in patients with spinal cord injury. *J Neurol Neurosurg Psychiatry* 1997;**62**:473–7.

11. Acute management of autonomic dysreflexia: adults with spinal cord injury presenting to health-care facilities. Consortium for spinal cord. *J Spinal Cord Med* 1997;**20**:284–308.

12. Chartier-Kastler E, Ruffion A. Démarche et bilan diagnostique en neuro-urologie. *Prog Urol* 2007;**17**:339–43.

13. Bladder management for adults with spinal cord injury: a clinical practice guideline for health-care providers. *J Spinal Cord Med* 2006;**29**:527–73.

14. Stohrer M, Blok B, Castro-Diaz D, et al. EAU guidelines on neurogenic lower urinary tract dysfunction. *Eur Urol* 2009;**56**:81–8.

15. Abrams P, Agarwal M, Drake M, et al. A proposed guideline for the urological management of patients with spinal cord injury. *BJU Int* 2008;**101**:989–94.

16. Alexander MS, Anderson KD, Biering-Sorensen F, et al. Outcome measures in spinal cord injury: recent assessments and recommendations for future directions. *Spinal Cord* 2009;**47**:582–91.

17. Thomassen SA, Johannesen IL, Erlandsen EJ, Abrahamsen J, Randers E. Serum cystatin C as a marker of the renal function in patients with spinal cord injury. *Spinal Cord* 2002;**40**:524–8.

18. Weld KJ, Dmochowski RR. Effect of bladder management on urological complications in spinal cord injured patients. *J Urol* 2000;**163**:768–72.

19. Chang SM, Hou CL, Dong DQ, Zhang H. Urologic status of 74 spinal cord injury patients from the 1976 Tangshan earthquake, and managed for over 20 years using the Crede maneuver. *Spinal Cord* 2000;**38**:552–4.

20. Hall MK, Hackler RH, Zampieri TA, Zampieri JB. Renal calculi in spinal cord-injured patient: association with reflux, bladder stones, and foley catheter drainage. *Urology* 1989;**34**:126–8.

21. Ost MC, Lee BR. Urolithiasis in patients with spinal cord injuries: risk factors, management, and outcomes. *Curr Opin Urol* 2006;**16**:93–9.

22. Lawrenson R, Wyndaele JJ, Vlachonikolis I, Farmer C, Glickman S. Renal failure in patients with neurogenic lower urinary tract dysfunction. *Neuroepidemiology* 2001;**20**:138–43.

23. Sekar P, Wallace DD, Waites KB, et al. Comparison of long-term renal function after spinal cord injury using different urinary management methods. *Arch Phys Med Rehabil* 1997;**78**:992–7.

24. Nicolle LE. Asymptomatic bacteriuria: review and discussion of the IDSA guidelines. *Int J Antimicrob Agents* 2006;**28**(Suppl 1):S42–8.

25. The prevention and management of urinary tract infections among people with spinal cord injuries. National Institute on Disability and Rehabilitation Research Consensus Statement. January 27–29, 1992. *J Am Paraplegia Soc* 1992;**15**:194–204.

26. Kass EH. Asymptomatic infections of the urinary tract. *Trans Assoc Am Physicians* 1956;**69**:56–64.

27. Esclarin De Ruz A, Garcia Leoni E, Herruzo Cabrera R. Epidemiology and risk factors for urinary tract infection in patients with spinal cord injury. *J Urol* 2000;**164**:1285–9.

28. Whiteneck GG, Charlifue SW, Frankel HL, et al. Mortality, morbidity, and psychosocial outcomes of persons spinal cord injured more than 20 years ago. *Paraplegia* 1992;**30**:617–30.

29. Cardenas DD, Hoffman JM, Kirshblum S, McKinley W. Etiology and incidence of rehospitalization after traumatic spinal cord injury: a multicenter analysis. *Arch Phys Med Rehabil* 2004;**85**:1757–63.

30. Hess MJ, Hess PE, Sullivan MR, Nee M, Yalla SV. Evaluation of cranberry tablets for the prevention of urinary tract infections in spinal cord injured patients with neurogenic bladder. *Spinal Cord* 2008;**46**:622–6.

31. Salomon J, Denys P, Merle C, et al. Prevention of urinary tract infection in spinal cord-injured patients: safety and efficacy of a weekly oral cyclic antibiotic (WOCA) programme with a 2 year follow-up – an observational prospective study. *J Antimicrob Chemother* 2006;**57**:784–8.

32. McGuire EJ, Savastano JA. Urodynamics and management of the neuropathic bladder in spinal cord injury patients. *J Am Paraplegia Soc* 1985;**8**:28–32.

33. Pannek J. Transitional cell carcinoma in patients with spinal cord injury: a high risk malignancy? *Urology* 2002;**59**:240–4.

34. Kaufman JM, Fam B, Jacobs SC, et al. Bladder cancer and squamous metaplasia in spinal cord injury patients. *J Urol* 1977;**118**:967–71.

35. Navon JD, Soliman H, Khonsari F, Ahlering T. Screening cystoscopy and survival of spinal cord injured patients with squamous cell cancer of the bladder. *J Urol* 1997;**157**:2109–11.

36. Hamid R, Bycroft J, Arya M, Shah PJ. Screening cystoscopy and biopsy in patients with neuropathic bladder and chronic suprapubic indwelling catheters: is it valid? *J Urol* 2003;**170**(2 Pt 1):425–7.

37. Yang CC, Clowers DE. Screening cystoscopy in chronically catheterized spinal cord injury patients. *Spinal Cord* 1999;**37**:204–7.

38. Ruffion A, De Sèze M, Denys P, Perrouin-Verbe B, Chartier-Kastler E. Suivi des vessies neurologiques du blesse medullaire et du patient porteur d'une myelomeningocele. Revue de la litterature et recommandations pratiques de suivi. *Pelv Perineol* 2006;**1**:304–23.

39. Costa P, Perrouin-Verbe B, Colvez A, et al. Quality of life in spinal cord injury patients with urinary difficulties. Development and validation of qualiveen. *Eur Urol* 2001;**39**:107–13.

40. Zahariou A, Karagiannis G, Papaioannou P, Stathi K, Michail X. The use of desmopressin in the management of nocturnal enuresis in patients with spinal cord injury. *Eura Medicophys* 2007;**43**:333–8.

41. Schurch B, Schmid DM, Stohrer M. Treatment of neurogenic incontinence with botulinum toxin A. *N Engl J Med* 2000;**342**:665.

42. Karsenty G, Denys P, Amarenco G, et al. Botulinum toxin A (Botox) intradetrusor injections in adults with neurogenic detrusor overactivity/neurogenic overactive bladder: a systematic literature review. *Eur Urol* 2008;**53**:275–87.

43. Giannantoni A, Mearini E, Del Zingaro M, Porena M. Six-year follow-up of botulinum toxin A intradetrusorial injections in patients with refractory neurogenic detrusor overactivity: clinical and urodynamic results. *Eur Urol* 2009;**55**:705–11.

44. Wyndaele JJ, Kovindha A, Madersbacher H, et al. Neurologic urinary and faecal incontinence. In: Abrams P, Cardozo L, Khoury S, Wein A, eds. *Incontinence*. Paris: Editions 21; 2009.

45. Sievert KD, Amend B, Gakis G, et al. Early sacral neuromodulation prevents urinary incontinence after complete spinal cord injury. *Ann Neurol* 2010;**67**:74–84.

46. Brindley GS. An implant to empty the bladder or close the urethra. *J Neurol Neurosurg Psychiatry* 1977;**40**:358–69.

47. Brindley GS. The actions of parasympathetic and sympathetic nerves in human micturition, erection and seminal emission, and their restoration in paraplegic

patients by implanted electrical stimulators. *Proc R Soc Lond* 1988;**235**:111–20.

48. Fowler CJ, Panicker JN, Drake M, et al. A UK consensus on the management of the bladder in multiple sclerosis. *J Neurol Neurosurg Psychiatry* 2009;**80**:470–7.

49. Game X, Karsenty G, Chartier-Kastler E, Ruffion A. Traitement de l'hyperactivite detrusorienne neurologique: enterocystoplasties. *Prog Urol* 2007;**17**:584–96.

50. Timoney AG, Shaw PJ. Urological outcome in female patients with spinal cord injury: the effectiveness of intermittent catheterisation. *Paraplegia* 1990;**28**:556–63.

51. Glickman S, Kamm MA. Bowel dysfunction in spinal-cord-injury patients. *Lancet* 1996;**347**:1651–3.

52. Courtois F, Mathieu C, Charvier K. Sexual rehabilitation for men with spinal cord injury: preliminary report on a behavioral strategy. *Sex Disabil* 2001;**19**:153–7.

53. Lombardi G, Macchiarella A, Cecconi F, Del Popolo G. Ten years of phosphodiesterase type 5 inhibitors in spinal cord injured patients. *J Sex Med* 2009;**6**:1248–58.

54. Soler JM, Previnaire JG, Denys P, Chartier-Kastler E. Phosphodiesterase inhibitors in the treatment of erectile dysfunction in spinal cord-injured men. *Spinal Cord* 2007;**45**:169–73.

55. Deforge D, Blackmer J, Garritty C, et al. Male erectile dysfunction following spinal cord injury: a systematic review. *Spinal Cord* 2006;**44**:465–73.

56. Brindley GS. Electroejaculation: its technique, neurological implications and uses. *J Neurol Neurosurg Psychiatry* 1981;**44**:9–18.

57. Soler JM, Previnaire JG, Plante P, Denys P, Chartier-Kastler E. Midodrine improves orgasm in spinal cord-injured men: the effects of autonomic stimulation. *J Sex Med* 2008;**5**:2935–41.

58. Patki P, Hamid R, Shah J, Craggs M. Fertility following spinal cord injury: a systematic review. *Spinal Cord* 2007;**45**:187.

59. Sipski ML, Alexander CJ, Rosen R. Sexual arousal and orgasm in women: effects of spinal cord injury. *Ann Neurol* 2001;**49**:35–44.

60. Komisaruk BR, Whipple B. Functional MRI of the brain during orgasm in women. *Annu Rev Sex Res* 2005;**16**:62–86.

61. Sipski ML, Rosen RC, Alexander CJ, Hamer RM. Sildenafil effects on sexual and cardiovascular responses in women with spinal cord injury. *Urology* 2000;**55**:812–5.

62. Forsythe E, Horsewell JE. Sexual rehabilitation of women with a spinal cord injury. *Spinal Cord* 2006;**44**:234–41.

Chapter 16

Spina bifida and tethered cord syndrome

Thomas M. Kessler and Gustav Kiss

Pathogenesis

Formation of the spinal cord and vertebral column begins at about the 18th day of gestation. Closure of the neural tube (differentiated from the ectoderm) proceeds in a caudal direction from the cephalad end and is complete by 35 days (Fig. 16.1). Disturbances of the neural tube are accompanied by malformations of the vertebral corpora, mostly closure defects of the bony arcs, explaining the collective term "spina bifida" (i.e. "split spine").

Spina bifida is one of the most common birth defects with a prevalence of 1–1.5 per 1000 births in the UK and Ireland [1]. Defective closure of the neural groove can be present as a hidden or an open lesion, i.e. spina bifida occulta and spina bifida aperta, respectively. Occult defects are covered by the meninges and skin; there may be a hairy area or a slight dimple on the lower back, or it may remain completely unnoticed. Other closed defects are marked by protrusions of different degree, but the malformation is coated with fat, bone, or membranes and skin. Beneath the covering layers is the cele, a cavity filled with meningeal and/or neural material (meningocele and/or myelomeningocele) (Fig. 16.2). Open lesions are very apparent and show a constant defect of the covering sheets. The leakage of CSF is an indicator of the severity of the abnormality and, because of the risk of central nervous system infection, indicates an immediate need for surgery.

The exact mechanisms resulting in closure or a dysraphic state are yet to be elucidated. The neural tube is formed by a sequence of events that is referred to as neurulation [2]. The brain and most of the spinal cord are formed by primary neurulation, which involves the shaping, folding and midline fusion of the neural plate. Primary neurulation extends caudally into the region of the future first to fifth sacral vertebrae. The most caudal portion of the spinal cord is formed by a distinct process called secondary neurulation, which does not include neural folding. Spina bifida is a defect of primary neurulation that results from failure of fusion in the caudal region of the neural tube (in contrast to anencephaly which results from failure of fusion in the cranial region of the neural tube).

The etiology of closure defects of the neural tube is supposed to be multifactorial, including both genetic and environmental factors. Considering genetic factors, most of the genes affecting these defects are in relation to folic acid metabolism, especially the "5,10-methylenetetrahydrofolate reductase gene" [3]. Thus, a deficit of folic acid in the early pregnancy period may be a major risk. Further known risks on the maternal side are diabetes mellitus, drug treatment of epilepsy with valproic acid [4] during pregnancy, and obesity.

The role of folic acid in the prevention of neural tube defects has been established since the early 1990s [5]. Maternal ingestion of 400 μg of folic acid per day in all women of child-bearing age can reduce the incidence of spina bifida by 50% [5]. It is now mandatory that enriched grain products be fortified with folic acid [6]. In the United Kingdom and Ireland, the yearly prevalence of neural tube defects declined, predating any periconceptional folic acid supplementation policy initiatives, from 4.5 per 1000 births in 1980 to 1–1.5 per 1000 in the 1990s. However, in the rest of Europe, the prevalence during the 1980s and thereafter was close to 1 per 1000 births [1]. These data suggest that the policy of simply recommending periconceptional supplementation of folic acid in planned pregnancies is not enough. Poor education regarding folate supplementation and the high rate of unplanned pregnancy has meant that the

Pelvic Organ Dysfunction in Neurological Disease: Clinical Management and Rehabilitation, ed. Clare J. Fowler, Jalesh N. Panicker & Anton Emmanuel. Published by Cambridge University Press. © Cambridge University Press 2010.

full potential of this preventative strategy has not been realized [7]. In addition, antibodies developed in response to increased folate ingestion may negate its beneficial effect [8].

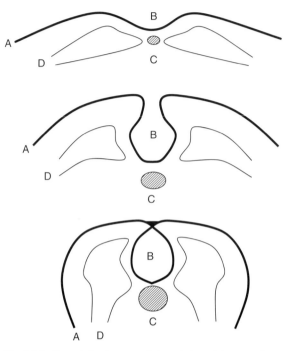

Fig. 16.1. Normal development of the spinal cord. A = ectoderm; B = neural tube; C = notochord; D = mesoderm.

While the likelihood of bladder, bowel and pelvic floor dysfunction depends on the severity of the lesion, the pattern of the dysfunction is determined by the level of the defect. Most spinal defects occur at the level of the lumbar vertebrae, with the sacral, thoracic and cervical areas, in decreasing order of frequency, less affected [9]. Dysraphic disturbances which affect the upper limbs are extremely rare and are accompanied mostly by fatal abnormities of the brain. In patients with lower spinal spina bifida the neurological findings can vary from the most discrete deficit to a complete paraplegia. Hydrocephalus has often been considered an almost inevitable sequel of myelomeningocele and shunt placement rates in the order of 80–90% are commonly quoted [10]. In addition, the Chiari II malformation (the features include elongated brainstem that extends into the cervical spinal canal, small fourth ventricle, tectal beaking and large massa intermedia) is present in almost all myelomeningocele patients and is symptomatic in between one-quarter and one-third [10]. In infants, central apnea and lower cranial nerve dysfunction are common manifestations whilst in the older child and young adult symptoms of foramen magnum impaction such as neck pain, headache and sensory disturbance in the limbs are more common [10]. It should be considered that the pelvic organ problems in spina bifida patients can also be part of a general physical deformity.

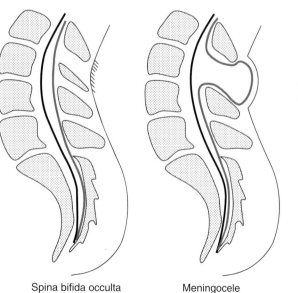

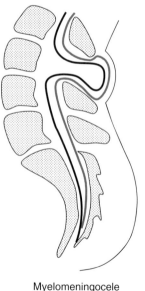

Fig. 16.2. Types of spina bifida.

Spina bifida occulta   Meningocele   Myelomeningocele

According to general neurological principles, spina bifida patients may suffer from central and peripheral lesions regarding bladder, bowel and pelvic floor (dys)function. Depending on the level of the neuronal defect, there is a malfunction of the first or the second motor-neuron, i.e. there are central or peripheral disconnections in somato-sensory and/or viscero-sensory pathways. Central lesions cause hyperreflexia and spasticity; peripheral lesions lead to areflexia and flaccid paresis. Somatic and visceral pathways show mostly, but not always, the same dysfunctional pattern: overactive detrusor and overactive (spastic) sphincter (pelvic floor) or underactive/acontractile detrusor and underactive/acontractile sphincter (pelvic floor). However, by contrast to the most traumatic spinal cord lesions, in spina bifida patients mixed dysfunctional patterns may occur, i.e. overactive detrusor with underactive/acontractile sphincter (pelvic floor) or underactive/acontractile detrusor with overactive (spastic) sphincter (pelvic floor). In these cases, the localization of the lesion is intraconal and affects the anterior and lateral horn of the spinal cord to a different extent.

Several centers have begun closing the defect in fetuses between 19 and 25 weeks of gestation in an attempt to improve the neurological defect in these children. It is estimated that more than 400 fetal operations have now been performed for spina bifida worldwide yet despite this growing experience, the technique remains of unproven benefit [11]. Although fetal surgery has not altered the incidence of abnormal findings on urodynamic assessment in the postnatal period [12], aqueduct obstruction and consequent hydrocephalus has not occurred at birth to the same incidence or extent [13]. Nevertheless, further research is needed to define the role of in utero interventions.

Urinary tract dysfunction

Introduction

Neurogenic bladder dysfunction in children with spina bifida can lead to secondary upper urinary tract deterioration and often causes chronic urinary incontinence [14]. Formerly, the preservation of renal function was the primary goal in the neuro-urological management of spina bifida patients but considering the impact on quality of life, efforts to promote urinary continence have become increasingly important. Continence is associated with better self-image and incontinent girls are at particularly high risk of poor self-esteem [15]. Urinary incontinence is a stress factor for these patients and even a small improvement in urinary continence may have a positive impact. Thus, reducing the frequency of incontinence or, even better, the achievement of continence is an important goal of urological medical care.

According to Verhoef et al. [16] urinary and fecal incontinence is common in young adults with spina bifida (61% and 34%, respectively) regardless of the bladder and bowel management they used. The majority of urinary and fecal incontinent patients perceived this as a problem (70% and 77%, respectively). Moreover, the authors of this study found that patients with a level of lesion at spinal cord L_5 or above were far more likely to be urinary and fecal incontinent than those with a level of lesion at spinal cord S_1 or below. However, patients with a level of lesion at spinal cord L_5 and above were also more likely to perceive urinary incontinence as a problem. Urinary incontinence in these patients has an underlying component of detrusor overactivity and/or poor bladder compliance, this being more common in patients with lower lesions and intact or at least partially intact sacral reflexes.

Assessment

Although some authors [17] have questioned the value of urodynamics shortly after birth and serially thereafter, most authors agree [18–20] that early urodynamics are a prerequisite for an adequate treatment strategy.

The Innsbruck approach [19, 21], based on more than 30 years of experience with spina bifida patients [22], is of early proactive conservative management, which improves upper urinary tract function and reduces the need for surgery in patients with myelomeningocele in the long term [19, 20]. The initial evaluation consists of a history, neuro-urological examination (especially including bulbocavernosus reflex, anal reflex and anal sphincter tone), urinalysis, urine culture, sonography of kidneys and bladder, as well as (video-)urodynamics. Patients undergo initial evaluation as early as possible, ideally at the day of birth or within two weeks after closure of an open spina bifida defect. Voiding cystourethrography and urodynamics are performed concurrently as videourodynamics. Patients at risk of upper urinary tract damage (low bladder compliance, intravesical pressure >40 cmH$_2$O, detrusor sphincter dyssynergia) and those with abnormal findings on imaging studies

257

(trabeculated bladder ± pseudodiverticula, vesico-ureteral reflux, dilated ureter, hydronephrosis, cortical thinning/scarring of renal parenchyma) undergo nuclear renal scan. Periodic reassessment with neuro-urological examination, urinalysis, urine culture, imaging studies and (video-)urodynamics is performed every three to six months up to age two years and at yearly intervals thereafter.

Treatment

For clinical practice the guidelines on neurogenic lower urinary tract dysfunction of the European Association of Urology [23] recommend the "Madersbacher classification" system (Chapter 4) [24]. Urodynamics together with clinical assessment of the anal/bulbocavernosus reflex allow definition of the dysfunctional pattern of the lower urinary tract: over- or underactivity of the detrusor and combination of sphincter (pelvic floor) dysfunction, the pattern not only determining the risk for upper urinary tract deterioration but also the chances of achieving urinary continence. In a retrospective study [21] of 123 spina bifida patients with a mean follow-up of 10 years, there was a significant difference in achieving continence or social dryness: more than 85% of patients with overactive (spastic) sphincter (pelvic floor) combined with overactive or underactive/acontractile detrusor became continent or socially dry, but only 57% and 74% of those with an underactive/acontractile sphincter (pelvic floor) combined with overactive or underactive/acontractile detrusor, respectively (Fig. 16.3). In addition, none of the patients with underactive/acontractile detrusor and overactive (spastic) sphincter (pelvic floor) underwent adjunctive incontinence surgery, compared to about 25% in the other groups.

Based on the pattern of dysfunction, our therapeutic strategy to preserve both upper and lower urinary tract function and to achieve urinary continence is determined as follows:

A. In patients with overactive detrusor and overactive (spastic) sphincter (pelvic floor), detrusor sphincter dyssynergia is the main problem and puts the upper urinary tract at risk due to low compliance and/or high intravesical pressures during the storage and voiding phase. On the other hand, sphincter (pelvic floor) overactivity provides urinary continence once detrusor overactivity is under control and regular bladder emptying is achieved by intermittent (self-)catheterization.

The therapeutic concept therefore is to convert the overactive into an underactive detrusor by antimuscarinic treatment and to assist or accomplish bladder emptying by intermittent (self-)catheterization. If this cannot be achieved by oral antimuscarinics, intradetrusor injections of botulinum neurotoxin type A (Chapter 6), bladder augmentation or rarely sphincterotomy (with the risk for even increased incontinence) or urinary diversions are considered (Chapter 7).

B. Overactive detrusor with underactive/acontractile sphincter (pelvic floor) results in detrusor overactivity incontinence combined with stress incontinence due to the decreased bladder outlet resistance. Antimuscarinics and sometimes also electrostimulation of the pelvic floor musculature in incomplete lesions help to restore urinary continence. However, in others with this pattern the implantation of an artificial urinary sphincter, sometimes combined with bladder augmentation, may be necessary (Chapter 7).

C. Underactive/acontractile detrusor with overactive (spastic) sphincter (pelvic floor) is best managed by intermittent (self-)catheterization. If the bladder is emptied regularly, the patient stays continent because of their active sphincter (pelvic floor) activity, as long as controlled fluid intake avoids "overflow incontinence." In patients with at least some sensation in the sacral dermatomes indicating functioning afferent fibers, at least one cycle of intravesical electrostimulation therapy may be considered to improve detrusor contractility and thereby bladder emptying.

D. Underactive/acontractile detrusor with underactive/acontractile sphincter (pelvic floor) is usually associated with stress urinary incontinence and is successfully treated by implantation of an artificial urinary sphincter combined with intermittent (self-)catheterization. Passive voiding by abdominal straining (Valsalva maneuver) or by suprapubic downwards compression of the lower abdomen (Credé maneuver) is not recommended as this creates unphysiologically high intravesical pressures, putting at risk the upper urinary tract and also causing a compression of the urethra and thus a functional obstruction leading to inefficient emptying. In some patients, intravesical electrostimulation may lead to improved bladder emptying (Chapter 7).

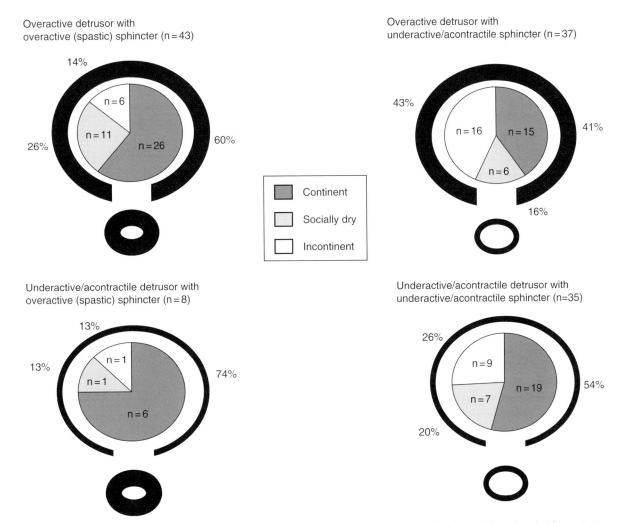

Overactive detrusor with overactive (spastic) sphincter (n = 43)

14%

n = 6

n = 11

n = 26

26%

60%

Overactive detrusor with underactive/acontractile sphincter (n = 37)

43%

n = 16

n = 15

n = 6

41%

16%

Continent

Socially dry

Incontinent

Underactive/acontractile detrusor with overactive (spastic) sphincter (n = 8)

13%

13%

n = 1

n = 1

n = 6

74%

Underactive/acontractile detrusor with underactive/acontractile sphincter (n=35)

26%

n = 9

n = 7

n = 19

54%

20%

Fig. 16.3. Urinary incontinence at the last follow-up in regard to the urodynamic pattern at initial evaluation. Reproduced with permission from [21].

Clean intermittent (self-)catheterization

While indwelling catheters have been used traditionally, clean intermittent (self-)catheterization, initially reported by Lapides et al. [25], has revolutionized the modern management of voiding dysfunction because of the significant decrease in urological complications. In children with spina bifida, parents and other caregivers carry out clean intermittent catheterization in the first 6–10 years of life. Thereafter, children with sufficient dexterity will take on this task. Clean intermittent self-catheterization was found a technique easily learned in one visit and mastered in a short time for most genitally sensate children [26]. Overall comfort with the technique was excellent, few problems were encountered and quality of life was comparable to that of normal children. In addition, most adult patients perceived clean intermittent self-catheterization as an easy and painless procedure that does not interfere with daily activities [27].

Antimuscarinic therapy

Seven antimuscarincs (i.e. darifenacin, fesoterodine, oxybutynin, propiverine, solifenacin, tolterodine and trospium chloride) with different dosages, formulations and routes of administration are currently used for treating overactive bladder (Chapter 6). In daily clinical practice, most currently used antimuscarinics for treating overactive bladder are often prescribed in (adolescent and adult) spina bifida patients, although there is a lack of well-designed randomized controlled trials in this specific neurological subpopulation. In addition, only oxybutynin has yet been registered for pediatric use. Thus, the role of newer antimuscarinics needs to be established, especially in the pediatric spina bifida population.

Intradetrusor injections of botulinum neurotoxin type A

In cases where antimuscarinic treatment fails and/or the medication is not tolerated, intradetrusor injections of botulinum neurotoxin type A are an alternative.

In systematic reviews [28, 29], botulinum neurotoxin type A has been found to be effective for treating neurogenic detrusor overactivity including myelomeningocele patients. In children [29], the underlying neurological disease was spina bifida in 93% and most were over two years of age. The most common amount of botulinum neurotoxin type A injected was 10–12 U/kg with a maximum dose of 300 U, usually as 30 injections of 10 U/ml into the bladder (excluding the trigone) under cystoscopic guidance and general anesthesia. Most of the studies reported a significant improvement in clinical (65–87% became completely dry) as well as urodynamic (in most studies mean maximum detrusor pressure was reduced to <40 cmH$_2$O and compliance was increased >20 ml/cmH$_2$O) variables, without major adverse events. Considering these findings, intradetrusor injections of botulinum neurotoxin type A appears to be a safe and minimally invasive procedure in children with spina bifida not responding to usual medical treatments, so that more invasive reconstructive surgery may be postponed or avoided. Although the literature of repeat intradetrusor injections of botulinum neurotoxin type A in spina bifida patients is very limited, repeat treatments seem to be as effective as the first [30, 31].

Surgical treatments

Surgical treatments in the spina bifida patient depend on the type of urinary tract dysfunction and do not differ from the procedures described in Chapter 7 for the general neurological patient.

Sexual dysfunction
Introduction

With the growing number of spina bifida children reaching adolescence and adulthood, sexuality is an increasingly important issue. However, few studies have critically assessed this and further investigations into sexuality, sex education, intimacy and treatments for sexual dysfunction and infertility in those with spina bifida are needed.

Sexual development depends on socialization and the ability of the child to make friends and discuss shared experiences and thoughts. Mental handicaps, poor manual dexterity, lack of education regarding normal and abnormal sexual function, invasion of personal privacy and overprotective parents often prevent independent behavior and, as a result, lead to poor understanding of sexual issues [32]. Spina bifida adolescents are often ignorant about sexuality issues and have not been told facts about reproductive life. Up to 23% of girls do not know about the hygienic management of menstruation [33]. The self-image in spina bifida adolescents was reported to be similar to that of their peers with the exception of the sexuality dimension, which was significantly below normal, especially in females [34].

Assessment

Assessment of sexual function in spina bifida patients is similar to that described in Chapter 10 for the general neurological patient, but there are some spina bifida-specific issues which should be considered when counseling patients and their parents about eventual sexual performance. In general, adult spina bifida patients have normal sexual desires and an interest in addressing these issues with healthcare providers. However, sexual education and access to intimacy are delayed compared to the general population [35, 36]. Sexual activity seems not to be related to gender, the level of urinary incontinence or the extent of physical disability but it appears more likely in patients with a lower level of neurological impairment [36]. In addition, patients with hydrocephalus are sexually less active and perceive more problems than those without [36, 37]. About 75% of men may achieve erections, but in some these may be merely reflexive in nature [38]. In women, reproductive function, which is under hormonal control, is generally not affected, whereas in males infertility is a common problem. Erectile dysfunction and infertility are related to the level of neurological lesion, with the best performance status in those with sacral lesions and intact reflexes. Men with lesions higher than T_{10} are at risk for azoospermia. Poor semen quality [39] and abnormal histology on testis biopsy (i.e. absence of germinal epithelium from the seminiferous tubules, which contain only Sertoli cells) [40] have been reported as reasons for infertility in males with spina bifida, in addition to erectile dysfunction.

Treatment

There is an almost complete lack of well-designed studies for treating sexual dysfunction in spina bifida patients. Thus extrapolations from the general neurological patient (Chapter 10) to the spina bifida patient are the best available. In the only trial to date in spina bifida patients, sildenafil was shown to be effective for treating erectile dysfunction in a prospective, blinded, randomized, placebo-controlled, dose-escalation, crossover study [41, 42].

In a case series of three spina bifida patients with absent penile sensibility [43], a newly designed neurological bypass procedure connecting the ilioinguinal nerve with the dorsal nerve of the penis resulted in glans sensibility and erogenous feeling. The new sensation appeared to contribute to the quality of the patient sexuality and sexual functioning as well as to the feeling of being a more normal and complete individual who is more conscious of the penis. If these results are reproducible and the benefits shown to be sustained, this new operation might become a valuable treatment option for spina bifida patients with absent penile sensitivity in the future.

Bowel dysfunction

Introduction

Bowel dysfunction is a major concern in spina bifida patients. It has a negative impact on quality of life and on social activities and this increases with advancing age [44]. Up to 34% of spina bifida patients suffer with fecal incontinence and more than 75% perceive this as having a negative impact on their lives [16]. Fecal incontinence causes odor and skin irritation, it increases dependence, impacts negatively on social interactions, lowers self-esteem and causes psychological problems [44, 45]. Poor bowel control is not associated with the attainment of urinary continence.

It is often related to fecal consistency, how rapidly the rectum refills after an evacuation, the sacral cord sensory and motor function, and reflex reactivity of the external anal sphincter [46].

Assessment

Until recently there was no specific instrument to measure the impact of bowel dysfunction on quality of life in spina bifida patients, but Nanigian et al. [47] have now designed a 51-item questionnaire, termed the "Fecal Incontinence and Constipation Quality of Life" (FIC QOL) measure, that is discriminative and evaluative. It specifically examines bowel issues that patients with spina bifida and their families encounter. The items are divided into seven quality-of-life factor groupings, including bowel program, dietary management, symptoms, travel and socialization, family relationships, caregiver emotional impact and financial impact. The FIC QOL questionnaire provides a valid and reliable tool to assess the effect of bowel care, fecal incontinence and constipation in spina bifida children and their caregivers [47] and is strongly recommended. If interventions are planned, stool diaries as well as manometric studies, enema tests and fecoflowmetry may be considered.

Treatment

Although most authors agree that regular and efficient bowel emptying in patients with spina bifida is important, the best method of attaining this objective is still uncertain. Since spina bifida patients are a heterogeneous group and since bowel dysfunction in this population includes both constipation and fecal incontinence, a uniform policy in treatment is not possible. Intake of a high-soluble fiber diet (fruit and vegetable fiber) and administration of laxatives are used in the prevention and treatment of constipation. Management of fecal incontinence is aimed at regular bowel emptying, achievable by stool diary, manual stool evacuation, or use of retrograde or antegrade enemas [48].

Most programs begin at about one year of age. The children are started on diets, i.e. fruits and bran, and on stool-softeners in older children. In addition, suppositories which help to evacuate the rectum are used and may train the lower bowel to fill and empty. At the age of about three years, bowel management can be performed successfully in the vast majority of patients with retrograde colonic enemas [49] although there may be difficulty in retaining the solution in the rectum when the anal sphincter muscle is lax. The Peristeen (Coloplast A/S, Denmark) transanal irrigation system is effective, easy to learn and safe and it also increases independence in spina bifida patients [50]. This system makes it possible for even immobilized children or children with poor hand function to perform the irrigation procedure without assistance from their parents or carers [50]. The catheter is inserted into the rectum and the balloon inflated to hold the catheter in place within the rectum while a tap-water enema is slowly administered with the manual pump. Subsequently, the balloon is deflated and the catheter removed, followed by bowel emptying of the enema and other bowel contents.

Biofeedback training seems to be no more effective than a conventional good bowel management program in attaining fecal continence [51]. Transrectal [52] and intravesical [53] electrostimulation may improve fecal incontinence. In patients with refractory constipation and fecal incontinence, the antegrade continence enema, initially described by Malone et al. [54], is an invaluable treatment option. The principles of antegrade colonic washout and the Mitrofanoff non-refluxing catheterizable channel (using the appendix vermiformis or, if this is unavailable, a small bowel segment) are combined to produce a continent catheterizable colonic stoma. Enemas consisting of tap water, polyethylene glycol or saline, sometimes in combination with mineral oil or bisacodyl, are instilled daily or every other day to evacuate the colon. Using the Malone antegrade continence enema, fecal continence rates over 80% are achieved [55]. Older children readily become independent in managing their bowel function leading to improved self-esteem and sociability [56].

Although sacral neuromodulation has improved fecal incontinence and constipation in some selected patients [57], there is no randomized trial in spina bifida patients so it remains to be shown if it is effective in this population.

Tethered cord syndrome

Tethered cord syndrome is defined as a stretch-induced functional disorder of the spinal cord with its caudal part anchored by inelastic structures restricting vertical movement [58]. This may be due to spina bifida (scar tissue) or be associated with spina bifida (thickening of the filum terminale attached to

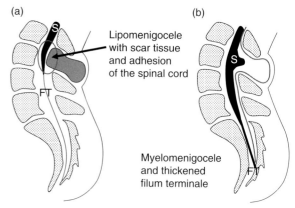

Fig. 16.4. Common causes of tethered cord. Abbreviations: S = spinal cord; FT = filum terminale. A. Scar tissue in the cele area. B. Thickened filum terminale.

the elongated spinal cord) (Fig. 16.4), or may be due to scar from prior non-spina-bifida surgery, fibrous or fibro-adipose filum terminale, bony or dural septum, or tumor. Symptoms and signs are back pain, leg weakness, foot deformity, scoliosis, sensory loss, lower urinary tract dysfunction and/or bowel dysfunction. Approximately 10–30% of children with repaired spina bifida will develop neurological deterioration related to tethered cord syndrome [59]. Lower urinary tract symptoms may not be present until the teenage years or later. However, without surgical release of a symptomatic tethered cord, 60% of children will experience further urological and orthopedic decline within five years [60]. The effect of untethering on lower urinary tract function is uncertain but we strongly advocate surgical release of a symptomatic tethered cord irrespective of age because this is beneficial in a majority of patients in maintaining or improving not only urological but also neurological and orthopedic disabilities at a relatively low risk of complications [61]. Nevertheless, it should be taken into account that in spina bifida patients with a ventriculo-peritoneal shunt, the most common cause of neurological changes is shunt malfunction [62] and most patients require two or three shunt revisions throughout childhood [63]. Shunt malfunction with consequent hydrocephalus may mimic the signs of tethered cord syndrome [61]. Considering that surgical untethering in a child with unrecognized shunt malfunction may have life-threatening consequences [64], shunt function must always be confirmed before surgical untethering [61].

Tethered cord syndrome has no typical urological dysfunction pattern. It often causes storage symptoms, more rarely voiding symptoms, and usually no sexual dysfunction. In a study by Giddens et al. [65], urgency (67%) and urgency incontinence (50%) were the most common complaints, and detrusor overactivity (72%) and detrusor sphincter dyssynergia (22%) the most common urodynamic findings. Treatment of lower urinary tract dysfunction due to tethered cord is guided by symptoms and based on the dysfunctional pattern of the lower urinary tract similar to spina bifida patients in general.

It is generally agreed that tethered cord syndrome may cause bowel dysfunction but the evidence from the literature is very limited [66, 67]. Poor voluntary control of the external anal sphincter and a hyperactive rectum have been suggested as major contributing factors to fecal incontinence in patients with tethered cord [67]. Fecodynamic studies allow early detection of neurogenic disturbances of the anorectum and may be beneficial for determination of the proper time for untethering surgery and also for monitoring in the postoperative follow-up [66, 67].

References

1. Busby A, Abramsky L, Dolk H, Armstrong B. Preventing neural tube defects in Europe: population based study. *BMJ* 2005;**330**:574–5.

2. Mitchell LE, Adzick NS, Melchionne J, et al. Spina bifida. *Lancet* 2004;**364**:1885–95.

3. Pacheco SS, Braga C, Souza AI, Figueiroa JN. Effects of folic acid fortification on the prevalence of neural tube defects. *Rev Saude Publica* 2009;**43**:565–71.

4. Defoort EN, Kim PM, Winn LM. Valproic acid increases conservative homologous recombination frequency and reactive oxygen species formation: a potential mechanism for valproic acid-induced neural tube defects. *Mol Pharmacol* 2006;**69**:1304–10.

5. Prevention of neural tube defects: results of the Medical Research Council Vitamin Study. MRC Vitamin Study Research Group. *Lancet* 1991; **338**:131–7.

6. U.S. Food and Drug Administration. Food standards: amendment of standards of identity for enriched grain products to require addition of folic acid. *Fed Reg* 1996;**61**:8781–97.

7. Busby A, Abramsky L, Dolk H, et al. Preventing neural tube defects in Europe: a missed opportunity. *Reprod Toxicol* 2005;**20**:393–402.

8. Rothenberg SP, da Costa MP, Sequeira JM, et al. Autoantibodies against folate receptors in women with a pregnancy complicated by a neural-tube defect. *N Engl J Med* 2004;**350**:134–42.

9. Bauer SB, Labib KB, Dieppa RA, Retik AB. Urodynamic evaluation of boy with myelodysplasia and incontinence. *Urology* 1977;**10**:354–62.

10. Thompson DN. Postnatal management and outcome for neural tube defects including spina bifida and encephalocoeles. *Prenat Diagn* 2009;**29**:412–9.

11. Sutton LN. Fetal surgery for neural tube defects. *Best Pract Res Clin Obstet Gynaecol* 2008;**22**:175–88.

12. Koh CJ, DeFilippo RL, Borer JG. Lower urinary tract function after fetal closure of myelomeningocele. *J Urol Suppl* 2003;**169**(Abstract 411).

13. Johnson MP, Sutton LN, Rintoul N, et al. Fetal myelomeningocele repair: short-term clinical outcomes. *Am J Obstet Gynecol* 2003;**189**:482–7.

14. Joseph DB. Bladder rehabilitation in children with spina bifida: state-of-the-"ART". *J Urol* 2005;**173**:1850–1.

15. Moore C, Kogan BA, Parekh A. Impact of urinary incontinence on self-concept in children with spina bifida. *J Urol* 2004;**171**:1659–62.

16. Verhoef M, Lurvink M, Barf HA, et al. High prevalence of incontinence among young adults with spina bifida: description, prediction and problem perception. *Spinal Cord* 2005;**43**:331–40.

17. Hopps CV, Kropp KA. Preservation of renal function in children with myelomeningocele managed with basic newborn evaluation and close followup. *J Urol* 2003;**169**:305–8.

18. Bauer SB. The management of the myelodysplastic child: a paradigm shift. *BJU Int* 2003;**92**(Suppl 1):23–8.

19. Kessler TM, Lackner J, Kiss G, Rehder P, Madersbacher H. Early proactive management improves upper urinary tract function and reduces the need for surgery in patients with myelomeningocele. *Neurourol Urodyn* 2006;**25**:758–62.

20. Dik P, Klijn AJ, van Gool JD, de Jong-de Vos van Steenwijk CC, de Jong TP. Early start to therapy preserves kidney function in spina bifida patients. *Eur Urol* 2006;**49**:908–13.

21. Kessler TM, Lackner J, Kiss G, Rehder P, Madersbacher H. Predictive value of initial urodynamic pattern on urinary continence in patients with myelomeningocele. *Neurourol Urodyn* 2006;**25**:361–7.

22. Madersbacher H. Development of the upper urinary tract in myelomeningocele and consequent urological care. *Int Urol Nephrol* 1975;**7**:13–22.

23. Stöhrer M, Castro-Diaz D, Chartier-Kastler E, et al. *EAU guidelines on neurogenic lower urinary tract dysfunction.* http://www.uroweb.org/fileadmin/ tx_eauguidelines/2009/Full/Neurogenic_LUTS.pdf. 2008:1–52.

24. Madersbacher H, Wyndaele JJ, Igawa Y, et al. Conservative management in neuropathic urinary incontinence. In: Abrams P, Khoury S, Wein A, eds. *Incontinence*. Second edn. Plymouth: Health Publications Ltd; 2002:697–754.

25. Lapides J, Diokno AC, Silber SJ, Lowe BS. Clean, intermittent self-catheterization in the treatment of urinary tract disease. *J Urol* 1972;**107**:458–61.

26. Alpert SA, Cheng EY, Zebold KF, Kaplan WE. Clean intermittent catheterization in genitally sensate children: patient experience and health related quality of life. *J Urol* 2005;**174**(4 Pt 2):1616–9.

27. Kessler TM, Ryu G, Burkhard FC. Clean intermittent self-catheterization: a burden for the patient? *Neurourol Urodyn* 2009;**28**:18–21.

28. Karsenty G, Denys P, Amarenco G, et al. Botulinum toxin A (Botox) intradetrusor injections in adults with neurogenic detrusor overactivity/neurogenic overactive bladder: a systematic literature review. *Eur Urol* 2008;**53**:275–87.

29. Game X, Mouracade P, Chartier-Kastler E, et al. Botulinum toxin-A (Botox) intradetrusor injections in children with neurogenic detrusor overactivity/neurogenic overactive bladder: a systematic literature review. *J Pediatr Urol* 2009;**5**:156–64.

30. Schulte-Baukloh H, Knispel HH, Stolze T, et al. Repeated botulinum-A toxin injections in treatment of children with neurogenic detrusor overactivity. *Urology* 2005;**66**:865–70.

31. Akbar M, Abel R, Seyler TM, et al. Repeated botulinum-A toxin injections in the treatment of myelodysplastic children and patients with spinal cord injuries with neurogenic bladder dysfunction. *BJU Int* 2007;**100**:639–45.

32. Joyner BD, McLorie GA, Khoury AE. Sexuality and reproductive issues in children with myelomeningocele. *Eur J Pediatr Surg* 1998;**8**:29–34.

33. Blum RW, Resnick MD, Nelson R, St Germaine A. Family and peer issues among adolescents with spina bifida and cerebral palsy. *Pediatrics* 1991;**88**:280–5.

34. Cartright DB, Joseph AS, Grenier CE. A self-image profile analysis of spina bifida adolescents in Louisiana. *J La State Med Soc* 1993; **145**:394–6, 399–402.

35. Game X, Moscovici J, Game L, et al. Evaluation of sexual function in young men with spina bifida and myelomeningocele using the International Index of Erectile Function. *Urology* 2006;**67**:566–70.

36. Lassmann J, Garibay Gonzalez F, Melchionni JB, Pasquariello PS, Jr., Snyder HM, 3rd. Sexual function in adult patients with spina bifida and its impact on quality of life. *J Urol* 2007;**178**(4 Pt 2):1611–4.

37. Verhoef M, Barf HA, Vroege JA, et al. Sex education, relationships, and sexuality in young adults with spina bifida. *Arch Phys Med Rehabil* 2005;**86**:979–87.

38. Bong GW, Rovner ES. Sexual health in adult men with spina bifida. *ScientificWorldJournal* 2007; 7:1466–9.

39. Reilly JM, Oates RD. Preliminary investigation of the potential fertility status of postpubertal males with myelodysplasia. *J Urol* 1992;**147**(75 A (abstract 150)).

40. Glass C, Soni B. ABC of sexual health: sexual problems of disabled patients. *BMJ* 1999;**318**:518–21.

41. Palmer JS, Kaplan WE, Firlit CF. Erectile dysfunction in spina bifida is treatable. *Lancet* 1999;**354**:125–6.

42. Palmer JS, Kaplan WE, Firlit CF. Erectile dysfunction in patients with spina bifida is a treatable condition. *J Urol* 2000;**164**(3 Pt 2):958–61.

43. Overgoor ML, Kon M, Cohen-Kettenis PT, et al. Neurological bypass for sensory innervation of the penis in patients with spina bifida. *J Urol* 2006;**176**:1086–90.

44. Krogh K, Lie HR, Bilenberg N, Laurberg S. Bowel function in Danish children with myelomeningocele. *APMIS Suppl* 2003;(109):81–5.

45. Lie HR, Lagergren J, Rasmussen F, et al. Bowel and bladder control of children with myelomeningocele: a Nordic study. *Dev Med Child Neurol* 1991;**33**:1053–61.

46. Younoszai MK. Stooling problems in patients with myelomeningocele. *South Med J* 1992;**85**:718–24.

47. Nanigian DK, Nguyen T, Tanaka ST, et al. Development and validation of the fecal incontinence and constipation quality of life measure in children with spina bifida. *J Urol* 2008;**180**(4 Suppl):1770–3.

48. Vande Velde S, Van Biervliet S, Van Renterghem K, et al. Achieving fecal continence in patients with spina bifida: a descriptive cohort study. *J Urol* 2007;**178**:2640–4.

49. de Jong TP, Chrzan R, Klijn AJ, Dik P. Treatment of the neurogenic bladder in spina bifida. *Pediatr Nephrol* 2008;**23**:889–96.

50. Lopez Pereira P, Salvador OP, Arcas JA, et al. Transanal irrigation for the treatment of neuropathic bowel dysfunction. *J Pediatr Urol* 2010; **6**:134–8.

51. Loening-Baucke V, Desch L, Wolraich M. Biofeedback training for patients with myelomeningocele and fecal incontinence. *Dev Med Child Neurol* 1988;**30**:781–90.

52. Palmer LS, Richards I, Kaplan WE. Transrectal electrostimulation therapy for neuropathic bowel dysfunction in children with myelomeningocele. *J Urol* 1997;**157**:1449–52.

53. Han SW, Kim MJ, Kim JH, et al. Intravesical electrical stimulation improves neurogenic bowel dysfunction

in children with spina bifida. *J Urol* 2004;**171** (6 Pt 2):2648–50.

54. Malone PS, Ransley PG, Kiely EM. Preliminary report: the antegrade continence enema. *Lancet* 1990;**336**:1217–8.

55. Bani-Hani AH, Cain MP, King S, Rink RC. Tap water irrigation and additives to optimize success with the Malone antegrade continence enema: the Indiana University algorithm. *J Urol* 2008; **180**(4 Suppl):1757–60.

56. Aksnes G, Diseth TH, Helseth A, et al. Appendicostomy for antegrade enema: effects on somatic and psychosocial functioning in children with myelomeningocele. *Pediatrics* 2002;**109**:484–9.

57. Mowatt G, Glazener C, Jarrett M. Sacral nerve stimulation for faecal incontinence and constipation in adults. *Cochrane Database Syst Rev* 2007(3):CD004464.

58. Yamada S, Won DJ, Yamada SM. Pathophysiology of tethered cord syndrome: correlation with symptomatology. *Neurosurg Focus* 2004;**16**(2):E6.

59. Brezner A, Kay B. Spinal cord ultrasonography in children with myelomeningocele. *Dev Med Child Neurol* 1999;**41**:450–5.

60. Phuong LK, Schoeberl KA, Raffel C. Natural history of tethered cord in patients with meningomyelocele. *Neurosurgery* 2002;**50**:989–93.

61. Bowman RM, Mohan A, Ito J, Seibly JM, McLone DG. Tethered cord release: a long-term study in 114 patients. *J Neurosurg Pediatr* 2009;**3**:181–7.

62. Dias MS, McLone DG. Hydrocephalus in the child with dysraphism. *Neurosurg Clin N Am* 1993; **4**:715–26.

63. Bowman RM, McLone DG, Grant JA, Tomita T, Ito JA. Spina bifida outcome: a 25-year prospective. *Pediatr Neurosurg* 2001;**34**:114–20.

64. Tomita T, McLone DG. Acute respiratory arrest. A complication of malformation of the shunt in children with myelomeningocele and Arnold-Chiari malformation. *Am J Dis Child* 1983;**137**:142–4.

65. Giddens JL, Radomski SB, Hirshberg ED, Hassouna M, Fehlings M. Urodynamic findings in adults with the tethered cord syndrome. *J Urol* 1999;**161**:1249–54.

66. Meyrat BJ, Vernet O, Berger D, de Tribolet N. Pre- and postoperative urodynamic and anorectal manometric findings in children operated upon for a primary tethered cord. *Eur J Pediatr Surg* 1993; **3**:309–12.

67. Kayaba H, Hebiguchi T, Itoh Y, et al. Evaluation of anorectal function in patients with tethered cord syndrome: saline enema test and fecoflowmetry. *J Neurosurg* 2003;**98**(3 Suppl):251–7.

17 Pelvic organ dysfunction following cauda equina damage

Simon Podnar and Clare J. Fowler

Structure of the cauda equina

The relationship between the numbering of the bony vertebrae and different levels of the cauda equina is sometimes the cause of confusion, particularly for patients who may be told "there has been damage to the sacral roots (S_2–S_4)" because of something which has happened at L_4–L_5. The problem may be further confounded by orthopedic surgeons and urologists referring to the vertebral level whereas neurosurgeons, neurologists and rehabilitationists tend to refer to the spinal cord level. The explanation lies in human developmental neuroanatomy.

During fetal development the spinal cord reaches adult length before the bony vertebral column but by the time of birth the vertebral structures have grown more and at birth the spinal cord ends opposite L_3. A few months after birth the cords ends opposite L_1 but the spinal nerves still exit through their original segmental foramina and the dorsal root ganglia remain at those segmentally determined levels. This means that, moving down the spinal cord, the dorsal and ventral roots increasingly elongate so that at the caudal end, the lumbar cistern is filled with the roots of L_2–S_4, collectively referred to as the "cauda equina" (Fig. 17.1). If the dura covering them is opened, the multiple, tightly packed pale thin roots look like a horse's tail.

According to the nineteenth century "Bell-Magendie law," anterior roots convey somatic and autonomic motor function and the posterior roots sensory information so there is a theoretical possibility that a partial injury to the cauda equina could result in a greater deficit of motor than sensory innervation [1] or vice versa. In practice it appears there may be minor exceptions to the Bell-Magendie law and some sensory fibers conveying pain may travel in the anterior roots. This becomes apparent when roots are separated into anterior and posterior for stimulation as when a "Brindley root stimulator" is implanted [2].

Table 17.1 shows the myotomes and Fig. 17.2 the dermatomes innervated by the lumbosacral roots. Based on these known facts, the expected deficits following injury to the cauda equina at different levels can be explained.

Although S_5 appears as a dermatome, albeit small and restricted to the perianal region (Fig. 17.2), the function and indeed the existence of an S_5 ventral, motor root are controversial. In very few instances of implanting a Brindley root stimulator was a significant functional S_5 root encountered, i.e. one which when stimulated produced a significant rise in bladder pressure. A recent published account of a microanatomical dissection of 17 cadaveric cauda equina showed that whereas all specimens had dorsal S_5 nerve roots (comprised usually of two rootlets), a ventral root was absent on one side in 25% and absent on both sides in 19% [3].

Brindley's observations on the effect of stimulation of S_4, S_3 and S_2 give a particularly valuable insight into the motor innervation provided by these roots and the data have been included in Table 17.1 [2]. An insufficiently well known fact is that the intrinsic foot muscles are innervated by S_1–S_3.

Epidemiology and causes of cauda equina damage

Damage to the cauda equina is not common. In a study performed at a national referral uro-neurophysiologic unit, an annual incidence rate of 3.4 per million and a prevalence of 8.9 per 100,000 population were

---

Pelvic Organ Dysfunction in Neurological Disease: Clinical Management and Rehabilitation, ed. Clare J. Fowler, Jalesh N. Panicker & Anton Emmanuel. Published by Cambridge University Press. © Cambridge University Press 2010.

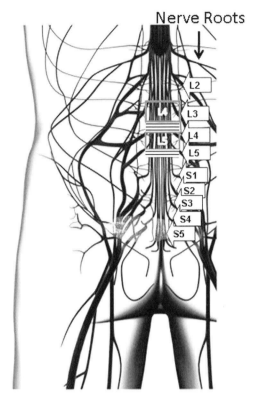

Nerve Roots

Fig. 17.1. Neural structures of the cauda equina and levels of injury from a central disc protrusion at L_4/L_5 (upper) and L_5/S_1 (lower). With permission from RF.Com/Science Photo Library.

Table 17.1. Myotomes and reflexes innervated by the lumbosacral roots

	Motor innervation	Reflexes
L_2	Hip flexors, thigh adductors	
L_3	Knee extensors	Knee jerk
L_4	Knee extensors and foot dorsiflexors	
L_5	Foot and toe dorsiflexors	
S_1	Foot and toe plantar flexors, intrinsic foot muscles	Ankle reflex
S_2	Calf muscles, gluteus medius, biceps femoris, pelvic floor, intrinsic foot muscles	
S_3	Urethral and anal sphincters, pelvic floor, intrinsic foot muscles	Bulbocavernosus reflex
S_4	Urethral and anal sphincters	

calculated [4]. Damage to the cauda equina was found to be most common in middle-aged men (41–50 years), while conus medullaris lesions were more common in young patients (<40 years) [4]. Table 17.2 lists the possible causes of damage to the cauda equina or conus medullaris causing cauda equina syndrome (CES), together with their annual incidence rates. Spinal fracture was the main etiology in young men (<40 years), disc herniations in middle-aged patients (40–60 years) and iatrogenic lesions (i.e. spinal stenosis surgery) in older patients (>60 years).

Acute causes of CES

Most commonly intervertebral disc material ("the nucleus pulposus") herniates dorsolaterally owing to weakness of posterior longitudinal ligaments in lateral positions, resulting in compression of single spinal roots and causing a simple radiculopathy. The most common radiculopathy is of L_5, caused by L_4–L_5 disc herniation. No change in pelvic organ function would be expected from such a lesion unless, to control pain, heavy opiate medication was needed, which commonly causes constipation, and impairs bladder emptying, leading even to urinary retention (see Chapter 19).

Rarely, however, disc material prolapses centrally at L_4/L_5 or L_5/S_1 levels causing compression of some (Figs 17.1, 17.3 and 17.4) or all of the lower lumbosacral roots within the spinal canal. Compression of the cauda equina occurs in ~0.12% of all herniated lumbar discs [4], and in ~2% of operated herniated lumbar discs [5]. So although an uncommon event, disc herniation is in fact the most common cause of CES [4].

The second most common cause of CES is spinal fracture, which most often occurs at L_1 and T_{12} vertebra level. This is an area of great mechanical stress due to transition from a rigid thoracic to a mobile lumbar spinal column. As a result, flexion-distraction and burst fractures are likely to occur in this region, causing damage to the tip of the spinal cord (i.e. conus medullaris) that contains sacral motor, sensory and autonomic parasympathetic neurons in the ventral, dorsal and intermediolateral gray matter horns, respectively. These injuries often result in a combination of upper and lower motor neuron deficits, may be more symmetric, and may be accompanied by less radicular pain than cauda equina damage due to disc herniations.

(a)

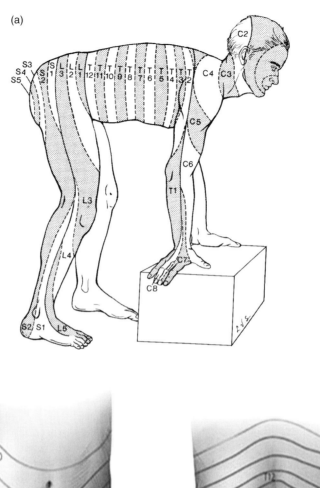

(b)

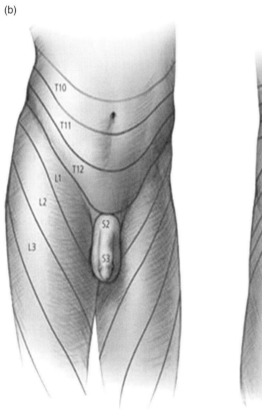
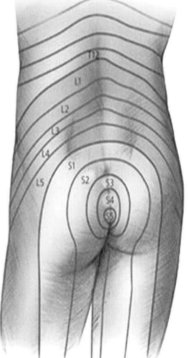

Fig. 17.2. A. "Quadruped" man. B. Details of sacral dermatomes.

Unfortunately, CES may also be iatrogenic and follow lumbar disc or spinal stenosis surgery. It appears that in patients with concomitant spinal stenosis

Table 17.2. Causes and the average annual incidence of cauda equina syndrome

Cause of cauda equina/ conus medullaris lesion	Average annual incidence per million*
Central prolapsed intervertebral disc (L$_4$/L$_5$, L$_5$/S$_1$)	1.8
Trauma – fractures and subluxation	1.5
Iatrogenic – following spinal surgery	0.6
Tumor – primary or metastatic	0.3
Spinal stenosis	
Infective – commonly TB	
Following spinal anesthesia	
Ischemic – spinal A-V malformation causing steal	

Note: *Data from [4]

who have only a partial (i.e. keyhole) laminectomy, there may be insufficient space to accommodate post-operative edema, with a resulting risk of cauda equina compression [7]. A post-operative hematoma should be suspected in all patients with severe post-operative pain and new numbness in the perianal region. Urgent imaging and surgical evacuation of hematoma may prevent permanent damage in these cases. Accidental tearing of the dura is also associated with damage to the sacral roots of the cauda equina, so that a "CSF leak" may be an indication that operative difficulties were encountered by the surgeon. More difficult to prevent is CES occurring after surgery for severe spinal stenosis (anteroposterior diameter <10 mm). This most often occurs in old patients (>65 years) and may be related to applied surgical technique [8].

Although very rare, CES has been described following central neuraxial block or various forms of spinal anesthesia [9]. A recent comprehensive audit in the UK by the Royal College of Anaesthetists estimated that the incidence of permanent damage to nerves or the spinal cord was 1 in 100,000 following central neuraxial block [10]. Details of the neurological deficits of all seven cases "with permanent harm"

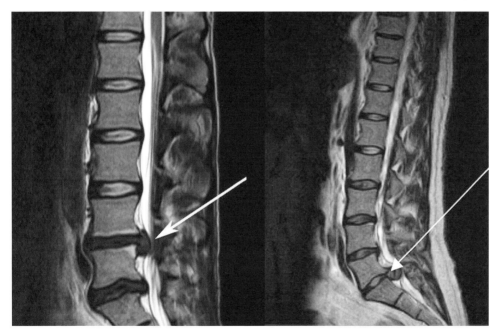

Fig. 17.3. Left: MRI scan showing compression of the cauda equina (arrow) due to a large posterior disc herniation at L$_4$/$_5$. Right: MRI scan showing a large disc herniation at L$_5$/S$_1$ (arrow) bulging posteriorly and compressing the cauda equina. From [6], with permission.

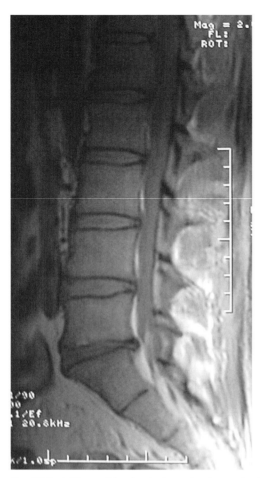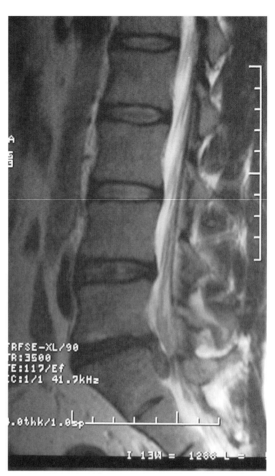

Fig. 17.4. A 40-year-old patient had occasional severe back pain for several years. After one such episode an MRI demonstrated small L_5/S_1 intervertebral disc protrusion (left). Three weeks before the second MRI (right) he had another episode of back pain, this time accompanied by a "hot sensation" in the left buttock and back of thigh. Two weeks later he noticed numbness and pins and needles affecting the left lateral border of his foot, posterior calf and thigh, and his perineum. He was unable to stand on his toes on that side. He had no bladder, bowel or sexual dysfunction. Due to a large disc sequester shown on the right MRI, the patient was referred to a neurosurgeon and operated on the next day. When reviewed a few weeks later his clinical picture resolved completely.

captured during the census period are not given but one illustrative case history is of a patient who developed severe archnoiditis and symptoms and signs of CES in addition to profound lower limb weakness. The comment on this CES case history is that "the delayed onset (of archnoiditis) would imply that a wrong drug or a contaminant was injected but there was no evidence for this" and no explanation was found.

Certainly injection of wrong drugs or preservatives has been implicated in other cases [10] although it is often very difficult to prove. Data from Swedish Pharmaceutical Insurance, an organization voluntarily supported by pharmaceutical companies to compensate patients who sustain injuries secondary to the side-effects of drugs, reported six cases of CES in the period between 1993 and 1997. The conclusion reached by the investigators was that these were due to the injection of hyperbaric (high-density) lignocaine, in most instances higher than the recommended dosage [11].

Causes of chronic CES

CES can present with a long history of chronic back pain with or without sciatica or with slow progression to numbness and urinary symptoms [6]. Such histories would be typical of a patient with a spinal tumor,

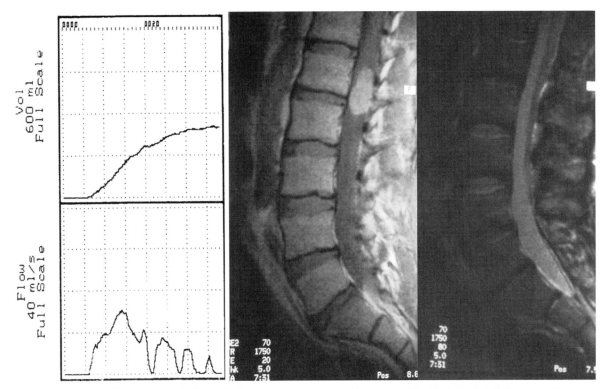

Fig. 17.5. A 41-year-old man was seen by five urologists on account of an unexplained post-void residual of 500 ml. He had urinary frequency and recurrent urinary infections but no neurological complaints. No urological abnormality could be found and there were normal findings on neurological examination, including perineal sensation. However, the penilo-cavernosus reflex (evoked by squeezing glans penis, and observing movement of the perineum) could not be elicited, and definite bilateral reinnervation changes were found on anal sphincter EMG. Uroflow study (left) shows intermittent urinary flow. The patient was sent to MRI, which demonstrated spinal canal ependymoma at L_1 vertebral level (middle). The tumor was resected (right), but he has to continue with intermittent self-catheterization due to persistent incomplete bladder emptying.

such as an ependymoma (Fig. 17.5) or schwannoma, which can cause external compression to the cauda equina or conus medullaris [12]. Occasionally astrocytomas of the spinal cord grow in the region of the conus medullaris [12]. Surgery for extramedullary tumors may lead to some improvement in clinical symptoms although recovery is rare, whereas surgery to remove an intramedullary tumor often leads to immediate deterioration of symptoms. Metastatic tumors may produce compression with rapidly progressive symptoms, usually accompanied with severe pain. A high index of suspicion and imaging studies are essential for optimal management of these patients.

The most common infective cause in developing countries is tuberculosis: Pott's disease, a tuberculous infection of the spine. This presents with back pain and the insidious onset of neurological symptoms [13].

Congenital or acquired stenosis of the lumbar spinal canal can produce symptoms of neurogenic claudication. Such patients describe increasing back and often leg pain, weakness and paresthesia during walking and stance. Walking on a slightly down-going surface makes problems worse. Symptoms are relieved by five to ten minutes of rest in a seated position. An unusual symptom of spinal stenosis was described in two men who experienced spontaneous penile erection on walking, together with numbness and tingling in the legs [14].

In a series of 100 women with a mean age of 58 years who had urinary retention, severe spinal canal stenosis was the fourth most common cause. The subgroup so affected were elderly women with a mean age of 71 years [15].

CES is also a recognized sequela of long-standing ankylosing spondylitis which characteristically causes dorsal arachnoid diverticula and bony erosions although the pathogenesis of the neural deficit is not known [16]. Urinary incontinence is a common presenting picture of this condition [17].

Presumably for hemodynamic reasons arteriovenous malformations in the thoracic region can present with a clinical picture predominantly of CES [18]. On clinical examination these patients often have a combination of the upper and lower motor neuron signs.

Acute motor and sensory symptoms

Acute compression of the cauda equina, commonly from a central disc protrusion, may cause sudden or rapidly progressive severe back pain with incapacitating pain radiating down the back of both legs. Prior to this the majority of patients will have experienced worsening back pain often with unilateral radicular symptoms, and some then describe an additional sudden worsening pain (Fig. 17.4).

Depending on the level of compression, dorsi or plantar flexion of the toes and feet may be affected (Table 17.1). At the same time patients also feel numbness and tingling in the saddle region, the back of the thighs and legs and the soles of the feet. Urinary retention is recognized as a critical feature in evolution of acute CES [19] and this in combination with the onset of saddle sensory loss and back pain should lead to urgent imaging study of the lumbosacral spine [20]. Although constipation is also very common, it often takes much longer to become apparent to patients and physicians; too long for optimal management of these patients [21].

However, acute CES may be difficult to recognize, as only a small proportion of patients (19%) present with the complete classical clinical picture of bilateral sciatica, motor and sensory sacral loss and bladder dysfunction. Of these, lower back pain, sacral sensory loss and urinary symptoms are the most robust presenting features of CES [20]. Probably due to these diagnostic difficulties and a wish to err on the side of caution, there was a high false-positive rate (45%) for suspected CES requiring urgent MRI by resident neurosurgeons [22]. An even more recent survey found that cases with and without abnormal imaging were almost indistinguishable [23].

Chronic motor and sensory symptoms

As with the acute condition, the symptoms of chronic CES depend on the level of the injury, which will determine the extent of the deficit. Following a complete lesion all neurological segments below the level of the lesion will be non-functional. Based on Table 17.1 it is apparent that damage at L_5 or S_1, the most common levels, will result in some leg weakness in combination with loss of pelvic organ function. Damage affecting L_5 root and below results in an inability to heel walk, and inclusion of S_1 root and roots below results in an inability to stand on the toes. Damage to S_2 and the roots below results in pelvic organ dysfunction without any impairment of mobility, which is something that patients report is particularly difficult to cope with since they have no obvious signs of disability to "accompany" their loss of ability to control the bladder and bowel.

The distribution of sensory loss is a good guide to the extent of root damage. This is usually bilateral but often asymmetric with an apparently larger number of roots affected on one side than the other. Indeed it is exceptional for there to be significant pelvic organ dysfunction without perianal sensory loss, this being observed in about 10% of patients with longstanding CES (Fig. 17.5) [1]. The mechanism of preserved touch and pinprick sensation in these patients, in spite of significant motor fiber damage to the same segments, is not clear. Animal studies have demonstrated a greater resistance to acute pressure damage of small- compared to large-diameter nerve fibers and equal susceptibility of large-diameter motor and sensory fibers [24]. This phenomenon goes some way to explaining patients with sensory loss but preserved pelvic organ function but not vice versa. Parasympathetic fibers within cauda equina are even thinner, and therefore might be even more resistant to compression than sensory fibers.

Pelvic organ dysfunction

The innervation of the lower bowel, bladder and genitals by sacral roots 2–4 means that dysfunction of all three of these organs is a feature of damage to the cauda equina. Which pelvic organ dysfunction the patient finds most troublesome – "is the bladder, bowel or sexual function loss which is worst?" – is unpredictable but must depend on the severity of neurological deficit, the individual's coping ability and their personal circumstances.

Professor Brindley's observations using implantation of the stimulator he devised on the effect of sacral root stimulation on pelvic organ function are

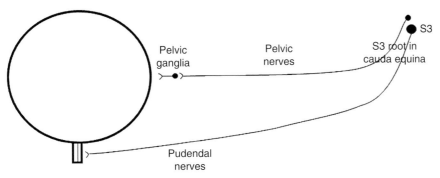

Fig. 17.6. Whereas sphincter denervation is a consequence of sacral root injury, root injury or damage to the pelvic nerves in the pelvis produces a "decentralized" bladder since the postganglionic innervation is intact.

highly relevant here [2]. Stimulation of S_3 had the most major effect on detrusor pressure rise, with S_2 and S_4 stimulation usually having a lesser effect. The rectum responded equally to stimulation of all three pairs of roots with waves of contraction despite continuous stimulation and the stimulation also had an effect on the pelvic colon, bringing feces down into the rectum. S_2 stimulation caused penile erection in the majority of men but without emission of semen. A similar but lesser effect was seen following stimulation of S_3. Several women reported that sacral anterior root stimulation caused vaginal lubrication.

Bladder

Urinary symptoms were reported to disturb daily life in 88% of men and 92% of women who had chronic CES [25].

Urinary retention in the acute situation is considered to be the most important clinical feature heralding the onset of CES. However, because these patients are often unable to void, and the compression of the sacral roots affects the motor neurons innervating the sphincter muscles, incontinence may also be a presenting symptom and is certainly a common feature of the chronic condition.

Although symptoms of disturbed bladder emptying were complaints of 95% of men and 92% of women, and urinary incontinence 56% and 71% respectively, urgency and frequency were also reported by 40% of men and 56% of women [25]. These subjective reports were only supported by the finding of detrusor overactivity in 21% of men but not in women. Differences in detrusor overactivity between men and women were probably caused by larger bladder capacities observed in men, because in men intrinsic

sphincter weakness is masked by obstructive anatomy of the urethra. However, Bors recognized long ago the existence of the "autonomous hyperactive bladder" seen following sacral root injury [26].

The occurrence of detrusor overactivity is difficult to understand according to the neurological concept of "upper and lower motor neuron" damage, the latter resulting in flaccid weakness. Although this thinking is appropriate when considering the innervation of the striated urethral sphincter, it cannot be applied to the motor innervation of the detrusor (Fig. 17.6). The S_2–S_4 roots contain the preganglionic parasympathetic fibers destined for ganglia in the pelvis, from which short postganglionic fibers originate to innervate the detrusor smooth muscle (Fig. 17.6). The bladder is innervated by both extramural and intramural ganglion cells [27] although the relative proportion of each type of ganglia is not known. Following loss of the parasympathetic innervation it was shown in cats that preganglionic sympathetic nerves reinnervated the parasympathetic ganglion cells [28] and bladder contractile activity could be induced by hypogastric nerve stimulation, a finding attributed to plasticity of the adrenergic innervation of the ganglia [28]. It seems likely that intrinsic activity of the smooth muscle driven by urothelial-detrusor mediated reflexes may also contribute (Chapter 1). So it is that low sacral cord or cauda equina lesions may produce an insensate "decentralised" bladder, with poor compliance or detrusor overactivity, as well as an underactive detrusor and urinary retention [25].

In patients with thoracolumbar fractures (the level of the conus medullaris), overactive bladder might be due to an upper motor neuron lesion [29]. It may also be a consequence of decentralization of the parasympathetic ganglia situated within the bladder wall

[30, 31], or irritation of the lower sacral roots (as a "positive symptom" of the nerve lesion). In patients with cauda equina lesions, preganglionic lesion to the parasympathetic fibers occurs. The classical bladder feature of such a lesion is low compliance [32]. Reduced bladder capacity was found on cystometry in 9% or men and 15% of women.

Bowel

Fecal incontinence, and even more commonly incontinence of flatus, are very frequent symptoms of chronic CES. Incontinence of flatus, a particularly embarrassing symptom with no other apparent disability, was reported by 80% of patients. Constipation is the most common bowel symptom and was reported by 68% of men and 93% of women [33]. However, most patients prefer to be constipated, because this reduces the risk of fecal incontinence, which is a much more disturbing and a socially isolating problem. Due to urine and fecal incontinence, about 21% of CES patients wear pads continuously, and another 14% occasionally [25].

Sexual dysfunction

Although often neglected by physicians, sexual dysfunction causes very significant frustration to patients with CES. The primary problem for the patient is diminished saddle sensation which includes impairment of genital sensation. Unfortunately, saddle sensation is also a symptom with very bad prognosis, as it recovers very poorly. In cauda equina lesions the central sensory axons between the dorsal root ganglia and the spinal cord are damaged: unlike the regrowth of axons into peripheral nerve, no such regrowth into the spinal cord occurs. The observation that cutting the dorsal roots at the conus (i.e. proximal to the dorsal root ganglia), rather than peripherally, produced a more permanent deafferentation is in keeping with this fundamental tenant.

Although impaired genital sensation reduces the desire for and some of the most rewarding features of sexual activity, in men erectile dysfunction is the major problem. This can vary from complete inability to obtain an erection, to inability to sustain an erection adequately to complete sexual activity. The result of impaired genital sensation and erectile dysfunction is orgasmic dysfunction, which was in fact the most common sexual dysfunction in men with CES [34].

Women with CES have similar problems with lost sensation and orgasmic dysfunction, but usually report diminished vaginal lubrication in response to psychogenic and genital stimulation [35].

Investigations

Acute CES is one of very few emergency conditions that affect the peripheral nervous system. A high level of suspicion is essential in every patient with back pain, saddle sensory loss and urinary symptoms [20, 22]. Careful clinical neurologic examination is needed in such patients, which includes motor, sensory and reflex testing of lower limbs, plus assessment of anal tone, perianal touch and pinprick, and in men the penilo-cavernosus reflex (Fig. 17.5) [4, 6, 21]. Measurement of the post-void residual urine volume is also valuable in this situation, either by catheterization or ultrasound. In patients with clinical abnormalities compatible with CES, urgent MRI of the lumbosacral spine is the investigation of choice [5, 6, 22]. In every case of suspected CES imaging studies should be performed as soon as possible.

In the chronic situation the reasoning and investigations are similar, but without the same urgency. When available, sacral electrodiagnostic studies, including anal sphincter EMG and penilo-/clitoro-cavernosus reflex measurements, are useful to demonstrate the existence of sacral root deficits and their severity [33]. Urological and proctological investigations are valuable in established cases of CES to assist in planning management (Chapters 1 and 2). Measurements of post-void residual urine, uro-flow measurements as well as filling and emptying cystometry all give valuable information about the underlying pathophysiology of the lower urinary tract [30, 33]. Likewise, colon transit studies using radio-opaque markers or radionuclide tracers can demonstrate the severity of constipation. Anal manometry reveals function of the pelvic floor relevant to anal continence and defecation.

Management

At acute presentation careful neurologic examination is needed, with emphasis on the lower sacral segments [6, 20] and urgent MRI of the lumbar spine. Although there is debate about the efficacy of timely surgical decompression, it is commonly accepted that early intervention is advisable, the optimum time being within 48 hours of the onset of definitive symptoms, because better outcomes of CES have been demonstrated with early compared to late intervention [36, 37]. Delays in CES diagnosis and decompression are among the most common causes of litigation in all spinal disorders [6, 21].

Insertion of a urinary catheter is needed to check for urinary retention and to drain the bladder. Further management will depend on the extent of nerve damage. Patients with mild lesions may only need a few days or weeks of intermittent bladder catheterizations but more severely affected patients or those with incontinence may require longer-term catheterization. Incomplete bladder emptying may be an aspect of bladder dysfunction [25] and the post-micturition residual volume should be checked. If this is more than 100 ml, patients should be taught clean intermittent self-catheterization, but because of the accompanying sphincter weakness many patients can void by straining. In general, men are more prone to incomplete emptying and women to urinary incontinence. Owing to the unpredictable nature of the bladder dysfunction in these patients [25], cystometry is valuable several months after CES has been established, particularly in patients with severe urinary symptoms.

Similarly, patients with severe lesions will be constipated with occasional fecal incontinence, particularly of liquid stools [33]. Therefore, CES patients generally prefer being mildly constipated. Patients are usually recommended to achieve bowel evacuation twice a week. Fecal incontinence is particularly difficult to manage. General measures for the management of constipation and fecal incontinence are described in Chapter 3.

Management of sexual dysfunction in CES patients is generally unsuccessful due to the sensory loss for which unfortunately there is no means of improvement. Erectile dysfunction can be improved by oral selective inhibitors of cGMP-specific phosphodiesterase type 5 (Chapter 4). Women with CES can become pregnant and deliver with no particular difficulties but theoretically vaginal delivery should be avoided to reduce potential damage to an already denervated pelvic floor.

Some patients may develop chronic neuropathic pain syndromes, which should be treated by appropriate medications, physiotherapy or acupuncture. Due to sensory loss patients should be, furthermore, warned against sitting on hot objects, because this can result in deep burns, so they should check the temperature of potentially hot objects by hand first. Orthoses for dropped foot may be needed, as may physiotherapy to aid what recovery is possible of lower limb dysfunction.

Peer support

Contact with other patients who have suffered CES and overcome many of the disabilities is often encouraging for the newly diagnosed and in many instances the internet offers opportunities to identify others who have been affected. Information from websites is certainly valuable:

- http://www.oldcity.org.uk/cauda_equina – website put up by Department of Uro-Neurology at the National Hospital for Neurology and Neurosurgery as a source of information about cauda equina injury
- Cauda Equina Syndrome Resource Center (www.caudaequina.org) – support group for people with cauda equina syndrome to share information about the condition
- BackPainExpert (www.backpainexpert.co.uk/CaudaEquinaSyndrome. html) – patient information site with articles written by invited experts
- Cauda Equina (http://orthoinfo.aaos.org/topic.cfm?topic=A00362) – information on the website of the American Academy of Orthopaedic surgeons
- Wikipedia (http://en.wikipedia.org/wiki/Cauda_equina) – part of the online editable encyclopedia Wikipedia; anyone may post comments or make changes.

Medicolegal aspects

Cauda equina syndrome is a rare condition, but its effects are serious, leading to profound physical and social disabilities. Litigation is common when the patient has residual symptoms [6] and claims relating to cauda equina syndrome tend to be expensive to settle. There are numerous reasons why CES generates medicolegal problems [21]. Indemnifiers for medicolegal claims in the UK frequently warn their members to be vigilant about this condition (www.mps.org.uk, UK Casebook 20, Spring 2003, 9).

Acknowledgement

The authors would like to thank Professor Giles S. Brindley for commenting on this chapter.

References

1. Podnar S. Saddle sensation is preserved in a few patients with cauda equina or conus medullaris lesions. *Eur J Neurol* 2007;**14**:48–53.

2. Brindley GS. The Ferrier lecture, 1986. The actions of parasympathetic and sympathetic nerves in human micturition, erection and seminal emission, and their restoration in paraplegic patients by implanted electrical stimulators. *Proc R Soc Lond B Biol Sci* 1988;**235**:111–20.

3. Hauck EF, Wittkowski W, Bothe HW. Intradural microanatomy of the nerve roots S1–S5 at their origin from the conus medullaris. *J Neurosurg Spine* 2008;**9**:207–12.

4. Podnar S. Epidemiology of cauda equina and conus medullaris lesions. *Muscle Nerve* 2007;**35**:529–31.

5. Gitelman A, Hishmeh S, Morelli BN, et al. Cauda equina syndrome: a comprehensive review. *Am J Orthop* 2008;**37**:556–62.

6. Lavy C, James A, Wilson-MacDonald J, Fairbank J. Cauda equina syndrome. *BMJ* 2009;**338**:b936

7. Jensen RL. Cauda equina syndrome as a postoperative complication of lumbar spine surgery. *Neurosurg Focus* 2004;**16**:e7.

8. Podnar S. Cauda equina lesions as a complication of spinal surgery. *Eur Spine J* 2010;**19**:451–7.

9. Aldrete JA. Neurologic deficits and arachnoiditis following neuroaxial anesthesia. *Acta Anaesthesiol Scand* 2003;**47**:3–12.

10. Cook TM, Counsell D, Wildsmith JA. Major complications of central neuraxial block: report on the Third National Audit Project of the Royal College of Anaesthetists. *Br J Anaesth* 2009;**102**:179–90.

11. Loo CC, Irestedt L. Cauda equina syndrome after spinal anaesthesia with hyperbaric 5% lignocaine: a review of six cases of cauda equina syndrome reported to the Swedish Pharmaceutical Insurance 1993–1997. *Acta Anaesthesiol Scand* 1999;**43**:371–9.

12. Bagley CA, Gokaslan ZL. Cauda equina syndrome caused by primary and metastatic neoplasms. *Neurosurg Focus* 2004;**16**:e3.

13. Moon MS. Tuberculosis of the spine. Controversies and a new challenge. *Spine (Phila Pa 1976)* 1997;**22**:1791–7.

14. Hopkins A, Clarke C, Brindley G. Erections on walking as a symptom of spinal canal stenosis. *J Neurol Neurosurg Psychiatry* 1987;**50**:1371–4.

15. Sakakibara R, Yamamoto T, Uchiyama T, et al. Is lumbar spondylosis a cause of urinary retention in elderly women? *J Neurol* 2005;**252**:953–7.

16. Bartelson JD, Cohen MD, Harrington TM. Cauda equina syndrome secondary to long-standing ankylosing spondylitis. *Ann Neurol* 1983;**14**:662–8.

17. Hassan I. Cauda equina syndrome in ankylosing spondylitis: a report of six cases. *J Neurol Neurosurg Psychiatry* 1976;**39**:1172–8.

18. Aminoff M, Logue V. Clinical features of spinal vascular malformations. *Brain* 1974;**97**:197–210.

19. DeLong WB, Polissar N, Neradilek B. Timing of surgery in cauda equina syndrome with urinary retention: meta-analysis of observational studies. *J Neurosurg Spine* 2008;**8**:305–20.

20. Jalloh I, Minhas P. Delays in the treatment of cauda equina syndrome due to its variable clinical features in patients presenting to the emergency department. *Emerg Med J* 2007;**24**:33–4.

21. Kostuik JP. Medicolegal consequences of cauda equina syndrome: an overview. *Neurosurg Focus* 2004;**16**:e8.

22. Bell DA, Collie D, Statham PF. Cauda equina syndrome: what is the correlation between clinical assessment and MRI scanning? *Br J Neurosurg* 2007;**21**:201–3.

23. Rooney A, Statham PF, Stone J. Cauda equina syndrome with normal MR imaging. *J Neurol* 2009;**256**:721–5.

24. Fowler TJ, Danta G, Gilliatt RW. Recovery of nerve conduction after a pneumatic tourniquet: observations on the hind-limb of the baboon. *J Neurol Neurosurg Psychiatry* 1972;**35**:638–47.

25. Podnar S, Trsinar B, Vodusek DB. Bladder dysfunction in patients with cauda equina lesions. *Neurourol Urodyn* 2006;**25**:23–31.

26. Bors E. Neurogenic bladder. *Urol Surv* 1957;**7**:177–250.

27. Dixon JS, Jen PY, Gosling JA. The distribution of vesicular acetylcholine transporter in the human male genitourinary organs and its co-localization with neuropeptide Y and nitric oxide synthase. *Neurourol Urodyn* 2000;**19**:185–94.

28. de Groat WC, Kawatani M. Reorganization of sympathetic preganglionic connections in cat bladder ganglia following parasympathetic denervation. *J Physiol* 1989;**409**:431–49.

29. Pavlakis AJ, Siroky MB, Goldstein I, Krane RJ. Neurourologic findings in conus medullaris and cauda equina injury. *Arch Neurol* 1983;**40**:570–3.

30. Hellstrom P, Kortelainen P, Kontturi M. Late urodynamic findings after surgery for cauda equina syndrome caused by a prolapsed lumbar intervertebral disk. *J Urol* 1986;**135**:308–12.

31. Fowler CJ. Neurological disorders of micturition and their treatment. *Brain* 1999;**122**:1213–31.

32. Hattori T, Yasuda K, Sakakibara R, et al. Micturitional disturbance in tumors of the lumbosacral area. *J Spinal Disord* 1992;**5**:193–7.

33. Podnar S. Bowel dysfunction in patients with cauda equina lesions. *Eur J Neurol* 2006;**13**:1112–7.

34. Podnar S, Oblak C, Vodusek DB. Sexual function in men with cauda equina lesions: a clinical and electromyographic study. *J Neurol Neurosurg Psychiatry* 2002;**73**:715–20.

35. Sipski ML, Alexander CJ, Rosen R. Sexual arousal and orgasm in women: effects of spinal cord injury. *Ann Neurol* 2001;**49**:35–44.

36. Shapiro S. Cauda equina syndrome secondary to lumbar disc herniation. *Neurosurgery* 1993;**32**:743–6.

37. Kennedy JG, Soffe KE, McGrath A, et al. Predictors of outcome in cauda equina syndrome. *Eur Spine J* 1999;**8**:317–22.

Neuromuscular disorders

Jalesh N. Panicker and Hadi Manji

Introduction

In general, pelvic organ dysfunction in patients with neuromuscular disorders is the result of damage to the pelvic nerves or when the autonomic nerves are involved as part of a more generalized neuropathy. The latter occurs in a limited number of conditions including diabetes mellitus, amyloid neuropathy (familial or acquired), porphyria and Guillain-Barre syndrome (GBS). In GBS, bladder and bowel symptoms are in fact a red flag indicating the clinician should consider a more central, spinal cord diagnosis. Bladder, bowel and sexual dysfunction in association with motor and sensory symptoms and signs will also be encountered in conditions that primarily involve the nerve roots (radiculopathies) in, for example, presentations with herpes varicella zoster and simplex, cytomegalovirus (CMV), Borrelia infections (Lyme disease) and in infiltrative conditions such as with lymphoma or sarcoidosis. Bladder, bowel and sexual dysfunction in purely muscular disorders are unusual and their presence would necessitate the search for an alternative etiology.

Neuropathies
Acquired neuropathies
Diabetes mellitus

Diabetes mellitus is the most common cause of peripheral neuropathy worldwide. Type 1 diabetes results from autoimmune pancreatic beta cell destruction and Type 2 from insulin resistance. These two categories were previously termed insulin-dependent (IDDM) and non-insulin-dependent (NIDDM) diabetes mellitus, respectively. Diabetic neuropathies can be classified into five categories [1] (Table 18.1). The most common

neuropathy is symmetrical distal neuropathy, which is a painful sensory neuropathy due to damage to the thinly myelinated Aδ-fibers and unmyelinated C-fibers. This presents with the so-called "small fiber" symptoms of burning, sharp stabbing pains and a sensation of walking on pebbles. Involvement of the larger, thickly myelinated Aß-fibers results in numbness, pins and needles and a sensation of tightness.

Although diabetic lower urinary tract dysfunction has been recognized since the mid-nineteenth century, it was first described in depth in the early twentieth century [2] and the term "diabetic cystopathy" was introduced by Frimodt-Moller [3, 4]. Because of the variety of tests employed, most epidemiological studies on the prevalence of diabetic autonomic neuropathy have focused on the incidence and prevalence of cardiac dysfunction. Studies looking at the prevalence of diabetic cystopathy found that 43–87% of Type 1 diabetics and 25% of Type 2 were affected. A Scandinavian study of patients with diabetes of 10 years' duration found a prevalence of 2–4 per 1000 in Type 1 and 1–3 per 1000 in Type 2. The correlation between diabetic cystopathy and peripheral neuropathy was 75–100%, and with nephropathy 30–40% [3]. There is evidence to suggest that incontinence is more prevalent amongst women with diabetes [5].

The pathophysiology of diabetic cystopathy is attributable to changes in the detrusor muscle, urothelium and innervation, along with changes in central neurological control [6]. Segmental demyelination has been demonstrated in the nerve fibers in the bladder wall and is a result of metabolic derangement of the Schwann cell. Axonal degeneration has also been demonstrated. Bladder wall biopsies on 14 patients with severe Type 1 diabetes revealed a decrease in acetylcholinesterase and increase in S100 staining when

Pelvic Organ Dysfunction in Neurological Disease: Clinical Management and Rehabilitation, ed. Clare J. Fowler, Jalesh N. Panicker & Anton Emmanuel. Published by Cambridge University Press. © Cambridge University Press 2010.

Table 18.1. Classification of diabetic neuropathies

Impaired glucose tolerance and hyperglycaemic neuropathy

Generalized neuropathies

Sensory – motor

Acute painful

Autonomic

Acute motor

Focal and multifocal neuropathies

Cranial

Thoracolumbar

Lumbosacral radiculoneuropathy (Bruns-Garland syndrome)

Focal neuropathy (entrapment and compression)

Superimposed chronic inflammatory demyelinating neuropathy (CIDP)

Hypoglycemic neuropathy

compared to controls, which were attributed to axonal degeneration and Schwann cell proliferation and regeneration [7]. Deficiency of axonal transport of nerve growth factor may be important in the genesis of diabetic neuropathy and possibly also cystopathy [8]. Urothelial dysfunction has been reported in rat models [9]. Abnormalities in bladder contractility have been demonstrated in rats with streptozotocin-induced diabetes [10].

Bladder dysfunction is likely to be multifactorial [11]. The onset of bladder dysfunction in diabetes is usually insidious and the classical picture is loss of sensation of bladder filling, decreased frequency of voiding, slowing of urinary stream, difficulty in voiding and incomplete emptying, often culminating in chronic retention. Peripheral neuropathy and the level of the glycosylated hemoglobin have been shown to be risk factors for voiding dysfunction [12]. Patients with diabetic cystopathy are prone to asymptomatic bacteriuria and recurrent urinary tract infections. A recent survey from a hospital-based diabetes clinic revealed the most bothersome lower urinary tract symptoms to be storage (overactive bladder) symptoms [12]. Bladder diary measurements have demonstrated that these symptoms are not due to polyuria, contrary to the prevailing view amongst

many patients and healthcare professionals [13]. A large observation study demonstrated that diabetics treated with insulin were more likely to have urge incontinence [14].

Urodynamic findings in diabetes are conflicting. While earlier studies have demonstrated impaired bladder sensation, increased cystometric capacity, reduced detrusor contractility and increased residual volumes, more recent studies have demonstrated detrusor overactivity, impaired contractility and poor compliance to be the most common findings [15]. The reason for detrusor overactivity is unknown, although it may be related to cerebrovascular disease associated with diabetes [16].

Management of diabetic cystopathy is on similar lines to those described in Chapters 5 and 6. In classical diabetic cystopathy, voiding dysfunction is more common and in early cases, bladder retraining and double voiding are usually sufficient. It is important to commence clean intermittent self-catheterization once the post-void residual becomes significantly elevated to reduce the risk of urinary tract infections [6].

Erectile dysfunction (ED) is a frequent co-morbidity and prevalence ranges from 9% in diabetic men aged 20–29 years to 95% in diabetic men >70 years [17]. The Massachusetts Male Aging study showed that up to 64% of men with treated diabetes had some degree of ED. Risk factors included control and duration of diabetes, the presence of neuropathy, retinopathy or nephropathy, and smoking [18]. More than 50% of men develop ED within 10 years of being diagnosed with diabetes [17]. Glycemic control is independently and inversely associated with ED [19]. ED is now increasingly considered a surrogate marker of endothelial dysfunction and has been shown to be associated with a marked increase in the metabolic syndrome, central adiposity and microangiopathy [20]. ED in diabetic men is due to a combination of factors – large and small vessel arteriosclerosis, autonomic neuropathy, anxiety and depression, and iatrogenic causes such as antihypertensive medications. ED in diabetic men responds less well to phosphodiesterase inhibitors (Fig. 10.2, p. 159), though a Cochrane review suggested that these medications do form a care that improves ED in diabetic men [21]. In addition to ED, retrograde ejaculation may occur due to sympathetic denervation of the internal urethral sphincter. Impaired testicular pain sensation is considered a sign of autonomic neuropathy.

Using history and a focused questionnaire (the Index of Female Sexual Function (IFSF)), one study found sexual dysfunction in 51% of young, otherwise healthy, diabetic women [22]. The pattern of sexual dysfunction has been recently characterized using questionnaires prepared from the DSM-IV (American Psychiatric Association Diagnostic and Statistical Manual) algorithm regarding sexual satisfaction and the Arizona Sexual Experience Scale (ASEX). The authors demonstrated that sex drive, arousal, vaginal lubrication, orgasm and sexual satisfaction were consistently reduced in diabetic women as compared to controls and that these changes were related to age and the duration of diabetes but occurred independently of body mass index (BMI) and glycemic control [23].

The gastrointestinal manifestations of diabetic autonomic neuropathy include abnormal esophageal motility, gastroparesis, diarrhea and constipation. The gastrointestinal tract dysfunction is more difficult to assess in the laboratory and the largest studies have focused on symptoms such as early satiety, fullness after meals and nausea, all of which are more common in both Type 1 and Type 2 diabetics compared to controls. Although delayed gastric emptying occurred in 30–50% of patients with longstanding diabetes in some studies [24, 25] others describe rapid gastric emptying in Type 2 diabetic patients [26]. Neither is specifically linked to autonomic neuropathy. Hyperglycemia itself may affect gastric and small bowel motility. Diabetic diarrhea may arise either due to rapid transit through the gastrointestinal tract or slow transit resulting in bacterial overgrowth. Diarrhea was found to be more prevalent in a study of Type 2 diabetics from Hong Kong [27], though not in two European studies [28, 29].

Diabetic patients with fecal incontinence have been shown to have increased thresholds of phasic external sphincter contraction compared to controls in addition to reduced resting and maximal voluntary anal sphincter pressures. Increased thresholds of conscious rectal sensation due to autonomic denervation may be a contributing factor by impairing the recognition of impending defecation [30]. Russo et al. found that acute hyperglycemia inhibits external anal sphincter function and decreases rectal compliance and may be another important factor contributing to fecal incontinence [31].

Guillain-Barre syndrome

Since the eradication of poliomyelitis, GBS is the most common cause of acute flaccid paralysis in the western world. The annual incidence is about 1.2–1.8 per 100,000. Typically, GBS presents as an acute monophasic symmetrical ascending radiculo-neuropathy with an emphasis on the motor rather than the sensory nerve fibers. There may in addition be involvement of respiratory muscles and cranial nerves. By definition, the nadir is reached within four weeks. Progression between four and eight weeks is termed subacute inflammatory demyelinating polyradiculoneuropathy (SIDP) and progression after eight weeks is termed chronic inflammatory demyelinating polyradiculoneuropathy (CIDP). Depending upon the neuroanatomical emphasis of the presentation, a range of disorders comes under the rubric of this syndrome (Table 18.2). Two-thirds of cases are associated with an antecedent infection which varies with geographical location. These include *Campylobacter jejuni*, *Cytomegalovirus*, Epstein Barr virus and *Mycoplasma pneumoniae*. The antecedent infection dictates the subtype of GBS – for example, *C. jejuni* infection is more likely to result in axonal GBS. As a consequence of the infection, a postinfectious autoimmune antibody response targets native peripheral nerve antigens – "molecular mimicry." Over 95% of cases of the Miller Fisher syndrome are associated with the pathogenic anti-GQ1b ganglioside antibody. In acute motor axonal neuropathy (AMAN), there are increased levels of antiganglioside GD1a, GM1 and GM1b antibodies. Despite modern treatment and improvement in intensive care facilities, the mortality rate remains static at 5% with nearly 20% of patients having persistent disability.

Autonomic dysfunction is a frequently overlooked complication but is important to identify, particularly in view of cardiac autonomic involvement. Approximately two-thirds of patients will have evidence of autonomic dysfunction [32]. Bladder, bowel and sexual dysfunction have been infrequently studied and in fact, the diagnostic criteria for GBS stipulate that bladder dysfunction is an exclusion criterion, since the important differential diagnosis is acute myelopathy, in which bladder dysfunction occurs commonly [33]. Furthermore, patients are frequently catheterized in order to maintain hygiene and monitor fluid balance. Concurrent medications, e.g. opiates and tricyclics, can affect bladder and bowel functions. However, the bladder complications are important to recognize since large post-micturition residuals will predispose patients to potentially life-threatening urinary tract infections and septicemia. In the largest study to date, Sakakibara et al. [34] studied 65 patients with definite GBS (clinically and neurophysiologically). Twenty-eight patients had acute inflammatory demyelinating polyneuropathy (AIDP) and 37 patients had AMAN. Urinary dysfunction was observed in 27.7% of cases, with 9.2% having urinary retention. Urinary dysfunction was more common in AIDP (39%) than in AMAN (19%). Other factors significantly associated with bladder symptoms were severity of motor weakness as assessed by the Hughes classification, bowel dysfunction (implicating the parasympathetic cholinergic system) and age. At follow-up, bladder symptoms ameliorated as the motor weakness improved. Importantly, there was no correlation between the presence of cardiovascular autonomic dysfunction (reflecting sympathetic adrenergic dysfunction) and bladder dysfunction. Urodynamic studies were performed within eight weeks of disease onset in nine patients. The findings were variable and demonstrated detrusor underactivity in two patients, detrusor overactivity in three patients, both detrusor overactivity and underactivity in five patients, non-relaxing sphincter in two patients, elevated post-void residuals in three patients, and reduced bladder sensation in one patient. These studies suggest that lower urinary tract dysfunction in GBS may arise from inflammatory changes affecting the pelvic parasympathic nerves. Detrusor overactivity, which implies a more central pathological mechanism, is more difficult to explain. One postulated mechanism is an inflammatory process attacking the inhibitory spinal cord interneurons [35]. The prevalence of ED is higher in men following GBS compared to the general population and is likely to be due to incomplete repair of the autonomic nerves of the pelvis [36].

There is even less data on bowel dysfunction in GBS. The most common manifestation is adynamic ileus, or pseudo-obstruction [37]. However, only five patients had additional evidence of cardiovascular autonomic abnormalities, suggesting once again a different pathological substrate. Apart from involvement of the sympathetic nerves within the lumbosacral plexus, other complicating variables include immobilization, mechanical ventilation and drug side-effects. Management of bowel complications is conservative, with judicial use of laxatives and enemas. Recovery usually coincides with motor improvement.

Acute idiopathic autonomic neuropathy

Bladder dysfunction is well recognized in acute idiopathic autonomic neuropathy (acute pandysautonomia). This condition is characterized by the acute onset of autonomic dysfunction and is thought to be due to lesions of the pre- and postganglionic sympathetic and parasympathetic fibers. Urinary retention and voiding difficulty are common and cystometry demonstrates detrusor areflexia. Bladder dysfunction tends to resolve earlier than other features of autonomic dysfunction such as orthostatic hypotension. ED and constipation are common as well [38].

Autoimmune autonomic ganglionopathy

Patients with autoimmune autonomic ganglionopathy present with rapid onset of severe autonomic failure, with orthostatic hypotension, gastrointestinal dysmotility, anhidrosis, bladder dysfunction, ED and sicca symptoms and may have circulating ganglionic acetylcholine receptor (AChR) antibodies. Bladder dysfunction generally manifests with voiding difficulty and incomplete emptying. Severity and distribution of autonomic dysfunction appear to depend upon the level of antibody titers [39].

Pure autonomic failure

Pure autonomic failure (PAF) is a degenerative postganglionic autonomic disorder. There is now evidence to suggest that the underlying basis is a synucleinopathy, with Lewy bodies confined primarily to the autonomic ganglia neurons [40]. Nocturia and voiding dysfunction are common and bladder emptying is often affected (Fig. 18.1). However, urodynamics may demonstrate detrusor overactivity in some patients [41]. Bladder dysfunction in PAF appears to be as common as, but less severe than, in MSA and this could possibly reflect slower progression of the disease [41]. ED and constipation are common.

Pelvic nerve injury

Injury to the pelvic nerves most often occurs in the setting of pelvic malignancy. Surgery for pelvic malignancy tends to require wide clearance for mitigating regional tumor spread and the autonomic nerves are intimately related to structures that often require excision. Bladder, bowel and sexual dysfunction are

		Time / Volume (mL)					Total Fluid intake	Episodes of leakage
Day 1 29 /7 /2009 Time out of bed (am)- 645 Time to bed (pm)- 10 PM	Time	6:45 AM	9:15 AM	11:30 AM	1:45 PM	3:00 PM	1600	None
	Volume	87	150	150	125	180		
	Time	3:35 PM	4:00 PM	4:35 PM	6:30 PM	9:35 PM		
	Volume	200	170	170	100	100		
	Time	11:10 PM	11:25 PM	12:20 AM	1:05 AM	2:10 AM		
	Volume	180	100	160	150	150		

Fig. 18.1. Bladder diary from a patient with pure autonomic failure demonstrating nocturnal polyuria (1345 ml during the daytime when awake and 827 ml during the night) and increased daytime and night-time frequency. The patient also had voiding dysfunction and had 300 ml post-void residual urine (not shown in the diary).

common following radical surgeries for malignancies arising from the cervix, bladder, prostate and rectum.

The organization of autonomic plexuses innervating the pelvic organs is shown in Chapter 1. The pathophysiology of bladder dysfunction following pelvic nerve injury is poorly understood. Complete transection of the pelvic plexuses is expected to decentralize rather than denervate the bladder, as many of the vesical ganglia are intramural and postganglionic fibers would thus be intact [42–44]. Thus, in addition to the expected dysfunction of voiding and impaired bladder emptying, features of detrusor overactivity may appear as well (Chapter 1). The pelvic plexus (inferior hypogastric plexus), superior hypogastric plexus, hypogastric nerves or pelvic splanchnic nerves may be damaged according to the site of surgery (Table 18.2). The pattern of damage depends upon the extent of surgery, which in turn would depend upon the site and spread of malignancy. Injury to the pudendal nerve may result in loss of the bulbocavernosus and anal reflexes. Table 18.2, compiled by the late Dr. Maas for a review article, lists the typical nerve damages that may occur during radical pelvic procedures [45].

Hysterectomy

Bladder dysfunction is a common side-effect after radical hysterectomy and an incidence as high as 42% has been reported. This most often manifests as bladder atonia resulting in voiding dysfunction [46]. However, changes are often of short duration and voiding functions may recover to baseline within six months [47]. Less commonly, hysterectomy for benign diseases may result in bladder dysfunctions. These include loss in filling sensation on cystometry, together with partial or complete sensory denervation of the bladder leading to an increase in bladder

capacity and secondary urinary retention [48]. Lower urinary tract dysfunction is often multifactorial and incontinence may be due to complications of the surgery, such as pelvic floor weakness, fistula formation or bladder injury as well. Adjuvant pelvic irradiation can result in nerve damage and also changes in the bladder resulting in a smaller capacity and detrusor overactivity. Anorectal dysfunction is uncommon following hysterectomy [49].

Sexual dysfunction is common following radical hysterectomy. Maas et al. used photoplethysmographic assessment of vaginal pulse amplitude to demonstrate abnormal vaginal blood flow response during sexual arousal in women following radical hysterectomy and concluded it might be related to denervation of the vagina [50]. An observational longitudinal study demonstrated that radical hysterectomy with pelvic lymphadenectomy for early-stage cervical cancer (stages I–IIa) had a negative effect on sexual function. Patients reported less vaginal lubrication, narrow/short vagina, labial hypoesthesia, dyspareunia and sexual dissatisfaction [51]. The negative impact on sexual interest and vaginal lubrication may persist even at 24 months after other symptoms of sexual dysfunction have resolved [52].

Techniques for nerve-sparing radical hysterectomy have evolved that aim to minimize damage to autonomic nerves and may be associated with less bladder, bowel and sexual dysfunction [53]. Overall vaginal blood flow has been shown to be better in patients undergoing nerve-sparing techniques, possibly due to less denervation of the vagina [54].

Cystectomy and prostatectomy

The findings from prospective observational studies suggest that sexual dysfunction is a prevalent problem

Table 18.2. Autonomic nerves that may be damaged during radical pelvic surgery

Surgery	Malignancy	Site of nerve damage	Typical nerve damage
Radical hysterectomy with lymphadenectomy	Cervical cancer	Uterosacral ligaments	Hypogastric nerve
		Cardinal ligaments	Pelvic plexus, pelvic splanchnic nerves
		Pelvic lymph node dissection	Pelvic splanchnic nerves
		Rectovaginal ligament/ vagina	Pelvic plexus
		Vesico-uterine ligaments	Pelvic plexus, vesical plexus
Radical cystectomy	Bladder cancer	Neurovascular bundle lateral to vagina or dorsolateral to prostate	Pelvic plexus
Radical prostatectomy	Prostate cancer	Neurovascular bundle dorsolateral to prostate	Pelvic plexus
Total mesorectal excision	Rectal cancer	Presacral mesorectal manipulation	Superior hypogastric plexus, hypogastric nerves
		Lateral ligament of rectum, lateral mesorectal manipulation	Pelvic plexus, pelvic splanchnic nerves

after radical cystectomy [55]. It commonly manifests with ED, decreased orgasm, insufficient lubrication, lack of sexual desire and dyspareunia. In females, clitoral devascularization may result from damage to the pelvic plexus near the lateral wall of the anterior vagina and removal of the distal urethra. Nerve-sparing radical cystectomy preserves sexual function and, in the case of orthotopic bladder substitution, results in better continence and reduced catheterization rates [56].

Damage to the cavernosal nerves is responsible for ED following radical prostatectomy. Injury to the pelvic nerve supply to the internal sphincter could be responsible for some cases of incontinence post-prostatectomy.

Abdominoperineal resection

Abdominoperineal resection for rectal cancer can be associated with voiding symptoms and ED. The etiology is likely to be nerve damage with an additional effect of radiotherapy [57]. Total mesorectal excision with autonomic nerve preservation does not impair urinary and sexual function [58].

HIV infection

Soon after the HIV pandemic started in 1981, it became apparent the nervous system was frequently affected by the opportunistic infections and tumors.

Subsequently, it was recognized that HIV itself can affect all areas of the central and peripheral nervous system with an HIV-associated dementia, vacuolar myelopathy, a distal sensory peripheral neuropathy and a myopathy. Pelvic organ dysfunction has, however, been poorly studied. Patients may develop voiding dysfunction and chronic retention due to lumbosacral polyradiculopathy. Prior to the introduction of the newer antiretroviral therapies in the 1990s, infection with *Cytomegalovirus* was the most common cause [59] and other causes include lymphomatous infiltration, syphilis or a herpetic radiculopathy due to herpes varicella zoster or simplex. Another pattern of lower urinary tract dysfunction is urge incontinence and detrusor external sphincter dyssynergia [60] in the context of vacuolar myelopathy.

Neurosyphilis

Neurosyphilis results from longstanding infection with *Treponema pallidum*. Bladder dysfunction is common, though most classically in tabes dorsalis. The predominant neurological manifestations are sensory ataxia and spontaneous lancinating pains. Voiding dysfunction occurs due to involvement of sacral posterior roots and the dorsal column of the spinal cord, resulting in loss of bladder sensation and significantly elevated post-void residual urine.

The bladder is atonic, though there may be some myogenic damage from chronic overdistension. Some patients may demonstrate detrusor overactivity and detrusor-sphincter dyssynergia [61, 62]. ED may occur as well.

Pudendal neuralgia

Pudendal neuralgia is the most common mononeuropathy affecting the perineum. It is a chronic perineal pain syndrome caused by injury to the pudendal nerve. Injury is usually unilateral and entrapment can occur at several points along the course of the nerve (Fig. 18.2). The most common site of entrapment is within the clamp formed between the sacrospinous and sacrotuberous ligaments [63].

The superficial course of the pudendal nerve makes it prone to compressive damage when cycling (Fig. 18.3). Other causes include trauma leading to fracture of the ischial spine, herpes simplex infection, tumors or endometriosis compressing the nerve, chemoradiation for rectal cancer, stretching of the pudendal nerve from chronic constipation and perineal descent, and iatrogenic causes from pudendal nerve blocks, pelvic surgeries and sacrospinous ligament fixation [64].

Patients present with neuropathic pain in the territory of some or all of the branches of the pudendal nerve (extending from the perianal region posteriorly to the penile/scrotal or clitoral/labial region anteriorly) (Fig. 18.4). Pain typically is aggravated by sitting and relieved by standing and may worsen as the day

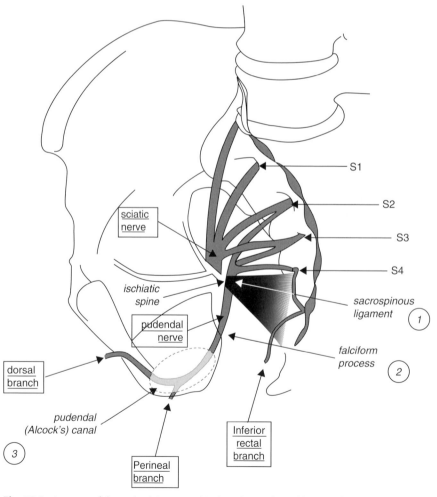

Fig. 18.2. Anatomy of the pudendal nerve and its branches and possible sites of entrapment (1–3). Redrawn, with permission, from *Clinical Neurophysiology* [63].

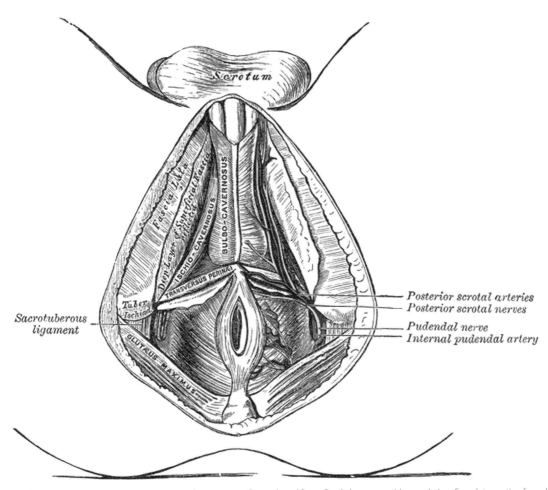

Fig. 18.3. Course of the pudendal nerve in the perineum. Reproduced from *Gray's Anatomy*, with permission. See plate section for color version.

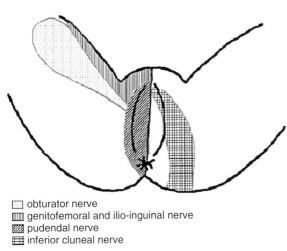

☐ obturator nerve
▥ genitofemoral and ilio-inguinal nerve
▨ pudendal nerve
▦ inferior cluneal nerve

Fig. 18.4. Cutaneous sensory innervation of the perineum. Redrawn with permission from *Neurourology and Urodynamics* [65].

proceeds. It is absent when recumbent or when sitting on a toilet seat [64]. Though initially remitting and relapsing, symptoms generally become chronic and persistent. Objective sensory impairment is unusual and presence of sensory loss often suggests a lesion of the sacral nerve roots rather than the pudendal nerve [65]. This may be due to sparing of the fibers for superficial sensations or due to overlapping dermatomes in the perineum which masks the sensory loss [65]. Other associated symptoms include a "foreign body" sensation in the rectum or vagina (sympathalgia), constipation, painful bowel movements and urinary frequency and urgency [65, 66]. Sexual dysfunction results from loss of libido due to pain, superficial dyspareunia and painful orgasms. There appears to be a predilection for involvement of larger-diameter sensory fibers [64]. A multidisciplinary working group

Table 18.3. Nantes criteria for diagnosing pudendal neuralgia [65]

Pain in the anatomical territory of the pudendal nerve
Pain worsened by sitting
Patient not woken at night by the pain
No objective sensory loss on clinical examination
Positive anesthetic pudendal nerve block

in France recently put forward diagnostic criteria for pudendal neuralgia (Table 18.3).

The diagnosis of pudendal nerve entrapment is essentially clinical and other causes for symptoms should be excluded. The clinical examination is generally normal. However there may be perineal hyperesthesia or allodynia and the pain may be replicated or worsened during vaginal or rectal digital pressure in the region of the ischial spine. CT scan serves to exclude other organic causes. MR neurography provides detailed views and localization of the site of nerve injury and may improve the specificity and success of treatment [67]. Though neurophysiology such as recording pudendal nerve motor terminal latency (PNMTL) and external anal sphincter or bulbocavernosus electromyography have been used (see Chapter 4), their role is limited and these tests are not recommended as part of the investigational workup. There are several reasons for this. Nerve entrapment initially results in axonal excitability and excessive ectopic spike discharges. This is followed by central sensitization, which plays an important role in maintaining chronic pain. These functional changes cannot be identified by clinical neurophysiology and only when entrapment is severe enough do abnormalities appear. Segmental demyelination results in conduction block with focal nerve conduction slowing and abnormal motor unit recruitment. At an advanced stage, axonal loss occurs. Also, these techniques investigate motor functions whereas symptoms and signs are mainly due to sensory dysfunction. Finally, these techniques are not useful in lesion localization. Hence neurophysiology has limited sensitivity and specificity in the diagnosis of pudendal nerve entrapment [63].

Conservative treatments for pudendal neuralgia include avoiding cycling, physical therapy and medications, such as gabapentin and amitryptiline. Pudendal nerve block performed either blindly or under CT guidance, C-arm fluoroscopy or, more recently, MR neurography, is successful in alleviating symptoms. Surgical nerve decompression may be an alternative if nerve compression is being suspected and there is only temporary or partial improvement after nerve blockade.

Inherited neuropathies
Familial amyloid polyneuropathy

Familial amyloid polyneuropathy (FAP) is a rare autosomal dominant neuropathy. It most commonly arises owing to mutation of the gene that encodes for the plasma protein transthyretin (TTR). The resulting aberrant protein, TTR Val30Met, is deposited as amyloid in all body tissues especially in the peripheral nerves, heart, kidneys and eyes. Rarely, FAP is due to deposition of aberrant apolipoprotein A1 or gelsolin protein. Neuropathy begins insidiously in the lower limbs and is characterized by painful dysesthesias and lancinating pains and is accompanied by loss of pain and temperature sensations (dissociated sensory loss) and mutilating acropathy. Motor involvement and large-fiber sensory loss can occur as the disease progresses.

Autonomic manifestations are common and may be the premonitory symptoms in nearly 25% of patients [68]. These include ED, orthostatic hypotension, bladder dysfunction, distal anhidrosis and abnormal pupils. Lower urinary tract symptoms generally appear early on and are present in 50% of patients within the first three years of the disease. Patients most often complain of difficulty in bladder emptying and incontinence [69]. Often, however, bladder dysfunction may be asymptomatic and uncovered only during investigations. Questionnaires such as the Compound Autonomic Dysfunction Test (CADT) are useful in identifying bladder, bowel and sexual dysfunction in FAP [70]. Bladder dysfunction is likely to be due to small nerve fiber damage and deposition of amyloid substance in the detrusor muscle [69]. Urodynamic studies have demonstrated reduced bladder sensations, underactive detrusor, poor urinary flow (Fig. 18.5) and opening of the bladder neck. There may be failure of relaxation of the smooth and striated sphincters as well. Bladder wall thickening may be seen on ultrasound scan. This tends to be progressive and may represent either amyloid deposition or detrusor hypertrophy secondary to functional obstruction [69]. Around 10% of patients with FAP type I may proceed to end-stage renal disease [71] and may complain of polyuria.

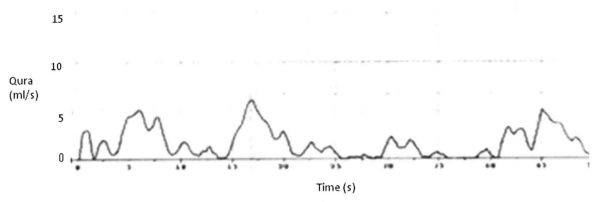

Fig. 18.5. Uroflow curve demonstrating poor urinary flow in a patient with FAP.

These patients tend to have a late onset of neuropathy. Patients should be followed up regularly as overdistension is likely to contribute to bladder dysfunction. In the early stage of disease, post-void residual urine will often be less than 100 ml and bladder scheduling and double voiding is often sufficient. However when bladder emptying deteriorates, intermittent catheterization is required.

Lower gastrointestinal dysfunction results in alternating constipation and diarrhea. This occurs concomitantly with other manifestations such as episodic nausea, vomiting and malnutrition. Anorectal physiology studies have demonstrated prolonged colonic transit time, low anal pressure at rest and loss of spontaneous phasic rectal contractions during squeeze, suggesting an enteric neuropathy [72]. Reduced libido and ED are common and phosphodiesterase inhibitors may have the adverse effect of accentuating orthostatic hypotension and should therefore be used with caution. One report, however, demonstrated dramatic improvement in erectile functions without causing hemodynamic changes [73].

Liver transplantation remains the only potentially curative treatment and gastrointestinal symptoms improve in about half of cases [68]. Studies suggest that bladder and sexual dysfunction do not improve following transplantation [74, 75], though there are anecdotal reports to the contrary [76]. Presence of urinary incontinence has been shown to be associated with high postoperative mortality [74].

Familial dysautonomia

Familial dysautonomia (FD), originally termed Riley-Day syndrome, is the best known and most studied of the hereditary sensory and autonomic neuropathies (HSAN) and is classified as HSAN type III. It has autosomal recessive inheritance and is associated with pervasive autonomic and small-fiber sensory dysfunction. Incontinence is well documented in women with FD and is most often related to stress. However, urgency and mixed incontinence may occur as well. Dry mouth becomes exacerbated when given antimuscarinics for managing overactive bladder symptoms. Women with FD may also have primary nocturnal enuresis or nocturia. Less often, they may have voiding dysfunction manifesting with hesitancy for micturition and high post-void residual volumes and are predisposed to recurrent urinary tract infections [77]. Renal functions tend to deteriorate with age and this could be related to renal hypoperfusion secondary to cardiovascular instability [78].

Charcot-Marie-Tooth disease

Lower urinary tract dysfunction is only occasionally described in Charcot-Marie-Tooth disease. It has been reported in a family with proximal lower limb weakness where it manifested as loss of bladder sensation and urinary retention with detrusor underactivity demonstrated in urodynamics [79]. ED and problems with sexuality are often under-reported [80, 81].

Porphyria

Porphyrias arise due to an acquired or inborn error of metabolism affecting the heme biosynthetic pathway. Neurological manifestations can occur in acute intermittent porphyria (AIP), variegate porphyria (VP), hereditary coproporphyria and δ-aminolevulinic acid dehydratase deficiency. Acute urinary retention and constipation may occur during an acute attack concomitant with other manifestations, such as abdominal pain, neuropsychiatric manifestations and peripheral motor neuropathy. Characteristically, urine changes dark red in color after exposure to sunlight.

Disorders of the neuromuscular junction

Widespread autonomic dysfunction occurs in Lambert-Eaton myesthenic syndrome (LEMS). This is associated with antibodies to voltage gated calcium channel (VGCC) of the P/Q-type and patients can manifest with ED, constipation and bladder dysfunction [82].

Lower urinary tract symptoms are rare in myasthenia gravis because of specificity of AChR antibodies to the neuromuscular junction. Voiding dysfunction has been reported and urodynamic studies have revealed detrusor underactivity in these patients. Voiding dysfunction may herald a new diagnosis of myasthenia or an exacerbation of the disease process [83]. The proposed mechanism is involvement of AChR in the detrusor muscle or pelvic ganglia [84]. Ganglionic AChR antibodies may be present in some patients [85]. Intestinal pseudo-obstruction has been reported in patients of myasthenia gravis with subacute autonomic failure. Bladder incontinence has been reported as a side-effect of anticholinesterase medications used in managing myesthenic symptoms [86], though in clinical practice this is rarely seen. Antimuscarinics can be safely used in myasthenia.

Muscle disorders
Muscular dystrophies

Bladder dysfunction is unusual in muscular dystrophies. Case series in boys with Duchenne muscular dystrophy (DMD) have reported detrusor overactivity in urodynamics and improvement in symptoms with antimuscarinic medications [87]. The exact mechanism is uncertain though it is likely to be due to a disturbance of neural control rather than severe myopathy of the detrusor or external sphincter. Severe scoliosis or complications of spinal fusion surgery may be contributory [88].

Myotonic dystrophy (MD) is an autosomal dominant disorder caused by unstable trinucleotide repeat expansions. Constipation is the most common bowel complaint, though the most burdensome and disabling bowel problem affecting MD patients is fecal incontinence. EMG has demonstrated myotonia and myopathic features of the striated external anal sphincter muscle, and histopathology demonstrates loss of muscle fibers and fibrosis in the smooth and striated anal sphincters and puborectalis muscles. Bowel incontinence is often refractory to treatment [89] and procainamide (300 mg twice a day) has been proposed as a treatment option [90]. Constipation is usually treated with prokinetics, laxatives and enemas. Bladder dysfunction is variable and less often reported, with detrusor overactivity or atonia being documented in urodynamics [91]. ED is more common in patients with larger trinucleotide repeat expansions and longer disease duration. Endocrinological abnormalities occurring in MD may be contributory [92].

Mitochondrial cytopathy

Mitochondrial neurogastrointestinal encephalomyopathy (MNGIE) is a rare autosomal recessive disorder characterized by gastrointestinal, extraocular, peripheral nerve and cerebral white matter involvement. The gastrointestinal disease manifests with intermittent diarrhea and pseudo-obstruction. Mitochondrial DNA abnormalities and/or thymidine phosphorylase mutations in the proper clinical setting are diagnostic [93]. Bowel dysmotility has also been reported in Wolfram syndrome (diabetes insipidus, diabetes mellitus, optic atrophy and deafness; acronym DIDMOAD) [94]. Lower urinary tract dysfunction has been described in both conditions, and the latter may be associated with dilated renal outflow tracts [94]. An autosomal recessive mitochondrial disorder manifesting with intestinal pseudo-obstruction and neurogenic bladder without central nervous system involvement has been described [95].

References

1. Llewelyn J, Tomlinson D, Thomas P. Diabetic neuropathies. In: Dyck P, Thomas P, eds. *Peripheral neuropathy*. Fourth edn. Philadelphia: Elsevier Saunders; 2005:1951–92.

2. Jordan W. Neuritic manifestations in diabetes mellitus. *Arch Intern Med* 1936;**57**:307–366.

3. Frimodt-Moller C. Diabetic cystopathy: epidemiology and related disorders. *Ann Intern Med* 1980;**92**(2 Pt 2): 318–21.

4. Frimodt-Moller C, Mortensen S. Treatment of diabetic cystopathy. *Ann Intern Med* 1980; **92**(2 Pt 2):327–8.

5. Lifford KL, Curhan GC, Hu FB, Barbieri RL, Grodstein F. Type 2 diabetes mellitus and risk of developing urinary incontinence. *J Am Geriatr Soc* 2005;**53**:1851–7.

6. Hill SR, Fayyad AM, Jones GR. Diabetes mellitus and female lower urinary tract symptoms: a review. *Neurourol Urodyn* 2008;**27**:362–7.

7. Van Poppel H, Stessens R, Van Damme B, Carton H, Baert L. Diabetic cystopathy: neuropathological examination of urinary bladder biopsies. *Eur Urol* 1988;**15**:128–31.

8. Sasaki K, Chancellor MB, Phelan MW, et al. Diabetic cystopathy correlates with a long-term decrease in nerve growth factor levels in the bladder and lumbosacral dorsal root ganglia. *J Urol* 2002; **168**:1259–64.

9. Yoshimura N, Chancellor MB, Andersson KE, Christ GJ. Recent advances in understanding the biology of diabetes-associated bladder complications and novel therapy. *BJU Int* 2005;**95**:733–8.

10. Longhurst PA, Belis JA. Abnormalities of rat bladder contractility in streptozotocin-induced diabetes mellitus. *J Pharmacol Exp Ther* 1986;**238**:773–7.

11. Yamaguchi C, Sakakibara R, Uchiyama T, et al. Overactive bladder in diabetes: a peripheral or central mechanism? *Neurourol Urodyn* 2007;**26**:807–13.

12. Fayyad AM, Hill SR, Jones G. Prevalence and risk factors for bothersome lower urinary tract symptoms in women with diabetes mellitus from hospital-based diabetes clinic. *Int Urogynecol J Pelvic Floor Dysfunct* 2009;**20**:1339–44.

13. Fayyad AM, Hill SR, Jones G. Urine production and bladder diary measurements in women with type 2 diabetes mellitus and their relation to lower urinary tract symptoms and voiding dysfunction. *Neurourol Urodyn* 2010;**29**:354–8.

14. Jackson RA, Vittinghoff E, Kanaya AM, et al. Urinary incontinence in elderly women: findings from the Health, Aging, and Body Composition Study. *Obstet Gynecol* 2004;**104**:301–7.

15. Kaplan SA, Te AE, Blaivas JG. Urodynamic findings in patients with diabetic cystopathy. *J Urol* 1995; **153**:342–4.

16. Ueda T, Yoshimura N, Yoshida O. Diabetic cystopathy: relationship to autonomic neuropathy detected by sympathetic skin response. *J Urol* 1997;**157**:580–4.

17. Vinik A, Richardson D. Erectile dysfunction in diabetes. *Diabetes Rev* 1998;**6**:16–33.

18. Feldman HA, Goldstein I, Hatzichristou DG, Krane RJ, McKinlay JB. Impotence and its medical and psychosocial correlates: results of the Massachusetts Male Aging Study. *J Urol* 1994;**151**:54–61.

19. Awad H, Salem A, Gadalla A, El Wafa NA, Mohamed OA. Erectile function in men with diabetes type 2: correlation with glycemic control. *Int J Impot Res* 2010;**22**:36–9.

20. Hermans MP, Ahn SA, Rousseau MF. Erectile dysfunction, microangiopathy and UKPDS risk in type 2 diabetes. *Diabetes Metab* 2009;**35**:484–9.

21. Vardi M, Nini A. Phosphodiesterase inhibitors for erectile dysfunction in patients with diabetes mellitus. *Cochrane Database Syst Rev* 2007(1):CD002187.

22. Erol B, Tefekli A, Ozbey I, et al. Sexual dysfunction in type II diabetic females: a comparative study. *J Sex Marital Ther* 2002;**28**(Suppl 1):55–62.

23. Fatemi SS, Taghavi SM. Evaluation of sexual function in women with type 2 diabetes mellitus. *Diab Vasc Dis Res* 2009;**6**:38–9.

24. Horowitz M, Harding PE, Maddox AF, et al. Gastric and oesophageal emptying in patients with type 2 (non-insulin-dependent) diabetes mellitus. *Diabetologia* 1989;**32**:151–9.

25. Ziegler D, Schadewaldt P, Pour Mirza A, et al. [13C] octanoic acid breath test for non-invasive assessment of gastric emptying in diabetic patients: validation and relationship to gastric symptoms and cardiovascular autonomic function. *Diabetologia* 1996;**39**:823–30.

26. Schwartz JG, Green GM, Guan D, McMahan CA, Phillips WT. Rapid gastric emptying of a solid pancake meal in type II diabetic patients. *Diabetes Care* 1996;**19**:468–71.

27. Ko GT, Chan WB, Chan JC, Tsang LW, Cockram CS. Gastrointestinal symptoms in Chinese patients with Type 2 diabetes mellitus. *Diabet Med* 1999; **16**:670–4.

28. Enck P, Rathmann W, Spiekermann M, et al. Prevalence of gastrointestinal symptoms in diabetic patients and non-diabetic subjects. *Z Gastroenterol* 1994;**32**:637–41.

29. Schvarcz E, Palmer M, Ingberg CM, Aman J, Berne C. Increased prevalence of upper gastrointestinal symptoms in long-term type 1 diabetes mellitus. *Diabet Med* 1996;**13**:478–81.

30. Caruana BJ, Wald A, Hinds JP, Eidelman BH. Anorectal sensory and motor function in neurogenic fecal incontinence. Comparison between multiple sclerosis and diabetes mellitus. *Gastroenterology* 1991;**100**:465–70.

31. Russo A, Botten R, Kong MF, et al. Effects of acute hyperglycaemia on anorectal motor and sensory

function in diabetes mellitus. *Diabet Med* 2004; **21**:176–82.

32. Zochodne DW. Autonomic involvement in Guillain-Barre syndrome: a review. *Muscle Nerve* 1994;**17**:1145–55.

33. Hughes RA, Cornblath DR. Guillain-Barre syndrome. *Lancet* 2005;**366**:1653–66.

34. Sakakibara R, Uchiyama T, Kuwabara S, et al. Prevalence and mechanism of bladder dysfunction in Guillain-Barre Syndrome. *Neurourol Urodyn* 2009;**28**:432–7.

35. Muller HD, Beckmann A, Schroder JM. Inflammatory infiltrates in the spinal cord of patients with Guillain-Barre syndrome. *Acta Neuropathol* 2003; **106**:509–17.

36. Burk K, Weiss A. Impotence after recovery from Guillain-Barre syndrome. *N J Med* 1998;**95**:31–4.

37. Burns TM, Lawn ND, Low PA, Camilleri M, Wijdicks EF. Adynamic ileus in severe Guillain-Barre syndrome. *Muscle Nerve* 2001;**24**:963–5.

38. Sakakibara R, Uchiyama T, Asahina M, et al. Micturition disturbance in acute idiopathic autonomic neuropathy. *J Neurol Neurosurg Psychiatry* 2004;**75**:287–91.

39. Gibbons CH, Freeman R. Antibody titers predict clinical features of autoimmune autonomic ganglionopathy. *Auton Neurosci* 2009;**146**:8–12.

40. Kaufmann H, Hague K, Perl D. Accumulation of alpha-synuclein in autonomic nerves in pure autonomic failure. *Neurology* 2001;**56**:980–1.

41. Sakakibara R, Hattori T, Uchiyama T, Asahina M, Yamanishi T. Micturitional disturbance in pure autonomic failure. *Neurology* 2000;**54**:499–501.

42. Thomas P. Pelvic plexus injury. In: Mundy A, Stephenson T, Wein A, eds. *Urodynamics, principles, practice and application*. Edinburgh: Churchill Livingstone; 1994.

43. Dixon JS, Gilpin SA, Gilpin CJ, Gosling JA. Intramural ganglia of the human urinary bladder. *Br J Urol* 1983;**55**:195–8.

44. Staskin DR, Parsons KF, Levin RM, Wein AJ. Bladder transection – a functional, neurophysiological, neuropharmacological and neuroanatomical study. *Br J Urol* 1981;**53**:552–7.

45. Rees PM, Fowler CJ, Maas CP. Sexual function in men and women with neurological disorders. *Lancet* 2007;**369**:512–25.

46. Artman LE, Hoskins WJ, Bibro MC, et al. Radical hysterectomy and pelvic lymphadenectomy for stage IB carcinoma of the cervix: 21 years experience. *Gynecol Oncol* 1987;**28**:8–13.

47. Chuang TY, Yu KJ, Penn IW, et al. Neurourological changes before and after radical hysterectomy in patients with cervical cancer. *Acta Obstet Gynecol Scand* 2003;**82**:954–9.

48. Everaert K, De Muynck M, Rimbaut S, Weyers S. Urinary retention after hysterectomy for benign disease: extended diagnostic evaluation and treatment with sacral nerve stimulation. *BJU Int* 2003; **91**:497–501.

49. Brooks RA, Wright JD, Powell MA, et al. Long-term assessment of bladder and bowel dysfunction after radical hysterectomy. *Gynecol Oncol* 2009; **114**:75–9.

50. Maas CP, ter Kuile MM, Laan E, et al. Objective assessment of sexual arousal in women with a history of hysterectomy. *BJOG* 2004;**111**:456–62.

51. Pieterse QD, Maas CP, ter Kuile MM, et al. An observational longitudinal study to evaluate miction, defecation, and sexual function after radical hysterectomy with pelvic lymphadenectomy for early-stage cervical cancer. *Int J Gynecol Cancer* 2006;**16**:1119–29.

52. Jensen PT, Groenvold M, Klee MC, et al. Early-stage cervical carcinoma, radical hysterectomy, and sexual function. A longitudinal study. *Cancer* 2004; **100**:97–106.

53. Dursun P, Ayhan A, Kuscu E. Nerve-sparing radical hysterectomy for cervical carcinoma. *Crit Rev Oncol Hematol* 2009;**70**:195–205.

54. Pieterse QD, Ter Kuile MM, Deruiter MC, et al. Vaginal blood flow after radical hysterectomy with and without nerve sparing. A preliminary report. *Int J Gynecol Cancer* 2008;**18**:576–83.

55. Zippe CD, Raina R, Shah AD, et al. Female sexual dysfunction after radical cystectomy: a new outcome measure. *Urology* 2004;**63**:1153–7.

56. Kessler TM, Burkhard FC, Studer UE. Clinical indications and outcomes with nerve-sparing cystectomy in patients with bladder cancer. *Urol Clin North Am* 2005;**32**:165–75.

57. Lange MM, Marijnen CA, Maas CP, et al. Risk factors for sexual dysfunction after rectal cancer treatment. *Eur J Cancer* 2009;**45**:1578–88.

58. Pocard M, Zinzindohoue F, Haab F, et al. A prospective study of sexual and urinary function before and after total mesorectal excision with autonomic nerve preservation for rectal cancer. *Surgery* 2002;**131**:368–72.

59. Cohen BA, McArthur JC, Grohman S, Patterson B, Glass JD. Neurologic prognosis of cytomegalovirus polyradiculomyelopathy in AIDS. *Neurology* 1993; **43**(3 Pt 1):493–9.

60. Gyrtrup HJ, Kristiansen VB, Zachariae CO, et al. Voiding problems in patients with HIV infection and AIDS. *Scand J Urol Nephrol* 1995;**29**:295–8.

61. Garber SJ, Christmas TJ, Rickards D. Voiding dysfunction due to neurosyphilis. *Br J Urol* 1990;**66**:19–21.

62. Hattori T, Yasuda K, Kita K, Hirayama K. Disorders of micturition in tabes dorsalis. *Br J Urol* 1990;**65**:497–9.

63. Lefaucheur JP, Labat JJ, Amarenco G, et al. What is the place of electroneuromyographic studies in the diagnosis and management of pudendal neuralgia related to entrapment syndrome? *Neurophysiol Clin* 2007;**37**:223–8.

64. Stav K, Dwyer PL, Roberts L. Pudendal neuralgia. Fact or fiction? *Obstet Gynecol Surv* 2009;**64**:190–9.

65. Labat JJ, Riant T, Robert R, et al. Diagnostic criteria for pudendal neuralgia by pudendal nerve entrapment (Nantes criteria). *Neurourol Urodyn* 2008;**27**:306–10.

66. Popeney C, Ansell V, Renney K. Pudendal entrapment as an etiology of chronic perineal pain: diagnosis and treatment. *Neurourol Urodyn* 2007;**26**:820–7.

67. Filler AG. Diagnosis and treatment of pudendal nerve entrapment syndrome subtypes: imaging, injections, and minimal access surgery. *Neurosurg Focus* 2009;**26**:E9.

68. Herlenius G, Wilczek HE, Larsson M, Ericzon BG. Ten years of international experience with liver transplantation for familial amyloidotic polyneuropathy: results from the Familial Amyloidotic Polyneuropathy World Transplant Registry. *Transplantation* 2004;**77**:64–71.

69. Andrade MJ. Lower urinary tract dysfunction in familial amyloidotic polyneuropathy, Portuguese type. *Neurourol Urodyn* 2009;**28**:26–32.

70. Denier C, Ducot B, Husson H, et al. A brief compound test for assessment of autonomic and sensory-motor dysfunction in familial amyloid polyneuropathy. *J Neurol* 2007;**254**:1684–8.

71. Lobato L. Portuguese-type amyloidosis (transthyretin amyloidosis, ATTR V30M). *J Nephrol* 2003;**16**:438–42.

72. Ito T, Sakakibara R, Ito S, et al. Mechanism of constipation in familial amyloid polyneuropathy: a case report. *Intern Med* 2006;**45**:1173–5.

73. Obayashi K, Ando Y, Terazaki H, et al. Effect of sildenafil citrate (Viagra) on erectile dysfunction in a patient with familial amyloidotic polyneuropathy ATTR Val30Met. *J Auton Nerv Syst* 2000;**80**:89–92.

74. Adams D, Samuel D, Goulon-Goeau C, et al. The course and prognostic factors of familial amyloid polyneuropathy after liver transplantation. *Brain* 2000;**123**(Pt 7):1495–504.

75. Holmgren G, Lundgren HE, Suhr OB. Successful pregnancies and fatherhood in familial amyloidotic polyneuropathy (FAP Val30Met) patients with liver transplantation. *Amyloid* 2004;**11**:125–9.

76. Stangou AJ, Hawkins PN. Liver transplantation in transthyretin-related familial amyloid polyneuropathy. *Curr Opin Neurol* 2004;**17**:615–20.

77. Saini J, Axelrod FB, Maayan C, Stringer J, Smilen SW. Urinary incontinence in familial dysautonomia. *Int Urogynecol J Pelvic Floor Dysfunct* 2003;**14**:209–13.

78. Axelrod FB. Familial dysautonomia. *Muscle Nerve* 2004;**29**:352–63.

79. Miura S, Shibata H, Kida H, et al. Hereditary motor and sensory neuropathy with proximal dominancy in the lower extremities, urinary disturbance, and paroxysmal dry cough. *J Neurol Sci* 2008;**273**:88–92.

80. Vinci P, Gargiulo P, Navarro-Cremades F. Sexuality in Charcot-Marie-Tooth disease. *Eura Medicophys* 2007;**43**:295–6.

81. Bird TD, Lipe HP, Crabtree LD. Impotence associated with the Charcot-Marie-Tooth syndrome. *Eur Neurol* 1994;**34**:155–7.

82. Waterman SA. Autonomic dysfunction in Lambert-Eaton myasthenic syndrome. *Clin Auton Res* 2001;**11**:145–54.

83. Sandler PM, Avillo C, Kaplan SA. Detrusor areflexia in a patient with myasthenia gravis. *Int J Urol* 1998;**5**:188–90.

84. Kaya C, Karaman MI. Case report: a case of bladder dysfunction due to myasthenia gravis. *Int Urol Nephrol* 2005;**37**:253–5.

85. Vernino S, Cheshire WP, Lennon VA. Myasthenia gravis with autoimmune autonomic neuropathy. *Auton Neurosci* 2001;**88**:187–92.

86. British National Formulary [online]. Available from: http://bnf.org/bnf/ [accessed 8 Sept 2009].

87. MacLeod M, Kelly R, Robb SA, Borzyskowski M. Bladder dysfunction in Duchenne muscular dystrophy. *Arch Dis Child* 2003;**88**:347–9.

88. Caress JB, Kothari MJ, Bauer SB, Shefner JM. Urinary dysfunction in Duchenne muscular dystrophy. *Muscle Nerve* 1996;**19**:819–22.

89. Abercrombie JF, Rogers J, Swash M. Faecal incontinence in myotonic dystrophy. *J Neurol Neurosurg Psychiatry* 1998;**64**:128–30.

90. Pelliccioni G, Scarpino O, Piloni V. Procainamide for faecal incontinence in myotonic dystrophy. *J Neurol Neurosurg Psychiatry* 1999;**67**:257–8.

91. Sakakibara R, Hattori T, Tojo M, et al. Micturitional disturbance in myotonic dystrophy. *J Auton Nerv Syst* 1995;**52**:17–21.

92. Antonini G, Clemenzi A, Bucci E, et al. Erectile dysfunction in myotonic dystrophy type 1 (DM1). *J Neurol* 2009;**256**:657–9.

93. Nishino I, Spinazzola A, Papadimitriou A, et al. Mitochondrial neurogastrointestinal encephalomyopathy: an autosomal recessive disorder due to thymidine phosphorylase mutations. *Ann Neurol* 2000; **47**:792–800.

94. Barrett TG, Bundey SE. Wolfram (DIDMOAD) syndrome. *J Med Genet* 1997;**34**:838–41.

95. Haftel LT, Lev D, Barash V, et al. Familial mitochondrial intestinal pseudo-obstruction and neurogenic bladder. *J Child Neurol* 2000;**15**:386–9.

Chapter 19

Urinary retention

Jalesh N. Panicker, Ranan DasGupta, Sohier Elneil and Clare J. Fowler

Introduction

Impairment of bladder emptying may manifest as complete or partial urinary retention, and be either acute or chronic. The conditions under which retention occur are many and varied, indicating there must be many different causes which effect the same end result.

Acute complete urinary retention is not uncommon following surgery irrespective of the operation site and is attributed to pain and the effects of postoperative analgesia, with full recovery of voiding when these effects wear off. Although complete retention can occur acutely, it may be due to a high post-void residual volume, of which the patient may or may not be aware. Partial retention may be discovered incidentally or as a result of investigation of a patient reporting the sensation of incomplete voiding in association with voiding difficulty or a poor stream. When a voiding disorder occurs in conjunction with detrusor overactivity, as commonly occurs with spinal cord disease, it may be conceptually helpful to think of the high residual volume as the result of "incomplete emptying."

Patients with retention may present to a urologist, uro-gynecologist or neurologist.

Causes of urinary retention

The underlying causes of urinary retention may be either structural or functional (Table 19.1).

Structural causes

Once a diagnosis has been made, most structural causes are amenable to surgical correction. Urological or gynecological assessment includes taking a history, genital and pelvic examination, and where indicated, urodynamic studies and possibly specialized imaging of the outflow tract. Urethrocystoscopy is then usually performed.

Mechanical causes in men generally result from an anatomical obstruction to the bladder outflow, due for example to an enlarged prostate gland, urethral stricture, or even a phimosis. Prolonged obstruction (chronic retention) can eventually result in detrusor "failure" or hypocontractility. As a general rule it is advisable for a man with a longstanding neurological condition to be investigated urologically before ascribing new bladder symptoms to his neurological disease: a urethral stricture may develop some years after prolonged catheterization during a period of unconsciousness or paralysis in intensive care.

In women, there is no specific diagnosis of bladder outlet obstruction, as occurs in the men. However, external factors can obstruct the urethra. These include urethral diverticulae, uterine and cervical fibroids and vaginal wall cysts.

Functional urinary retention with associated neurological dysfunction

Spinal cord disease is a common cause of incomplete bladder emptying although this usually occurs in combination with detrusor overactivity so that the clinical picture is dominated by urgency incontinence. Sometimes, however, the impaired emptying may be the more prominent part of the disorder, resulting occasionally in complete retention. An acute spinal cord injury causing "spinal shock" will result in detrusor areflexia lasting some weeks (Chapter 15). Be the spinal cord pathology causing bladder dysfunction acute or chronic, its other neurological features will be readily apparent: it is extremely unusual for a spinal lesion to cause bladder dysfunction without

Pelvic Organ Dysfunction in Neurological Disease: Clinical Management and Rehabilitation, ed. Clare J. Fowler, Jalesh N. Panicker & Anton Emmanuel. Published by Cambridge University Press. © Cambridge University Press 2010.

Table 19.1. Causes for urinary retention

Mechanical (anatomical)		
	Congenital malformations	Posterior urethral valves
	Tumors	Prostate and bladder
		Gynaecological, e.g. leiomyomas, pregnancy, vaginal wall cysts
		Urethral, e.g. urethral diverticulum or cysts
	Stenosis and strictures	Urethral stricture, bladder neck stenosis
	Calculi	Bladder or urethral
	Urogenital prolapse	
Functional *Neurological causes*		
	Detrusor external sphincter dyssynergia and poorly sustained detrusor contraction	Spinal cord injury or disease
	Detrusor areflexia or hypocontractility	Multiple system atrophy
		Lesion of conus medullaris or spinal roots
		Pure autonomic failure
		Radical pelvic surgery
Non-neurological causes		
	Primary failure of urethral sphincter relaxation	Fowler's syndrome (FS)
	Medication	Anticholinergic drugs or those with anticholinergic activity
		Opiates
	Primary detrusor myogenic failure	

there being long tract signs on neurological examination. Normal lower limb-evoked potentials may be reassuring, as will a normal MRI of the spine, an investigation which is frequently performed but rarely reveals unsuspected abnormalities in this context.

Incomplete bladder emptying has been identified as a feature that can be used to distinguish between MSA and Parkinson's disease [1] and an increasing post-micturition residual volume has been demonstrated as disease progresses in MSA [2] (Chapter 13). Just occasionally complete urinary retention can be a presenting symptom of MSA, although on careful clinical examination other neurological features will be apparent.

The neurological concept of "upper" and "lower motor neuron" lesion, which is fundamental for understanding neurogenic skeletal muscle weakness, is not directly applicable to neurogenic bladder disorders. Whereas damage to an anterior horn cell in the cord or its motor axon in a ventral root or peripheral nerve will result in denervated striated muscle and flaccid paralysis, a sacral root lesion does not produce detrusor denervation. This is because the S_2–S_4 roots contain the preganglionic parasympathetics destined for ganglia in the pelvis from which short postganglionic fibers originate to innervate the detrusor smooth muscle (Chapter 1) (Fig. 19.1).

So it is that subsacral cord or cauda equina lesions (Chapters 15 and 17) produce an insensate "decentralized" bladder which may exhibit poor compliance or detrusor overactivity, presumably due to preserved

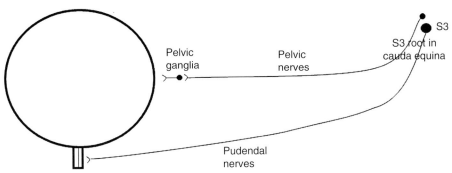

Fig. 19.1. Whereas sphincter denervation is a consequence of sacral root injury, root injury or damage to the pelvic nerves in the pelvis produces a "decentralized" bladder since the postganglionic innervation is intact.

urothelial-detrusor reflexes and continuing intact sympathetic innervation, rather than an acontractile detrusor and urinary retention. Retention can, however, result from damage to the ganglia as may occur in the condition of pure autonomic failure with ganglionic autoantibodies, or surgical damage to the ganglia and postganglionic fibers during radical pelvic surgery (Chapter 18). Incomplete emptying or complete retention can also result from the small fiber involvement of diabetic or amyloid neuropathy which may affect the pre- and postganglionic innervation (Chapter 18).

What may either be a neuropathy confined to the visceral innervation, or in infants a myopathy, can cause "visceral enteropathy." This can present as chronic idiopathic pseudo-obstruction (CIPO), a rare syndrome characterized by gross distension of predominantly the small bowel without any anatomical or mechanical obstruction. Bladder dysfunction has been reported in 10–69% of patients with CIPO [3–5]. Urodynamic investigations reveal similar changes to those seen in diabetic cystopathy including detrusor hypocontractilty, increased residual volume and decreased bladder sensation [3]. Many are able to void with the Valsalva maneuver or using catheters.

In men, there is an uncommon condition where painless urinary retention presents without a mechanical cause or associated neurological disorder. They have neither accompanying constipation nor sexual dysfunction and extensive investigation fails to reveal any underlying abnormality. It has been speculatively proposed that this disorder is due to some abnormality of the intrinsic afferent innervation, possibly loss of the "myofibroblast" or interstitial cells, thought to be an integral part of the bladder stretch-sensing mechanism [6], although any evidence for this is currently lacking. Presumably, this same condition makes up a proportion of the women with unexplained urinary retention.

Fowler's syndrome (FS)

Urinary retention in young women in whom no urological, gynecological or neurological abnormality can be identified present a diagnostic dilemma. Women experiencing otherwise unexplained urinary retention are more numerous than men and in a young woman a primary failure of sphincter relaxation (FS) should be suspected. Previously, isolated urinary retention in young women in whom no abnormalities on routine tests could be found was purported to be of psychogenic or hysterical origin [7–13], although a disorder of sphincter relaxation in young women has been recognized for several years. Moore observed urethral sphincter hypertrophy during cystoscopy in a series of women with voiding dysfunction [14] and Raz observed elevated urethral closure pressures in a group of young women with urinary retention and postulated that their retention was due to spasticity of the striated urethral sphincter or pelvic floor [15]. Fowler and colleagues then recorded myotonia-like electromyographic (EMG) activity in the striated urethral sphincter of women presenting with urinary retention [16] and proposed that the urinary retention was due to a primary impairment of sphincter relaxation [17].

Although the EMG activity sounds superficially like myotonia, detailed analyses show that the characteristic descending sound is due to a decelerating component of a complex repetitive discharge [18] (Fig. 19.2A). When a number of generators of this type of activity are heard, the sound has been likened

(a)

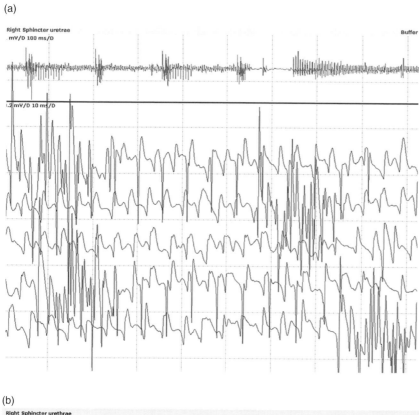

(b)

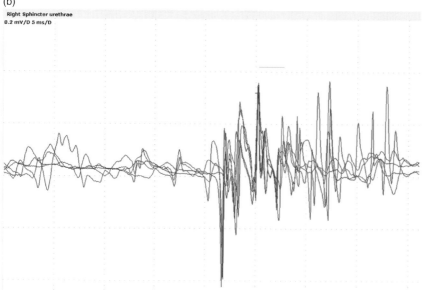

Fig. 19.2. Electromyographic recording from the striated urethral sphincter of a woman in complete urinary retention. A. "Decelerating burst." B. "Complex repetitive discharge." When heard over the audio output of the EMG machine, it is likened to the sound of helicopters.

to that of underwater recordings of whale song [19]. Complex repetitive discharges without deceleration produce a sound like helicopters over the audio-amplifier of the EMG machine (Fig. 19.2B). Jitter analysis of the components of the complex repetitive discharges shows that this is so low that it must be due to ephaptic transmission between muscle fibers [18] generating repetitive, circuitous self-excitation. It is this abnormal activity which is thought to prevent relaxation of the sphincter and cause urinary retention or voiding dysfunction [18]. Other studies have demonstrated an association between complex repetitive discharges and increased post-void residual urine [20] and voiding dysfunction [21].

At the time of the original description of FS, many of the patients were observed to be hirsute, obese and to have menstrual irregularities and there appeared to be a clinical association with polycystic ovaries (PCO) [17]. This association is now no better understood than when the observation was first made, and although the coincidence of PCO and retention is by no means inevitable, a hormonal basis for the EMG abnormality seems likely and it has been proposed that it is the result of a hormonally dependent channelopathy [22]. The same type of sphincter disorder has not been found in men with otherwise unexplained retention. According to the recent work of O'Connell and colleagues [23] the distal urethra is a constituent part of the clitoris, forming the "clitoro-urethrovaginal complex" [24] and clearly the distal urethra has major sex-determined attributes.

Clinical features and investigations

A retrospective study by Swinn et al. defined the characteristic features of FS [25]. Patients are typically young post-menarche females who become unable to void and present with painless urinary retention, having a demonstrated residual volume exceeding 1 l at some stage in the evolution of their disorder (Table 19.2). Although they may experience pain if bladder distension becomes extreme, they do not report the expected urgency at such a large bladder capacity. Straining does not help emptying and intuitively women feel they must promote sphincter relaxation to void by whatever means they can.

The women often report that there has been an antecedent event prior to the onset of their retention, such as an obstetric, gynecological or urological

Table 19.2. Fowler's syndrome: clinical features and laboratory findings

Clinical history	Female
	Aged between onset of menarche and menopause
	No evidence of urological, gynecological or neurological disease
	Retention with a volume in excess of 1000 ml
	No sense of urinary urgency despite high bladder volumes
	Straining does not help emptying
	Sense of "something gripping" or difficulty on removing catheter
	No history of urological abnormalities in childhood or associated abnormalities of the urinary tract
	Association with polycystic ovarian syndrome and endometriosis
Laboratory findings	Raised urethral pressure (>50% expected value for age)
	Increased sphincter volume (>1.8 ml on USS assessment)
	Characteristic urethral sphincter EMG

surgical procedure using regional or general anesthesia. That the surgical procedure can be distant from the pelvis and as minor as wisdom teeth extraction suggests the significant factor is the general anesthetic. In some cases it is possible to elicit a prior history of poor voiding with an interrupted flow with which the woman may have been unconcerned but indicating at least some pre-existing abnormality. Why then a transient event such as a general anesthetic should precipitate retention which does not resolve remains unknown and has undoubtedly been the cause of a number of medicolegal problems.

If a trial without a catheter fails, the woman is usually introduced to clean intermittent self-catheterization and her loss of sensation of urgency and their large capacity mean she can go for long intervals without catheterizing. However, catheterization is often painful, particularly on removing the catheter, with many women complaining of a sensation of "something gripping" as the catheter is withdrawn. The discomfort with self-catheterization appears to be much greater for these women than is reported by similarly aged young women with multiple sclerosis and it is not uncommon for the difficulties to be so extreme that a suprapubic catheter is required. This is clearly a thoroughly unsatisfactory arrangement for an otherwise healthy young woman.

Routine cystometry demonstrates a large-capacity bladder without the usual sensations during the filling phase, and filling is often stopped at 500 ml on grounds of safety although the subject's capacity is much greater. The patient is then unable to initiate voiding and no rise in detrusor pressure observed.

The diagnostic investigation is urethral sphincter EMG using a concentric needle electrode (see Chapter 4), to detect the abnormality previous described. However, despite paraurethral injection of local anesthetic first, which may itself be painful, this test is uncomfortable and furthermore the information obtained is qualitative rather than quantitative: "is there or is there not abnormal EMG activity?" It provides only limited information about the severity of abnormality and expected resulting dysfunction, and it is sometimes difficult to be sure that "sufficient abnormality" has been found to account for a woman's complete urinary retention. The urethral pressure does however give insight into the functional abnormality. Using an infusion technique (withdrawal of an 8 Fr urethral catheter at 2 mm/s while infusing saline at 2 ml/min), maximum urethral closure pressure (MUCP) can be measured (Fig. 19.3) and typically women with FS are found to have resting values in excess of 100 cm of water [26]. The formula of 92 – age (in years) is used to derive the expected pressure, based on the work of Edwards and Malvern [27]. Wiseman et al. [28] also proposed that ultrasound measurement of sphincter volume was helpful to detect the hypertrophy of the striated sphincter resulting from sustained overactivity; but operator variability in this measurement has restricted its usefulness in the diagnostic algorithm for these patients.

Pathogenesis of retention

Initially the findings seemed to suggest that urinary retention in these young women was simply the result of chronic outflow obstruction owing to poor sphincter relaxation. However the restoration of detrusor

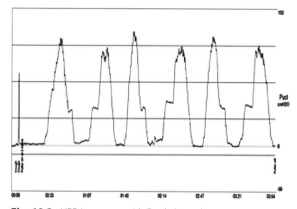

Fig. 19.3. UPP in woman with Fowler's syndrome.

contractions following sacral neuromodulation (SNM) and the evidence from functional brain imaging suggests the underlying mechanism of the retention is more complicated. That contraction of the striated urethral sphincter can inhibit detrusor contraction and suppress bladder afferents is known from animal experiments [29], although this has been little studied as it is a difficult phenomenon to investigate in animals. We do know that in health, urethral afferents are hard-wired in the spinal cord to suppress sensation, inhibit bladder activity and moderate ascending bladder signals [30] (Chapter 1). This is the neural basis for the "pro-continence reflex" whereby voluntary contraction of the sphincter reduces urgency, and it is enhancement of this reflex that is the basis for physiotherapy exercises to encourage pelvic floor contractions to control urgency incontinence. Feed forward from the guarding reflex may further activate the pro-continence reflex in health, both mechanisms combining to maintain bladder control as the bladder fills. In FS it is hypothesized that extreme involuntary sphincter contraction results in accentuation of the pro-continence reflex to the point that bladder sensation is suppressed and detrusor contraction completely inhibited. Certainly an absence of sensation with gross bladder filling is characteristic of this condition and further implies that signals from the bladder reaching the brain are abnormally weak. The recent surprising results of an fMRI research study provide confirmation of this hypothesis [31].

Repeated bladder filling and emptying of only 50 ml at the baseline "bladder empty" condition showed widespread negative responses to bladder infusion (appearing blue in Fig. 19.4) in six women

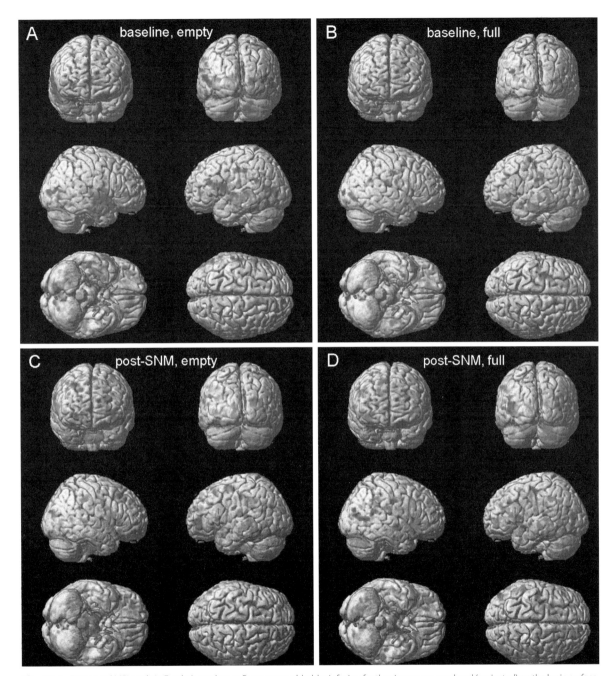

Fig. 19.4. Functional MRI study in Fowler's syndrome. Responses to bladder infusion for the six women, rendered (projected) on the brain surface. Red = activation; blue = negative response. A. Session at baseline with a near-empty bladder. B. at baseline with a full bladder. C. After SNM and a near-empty bladder. D. After SNM and a full bladder. Positive responses (red) indicate activation by bladder infusion. Negative responses (blue) indicate that the fMRI signal is smaller during infusion than during withdrawal. For the session at baseline with an empty bladder (Fig. 19.2A), the brain responses to bladder infusion (relative to withdrawal) were almost exclusively negative. See plate section for color version.

with FS, quite different from the activations seen in "normal" individuals. Negative responses indicate that the fMRI signal is smaller during infusion than during withdrawal, the interpretation of this finding being that bladder filling in these women elicits abnormally strong urethral afferent signals that inhibit bladder afferent activity reducing input to (and so deactivating) the periaqueductal gray (PAG)

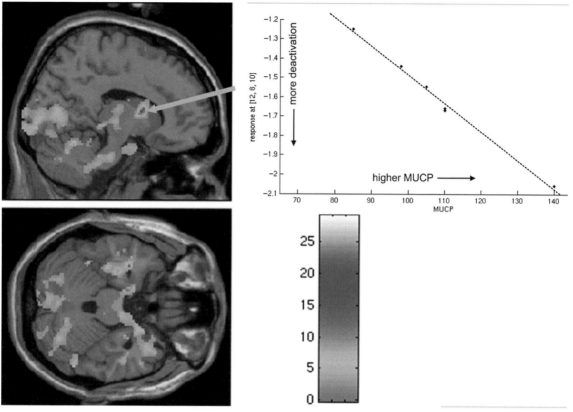

Fig. 19.5. Correlation between the defect in the interoception of filling, i.e. an abnormal negative response, and the maximum urethral closure pressure (MUCP), a proxy measure of the abnormality of sphincter activity, in the individual subjects. See plate section for color version.

and higher centers. Furthermore a correlation was demonstrated between the defect in the interoception of filling (i.e. the abnormal negative responses) and the maximum urethral closure pressure, a proxy measure of the abnormality of sphincter activity, in the individual subjects (Fig. 19.5).

Our understanding of the mechanism of action of SNM in FS has developed through a number of experimental approaches including urodynamics, electrophysiological, brain imaging and clinical observation. An elegant demonstration of the restoration of sensation and its timing in relation to the start of neuromodulation was described by Swinn et al. Within hours of switching on the stimulator for SNM, bladder sensations return and the woman is able to void again. In a study that measured the voided volumes and the post-micturition residual volumes before and after the onset of neuromodulation, there continued to be increased volumes voided

(and concomitant decreased residual volume) over 48–72 hours [32] (Fig. 19.6).

A study by DasGupta and Fowler included assessment of striated sphincter EMG and MUCP before and after SNM, and showed no overall change in these parameters in women with restored voiding [33]. Urodynamic data from that study showed that the restoration of voiding is not due to changes in sphincter overactivity but an improvement in detrusor contractility: a surrogate measurement of "work done" by the detrusor suggested that the restored voiding was achieved by overcoming obstructed bladder outflow.

A PET study suggested SNM probably restored voiding in women with FS by resetting brainstem function [34]. What was demonstrated with PET imaging was that with SNM afferent activity reached the midbrain [34], and more recently with functional magnetic resonance imaging (fMRI) [31] it reached

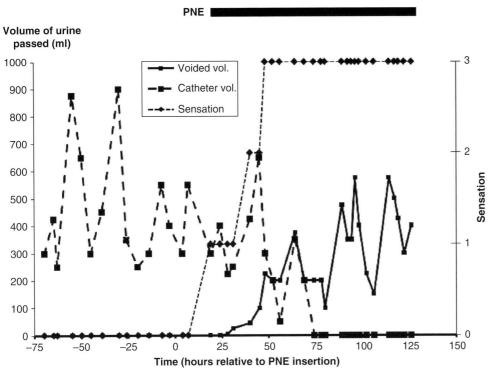

Fig. 19.6. Within hours of switching on the stimulator for sacral neuromodulation (SNM) bladder sensations return and the woman is able to void again. A study that measured the voided volumes and the post-micturition residual volumes before and after the onset of neuromodulation showed that there continued to be increased volumes voided (and concomitant decrease in residual volume) over 48–72 hours. From [32], with permission.

the PAG (Fig. 19.7). It is therefore hypothesized that SNM blocks the urethral inhibition of afferent information flow from the bladder, thus re-enabling voiding.

Opiates and voiding dysfunction

Although the theory outlined above provides the main basis for understanding urinary retention in young women with FS, the role of medication in causing retention, opiates in particular, has recently become the focus of attention. Drugs with anticholinergic activity (e.g. antipsychotic drugs, antidepressant agents and anticholinergic respiratory agents), α-adrenoceptor agonists, benzodiazepines, nonsteroidal anti-inflammatory drugs (NSAIDs) and calcium channel antagonists [35] are well known to affect voiding but we have recently become increasingly aware of the effect of opiates in causing a failure to void. Although notorious as a potent cause of constipation, the role of opiates as a cause of urinary retention seems to be less well recognized. Previous

studies have demonstrated significant urodynamic findings in patients receiving intrathecal and intravenous opiates, including impaired bladder sensation, detrusor hypocontractility and increased bladder capacity with normal urethral pressures [36, 37]. The effect may be dose-related as evidenced by the increased risk of postoperative retention with patient-controlled analgesia as compared to intramuscular opioids [38]. Tramadol in particular has been shown to have a potent effect in reducing detrusor overactivity in experimental animal models [39, 40]. The Netherlands Pharmacovigilance Foundation reported five cases where there was a temporal association between transient voiding dysfunction or urinary retention with the use of tramadol [41]. Animal studies suggest that the activation of μ opioid receptors in the PAG region of the midbrain inhibit detrusor contractions, thus resulting in urinary retention [42]. Both men and women taking these medications are similar to women with FS in that they lack sensations of urgency but by contrast they can usually empty to completion.

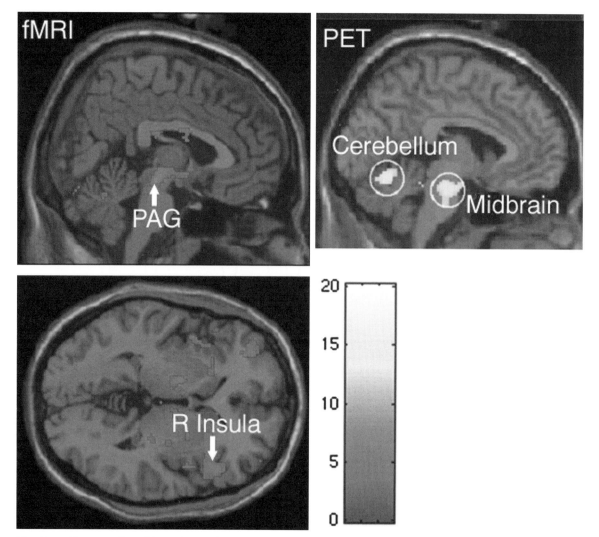

Fig. 19.7. PET imaging showed that with SNM afferent activity reached the midbrain [34] and more recently with functional magnetic resonance imaging (fMRI) [31] the PAG and right insula showed activation. Reproduced with permission. See plate section for color version.

The effect of these medications on a patient with "incomplete" FS is not clear but it may well be synergistic and precipitate complete retention. In a prospective study of 61 referrals to our department for investigation and management of urinary retention, the cause could be identified in only 19. However, 24 of the 61 patients were using significant doses of opiates and in 34 of them, no other cause for urinary retention could be identified [43] (Fig. 19.8). This recent observation explains a longstanding difficulty for the originator of FS which has been the defence of the proposal that there is an organic cause for urinary retention in young women who do not

have neurological or urological disease, some of whom have personality traits which many medical practitioners regard as "manipulative or immature." This has led to the observation that "Fowler's syndrome does not keep good company." In retrospect women taking high doses of opiates almost certainly comprised a cohort of such cases and the possibility that the effect of opiates is to accentuate the pathophysiological consequences of an overactive sphincter may explain why 29% of those diagnosed with FS on the basis of abnormal sphincter EMG and an elevated MUCP were also taking opiates [43] (Fig. 19.8).

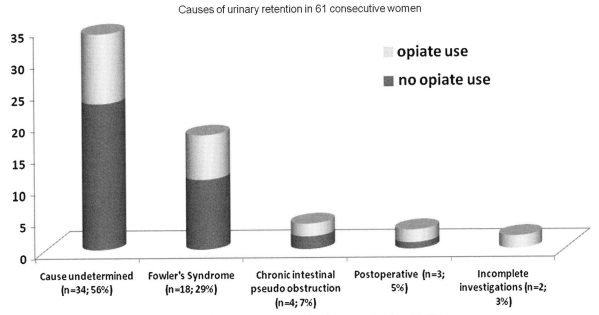

Fig. 19.8. Opiate use in a prospective study of women presenting with urinary retention (n = 61) [43].

Recently, Elneil et al. performed a retrospective analysis of the outcome of "two-stage" sacral neuro-modulation in treating 100 women with chronic urinary retention, 25 of whom were on opiate medications prescribed by their general practitioners or pain physicians for symptomatic management of chronic back, pelvic or abdominal pain. Eight of these women had been diagnosed with FS on the basis of their history, a raised UPP and abnormal sphincter EMG and a further eight had a suitable history and raised UPP but had not had a sphincter EMG test.

It is now being hypothesized that FS results in excessive levels of endogenous encephalins, possibly at the level of the sacral spinal cord [43], and that in some patients this may be compounded by the effect of exogenous opiates. Sacral neuromodulation, but not pudendal nerve stimulation, somehow success-fully counteracts that pathological condition.

Outcomes of SNM

In the analysis of our initial cohort of 60 women who underwent percutaneous nerve evaluation (PNE) and subsequent implant, when followed up with a mean interval of 7 years, 70% were voiding spontaneously [44]. This is in keeping with the findings from other centers of the longer-term efficacy of SNM as a treatment for non-obstructive retention, van Voskuilen

et al. showing 76.2% efficacy at 70.5 months [45] and Elhilali et al. showing efficacy of 78% at 77 months [46]. Importantly, De Ridder and colleagues showed that women with urinary retention due to FS had a better outcome from SNM at five years than those without an abnormal sphincter EMG (72% vs. 46%) [47]. Our results were similar, with 78% versus 43% efficacy, respectively [44].

Having changed to the "two-stage" procedure (see Chapter 7) in 2004, a recent, medium-term follow-up of 100 women showed that the efficacy of the first stage of the implant was 81% and an abnormal sphincter EMG was a predictor for responsiveness [48]. Stage 2 was carried out in 77 patients and complete voiding was restored in 54 patients, improved bladder emptying in 9 patients but failure in 14 patients. Of the 77 women, only 49 had had sphincter EMG but all had had UPP measurement. An elevated UPP was found to predict a good response to stage 2 but the EMG findings were inadequately powered to demonstrate an effect. A new surgical intervention was required in 40 patients either because of leg pain or pain in relation to the battery site, lead displacement or fracture, loss of efficacy or battery site infection.

As mentioned above, 25% of this cohort was being treated with opiates but the use of opiates was shown to have no effect on the outcome of stage 1 or stage

2, nor was it a determining factor for the need for revision surgery. A deduction that can be made from the observation that those taking and those not taking opiates had a comparable response to SNM suggests that its mechanism of action is likely to involve an anti-inhibitory effect of neurotransmitters common in both groups, possibly at opiate receptors in the cord or PAG. Recently Chen et al. [49] have demonstrated that the inhibitory effect of pudendal nerve stimulation on bladder reflexes in experimental cats can be influenced by naloxone, suggesting an inhibitory role of endogenous opioids as a mediator for the stimulation effect. However, pudendal nerve stimulation at standard frequencies has been found not to be effective in restoring voiding in women with retention (personal communication, Dr. Spinelli), suggesting that pudendal nerve stimulation and sacral neuromodulation produce a fundamentally different effect on the neural control of micturition. It is postulated that SNM may specifically counteract an excessive level of endogenous, and sometimes additional exogenous, opiate transmitters.

Management of chronic urinary retention and SNM

The alternatives for management of chronic urinary retention in women are limited. Many patients are treated with α-blockers, urethral dilatation or urethrotomy with little long-term success. Working on the principle that a phosphodiesterase inhibitor might increase nitric oxide availability in the sphincter and thus improve sphincter relaxation, we treated five women with FS in a placebo-controlled trial with sildenafil but unfortunately without benefit [50]. Although an early study of the effect of injection of botulinum toxin into the striated urethral sphincter [51] failed to restore voiding in women with FS, there is some evidence that this is an intervention worth revisiting.

Whilst no pharmacological has yet been discovered to be effective, many women face the prospect of indefinite, often uncomfortable intermittent catheterization or a permanent drainage procedure (either an indwelling catheter or a surgical urinary diversion procedure). This is an unsatisfactory solution for young women and their problem is commonly compounded by a deep dissatisfaction because they may have had no explanation as to why they continue to have chronic urinary retention. With increasing

access to the internet, more patients and their relatives are becoming aware that SNM is an intervention that can restore voiding for some and they naturally seek out the opportunity to be treated by this intervention. The result is that both women and men with chronic retention are being referred to centers that offer this treatment, although only a small proportion may be considered suitable.

That SNM restores voiding in FS is well established [32], its long-term efficacy has been shown to be greatest in women with FS [47], and furthermore we now have a scientific basis for understanding how it works in this condition [31, 34]. The efficacy of SNM in other causes of retention (most of which are of unknown cause) is much less certain [52]. This presents a problem when counseling patients, although many centres operate a policy that it is reasonable to carry out a PNE, or nowadays more likely stage 1 with tined lead, to test for efficacy in each individual wishing to be considered for long-term SNM. Certainly the indications for SNM seem to be widening and its effect in men with non-surgical urinary retention deserves further investigation.

Selection of patients with retention for SNM

It is assumed that patients have had structural or neurological diagnosis excluded or at least uncovered. Although a diagnosis of FS is now established as a predictor for a good outcome for SNM [32, 47, 48], sphincter needle EMG is not an easy test for the patient or electromyographer and the test is not widely performed outside academic centers. However, urethral pressure profile is a standard urodynamic investigation and it is recommended that this is more widely used in the preoperative assessment of women with retention. It will be elevated in women with a primary disorder of sphincter relaxation (i.e. FS) but abnormally low in women who have urinary retention as a result of a damage to innervation of the sphincter and detrusor. Consideration of patients taking opiates, which may either be the cause alone or a contributing factor to urinary retention [43], is a difficulty. Clearly if the dosage is such that the medication appears to affecting daily function or addictive behaviour patterns are evident, then steps to stop or reduce it, although difficult to achieve, would seem to be a better medical approach than SNM.

Since SNM it is a resource-intensive procedure requiring a number of hospital visits and an expensive implant, patients should be selected carefully for their ability to understand the implications of what the treatment involves and their own capability to manage possible adverse events.

References

1. Hahn K, Ebersbach G. Sonographic assessment of urinary retention in multiple system atrophy and idiopathic Parkinson's disease. *Mov Disord* 2005;**20**:1499–502.

2. Ito T, Sakakibara R, Yasuda K, et al. Incomplete emptying and urinary retention in multiple-system atrophy: when does it occur and how do we manage it? *Mov Disord* 2006;**21**:816–23.

3. Lapointe SP, Rivet C, Goulet O, Fekete CN, Lortat-Jacob S. Urological manifestations associated with chronic intestinal pseudo-obstructions in children. *J Urol* 2002;**168**(4 Pt 2):1768–70.

4. Mousa H, Hyman PE, Cocjin J, Flores AF, Di Lorenzo C. Long-term outcome of congenital intestinal pseudoobstruction. *Dig Dis Sci* 2002;**47**:2298–305.

5. Vargas JH, Sachs P, Ament ME. Chronic intestinal pseudo-obstruction syndrome in pediatrics. Results of a national survey by members of the North American Society of Pediatric Gastroenterology and Nutrition. *J Pediatr Gastroenterol Nutr* 1988;**7**:323–32.

6. Wiseman OJ, Fowler CJ, Landon DN. The role of the human bladder lamina propria myofibroblast. *BJU Int* 2003;**91**:89–93.

7. Knox S. Psychogenic urinary retention after parturition resulting in hydronephrosis. *Br Med J* 1960;**2**:1422–4.

8. Margolis GJ. A review of literature on psychogenic urinary retention. *J Urol* 1965;**94**:257–8.

9. Allen TD. Psychogenic urinary retention. *South Med J* 1972;**65**:302–4.

10. Barrett DM. Psychogenic urinary retention in women. *Mayo Clin Proc* 1976;**51**:351–6.

11. Montague DK, Jones LR. Psychogenic urinary retention. *Urol* 1979;**13**:30–5.

12. Bird JR. Psychogenic urinary retention. *Psychother Psychosom* 1980;**34**:45–51.

13. Bassi P, Zattoni F, Aragona F, et al. La retention psychogene d'urine chez la femme: aspects diagnostiques et therapeutiques. *J d'Urologie* 1988;**94**:159–62.

14. Moore T. Bladder-neck obstruction in women. *Proc R Soc Med* 1953;**46**:558–64.

15. Raz S, Smith RB. External sphincter spasticity syndrome in female patients. *J Urol* 1976;**115**:443–6.

16. Fowler CJ, Kirby RS. Abnormal electromyographic activity (decelerating bursts and complex repetitive discharges) in the striated muscle of the urethral sphincter in 5 women with persisting urinary retention. *Br J Urol* 1985;**57**:69–70.

17. Fowler CJ, Christmas TJ, Chapple CR, et al. Abnormal electromyographic activity of the urethral sphincter, voiding dysfunction, and polycystic ovaries: a new syndrome? *BMJ* 1988;**297**:1436–8.

18. Fowler CJ, Kirby RS, Harrison MJ. Decelerating burst and complex repetitive discharges in the striated muscle of the urethral sphincter, associated with urinary retention in women. *J Neurol Neurosurg Psychiatry* 1985;**48**:1004–9.

19. Butler WJ. Pseudomyotonia of the periurethral sphincter in women with urinary incontinence. *J Urol* 1979;**122**:838–40.

20. Jensen D, Stien R. The importance of complex repetitive discharges in the striated female urethral sphincter and male bulbocavernosus muscle. *Scand J Urol Nephrol Suppl* 1996;**179**:69–73.

21. FitzGerald MP, Blazek B, Brubaker L. Complex repetitive discharges during urethral sphincter EMG: clinical correlates. *Neurourol Urodyn* 2000;**19**:577–83.

22. Fowler CJ, Dasgupta R. Electromyography in urinary retention and obstructed voiding in women. *Scand J Urol Nephrol Suppl* 2002:55–8.

23. O'Connell HE, Hutson JM, Anderson CR, Plenter RJ. Anatomical relationship between urethra and clitoris. *J Urol* 1998;**159**:1892–7.

24. O'Connell HE, DeLancey JO. Clitoral anatomy in nulliparous, healthy, premenopausal volunteers using unenhanced magnetic resonance imaging. *J Urol* 2005;**173**:2060–3.

25. Swinn MJ, Wiseman O, Lowe E, Fowler CJ. The cause and natural history of isolated urinary retention in young women. *J Urol* 2002;**167**:151–6.

26. Wiseman OJ, Swinn MJ, Brady CM, Fowler CJ. Maximum urethral closure pressure and sphincter volume in women with urinary retention. *J Urol* 2002;**167**:1348–51.

27. Edwards L, Malvern J. The urethral pressure profile: theoretical considerations and clinical application. *Br J Urol* 1974;**46**:325–36.

28. Wiseman OJ, Swinn MJ, Brady CM, Fowler CJ. Maximum urethral closure pressure and sphincter volume in women in retention. *J Urol* 2002;**167**:367–71.

29. de Groat WC, Fraser MO, Yoshiyama M, et al. Neural control of the urethra. *Scand J Urol Nephrol Suppl* 2001;**35**:35–43.

30. Fowler CJ, Griffiths D, de Groat WC. The neural control of micturition. *Nat Rev Neurosci* 2008;**9**:453–66.

31. Kavia R, Dasgupta R, Critchley H, Fowler C, Griffiths D. A functional magnetic resonance imaging study of the effect of sacral neuromodulation on brain responses in women with Fowler's syndrome. *BJU Int* 2010;**105**:366–72.

32. Swinn MJ, Kitchen ND, Goodwin RJ, Fowler CJ. Sacral neuromodulation for women with Fowler's syndrome. *Eur Urol* 2000;**38**:439–43.

33. DasGupta R, Fowler CJ. Urodynamic study of women in urinary retention treated with sacral neuromodulation. *J Urol* 2004;**171**:1161–4.

34. Dasgupta R, Critchley HD, Dolan RJ, Fowler CJ. Changes in brain activity following sacral neuromodulation for urinary retention. *J Urol* 2005;**174**:2268–72.

35. Verhamme KM, Sturkenboom MC, Stricker BH, Bosch R. Drug-induced urinary retention: incidence, management and prevention. *Drug Saf* 2008; **31**:373–88.

36. Malinovsky JM, Le Normand L, Lepage JY, et al. The urodynamic effects of intravenous opioids and ketoprofen in humans. *Anesth Analg* 1998;**87**:456–61.

37. Kuipers PW, Kamphuis ET, van Venrooij GE, et al. Intrathecal opioids and lower urinary tract function: a urodynamic evaluation. *Anesthesiology* 2004;**100**:1497–503.

38. Petros JG, Realica R, Ahmad S, Rimm EB, Robillard RJ. Patient-controlled analgesia and prolonged ileus after uncomplicated colectomy. *Am J Surg* 1995; **170**:371–4.

39. Pandita RK, Pehrson R, Christoph T, Friderichs E, Andersson KE. Actions of tramadol on micturition in awake, freely moving rats. *Br J Pharmacol* 2003; **139**:741–8.

40. Pehrson R, Andersson KE. Tramadol inhibits rat detrusor overactivity caused by dopamine receptor stimulation. *J Urol* 2003;**170**:272–5.

41. Meyboom RH, Brodie-Meijer CC, Diemont WL, van Puijenbroek EP. Bladder dysfunction during the use of tramadol. *Pharmacoepidemiol Drug Saf* 1999;**8** (Suppl 1):S63–4.

42. Matsumoto S, Levendusky MC, Longhurst PA, Levin RM, Millington WR. Activation of mu opioid receptors in the ventrolateral periaqueductal gray inhibits reflex micturition in anesthetized rats. *Neurosci Lett* 2004;**363**:116–9.

43. Panicker J, Khan S, Kessler T, et al. The possible role of opiates in women with urinary retention. Observations from a prospective clinical study. 39th Annual Meeting of the International Continence Society (ICS). San Francisco; 2009.

44. Datta SN, Chaliha C, Singh A, et al. Sacral neurostimulation for urinary retention: 10-year experience from one UK centre. *BJU Int* 2008;**101**:192–6.

45. Van Voskuilen AC, Oerlemans DJ, Weil EH, van den Hombergh U, van Kerrebroeck PE. Medium-term experience of sacral neuromodulation by tined lead implantation. *BJU Int* 2007;**99**:107–10.

46. Elhilali MM, Khaled SM, Kashiwabara T, Elzayat E, Corcos J. Sacral neuromodulation: long-term experience of one center. *Urology* 2005;**65**:1114–7.

47. De Ridder D, Ost D, Bruyninckx F. The presence of Fowler's syndrome predicts successful long-term outcome of sacral nerve stimulation in women with urinary retention. *Eur Urol* 2007;**51**:229–33.

48. Elneil S, Khan S, Kavia RBC et al. Two-stage sacral neuromodulation for chronic urinary retention in women: outcome and response prognostic factors. In prepration.

49. Chen ML, Shen B, Wang J et al. Influence of naloxone on inhibitory predendal-to-bladder reflex in cats. *Exp Neurol* 2010;**224**:282–91.

50. Datta SN, Kavia RB, Gonzales G, Fowler CJ. Results of double-blind placebo-controlled crossover study of sildenafil citrate (Viagra) in women suffering from obstructed voiding or retention associated with the primary disorder of sphincter relaxation (Fowler's syndrome). *Eur Urol* 2007;**51**:489–97.

51. Fowler CJ, Betts CD, Christmas TJ, Swash M, Fowler CG. Botulinum toxin in the treatment of chronic urinary retention in women. *Br J Urol* 1992;**70**:387–9.

52. Jonas U, Fowler CJ, Chancellor MB, et al. Efficacy of sacral nerve stimulation for urinary retention: results 18 months after implantation. *J Urol* 2001;**165**:15–9.

Appendix 1: Management algorithms

Evaluation and management of lower urinary tract dysfunction

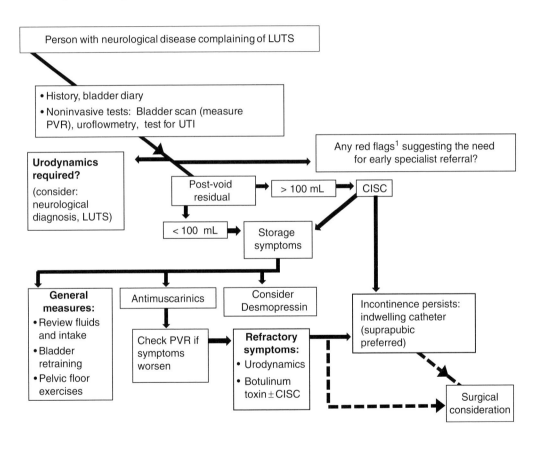

---

[1] Red flags suggesting the need for specialist referral: frequent urinary tract infections; haematuria; evidence of impaired renal function; pain thought to be arising from the upper or lower urinary tract; suspicion of concomitant urological/urogynecological condition, e.g., prostate enlargement, stress incontinence, fistula; symptoms refractory to medical management; consideration for intradetrusor injections of Botulinum toxin A; need for suprapublic catheterization; rare consideration of surgery (e.g., ileocystoplasty, ileal conduit).

Evaluation and management of sexual dysfunction

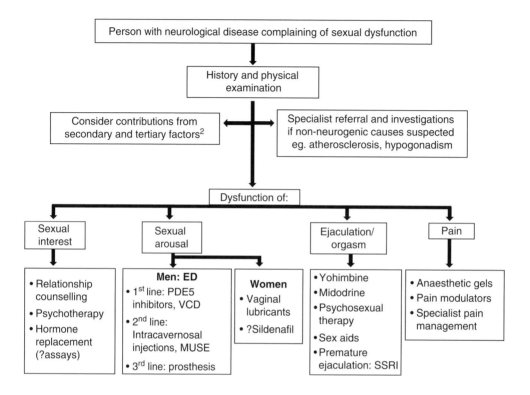

Person with neurological disease complaining of sexual dysfunction

↓

History and physical examination

Consider contributions from secondary and tertiary factors[2]

Specialist referral and investigations if non-neurogenic causes suspected eg. atherosclerosis, hypogonadism

↓

Dysfunction of:

Sexual interest
- Relationship counselling
- Psychotherapy
- Hormone replacement (?assays)

Sexual arousal

Men: ED
- 1st line: PDE5 inhibitors, VCD
- 2nd line: Intracavernosal injections, MUSE
- 3rd line: prosthesis

Women
- Vaginal lubricants
- ?Sildenafil

Ejaculation/ orgasm
- Yohimbine
- Midodrine
- Psychosexual therapy
- Sex aids
- Premature ejaculation: SSRI

Pain
- Anaesthetic gels
- Pain modulators
- Specialist pain management

[2] Factors contributing to sexual dysfunction: secondary factors – fatigue; difficulties in attention and concentration; bladder/bowel incontinence; physical immobility: muscle weakness, leg spasms; dysesthesia/allodynia; other factors: incoordination, tremor, pain; medications: antidepressants, baclofen, gabapentin; presence of urethral indwelling catheter; tertiary factors – depression; anxiety; anger, guilt and fear; altered self-image, low self-esteem; relationship with the partner, change in family role.

Algorithm for neurogenic bowel evaluation and management

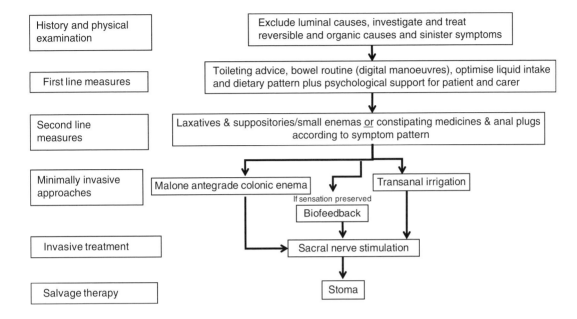

Algorithm for constipation

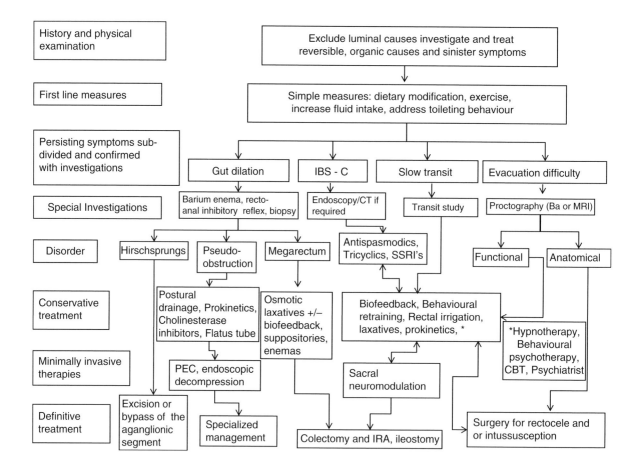

History and physical examination

Exclude luminal causes investigate and treat reversible, organic causes and sinister symptoms

First line measures

Simple measures: dietary modification, exercise, increase fluid intake, address toileting behaviour

Persisting symptoms sub-divided and confirmed with investigations

Gut dilation | IBS - C | Slow transit | Evacuation difficulty

Special Investigations

Barium enema, recto-anal inhibitory reflex, biopsy | Endoscopy/CT if required | Transit study | Proctography (Ba or MRI)

Disorder

Hirschsprungs | Pseudo-obstruction | Megarectum | Antispasmodics, Tricyclics, SSRI's | Functional | Anatomical

Conservative treatment

Postural drainage, Prokinetics, Cholinesterase inhibitors, Flatus tube | Osmotic laxatives +/− biofeedback, suppositories, enemas | Biofeedback, Behavioural retraining, Rectal irrigation, laxatives, prokinetics, * | *Hypnotherapy, Behavioural psychotherapy, CBT, Psychiatrist

Minimally invasive therapies

PEC, endoscopic decompression | Sacral neuromodulation

Definitive treatment

Excision or bypass of the aganglionic segment | Specialized management | Colectomy and IRA, ileostomy | Surgery for rectocele and or intussusception

Algorithm for fecal incontinence

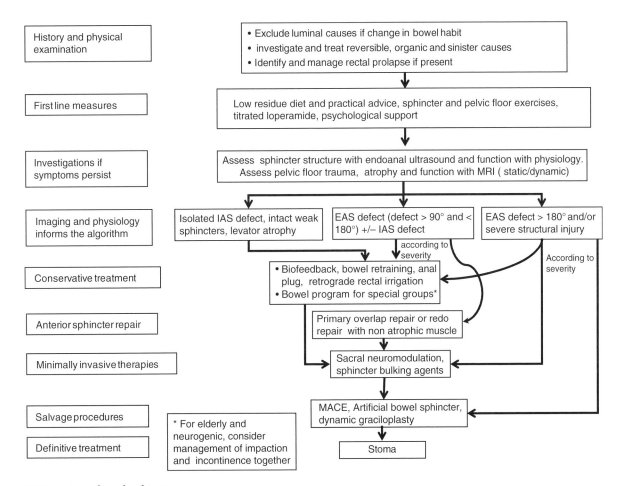

History and physical examination
- Exclude luminal causes if change in bowel habit
- investigate and treat reversible, organic and sinister causes
- Identify and manage rectal prolapse if present

First line measures
Low residue diet and practical advice, sphincter and pelvic floor exercises, titrated loperamide, psychological support

Investigations if symptoms persist
Assess sphincter structure with endoanal ultrasound and function with physiology. Assess pelvic floor trauma, atrophy and function with MRI (static/dynamic)

Imaging and physiology informs the algorithm
Isolated IAS defect, intact weak sphincters, levator atrophy
EAS defect (defect > 90° and < 180°) +/– IAS defect
EAS defect > 180° and/or severe structural injury

according to severity

According to severity

Conservative treatment
- Biofeedback, bowel retraining, anal plug, retrograde rectal irrigation
- Bowel program for special groups*

Anterior sphincter repair
Primary overlap repair or redo repair with non atrophic muscle

Minimally invasive therapies
Sacral neuromodulation, sphincter bulking agents

Salvage procedures
MACE, Artificial bowel sphincter, dynamic graciloplasty

Definitive treatment
* For elderly and neurogenic, consider management of impaction and incontinence together

Stoma

IAS = internal anal sphincter;
EAS = external anal sphincter

311

Appendix 2: Surveys and questionnaires

Urogenital Distress Inventory 6 (1)

DO YOU EXPERIENCE ANY URINARY INCONTINENCE? YES ———NO———

Please circle the number that best describes what you are feeling. Use the following as your guide.

(0) Not at All
(1) Slightly
(2) Moderately
(3) Greatly

Do you experience, and if so, how much are you bothered by:

Frequent urination? (0) (1) (2) (3)

Urine leakage related to the feeling of urgency? (0) (1) (2) (3)

Urine leakage related to physical activity, coughing or sneezing? (0) (1) (2) (3)

Small amounts of urine leakage? (0) (1) (2) (3)

Difficulty emptying your bladder? (0) (1) (2) (3)

Pain or discomfort in the lower abdomen or genital area? (0) (1) (2) (3)

Incontinence Impact Questionnaire 7 (1)

Please circle the number that best describes what you are feeling. Use the following as your guide.

(0) Not at All
(1) Slightly
(2) Moderately
(3) Greatly

Has urine leakage affected your ability to do household chores (cooking, cleaning, laundry, etc.)? (0) (1) (2) (3)

Has urine leakage affected your physical recreation such as walking, swimming or other exercise? (0) (1) (2) (3)

Has urine leakage affected your entertainment activities (movies, concerts, etc.)? (0) (1) (2) (3)

Has urine leakage affected your ability to travel by car or bus more than 30 minutes from home? (0) (1) (2) (3)

Has urine leakage affected your participation in social activities outside your house? (0) (1) (2) (3)

Has urine leakage affected your emotional health (nervousness, depression, etc.)? (0) (1) (2) (3)

Has urine leakage affected your feeling frustrated? (0) (1) (2) (3)

International Prostate Symptom Score (IPSS) (2)

	Not at all	Less than 1 time in 5	Less than half the time	About half the time	More than half the time	Almost always	Your score
Incomplete emptying Over the past month, how often have you had a sensation of not emptying your bladder completely after you finish urinating?	0	1	2	3	4	5	
Frequency Over the past month, how often have you had to urinate again less than two hours after you finished urinating?	0	1	2	3	4	5	
Intermittency Over the past month, how often have you found you stopped and started again several times when you urinated?	0	1	2	3	4	5	
Urgency Over the last month, how difficult have you found it to postpone urination?	0	1	2	3	4	5	
Weak stream Over the past month, how often have you had a weak urinary stream?	0	1	2	3	4	5	
Straining Over the past month, how often have you had to push or strain to begin urination?	0	1	2	3	4	5	

	None	1 times	2 times	3 times	4 times	5 times or more	Your score
Nocturia Over the past month, how many times did you most typically get up to urinate from the time you went to bed until the time you got up in the morning?	0	1	2	3	4	5	

Total IPSS score

Quality of life due to urinary symptoms	Delighted	Pleased	Mostly satisfied	Mixed – about equally satisfied and dissatisfied	Mostly dissatisfied	Unhappy	Terrible
If you were to spend the rest of your life with your urinary condition the way it is now, how would you feel about that?	0	1	2	3	4	5	6

Total score: 0–7 Mildly symptomatic; 8–19 moderately symptomatic; 20–35 severely symptomatic.

Urinary Symptom Profile – USP©(3)

- Before starting the questionnaire, please fill in today's date:

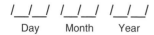

The following questions concern the intensity and frequency of urinary symptoms that you have had over the past 4 weeks.

To answer the following questions, please tick the box which best applies to you. There are no "right" or "wrong" answers. If you are not quite sure how to answer, choose the answer which best applies to you.

Please answer this questionnaire somewhere quiet and preferably on your own. Take as long as you need to fill it in.

Once you have finished, put the questionnaire into the envelope provided and hand it to your doctor.

Thank you for your cooperation.

You may sometimes experience urine leaks during physical effort. This effort could be strenuous (such as doing sport or having a violent coughing fit), moderate (climbing or coming down the stairs) or even light (walking or changing position).

1. Over the past 4 weeks, please specify the number of times a week you have had leaks during physical effort:

Please tick one box for each of the lines 1a, 1b and 1c.

Over the past 4 weeks and under everyday conditions of social, professional or family life:

	No urine leaks	Less than one urine leak a week	Several urine leaks a week	Several urine leaks a day
1a. During **strenuous** physical effort	$\square_0$	$\square_1$	$\square_2$	$\square_3$
1b. During **moderate** physical effort	$\square_0$	$\square_1$	$\square_2$	$\square_3$
1c. During **light** physical effort	$\square_0$	$\square_1$	$\square_2$	$\square_3$

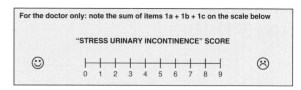

For the doctor only: note the sum of items 1a + 1b + 1c on the scale below

"STRESS URINARY INCONTINENCE" SCORE

☺ 0 1 2 3 4 5 6 7 8 9 ☹

2. How many times a week have you had to rush to the toilet to urinate because you urgently needed to go?

$\square_0$ Never	$\square_1$ Less than once a week	$\square_2$ Several times a week	$\square_3$ Several times a day

3. When you have had an urgent need to urinate, for how many minutes on average have you been able to hold on?

$\square_0$ More than 15 minutes	$\square_1$ From 6 to 15 minutes	$\square_2$ From 1 to 15 minutes	$\square_3$ Less than 1 minute

4. How many times a week have you experienced a urine leak preceded by an urgent need to urinate that you were unable to control?

$\square_0$ Never	$\square_1$ Less than once a week	$\square_2$ Several times a week	$\square_3$ Several times a day

4a. In the above case, what kind of leaks did you have?

$\square_0$ No leaks in this case	$\square_1$ A few drops	$\square_2$ Light leaks	$\square_3$ Heavy leaks

5. During the day, in general, how long elapsed between urinating?

$\square_0$ 2 hours or more	$\square_1$ Between 1 and 2 hours	$\square_2$ Between 30 minutes and 1 hour	$\square_3$ Less than 30 minutes

6. How many times on average have you been woken up during the night by a need to urinate?

$\square_0$ Never or once	$\square_1$ Twice	$\square_2$ 3 or 4 times	$\square_3$ More than 4 times

7. How many times a week have you had a urine leak while asleep or have you woken up wet?

$\square_0$	$\square_1$	$\square_2$	$\square_3$
Never	Less than once a week	Several times a week	Several times a day

> **For the doctor only: note the sum of items 2 + 3 + 4 + 4a + 5 + 6 + 7 on the scale below**
>
> **"OVERACTIVE BLADDER" SCORE**
>
> ☺ ├─┼─┤ ☹
>
> 0 1 2 3 4 5 6 7 8 9 10 11 12 13 14 15 16 17 18 19 20 21

8. How would you describe your usual urination over these past 4 weeks?

$\square_0$	$\square_1$	$\square_2$	$\square_3$
Normal	Needed to push with abdominal (stomach) muscles or lean forward (or required a change of position) to urinate	Needed to press on the lower stomach with my hands	Used a catheter

9. In general, how would you describe your urine flow?

$\square_0$	$\square_1$	$\square_2$	$\square_3$
Normal	Weak	Drop by drop	Used a catheter

10. In general, how has your urination been?

$\square_0$	$\square_1$	$\square_1$	$\square_2$	$\square_3$
Normal and quick	Difficult to start, then normal	Easy at first but slow to finish	Very slow from start to finish	Used a catheter

> **For the doctor only: note the sum of items 8 + 9 + 10 on the scale below**
>
> **"LOW STREAM" SCORE**
>
> ☺ ├─┼─┼─┼─┼─┼─┼─┼─┼─┤ ☹
>
> 0 1 2 3 4 5 6 7 8 9

Please check that you have answered all the questions.

Thank you for your cooperation

Center N° ⌴⌴⌴   Visit N° ⌴⌴⌴
Patient N°   Patient's initials ⌴⌴⌴

315

SF-Qualiveen© (4)

How to answer the questionnaire:

The following questions are about the bladder problems you may have and how you deal and live with them.

Please fill in this questionnaire in a quiet place and preferably on your own. Take the time you need. There are no right or wrong answers. If you are not sure how to answer a question, choose the answer which best applies to you. Please note that your answers will remain strictly anonymous and confidential.

When answering the questions, think about how you pass urine at present.

Thank you for your participation.

- Before filling in this questionnaire, please write today's date:

/__/__/ /__/__/ /__/__/
Day   Month   Year

THE INFORMATION CONTAINED IN THIS QUESTIONNAIRE IS STRICTLY ANONYMOUS AND CONFIDENTIAL

YOUR BLADDER PROBLEMS AND HOW YOU PASS URINE AT PRESENT:

Please answer all the questions by ticking the appropriate box.

	Not at all	Slightly	Moderately	Quite a bit	Extremely
1. In general, do your bladder problems complicate your life?	$\square_0$	$\square_1$	$\square_2$	$\square_3$	$\square_4$
2. Are you bothered by the time spent passing urine or realizing catheterization	$\square_0$	$\square_1$	$\square_2$	$\square_3$	$\square_4$
3. Do you worry about your bladder problems worsening	$\square_0$	$\square_1$	$\square_2$	$\square_3$	$\square_4$
4. Do you worry about smelling of urine	$\square_0$	$\square_1$	$\square_2$	$\square_3$	$\square_4$
5. Do you feel worried because of your bladder problems	$\square_0$	$\square_1$	$\square_2$	$\square_3$	$\square_4$
6. Do you feel embarrassed because of your bladder problems	$\square_0$	$\square_1$	$\square_2$	$\square_3$	$\square_4$
	Never	Rarely	From time to time	Often	Always
7. Is your life regulated by your bladder problems?	$\square_0$	$\square_1$	$\square_2$	$\square_3$	$\square_4$
8. Can you go out without planning anything in advance?	$\square_0$	$\square_1$	$\square_2$	$\square_3$	$\square_4$

Thank you for valuable help

Center N° ⌴⌴

Patient No.

Patient's initials ⌴⌴

Calculation grid for scores of SF-Qualiveen

	Qualiveen domain scores							
	Bother with limitations		**Fears**		**Feeling**		**Frequency of limitations**	
	#	answ	#	answ	#	answ	#	answ
	1	_____	3	_____	5	_____	7	_____
	2	_____	4	_____	6	_____	8	_____
Sum of items	=	_____	=	_____	=	_____	=	_____
Divide by	÷	2	÷	2	÷	2	÷	2
Score	=	_____	=	_____	=	_____	=	_____

SF-Qualiveen overall score		
	Scores	
Bother with limitations	_____	
Fears	_____	
Feeling	_____	
Frequency of limitations	_____	
Sum of scores	=	_____
Divide by	÷	4
SF-Qualiveen overall score	=	_____

#:number of the item
answ: answer recorded for the item

International Index of Erectile Function (IIEF) (5)

These questions ask about the effects that your erection problems have had on your sex life over the last four weeks. Please try to answer the questions as honestly and as clearly as you are able. Your answers will help your doctor to choose the most effective treatment suited to your condition. In answering the questions, the following definitions apply:

- sexual activity includes intercourse, caressing, foreplay and masturbation
- sexual intercourse is defined as sexual penetration of your partner
- sexual stimulation includes situations such as foreplay, erotic pictures, etc.
- ejaculation is the ejection of semen from the penis (or the feeling of this)
- orgasm is the fulfilment or climax following sexual stimulation or intercourse.

		Over the past 4 weeks:	Please check one box only
☐	Q1	How often were you able to get an erection during sexual activity?	0 No sexual activity 1 Almost never or never 2 A few times (less than half the time) 3 Sometimes (about half the time) 4 Most times (more than half the time) 5 Almost always or always
☐	Q2	When you had erections with sexual stimulation, how often were your erections hard enough for penetration?	0 No sexual activity 1 Almost never or never 2 A few times (less than half the time) 3 Sometimes (about half the time) 4 Most times (more than half the time) 5 Almost always or always
☐	Q3	When you attempted intercourse, how often were you able to penetrate (enter) your partner?	0 Did not attempt intercourse 1 Almost never or never 2 A few times (less than half the time) 3 Sometimes (about half the time) 4 Most times (more than half the time) 5 Almost always or always
☐	Q4	During sexual intercourse, how often were you able to maintain your erection after you had penetrated (entered) your partner?	0 Did not attempt intercourse 1 Almost never or never 2 A few times (less than half the time) 3 Sometimes (about half the time) 4 Most times (more than half the time) 5 Almost always or always
☐	Q5	During sexual intercourse, how difficult was it to maintain your erection to completion of intercourse?	0 Did not attempt intercourse 1 Extremely difficult 2 Very difficult 3 Difficult 4 Slightly difficult 5 Not difficult

	Over the past 4 weeks:	**Please check one box only**
☐ Q6	How many times have you attempted sexual intercourse?	0 No attempts 1 One to two attempts 2 Three to four attempts 3 Five to six attempts 4 Seven to ten attempts 5 Eleven or more attempts
☐ Q7	When you attempted sexual intercourse, how often was it satisfactory for you?	0 Did not attempt intercourse 1 Almost never or never 2 A few times (less than half the time) 3 Sometimes (about half the time) 4 Most times (more than half the time) 5 Almost always or always
☐ Q8	How much have you enjoyed sexual intercourse?	0 No intercourse 1 No enjoyment at all 2 Not very enjoyable 3 Fairly enjoyable 4 Highly enjoyable 5 Very highly enjoyable
☐ Q9	When you had sexual stimulation or intercourse, how often did you ejaculate?	0 No sexual stimulation or intercourse 1 Almost never or never 2 A few times (less than half the time) 3 Sometimes (about half the time) 4 Most times (more than half the time) 5 Almost always or always
☐ Q10	When you had sexual stimulation or intercourse, how often did you have the feeling of orgasm or climax?	1 Almost never or never 2 A few times (less than half the time) 3 Sometimes (about half the time) 4 Most times (more than half the time) 5 Almost always or always
☐ Q11	How often have you felt sexual desire?	1 Almost never or never 2 A few times (less than half the time) 3 Sometimes (about half the time) 4 Most times (more than half the time) 5 Almost always or always
☐ Q12	How would you rate your level of sexual desire?	1 Very low or none at all 2 Low 3 Moderate 4 High 5 Very high
☐ Q13	How satisfied have you been with your overall sex life?	1 Very dissatisfied 2 Moderately dissatisfied 3 Equally satisfied & dissatisfied 4 Moderately satisfied 5 Very satisfied

	Over the past 4 weeks:	Please check one box only
☐ Q14	How satisfied have you been with your <u>sexual relationship</u> with your partner?	1 Very dissatisfied 2 Moderately dissatisfied 3 Equally satisfied & dissatisfied 4 Moderately satisfied 5 Very satisfied
☐ Q15	How do you rate your <u>confidence</u> that you could get and keep an erection?	1 Very low 2 Low 3 Moderate 4 High 5 Very high

Female Sexual Function Index (FSFI) (6)

INSTRUCTIONS: These questions ask about your sexual feelings and responses <u>during the past 4 weeks.</u> Please answer the following questions as honestly and clearly as possible. Your responses will be kept completely confidential. In answering these questions the following definitions apply:

<u>Sexual activity</u> can include caressing, foreplay, masturbation and vaginal intercourse.

<u>Sexual intercourse</u> is defined as penile penetration (entry) of the vagina.

<u>Sexual stimulation</u> includes situations like foreplay with a partner, self-stimulation (masturbation), or sexual fantasy.

CHECK <u>ONLY</u> ONE BOX PER QUESTION.

<u>Sexual desire</u> or <u>interest</u> is a feeling that includes wanting to have a sexual experience, feeling receptive to a partner's sexual initiation, and thinking or fantasizing about having sex.

1. Over the past 4 weeks, how **often** did you feel sexual desire or interest?
   - ☐ Almost always or always
   - ☐ Most times (more than half the time)
   - ☐ Sometimes (about half the time)
   - ☐ A few times (less than half the time)
   - ☐ Almost never or never

2. Over the past 4 weeks, how would you rate your **level** (degree) of sexual desire or interest?
   - ☐ Very high
   - ☐ High
   - ☐ Moderate
   - ☐ Low
   - ☐ Very low or none at all

   Sexual arousal is a feeling that includes both physical and mental aspects of sexual excitement. It may include feelings of warmth or tingling in the genitals, lubrication (wetness) or muscle contractions.

3. Over the past 4 weeks, how **often** did you feel sexually aroused ("turned on") during sexual activity or intercourse?
   - ☐ No sexual activity
   - ☐ Almost always or always
   - ☐ Most times (more than half the time)
   - ☐ Sometimes (about half the time)
   - ☐ A few times (less than half the time)
   - ☐ Almost never or never

4. Over the past 4 weeks, how would you rate your level of sexual arousal ("turn on") during sexual activity or intercourse?
   - ☐ No sexual activity
   - ☐ Very high
   - ☐ High
   - ☐ Moderate
   - ☐ Low
   - ☐ Very low or none at all

5. Over the past 4 weeks, how **confident** were you about becoming sexually aroused during sexual activity or intercourse?
   - ☐ No sexual activity
   - ☐ Very high confidence
   - ☐ High confidence
   - ☐ Moderate confidence
   - ☐ Low confidence
   - ☐ Very low or no confidence

6. Over the past 4 weeks, how **often** have you been satisfied with your arousal (excitement) during sexual activity or intercourse?
   - ☐ No sexual activity
   - ☐ Almost always or always
   - ☐ Most times (more than half the time)
   - ☐ Sometimes (about half the time)
   - ☐ A few times (less than half the time)
   - ☐ Almost never or never

7. Over the past 4 weeks, how **often** did you become lubricated ("wet") during sexual activity or intercourse?
   - ☐ No sexual activity
   - ☐ Almost always or always
   - ☐ Most times (more than half the time)
   - ☐ Sometimes (about half the time)
   - ☐ A few times (less than half the time)
   - ☐ Almost never or never

8. Over the past 4 weeks, how **difficult** was it to become lubricated ("wet") during sexual activity or intercourse?
   - ☐ No sexual activity
   - ☐ Extremely difficult or impossible
   - ☐ Very difficult
   - ☐ Difficult
   - ☐ Slightly difficult
   - ☐ Not difficult

9. Over the past 4 weeks, how often did you **maintain** your lubrication ("wetness") until completion of sexual activity or intercourse?
   - ☐ No sexual activity
   - ☐ Almost always or always
   - ☐ Most times (more than half the time)
   - ☐ Sometimes (about half the time)
   - ☐ A few times (less than half the time)
   - ☐ Almost never or never

10. Over the past 4 weeks, how **difficult** was it to maintain your lubrication ("wetness") until completion of sexual activity or intercourse?
    - ☐ No sexual activity
    - ☐ Extremely difficult or impossible
    - ☐ Very difficult
    - ☐ Difficult
    - ☐ Slightly difficult
    - ☐ Not difficult

11. Over the past 4 weeks, when you had sexual stimulation or intercourse, how **often** did you reach orgasm (climax)?
    - ☐ No sexual activity
    - ☐ Almost always or always
    - ☐ Most times (more than half the time)
    - ☐ Sometimes (about half the time)
    - ☐ A few times (less than half the time)
    - ☐ Almost never or never

12. Over the past 4 weeks, when you had sexual stimulation or intercourse, how **difficult** was it for you to reach orgasm (climax)?
    - ☐ No sexual activity
    - ☐ Extremely difficult or impossible
    - ☐ Very difficult
    - ☐ Difficult
    - ☐ Slightly difficult
    - ☐ Not difficult

13. Over the past 4 weeks, how **satisfied** were you with your ability to reach orgasm (climax) during sexual activity or intercourse?
    - ☐ No sexual activity
    - ☐ Very satisfied
    - ☐ Moderately satisfied
    - ☐ About equally satisfied and dissatisfied
    - ☐ Moderately dissatisfied
    - ☐ Very dissatisfied

14. Over the past 4 weeks, how **satisfied** have you been with the amount of emotional closeness during sexual activity between you and your partner?
    - ☐ No sexual activity
    - ☐ Very satisfied
    - ☐ Moderately satisfied
    - ☐ About equally satisfied and dissatisfied
    - ☐ Moderately dissatisfied
    - ☐ Very dissatisfied

15. Over the past 4 weeks, how **satisfied** have you been with your sexual relationship with your partner?
    - ☐ Very satisfied
    - ☐ Moderately satisfied
    - ☐ About equally satisfied and dissatisfied
    - ☐ Moderately dissatisfied
    - ☐ Very dissatisfied

16. Over the past 4 weeks, how **satisfied** have you been with your overall sexual life?
    - ☐ Very satisfied
    - ☐ Moderately satisfied
    - ☐ About equally satisfied and dissatisfied
    - ☐ Moderately dissatisfied
    - ☐ Very dissatisfied

17. Over the past 4 weeks, how **often** did you experience discomfort or pain <u>during</u> vaginal penetration?
    - ☐ Did not attempt intercourse
    - ☐ Almost always or always
    - ☐ Most times (more than half the time)
    - ☐ Sometimes (about half the time)
    - ☐ A few times (less than half the time)
    - ☐ Almost never or never

18. Over the past 4 weeks, how **often** did you experience discomfort or pain <u>following</u> vaginal penetration?
    - ☐ Did not attempt intercourse
    - ☐ Almost always or always
    - ☐ Most times (more than half the time)
    - ☐ Sometimes (about half the time)
    - ☐ A few times (less than half the time)
    - ☐ Almost never or never

19. Over the past 4 weeks, how would you rate your **level** (degree) of discomfort or pain during or following vaginal penetration?

☐ Did not attempt intercourse
☐ Very high

☐ High
☐ Moderate
☐ Low
☐ Very low or none at all

Sexual Compulsivity Scale (7)

A number of statements that some people have used to describe themselves are given below. Read each statement and then circle the number to show how well you believe the statement describes you.

	Not at all like me	Slightly like me	Mainly like me	Very Much like me
1. My sexual appetite has gotten in the way of my relationships.	1	2	3	4
2. My sexual thoughts and behaviors are causing problems in my life.	1	2	3	4
3. My desires to have sex have disrupted my daily life.	1	2	3	4
4. I sometimes fail to meet my commitments and responsibilities because of my sexual behaviors.	1	2	3	4
5. I sometimes get so horny I could lose control.	1	2	3	4
6. find myself thinking about sex while at work.	1	2	3	4
7. I feel that sexual thoughts and feelings are stronger than I am.	1	2	3	4
8. I have to struggle to control my sexual thoughts and behavior.	1	2	3	4
9. I think about sex more than I would like to.	1	2	3	4
10. It has been difficult for me to find sex partners who desire having sex as much as I want to.	1	2	3	4

To Score: Add items that have responses and divide by number of items responded.

The Neurogenic Bowel Dysfunction (NBD) score (8)

The number of points given for each possible answer is given in parenthesis.

How often do you open your bowels?
Daily $\square_{(0)}$ 2–6 times every week$\square_{(1)}$ Less than once a week $\square_{(6)}$

How long does it take to open your bowels? 0–30 min$\square_{(0)}$ 31–60 min$\square_{(3)}$ More than 1 hour $\square_{(7)}$

Do you suffer from uneasiness, headache or perspiration whilst opening your bowels? No $\square_{(0)}$ Yes $\square_{(2)}$

Do you regularly use tablet laxatives for constipation? No $\square_{(0)}$ Yes $\square_{(2)}$

Do you regularly use liquid laxatives for constipation? No $\square_{(0)}$ Yes $\square_{(2)}$

Do you stimulate defecation by putting a finger in your back passage?
Less than once a week $\square_{(0)}$ Once or more every week $\square_{(6)}$

How often are you incontinent of feces?
Less than once a month $\square_{(0)}$ 1–4 times every month $\square_{(6)}$
1–6 times every week $\square_{(7)}$ Daily $\square_{(13)}$

Do you take medication for fecal incontinence? No $\square_{(0)}$ Yes $\square_{(4)}$

Do you suffer from flatus incontinence? No $\square_{(0)}$ Yes $\square_{(2)}$

Do you have problems with your anal skin? No $\square_{(0)}$ Yes $\square_{(3)}$

Total NBD score (range 0–47) ——— points

NBD score	Bowel dysfunction
0–6	Very minor
7–9	Minor
10–13	Moderate
14 or more	Severe

References

1. Uebersax JS, Wyman JF, Shumaker SA, McClish DK, Fantl JA. Short forms to assess life quality and symptom distress for urinary incontinence in women: the Incontinence Impact Questionnaire and the Urogenital Distress Inventory. Continence Program for Women Research Group. *Neurourol Urodyn* 1995;**14**:131–9.

2. Barry MJ, Fowler FJ, Jr., O'Leary MP, et al. The American Urological Association symptom index for benign prostatic hyperplasia. The Measurement Committee of the American Urological Association. *J Urol* 1992;**148**:1549–57.

3. Haab F, Richard F, Amarenco G, et al. Comprehensive evaluation of bladder and urethral dysfunction symptoms: development and psychometric validation of the Urinary Symptom Profile (USP) questionnaire. *Urology* 2008;**71**:646–56.

4. Bonniaud V, Bryant D, Parratte B, Guyatt G. Development and validation of the short form of a urinary quality of life questionnaire: SF-Qualiveen. *J Urol* 2008;**180**:2592–8.

5. Rosen RC, Riley A, Wagner G, et al. The international index of erectile function (IIEF): a multidimensional scale for assessment of erectile dysfunction. *Urology* 1997;**49**:822–30.

6. Rosen R, Brown C, Heiman J, et al. The Female Sexual Function Index (FSFI): a multidimensional self-report instrument for the assessment of female sexual function. *J Sex Marital Ther* 2000;**26**:191–208.

7. Kalichman SC, Rompa D. Sexual sensation seeking and sexual compulsivity scales: reliability, validity, and predicting HIV risk behavior. *J Pers Assess* 1995;**65**:586–601.

8. Krogh K, Christensen P, Sabroe S, Laurberg S. Neurogenic bowel dysfunction score. *Spinal Cord* 2006;**44**:625–31.

Index